Controversy
in Obstetrics
and Gynecology
II

Edited by

DUNCAN E. REID, M.D.

Late Clinical Professor of Obstetrics and Gynecology
University of Arizona College of Medicine

and

C. D. CHRISTIAN, M.D.

Professor and Head of the Department
of Obstetrics and Gynecology
University of Arizona College of Medicine

W. B. SAUNDERS COMPANY

PHILADELPHIA · LONDON · TORONTO 1974

W. B. Saunders Company: West Washington Square
Philadelphia, PA 19105

12 Dyott Street
London, WC1A   1DB

833 Oxford Street
Toronto, Ontario M8Z 5T9, Canada

Controversy in Obstetrics
and Gynecology II

ISBN   0-7216-7528-X

Print No: 9   8   7   6   5   4   3   2   1

Contributors

LEONARD A. AARO, M.D., Associate Professor of Obstetrics and Gynecology, Mayo Medical School. Consultant, Department of Obstetrics and Gynecology, Mayo Clinic and Mayo Foundation, Rochester, Minnesota.

WILLARD M. ALLEN, M.D., Professor of Obstetrics and Gynecology, University of Maryland. Obstetrician and Gynecologist, University of Maryland Hospital, Baltimore, Maryland.

HASSAN AMIRIKIA, M.D., F.A.C.O.G., Instructor, Wayne State University School of Medicine, Department of Gynecology-Obstetrics. Hutzel Hospital, Harper Hospital, Detroit General Hospital, Detroit, Michigan.

GAIL V. ANDERSON, M.D., Professor of Obstetrics and Gynecology and Professor and Chairman, Department of Emergency Medicine, University of Southern California School of Medicine. Director, Department of Emergency Medicine, Los Angeles County–University of Southern California Medical Center, Los Angeles, California.

DAVID L. BARCLAY, M.D., Professor and Chairman, Department of Obstetrics and Gynecology, University of Arkansas Medical Center, Little Rock, Arkansas.

TOM P. BARDEN, M.D., Associate Professor, Obstetrics and Gynecology and Pediatrics, University of Cincinnati Medical Center. Attending Obstetrician and Gynecologist, University of Cincinnati Medical Center, Cincinnati, Ohio.

ROBERT H. BARTER, M.D., Professor, Obstetrics and Gynecology, George Washington School of Medicine, Washington, D.C.

WILLIAM S. BAZLEY, M.D., Assistant Professor (Clinical), University of Florida College of Medicine, Gainesville, Florida.

CLAYTON T. BEECHAM, M.D., Senior Consultant, Gynecology and Obstetrics, Geisinger Medical Center, Danville, Pennsylvania.

JACKSON B. BEECHAM, M.D., Senior Resident, Obstetrics and Gynecology, University of Vermont Medical Center, Burlington, Vermont.

S. J. BEHRMAN, M.D., F.R.C.O.G., Professor of Obstetrics and Gynecology, University of Michigan Medical School, Ann Arbor, Michigan.

FRITZ K. BELLER, M.D., Universitaets Frauenklinik, Muenster, Germany.

KURT BENIRSCHKE, M.D., Professor of Reproductive Medicine, University of California at San Diego. University Hospital, San Diego, California.

EDWARD H. BISHOP, M.D., Professor of Obstetrics and Gynecology, School of Medicine, University of North Carolina. Attending Obstetrician and Gynecologist, North Carolina Memorial Hospital, Chapel Hill, North Carolina.

EDWARD T. BOWE, M.D., Assistant Professor of Obstetrics and Gynecology, College of Physicians and Surgeons, Columbia University. Assistant Attending Obstetrician and Gynecologist, Sloane Hospital, Columbia–Presbyterian Medical Center, New York, New York.

WATSON A. BOWES, Jr., M.D., Associate Professor, University of Colorado Medical School. University of Colorado Medical Center, Denver, Colorado.

JOHN I. BREWER, M.D., Ph.D., Professor and Chairman, Department of Obstetrics and Gynecology, Northwestern University Medical School. Chief, Obstetrics and Gynecology, Northwestern Memorial Hospital, Chicago, Illinois.

R. CLAY BURCHELL, M.D., Clinical Professor, University of Vermont School of Medicine, Associate Professor, University of Connecticut Health Center. Senior Attending Staff, Director of Obstetrics and Gynecology, Hartford Hospital, Hartford, Connecticut.

DOUGLAS E. CANNELL, M.B., B.Sc.(Med.), F.R.C.S.(C.), F.R.C.O.G., F.A.C.O.G., LL.D., Professor Emeritus, Department of Obstetrics and Gynaecology, University of Toronto. Honorary Consultant, Toronto General Hospital, Hospital for Sick Children, Wellesley Hospital, Consultant, Toronto East General and Orthopaedic Hospital, Toronto, Ontario.

VINCENT J. CAPRARO, M.D., Clinical Professor of Gynecology-Obstetrics, State University of New York at Buffalo. Chief, Division of Pediatric and Adolescent Gynecology, Buffalo Children's Hospital, Buffalo, New York.

DAVID CHARLES, M.D., Professor and Chairman of Obstetrics and Gynecology, Boston University School of Medicine, Boston, Massachusetts.

S. Y. CHEN, M.D., Associate, Department of Obstetrics and Gynecology, Mount Sinai School of Medicine of the City University of New York. Assistant Attending Obstetrician and Gynecologist, Mount Sinai Hospital, New York, New York.

JOSEPH CHEUNG, M.D., M.R.C.O.G., F.A.C.O.G., Attending Obstetrician and Gynecologist, California Hospital Medical Center, Los Angeles, California.

ARTHUR CHRIS CHRISTAKOS, M.D., Associate Professor of Obstetrics and Gynecology and Community Health Sciences, Duke University Medical School, Durham, North Carolina.

LUIS A. CIBILS, M.D., Mary Campau Ryerson Professor of Obstetrics and Gynecology, University of Chicago. Consultant Obstetrician and Gynecologist, University of Chicago and The Chicago Lying-In Hospital, Chicago, Illinois.

JAMES J. CORRIGAN, Jr., M.D., Associate Professor of Pediatrics, University of Arizona College of Medicine. Attending Hematologist, University of Arizona Medical Center, Consultant, Tucson Medical Center and St. Joseph's Hospital, Tucson, Arizona.

MARION CARLYLE CRENSHAW, Jr., M.D., E.C. Hamblen Professor of Reproductive Biology and Family Planning, and Assistant Professor of Pediatrics, Duke University Medical Center. Co-Director, Division of Perinatal Medicine, Duke University Medical Center, Durham, North Carolina.

JOHN F. CRIGLER, Jr., M.D., Associate Professor of Pediatrics, Children's Hospital Medical Center, Harvard Medical School. Chief, Division of Endocrinology, Department of Medicine, and Director, Clinical Research Center, Children's Hospital Medical Center, Boston, Massachusetts.

WILLIAM E. CRISP, M.D., Clinical Associate, University of Arizona College of Medicine. Chairman, Department of Obstetrics and Gynecology, Maricopa County Hospital, Phoenix, Arizona.

MICHAEL J. DALY, M.D., Professor and Chairman, Department of Obstetrics and Gynecology, Temple University Health Sciences Center, Philadelphia, Pennsylvania.

JOHN R. DAVIS, M.D., Associate Professor of Pathology, University of Arizona College of Medicine. Chief, Anatomic Pathology Section, Arizona Medical Center, Tucson, Arizona.

RUSSELL RAMON de ALVAREZ, M.D., F.A.C.S., F.A.C.O.G., Chairman Emeritus of Obstetrics and Gynecology, Temple University School of Medicine, Philadelphia, Pennsylvania. First Chairman and Professor of Obstetrics and Gynecology, University of Washington Health Sciences Center, Seattle, Washington.

WAYNE H. DECKER, M.D., Associate Clinical Professor of Obstetrics and Gynecology, New York University Medical College. Surgeon-in-Chief, New York Fertility Research Foundation. Associate Attending Obstetrician-Gynecologist, University Hospital, New York, New York.

WILLIAM DROEGEMUELLER, M.D., Associate Professor, University of Colorado Medical School. University of Colorado Medical Center, Denver, Colorado.

RAPHAEL B. DURFEE, M.D., Professor of Obstetrics and Gynecology, University of Oregon Medical School. Staff, University of Oregon Medical School Hospitals and Clinics, Good Samaritan Hospital, U.S. Veterans Hospital, Portland, Oregon.

CHARLES L. EASTERDAY, M.D., Associate Clinical Professor of Obstetrics and Gynecology, Harvard Medical School. Senior Obstetrician-Gynecologist, Boston Hospital for Women, Boston, Massachusetts.

THOMAS R. ECKMAN, M.D., F.A.C.O.G., Assistant Professor of Gynecology and Obstetrics, Emory University Medical School. Deputy Chief of Obstetrics and Gynecology, Crawford W. Long Hospital, Atlanta, Georgia.

T. N. EVANS, M.D., Professor and Chairman, Department of Gynecology-Obstetrics, Wayne State University School of Medicine. Director, C. S. Mott Center for Human Growth and Development. Chief of Gynecology-Obstetrics, Hutzel Hospital, Harper Hospital, and Detroit General Hospital; Consultant, Sinai Hospital, William Beaumont Hospital, and Children's Hospital, Detroit, Michigan.

MARTIN FARBER, M.D., Assistant Professor of Obstetrics and Gynecology, Tufts University School of Medicine. Assistant Gynecologist, New England Medical Center Hospital, Boston, Massachusetts.

ERNEST W. FRANKLIN, III, M.D., Associate Professor of Gynecology and Obstetrics, Emory University School of Medicine. Director, Division of Gynecologic Oncology, Emory University Clinic and Hospital, Grady Memorial Hospital, Atlanta, Georgia.

JAMES H. FREEL, M.D., Instructor, Department of Obstetrics and Gynecology, Cornell University Medical School. Assistant Attending Surgeon, Gynecology Service, Memorial Hospital for Cancer and Allied Diseases, Assistant Attending Obstetrician and Gynecologist, New York Hospital, New York, New York, Consultant, Department of Obstetrics and Gynecology, North Shore Hospital, Manhasset, New York.

ROGER K. FREEMAN, M.D., Associate Professor and Chief, Section of Obstetrics, Department of Obstetrics and Gynecology, University of Southern California School of Medicine. Los Angeles County–University of Southern California Medical Center, Los Angeles, California.

MARY ANNA FRIEDERICH, M.D., Associate Professor in Obstetrics-Gynecology and Psychiatry, University of Rochester School of Medicine and Dentistry, and Strong Memorial Hospital. Senior Associate Obstetrician and Gynecologist and Psychiatrist, Strong Memorial Hospital, Rochester, New York.

FREDRIC D. FRIGOLETTO, Jr., M.D., Assistant Professor of Obstetrics and Gynecology, Harvard Medical School. Obstetrician-Gynecologist, Boston Hospital for Women, Boston, Massachusetts.

HARLAN RAYMOND GILES, M.D., Assistant Professor and Head of Division of Perinatal Medicine, Department of Obstetrics and Gynecology, University of Arizona School of Medicine. Attending Physician, Pima County Hospital, Tucson, Arizona.

DONALD PETER GOLDSTEIN, M.D., Assistant Clinical Professor of Obstetrics and Gynecology, Harvard Medical School. Obstetrician-Gynecologist, Boston Hospital for Women, Associate in Surgery (Gynecology), Peter Bent Brigham Hospital, Chief of Gynecology, Children's Hospital Medical Center, Director, New England Trophoblastic Disease Center, Boston, Massachusetts.

MYRON GORDON, M.D., Associate Professor, Obstetrics and Gynecology, New York Medical College. Chief of Service, Obstetrics and Gynecology, Metropolitan Hospital Center, Attending Obstetrician and Gynecologist, Flower and Fifth Avenue Hospitals, New York, New York.

THOMAS H. GREEN, Jr., M.D., Associate Clinical Professor of Gynecology, Harvard Medical School. Associate Visiting Surgeon, Massachusetts General Hospital, Boston, Massachusetts.

S. B. GUSBERG, M.D., D.Sci., Professor and Chairman of Obstetrics and Gynecology, Mount Sinai School of Medicine of the City University of New York. Director, Obstetrician and Gynecologist-in-Chief, Mount Sinai Hospital, New York, New York.

C. D. HAAGENSEN, M.D., Professor Emeritus of Clinical Surgery, College of Physicians and Surgeons, Columbia University. Columbia-Presbyterian Medical Center, New York, New York.

DWAIN D. HAGERMAN, M.D., Professor of Obstetrics and Gynecology and Professor of Biochemistry, University of Colorado School of Medicine. Colorado General Hospital, Denver, Colorado.

CHARLES B. HAMMOND, M.D., Associate Professor, Department of Obstetrics and Gynecology, Duke University Medical Center, Durham, North Carolina.

FREDERICK W. HANSON, M.D., Assistant Professor, Department of Obstetrics and Gynecology, University of California at Davis, School of Medicine. Staff, Sacramento Medical Center, Sacramento, California; Courtesy Staff, San Joaquin General Hospital, Stockton, California.

STEPHEN J. HEALEY, M.D., Instructor in Surgery, Harvard Medical School and Tufts Medical School. Senior Associate in Surgery, Peter Bent Brigham Hospital; Surgeon, Boston Hospital for Women, Boston, Massachusetts.

M. WAYNE HEINE, M.D., Professor of Obstetrics and Gynecology, University of Arizona School of Medicine. Consultant, Tucson Medical Center, Pima County Hospital, St. Joseph's Hospital, and Davis Monthan AFB Hospital, Tucson, Arizona.

C. PAUL HODGKINSON, M.D., M.S. (Ob.-Gyn.), Adjunct Professor of Gynecology and Obstetrics, Wayne State University; Clinical Professor of Gynecology and Obstetrics, University of Michigan. Chairman, Department of Gynecology and Obstetrics, Henry Ford Hospital, Detroit, Michigan.

JOHN W. HUFFMAN, M.D., Professor of Obstetrics and Gynecology, Emeritus, Northwestern University Medical School; Professor of Gynecology, Cook County Graduate School of Medicine. Attending Gynecologist, Passavant Memorial Hospital, Attending Gynecologist and Head of Division of Gynecology, Emeritus, Children's Memorial Hospital, Chicago, Illinois.

L. STANLEY JAMES, M.D., Professor of Pediatrics, College of Physicians and Surgeons, Columbia University. Attending Pediatrician, Babies Hospital, Columbia–Presbyterian Medical Center, New York, New York.

JOHN BRIGHAM JOSIMOVICH, M.D., Professor of Obstetrics and Gynecology, University of Pittsburgh School of Medicine. Magee-Women's Hospital, Pittsburgh, Pennsylvania.

JOHN L. JUERGENS, M.D., Associate Professor of Medicine, Mayo Medical School. Consultant, Division of Cardiovascular Diseases and Internal Medicine, Mayo Clinic and Mayo Foundation, Rochester, Minnesota.

NATHAN KASE, M.D., Professor and Chairman, Department of Obstetrics and Gynecology, Yale University School of Medicine. Chief of Service, Obstetrics-Gynecology, Yale–New Haven Hospital, New Haven, Connecticut.

ANTHONY HENRY LABRUM, M.D., Associate Professor, Obstetrics-Gynecology and Psychiatry, University of Rochester School of Medicine and Dentistry, and Strong Memorial Hospital. Senior Associate Obstetrician-Gynecologist, University of Rochester, and Strong Memorial Hospital, Rochester, New York.

ROBERT LANDESMAN, M.D., Clinical Professor of Obstetrics and Gynecology, Cornell University Medical College. Director of Obstetrics and Gynecology, Jewish Memorial Hospital, Attending Obstetrician-Gynecologist, New York Hospital, New York, New York.

JOHN M. LEVENTHAL, M.D., Clinical Instructor of Obstetrics and Gynecology, Harvard Medical School. Assistant Obstetrician and Gynecologist, Boston Hospital for Women, Boston, Massachusetts.

GEORGE C. LEWIS, Jr., M.D., Professor, Thomas Jefferson University Medical College. Staff, Jefferson Hospital; Consultant, Lankenau Hospital, American Oncologic Hospital, and U.S. Naval Hospital, Philadelphia, Pennsylvania.

JOHN L. LEWIS, Jr., M.D., Professor of Obstetrics and Gynecology, Cornell University Medical College. Chief, Gynecology Service, Department of Surgery, Memorial Sloan-Kettering Cancer Center, New York, New York.

MILAGROS A. MACASAET, M.D., Assistant Professor, Department of Obstetrics and Gynecology, State University of New York Downstate Medical Center. Attending Physician, State University Hospital and Kings County Hospital Center, Brooklyn, New York.

DONALD G. McKAY, M.D., Professor of Pathology, University of California at San Francisco. Chief of Pathology, San Francisco General Hospital, San Francisco, California.

RICHARD F. MATTINGLY, M.D., F.A.C.O.G., Professor and Chairman, Department of Gynecology and Obstetrics, Medical College of Wisconsin. Milwaukee County General Hospital, Milwaukee, Wisconsin.

ABE MICKAL, M.D., Professor and Head, Obstetrics and Gynecology, Louisiana State University School of Medicine. Senior Visiting Surgeon, Obstetrician and Gynecologist-in-Chief, Charity Hospital of Louisiana. Active Staff, Southern Baptist Hospital, New Orleans, Louisiana.

DANIEL R. MISHELL, Jr., M.D., Professor and Associate Chairman, Department of Obstetrics and Gynecology, University of Southern California School of Medicine. Associate Chief of Professional Services, Women's Hospital, Los Angeles County–University of Southern California Medical Center, Los Angeles, California.

GEORGE W. MITCHELL, Jr., M.D., Professor of Obstetrics and Gynecology and Chairman of the Department, Tufts University School of Medicine. Gynecologist-in-Chief, New England Medical Center Hospital, Boston, Massachusetts.

MAMDOUH MOUKHTAR, M.D., B.Sc.OXON, F.R.C.S., M.R.C.O.G., F.A.C.O.G., Assistant Professor of Obstetrics and Gynecology, Albert Einstein College of Medicine. Attending Physician, Abraham Jacobi Hospital and Bronx–Lebanon Hospital, New York, New York.

JAMES H. NELSON, Jr., M.D., Professor and Chairman, Department of Obstetrics and Gynecology, State University of New York Downstate Medical Center. Obstetrician and Gynecologist-in-Chief, State University Hospital and Kings County Hospital Center, Brooklyn, New York.

KENNETH R. NISWANDER, M.D., Professor and Chairman, Obstetrics and Gynecology, University of California at Davis. Chief, Obstetrics and Gynecology, University of California at Davis, Sacramento Medical Center, Sacramento, California.

JON M. PASSMORE, M.D., Instructor of Obstetrics and Gynecology, Temple University School of Medicine, Philadelphia, Pennsylvania. Holy Cross Hospital, Taos, New Mexico.

ERLE E. PEACOCK, Jr., M.D., Professor and Chairman, University of Arizona College of Medicine. Chief of Surgical Services, University of Arizona Medical Center, Tucson, Arizona.

JACK W. PEARSON, M.D., Professor of Obstetrics and Gynecology, Indiana University School of Medicine. Chairman, Department of Obstetrics and Gynecology, Columbia–Presbyterian Medical Center, New York, New York.

OTTO C. PHILLIPS, M.D., Clinical Professor of Anesthesiology, University of Pittsburgh. Chief, Division of Anesthesiology, Western Pennsylvania Hospital, Pittsburgh, Pennsylvania.

EDWARD J. QUILLIGAN, M.D., Professor and Chairman, Department of Obstetrics and Gynecology, University of Southern California School of Medicine. Chief of Professional Services, Women's Hospital, Los Angeles County–University of Southern California Medical Center, Los Angeles, California.

BROOKS RANNEY, M.S., M.D., Professor and Chairman, Department of Obstetrics and Gynecology, University of South Dakota School of Medicine. Chairman, Departments of Obstetrics and Gynecology, The Yankton Clinic, Sacred Heart Hospital, Yankton State Hospital, Yankton, South Dakota.

HENRY R. REY, M.S.E.E., Staff Associate, Department of Obstetrics and Gynecology, Columbia–Presbyterian Medical Center, New York, New York.

J. W. RODDICK, Jr., M.D., Professor and Chairman, Department of Obstetrics and Gynecology, Southern Illinois University School of Medicine, Springfield, Illinois.

SEYMOUR L. ROMNEY, M.D., Professor of Obstetrics and Gynecology, Albert Einstein College of Medicine. Attending Physician, Abraham Jacobi Hospital, New York, New York.

MORTIMER G. ROSEN, M.D., Associate Professor and Director of Research, Department of Obstetrics and Gynecology, University of Rochester School of Medicine and Dentistry, Rochester, New York.

KEITH P. RUSSELL, M.D., F.A.C.O.G., Clinical Professor of Obstetrics and Gynecology, University of Southern California School of Medicine. Senior Attending Obstetrician-Gynecologist, California Hospital Medical Center, Los Angeles, California.

PHILLIP H. RYE, M.D., Assistant Professor, Obstetrics and Gynecology, Louisiana State University Medical School. Visiting Surgeon, Charity Hospital of Louisiana. Active Staff, Southern Baptist Hospital, New Orleans, Louisiana.

HILTON A. SALHANICK, Ph.D., M.D., Frederick L. Hisaw Professor of Reproductive Physiology, Harvard School of Public Health, and Professor of Obstetrics and Gynecology, Harvard Medical School. Senior Obstetrician and Gynecologist, Boston Hospital for Women, Boston, Massachusetts.

WILLIAM C. SCOTT, M.D., M.S.(Ob.-Gyn.), Associate Professor, Department of Obstetrics and Gynecology, University of Arizona School of Medicine. Attending Physician, Arizona Medical Center and Pima County Hospital. Consulting Staff, Tucson Medical Center, St. Joseph's Hospital, Palo Verde Hospital, Tucson, Arizona.

RICHARD S. SHELDON, M.D., Assistant Professor of Obstetrics and Gynecology, Mayo Medical School. Consultant, Department of Obstetrics and Gynecology, Mayo Clinic and Mayo Foundation, Rochester, Minnesota.

ALFRED I. SHERMAN, M.D., Professor of Obstetrics and Gynecology, Wayne State University School of Medicine. Chairman, Department of Obstetrics and Gynecology, Sinai Hospital of Detroit, Detroit, Michigan.

ROBERT L. SHIRLEY, M.D., Assistant Clinical Professor, Harvard Medical School. Obstetrician-Gynecologist, Boston Hospital for Women, Boston, Massachusetts.

BRADLEY E. SMITH, M.D., Professor of Anesthesiology, Vanderbilt University. Chief Anesthesiologist, Vanderbilt Hospital, Nashville, Tennessee.

GEORGE V. SMITH, M.D., Professor of Gynecology, Emeritus, Harvard Medical School. Gynecologist, Boston Hospital for Women, Boston, Massachusetts.

MORTON A. STENCHEVER, M.D., Professor and Chairman, Department of Obstetrics and Gynecology, University of Utah College of Medicine. Chief Attending Obstetrician, University Medical Center, Salt Lake City, Utah.

ROBERT ALAN STOOKEY, M.D., Chief Resident, Obstetrics-Gynecology Department, Strong Memorial Hospital, University of Rochester School of Medicine and Dentistry, Rochester, New York.

E. STEWART TAYLOR, M.D., Professor and Chairman, Department of Obstetrics and Gynecology, University of Colorado School of Medicine. Colorado General Hospital, Denver, Colorado.

ALLAN B. WEINGOLD, M.D., Professor and Assistant Director, Obstetrics and Gynecology, New York Medical College. Visiting Physician, Obstetrics and Gynecology, Metropolitan Hospital Center. Attending Obstetrician and Gynecologist, Flower and Fifth Avenue Hospitals, New York, New York.

JESS BERNARD WEISS, M.D., Assistant Professor of Anaesthesia, Boston Hospital for Women, Harvard Medical School. Senior Anesthesiologist and Director of Clinical Services, Boston Hospital for Women, Boston, Massachusetts.

GEORGE D. WILBANKS, M.D., Professor, Rush Medical College. Chairman, Department of Obstetrics and Gynecology, Rush-Presbyterian–St. Luke's Medical Center, Chicago, Illinois.

EDWARD J. WILKINSON, M.D., F.A.C.O.G., Assistant Professor, Department of Gynecology and Obstetrics, Medical College of Wisconsin. Milwaukee County General Hospital, Milwaukee, Wisconsin.

TIFFANY J. WILLIAMS, M.D., Associate Professor of Obstetrics and Gynecology, Mayo Medical School. Consultant, Department of Surgery, Mayo Clinic and Mayo Foundation, Rochester, Minnesota.

Preface

Obstetrics and Gynecology as now practiced encompasses in very great measure the medical supervision of the female patient and responsibility for the welfare of the fetus and newborn. With the creditable reduction in maternal mortality during the past three decades, emphasis is now being placed on quality of life—obviously this must begin at the beginning.

This broadening of the medical assignments for obstetrics and gynecology in the delivery of health care presents several areas of controversy. Furthermore, one of the hallmarks of medicine in recent decades has been the rapid expansion of knowledge in nearly all areas, which in itself often leads to controversies by those regarded as authorities in their special fields of interest and investigation. These individuals must therefore communicate and document their observations and findings that have particular clinical relevance to those physicians whose major concern and activity are directed toward the daily care of patients. The authorities who have contributed to this book have attempted to do this and we are grateful for their efforts.

The topics selected represent the broad spectrum of obstetrics and gynecology. Specifically and in brief, these include the physical development and metabolic function of the reproductive system, including the breast, and the many facets of neoplasia of these structures. It is our hope that the information and authoritative opinions expressed may prove useful and helpful to the student, resident, and practicing physician.

Department members Drs. William Scott and Wayne Heine have lent consultative assistance and sympathetic support. Miss Carol Ann De Gilio has provided enthusiastically and patiently the necessary secretarial assistance. Finally, we are most indebted to our editor, Mr. John Dusseau, who has been his usual tranquil self during this travail and has assisted in many ways, giving unstintingly of his time and publishing experience.

Duncan E. Reid

C. D. Christian

Contents

1

Identification and Management of Intrauterine Growth Retardation

Alternative Points of View:

By Harlan R. Giles and Carlyle Crenshaw, Jr.

By Watson A. Bowes, Jr., and William Droegemueller

By Fredric D. Frigoletto, Jr.

Editorial Comment

Identification and Management
of Intrauterine Growth Retardation

HARLAN R. GILES
University of Arizona Medical Center

CARLYLE CRENSHAW, JR.
Duke University Medical Center

For more than a decade, it has been appreciated that infants born with low birth weight suffer a high incidence of severe physical and mental handicaps. Many of these impairments do not become evident for months to years after birth. Recent studies which differentiate between infants of low birth weight for gestational age and purely premature infants consistent in size for gestational age would indicate a similar, if not greater, risk of sequelae in the former. Increased awareness of this problem on the part of the physician and improved methods for determining fetal status have facilitated the recognition of the growth retarded fetus.

One of the major problems in the identification of intrauterine growth retardation is the lack of a uniform definition agreed upon by perinatologists. Various terminologies such as "small for dates," "fetal malnutrition," "pseudo-prematurity," "dysmaturity," "placental insufficiency," and "chronic fetal distress" have been assigned, almost interchangeably, to designate infants with birth weights significantly below the mean for gestational age. It is hardly surprising, therefore, to find no uniform recommendations for the diagnosis and management of the disorder.

At our institutions we utilize the criteria established by Gruenwald[1] to correlate infant weight with gestational age. When the birth weight is less than two standard deviations below the mean weight expected for gestational age, the diagnosis is fetal growth retardation. To include in this category all infants whose birth weights are below the tenth percentile would increase the incidence of the disorder without contributing to the solution of the problem. Moreover, in order to separate intrauterine growth retardation from the pure dysmaturity syndrome, Szalay[2] requires, in addition to the weight criterion, an appropriate reduction in infant height or length.

When the menstrual date is uncertain, physical examination of the newborn may provide a reasonably accurate estimation of true gestational age. Clinical correlatives, such as the appearance of sole creases, the amount of ear lobe cartilage, and the degree of testicular descent, may be utilized with equal validity in the growth retarded infant.

Unfortunately, the diagnosis of intrauterine growth retardation after birth does little to alter the high perinatal morbidity and mortality rates associated with the disorder. The following discussion describes the antepartum recognition, evaluation, and management of the fetus at risk.

Etiology

Although the etiology of intrauterine growth retardation is as yet poorly understood, the concept of prolonged fetal hypoxia or malnutrition, or both, forms the basis of many hypotheses. At best there is a definite association between the failure of the fetus to grow and certain clinical states. In a significant percentage of patients the disorder must be classified as idiopathic, at least for the present.

The association of intrauterine growth retardation with the hypertensive vascular diseases, the acute toxemias, chronic renal disease, and certain patients with diabetes mellitus is unequivocal. The disorder is frequently encountered in infants of patients with collagen diseases, sickling disorders, drug addiction, and cyanotic heart disease.

Genetic factors may account for a small percentage of infants observed to be growth retarded in weight and height. Such chromosomal aberrations as the trisomies 13-15, 18, and 21 are representative examples. In other patients, developmental anomalies such as anencephaly or phocomelia may be the unfortunate explanation for the subnormal intrauterine growth pattern. However, inherited factors have been documented and should be considered in only a small minority of infants with intrauterine growth retardation.

External influences, similarly, play a minor role in the spectrum of pathogenesis in infants who are small for gestational age. Maternal cigarette smoking, living at high altitudes, and low socioeconomic status, while unequivocally related to a reduction of fetal weight, rarely produce infants who fall two standard deviations below the expected mean weight or height for gestational age. A smaller number of instances of intrauterine growth retardation are ascribed to various chemical or minor irradiation insults.

Chronic intrauterine infectious processes, such as rubella, herpes simplex, syphilis, toxoplasmosis, and cytomegalic inclusion disease have often been implicated as etiologic agents for the growth retarded fetus. The effect of such pathogens is proportional to the duration of the infection in utero. The fetuses with the worst prognosis are those infected in the first trimester.

The single leading factor responsible for intrauterine growth retardation in the majority of fetuses is chronic fetal malnutrition. This malnutrition may result from inadequacies in the composition of maternal blood, reduction of uteroplacental blood flow, or impaired placental transport.

Rapid cell growth and division make the fetus particularly susceptible to nutritional stresses. Animal studies have repeatedly confirmed both a diminished rate of fetal cell division and a permanent reduction in cell number for most organ systems in fetuses deprived of essential nutrients, such as glucose and amino acids.[3] The product may be a runt which, despite nutritional abundance in the neonatal period, may never attain the weight of his litter mates. However, it is of interest that in the human, chronic reduction of maternal protein intake and chronic maternal ketonuric states from starvation have seldom been linked with severe intrauterine growth retardation. Human fetuses with this syndrome have been shown to have a normal complement of cells, with a reduction only in cell size. This would afford a good prognosis for correction of the growth pattern in the neonatal period. Apparently, fetal nutrition is minimally impaired unless there is either drastic reduction of caloric intake or an associated compromise of the fetomaternal circulation.

The relationship of ischemia or chronic hypoxia to progressive fetal stunting has been amply demonstrated in experiments compromising the uteroplacental vasculature in rats.[4] This might serve to explain the association between intrauterine growth retardation and chronic retroplacental bleeding or the circumvallate placenta. Placentas of growth retarded infants are generally small and may contain multiple placental infarcts. Correlation of intrauterine growth retardation with human vascular disorders has been facilitated by documentation of obliterative and degenerative lesions in spiral vessels of the decidua. These changes reflect a diminished uteroplacental blood flow and presumably a decrease in placental transport.

Diagnosis

The initial suspicion that intrauterine growth retardation is or might be present depends upon the physician's awareness of the problem, a complete medical and obstetrical history, a thorough physical examination, and meticulous prenatal care.

The history of hypertension, diabetes mellitus, renal disease, sickle cell disease, collagen disorder, or cyanotic heart disease in the mother places the fetus in a high risk category for intrauterine growth retardation. The obstetrical history provides information regarding previous pregnancies, complications, and gestational age-weight relationships. The patient must be questioned carefully by the physician to determine the regularity of menses and to ascertain that the last menstrual period was indeed a normal one. For gestations greater than 20 weeks, the date of quickening should be recorded, although the calculation of gestational age from the date of quickening can be misleading in individual patients.

Perhaps the most important aspect of the initial visit concerns the estimation of gestational age from uterine size. Although this can be accurate up to 30 weeks gestation, it is more accurate during the first 12 weeks. The initial examination and establishment of gestational age should be performed by an experienced obstetrician-gynecologist.

Estimations of gestational age from uterine fundal height can be quite deceptive. However, the rule of thumb that "between 16 and 30 weeks of gestation, the fundal height in centimeters above the symphysis pubis is equal to gestational age in weeks" is clinically helpful, particularly if the patient is repeatedly examined by the same physician. During the course of prenatal care failure of uterine growth or any discrepancy between uterine size and gestational age by menstrual dates should be noted. Patients with size-date discrepancies in excess of three weeks should be suspected of having intrauterine growth retardation.

It has been shown that intrauterine growth can be followed by extrapolating ultrasonic measurements of the fetal biparietal and thoracic diameters to fetal weight.[5] Results of such measurements have been found to be both reproducible and reliable. By ultrasonic examination, fetuses who fail to exhibit a normal progressive increase in size over a two week interval should be diagnosed as growth retarded.

Management

All patients suspected of having the syndrome of intrauterine growth retardation should be transferred to a "high risk" perinatal clinic staffed by experienced obstetrician-gynecologists, neonatologists, anesthesiologists, and internists. In this setting, each patient is followed by an individual clinician, with immediate consultative assistance available from the team. Follow-up examinations are performed no less frequently than every two weeks for the first 20 weeks of gestation and at weekly intervals thereafter.

Currently, except for correcting underlying maternal illnesses or nutritional deficiencies, there are no clinically acceptable methods for improving the growth, development, or health of the fetus in utero. The primary difficulty in the management of the patient with intrauterine growth retardation lies in arbitrating chronic fetal distress against the risk of delivering an immature infant who is ill-equipped for survival.

After the thirtieth week of gestation, the 24 hour urinary estriol excretion rate is monitored weekly. More frequent monitoring of this parameter is recommended by some investigators. Whereas depression of the absolute 24 hour estriol excretion rate may be encountered in some supposedly normal patients, the physician nevertheless should expect a progressive increase in estriol values as gestation advances. Patients who demonstrate at least a fifty per cent reduction in estriol excretion from the previous determination or those whose excretion rate is less than 10 mg. per 24 hours should be monitored daily. This precaution will separate spuriously low values from those associated with chronic fetal distress. If there is persistence of abnormal estriol excretion, maturity of the fetus must be documented before the pregnancy is terminated.

Because of the myriad difficulties inherent in the collection, assay, and interpretation of urinary estriols, other methods for establishing the health of the fetus in utero are being investigated. These include serum estrogen, heat-stable alkaline phosphatase, and human chorionic somatotropin (HCS or placental lactogen). Our experience with the use of heat-stable alkaline phosphatase in 750 patients followed serially revealed poor correlation with fetal status; consequently, this assay has been discontinued.[6] Our experience with total serum estrogens and serum estriol appears to be more promising. The results of studies by other investigators would indicate that serial estimations of human chorionic somatotropin provide a useful appraisal of placental function. Further clinical experience is needed before these methods can be recommended routinely.

Beginning as early as the thirty-second week of gestational age, efforts are made to document fetal maturity. The most accurate assessment is accomplished by examination of the amniotic fluid via amniocentesis. The presence of meconium in the amniotic fluid presents a grave prognosis, and immediate delivery by an expeditious route becomes mandatory. Whereas the amniotic fluid can be examined for meconium by amnioscopy, the cervix rarely is sufficiently dilated at this stage in gestation to permit the application of this technique.

Samples of amniotic fluid are sent for determination of creatinine concentration and lecithin/sphingomyelin ratios. Since various criteria and standards are described in the literature, each laboratory should specify the indicators of maturity it uses. In our laboratory, creatinine concentrations in excess of 1.5 mg. per 100 ml. are indicative of a fetus of at least 36 weeks' gestational age or 2500 grams.[7] Values less than 1.5 mg. per 100 ml., however, do not indicate necessarily an immature fetus.

Determination of lecithin/sphingomyelin ratios by the method of Gluck[8] is a valuable adjunct for assessing the ability of the fetus to survive outside the uterus. Fetal pulmonary maturity is virtually assured with lecithin/sphingomyelin ratios in excess of 2:1. It is of interest and must be appreciated that some of the etiologic factors responsible for intrauterine growth retardation, such as hypertension, chronic renal disease, and toxemia, may be associated with precocious maturation of the fetal respiratory system. Our experience with the use of absolute concentrations of lecithin in the amniotic fluid and with the "shake test" is relatively limited but these methods do not appear to be as useful as the lecithin/sphingomyelin ratio.

Nile blue staining of fetal fat cells in the amniotic fluid has been employed by us, but was found to be less reliable than creatinine concentrations. Combined results utilizing "fat cell" counts plus creatinine values similarly were inferior to creatinine concentrations alone for predicting fetal maturity.

Although delay in interosseous development may be associated with intrauterine growth retardation, the X-ray examination of the maternal abdomen still serves as a reliable indicator of fetal maturity when distal femoral or proximal tibial epiphyses are present. Ancillary information regarding fetal size and the presence of certain fetal abnormalities also may be obtained by X-ray.

Delivery

In the presence of indicators of fetal jeopardy or evidence for fetal maturity, delivery should be accomplished without delay by the most appropriate method to insure maximum safety to the fetus.

Vaginal delivery is attempted in those patients in whom labor is judged to be easily initiated, as determined by pelvic evaluation. If the cervix is soft, partially effaced, and dilated, and the presenting part is low in the pelvis, the membranes are gently stripped away from the lower uterine segment. A graduated intravenous infusion of oxytocin is administered via an infusion pump. Amniotomy alone, or in conjunction with oxytocin infusion, often is performed to facilitate labor.

Continuous fetal heart monitoring, either external or internal, is employed throughout the labor process. Sustained, severe fetal bradycardia, tachycardia, or persistent late deceleration patterns demand operative intervention. The recently described ominous fetal heart rate pattern of the "silent baseline" is coming under closer scrutiny.

If induction of labor cannot be accomplished readily, if there are complications of labor, or if there is evidence of superimposed acute fetal distress, we do not hesitate to employ cesarean section as the preferred method of delivery.

Regardless of the mode of delivery, pediatric colleagues who have assisted in the management and delivery decisions should be present in the delivery suite. The occurrence of neonatal acidosis,[9] hypoglycemia,[10] hypocalcemia, and pulmonary hemorrhage in the growth retarded neonate is well established. Anticipation and early preparation for management of these complications is mandatory.

Summary

Figure 1-1 summarizes the diagnosis and management of patients suspected of having a fetus who may be growth retarded.

Through increased physician awareness, more compulsive prenatal care, improved maternal health, innovative diagnostic methodology, and superior neonatal care, a reduction of perinatal morbidity and mortality rates associated with intrauterine growth retardation can be achieved.

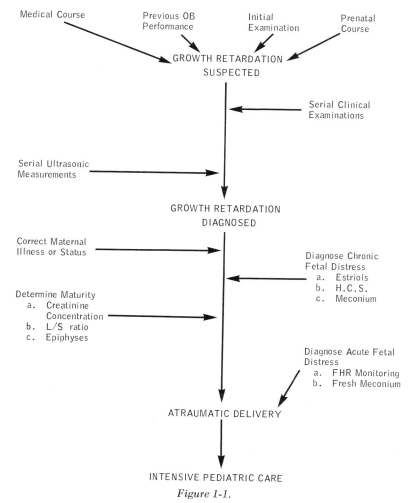

Figure 1-1.

REFERENCES

1. Gruenwald, P.: Growth of the human fetus. Amer. J. Obstet. Gynec. *94*:1112, 1966.
2. Szalay, G. C.: Intrauterine growth retardation versus Silver's syndrome. J. Pediat. *64*:234, 776, 1964.
3. Bard, H.: Intrauterine growth retardation. Clin. Obstet. Gynec. *13*:511–525, 1970.
4. Wigglesworth, J. S.: Foetal growth retardation. Brit. Med. Bull. *22*:13–15, 1966.
5. Gottesfeld, K.: Personal communication.
6. Magendantz, H., and Crenshaw, C.: Unpublished data.
7. Wyatt, T. H., Halbert, D. R., and Crenshaw, C.: Estimation of fetal weight by cytological examination and creatinine determination of amniotic fluid. Obstet. Gynec. *34*:772, 1969.
8. Gluck, L., Kulovich, M. V., Borer, R. C., Jr., *et al.*: Diagnosis of the respiratory distress syndrome by amniocentesis. Amer. J. Obstet. Gynec. *109*:440–445, 1971.
9. Low, J. S., Boston, R. W., and Pancham, S. R.: Fetal asphyxia during the intrapartum period in intrauterine growth retarded infants. Amer. J. Obstet. Gynec. *113*:351, 1972.
10. Crenshaw, C.: Fetal glucose metabolism. Clin. Obstet. Gynec. *13*:583, 1970.

Identification and Management
of Intrauterine Growth Retardation

WATSON A. BOWES, JR., and WILLIAM DROEGEMUELLER
University of Colorado Medical School

The concept of intrauterine growth retardation was introduced by McBurney in 1947.[1] In a paper presented to the Pacific Coast Society of Obstetrics and Gynecology, McBurney—somewhat apologetically—described a number of cases in which he was convinced that the duration of gestation was 38 weeks or more, but the infants weighed less than 2500 grams. He objected to the insistence that these were premature infants when the sole criterion was weight. In his study, approximately one per cent of all infants born were in this group of term babies weighing less than 2500 grams, and the associations between this syndrome, maternal vascular disease, and fetal anomalies were emphasized. He cautioned that the risk of fetal death is increased and suggested that if born alive and without anomalies, these babies fare well in the newborn nursery. Little else was reported about this syndrome for 10 years, until the papers of Lubchenco[2] and Gruenwald[3] called attention to babies who were born with weights well below the norm for their gestational age. Since the publication of these papers, there has been a keen interest in this syndrome, which has been called intrauterine growth retardation, fetal malnutrition, placental insufficiency, the dysmaturity syndrome, the "small for dates" baby, "small for gestational age," and so forth.[4,5,6]

There are at least five controversies that surround the issue of intrauterine growth retardation. The problems are as follows:

1. What are the standards for intrauterine growth retardation?

2. What causes intrauterine growth retardation?

3. How dangerous is intrauterine growth retardation to the fetus and to the newborn?

4. Can the fetus with intrauterine growth retardation be detected prior to birth?

5. Can the outcome of intrauterine growth retardation for either the fetus or the newborn be significantly altered by changes in management of the pregnancy?

We have partial answers for all of these questions, but despite the extensive literature that has accumulated about this problem and our own investigations of human fetal growth retardation, the syndrome is still shrouded in mystery, ambiguities, and disagreements.

WHAT ARE THE STANDARDS FOR INTRAUTERINE GROWTH RETARDATION?

Battaglia and Lubchenco[7] have described babies small for their gestational age as those below the tenth percentile as defined by birth weights and gestational age of 14,000 infants born at the University of Colorado Medical Center (Figure 1-2). This definition has been adopted by many investigators in their reports of the same problem. Gruenwald,[8] who published one of the original reports describing the effects of intrauterine growth retardation, used the definition of two standard deviations below the norm. This definition, too, has been accepted by many investigators. It is important to remember that these criteria define different groups of babies in any individual population. Using two standard deviations below the norm identifies only the babies in the third percentile or lower. Consequently, one will be dealing with a much smaller number of babies who, presumably, have much more severe fetal growth retardation than the total group described by Lubchenco. In Aberdeen, Scotland, Thomson and his colleagues[9] have demonstrated the effect of parity, maternal height, sex of the infant, and social class on intrauterine growth curves. Their work shows that the mean weight for girls at any gestational age is significantly lower than that for boys. Consequently, any definition that does not take this sex difference into account will result in the inclusion of a greater number of females than males in the group. This same phenomenon results in a larger percentage of complications in boys. Most reports of intrauterine growth retardation do not take into account these factors, mentioned by Thomson and his co-workers.

Studies done on different populations have demonstrated that there is a geographic and racial difference in intrauterine growth retardation.[7,8,9,10,11] Babies in Sweden whose birth weights are below the tenth percentile as a group will be larger infants than small for gestational age babies born in Denver. Tanner has summarized the dilemma of the description of intrauterine growth patterns.[12]

Prior to the introduction of ultrasound, it was virtually impossible to measure chronologically the accurate growth (either in length or in weight) of a fetus in utero. Therefore, all of the growth curves constructed were based upon data of babies born at various gestational ages. For those babies born with less than 37 weeks' gestation, the abnormal condition which resulted in premature labor might also have significantly affected intrauterine growth. Finally, the gestational ages used in determining the growth curves were obtained from histories of the last menstrual period. Many of the reports have attempted to exclude any questionable menstrual dates, but this does not take into account the well-known significant variation in date of ovulation following the last menstrual period.

Despite these inconsistencies and reservations, there is a group of babies whose birth weights are well below the norm for that particular gestational age, for whom the duration of gestation has been well documented. We have used Lubchenco's definition of babies below the tenth percentile for weight and have not made corrections for sex, maternal height, social class, or race (Figure 1-2). In the day to day management of these pregnancies and of the newborns. all of these factors are taken into consideration.

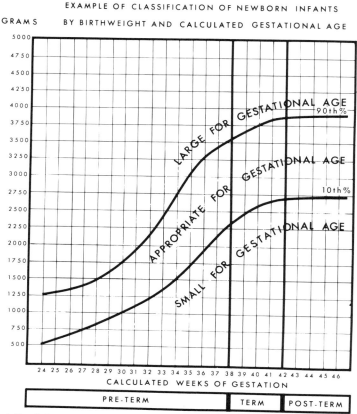

UNIVERSITY OF COLORADO MEDICAL CENTER
EXAMPLE OF CLASSIFICATION OF NEWBORN INFANTS
BY BIRTHWEIGHT AND CALCULATED GESTATIONAL AGE

Figure 1-2. Intrauterine growth curves estimated from live-born birth weights at 24 to 42 weeks of gestation. (From Battaglia, F. C., and Lubchenco, L. O.: A practical classification of newborn infants by weight and gestational age. J. Pediatr. *71*:159–163, 1967.)

What causes intrauterine growth retardation?

Babies who are small for gestational age will vary from 2 per cent to 8 per cent of the total population, depending upon the definition used. Within this group, approximately 10 per cent will have occurred in a multiple gestation, 10 to 20 per cent of the babies will have congenital anomalies or congenital infections, 20 to 30 per cent will be infants born to mothers who suffer chronic vascular, renal, or collagen diseases, and 40 to 60 per cent of the babies will be products of essentially normal pregnancies. In many studies, these babies have been considered as a single group, although clearly the mortality and morbidity rates will vary considerably, depending upon the underlying condition. As one would expect, the perinatal mortality is highest among those babies with fetal malformations or intrauterine infections.

Naeye studied organ and cellular development in autopsy material from fetuses and newborns whose birth weights were two or more standard deviations below the mean for their gestational age.[13] In 11 such infants, he found subnormal amounts of cytoplasm in cells and compared this with similar findings in infants dying of alimentary malnutrition. In 6 cases, the placenta was markedly subnormal in size, and in two other infants there were partial placental separations with retroplacental hemorrhage. These findings suggest a placental abnormality restricting normal fetal nutrition. The same investigator, studying organ and cellular development in small for gestational age infants with chromosomal abnormalities, found that reduction in organ weight resulted from a subnormal number of cells in many body organs.[14] Clearly, there may be several different mechanisms for intrauterine growth retardation.

We have found that in multiparous mothers whose pregnancies are normal except for the birth of a small for dates baby, 50 per cent had previously given birth to a similarly affected infant. This suggests either a variation of the norm, a congenital predisposition to have small infants, or an underlying disorder restricting fetal growth, which is too subtle for current detection. Ounsted[15] pointed out that most infants whose weights are two standard deviations below the norm for gestational age have siblings with low birth weights, and rarely will they have a sibling who is large for its gestational age.

How dangerous is intrauterine growth retardation to the fetus and newborn?

The risk of antepartum death for intrauterine growth retardation is not well known. The time of fetal death, the effects of maceration and of the interval to delivery on fetal weight, and the inaccurate recording in cases of antepartum death have all played a role in obscuring the hazards of intrauterine death. The danger is recognized to be greater in cases of severe fetal growth retardation than in cases of normal intrauterine development.[5,7,16,17] All forms of severe hypertensive, vascular, and renal disease, including chronic hypertensive disease, lupus erythematosus, diabetes mellitus, and preeclampsia have been associated with an increased risk of antepartum fetal death, and all are known frequently to produce babies who are small for gestational age. What is not so clearly established is the risk of fetal death for the small for dates baby in an otherwise normal pregnancy.

There is little doubt that small for dates babies are at greater risk for fetal and neonatal death than their counterparts of similar gestational age with normal growth. The perinatal mortality in these infants is between 10 and 14 per 100 live births and increases substantially with the degree of growth retardation.[5,7,17] In the Newborn Service at our hospital, 30 per cent of all deaths are among the small for gestational age infants.[4] The mortality risk for these infants is higher at all stages of development, although the specific antenatal and intrapartum death rates have been less well documented than the risk of neonatal death. Forty per cent of the perinatal mortality in these infants can be accounted for by major congenital anomalies.[18]

Fetal deaths during labor or immediately after birth have been shown to be five times more common in cases of intrauterine growth retardation. It is our impression that babies with intrauterine growth retardation, irrespective of the etiology, will demonstrate clear signs of fetal distress during labor in about 30 per cent of cases, and our cesarean section rates with these infants is correspondingly high.

One of the most difficult questions to answer at the present time is the long-term prognosis for intrauterine growth retardation. Many of the studies on low birth weight infants have not separated the premature infants from the small for dates babies. From the point of view of management of the pregnancy, it would be most useful to know if low birth weight babies with a longer gestation have a better prognosis than those of similar weight but of shorter gestation. Specific evidence to confirm or refute such an impression is lacking. Babson's work on growth of infants shows that small for dates babies have growth curves during the first year which parallel in weight and length those of normal controls, but there is no "catching-up" during this time. Beargie and his co-workers found, in a 13 to 53 month follow-up exam of small for dates newborns, that 28 of 45 babies had exceeded the tenth percentile in height and weight.[20] Using both the James and the Denver Developmental screening tests, investigators found that 9 of the 45 infants did not perform at their chronological age level in two or more areas. Weiner's study on intellectual development related to birth weight and gestational age in 8 to 10 year olds suggests that for low birth weight infants, gestational age at birth has little affect on IQ levels.[21] The studies of Drillien indicate that babies with intrauterine growth retardation born to low-income families have poorer long-term development records than babies with weights that are similar but appropriate for their gestational ages.[22] However, small for dates babies born to high-income families did much better than control premature infants of similar birth weights.

Recently, Lubchenco and her co-workers have demonstrated a remarkable decrease in the incidence of significant handicaps in long-term follow-up of low birth weight babies who have been treated in an intensive care nursery.[23] These data suggest that the early recognition and prompt correction of dehydration, hypoglycemia, hypothermia, or other problems encountered by the low birth weight infants will significantly alter the prospects of future development in these babies. Nevertheless, many of the questions about the relationship of specific antepartum complications (e.g., chronic hypertension, chronic renal disease, preeclampsia, or maternal malnutrition) to long-term development are not known.

CAN THE FETUS WITH INTRAUTERINE GROWTH RETARDATION BE DETECTED PRIOR TO BIRTH?

With the increasing interest surrounding intrauterine growth retardation and the possibility that antepartum management may play a role in reducing the antenatal morbidity and mortality rates, there is a need to recognize the disorder prior to the infant's arrival in the nursery. Beard and Roberts recently reported the efforts of their clinic in making the diagnosis of fetal growth compromise.[24] The results showed their diagnostic accuracy to be 65 per cent. Among 41 patients suspected of having small for dates babies, 12 were above the tenth percentile for weight at birth. They did not comment on the number of small for dates babies who were born without having been suspected in the antepartum period. Brush and co-workers have alluded to the difficulty in detecting intrauterine growth retardation by clinical means in the antepartum period, and found that screening all patients with a single urinary pregnanediol determination was only slightly more selective.[25]

We have encountered similar problems. With two staff physicians reviewing all records in the prenatal clinic to detect patients with evidence of fetal growth retardation, we were able in a one year period to correctly detect approximately 50 per cent of those babies born small for their gestational age. Conversely, more than half of those patients whom we suspected of having fetal growth retardation subsequently delivered babies whose weights were appropriate for their gestational ages. Our primary clinical tool for the detection of intrauterine growth retardation is the McDonald measurement, performed by stretching a centimeter tape from the symphysis pubis over the abdomen to the most superior portion of the uterine fundus. If, between 20 to 34 weeks' gestation, this measurement was 4 cm. less than the week of gestation, intrauterine growth retardation was suspected. Any other patient thought to have inadequate uterine growth by members of the house staff was also investigated as a possible candidate for the syndrome.

Some of the patients delivering infants with unsuspected and hence undiagnosed fetal growth retardation as defined by Lubchenco (Figure 1-2) had been followed in outlying clinics by many different physicians, or had no prenatal care whatsoever. Discouragingly, a surprising number had been followed in our own clinic and to the best of our appraisal had normal uterine growth. In short, we have found the antenatal detection of fetal growth retardation to be a frustrating endeavor. Many cases will become apparent only in labor or even in the nursery before the syndrome is confirmed.

In our clinic, any patient suspected of having the syndrome of fetal growth retardation as indicated by a lag in normal uterine enlargement is evaluated with serial ultrasound examination of the fetus. This technique has sharpened our diagnostic acumen remarkably. Rarely did we find that a baby whose biparietal diameter was consistently near the norm published by Thompson and his co-workers (Figure 1-3)[26] was, in fact, small for gestational age at the time of birth. Undoubtedly, the use of ultrasound determination of the biparietal diameter in all pregnancies would be a more precise technique for screening patients for abnormal fetal growth, but the expense and time required are substantial.

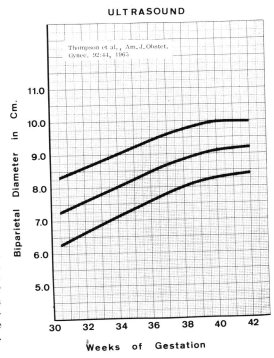

ULTRASOUND

Thompson et al., Am. J. Obstet. Gynec. 92:44, 1965

Biparietal Diameter in Cm.

Weeks of Gestation

Figure 1-3. Growth of biparietal diameter measured by ultrasound from 31 to 42 weeks of gestation. The lines represent the upper median, and lower limits of growth, respectively. (From Thompson, H. E., *et al.*: Fetal development as determined by ultrasonic pulse echo techniques. Amer. J. Obstet. Gynec. 92:44–52, 1965.)

CAN THE OUTCOME OF INTRAUTERINE GROWTH RETARDATION FOR EITHER THE FETUS OR THE NEWBORN BE SIGNIFICANTLY ALTERED BY CHANGES IN MANAGEMENT OF THE PREGNANCY?

Usher has thrown down the gauntlet to the obstetricians. In an article entitled "Clinical and Therapeutic Aspects of Fetal Nutrition," he advises that "Reduction of mortality and long-term disability is predominately the role of the obstetricians, who must learn to recognize these infants early and deliver them before irremediable damage has been done."[5] This philosophy has convinced some obstetricians that the dangers to the fetus from intrauterine growth retardation increase substantially after 37 weeks' gestation and that pregnancy should be terminated at that time. For several reasons we believe this is a more wasteful approach than selective delivery in cases that demonstrate evidence of fetal distress, cautiously anticipating spontaneous labor in the remainder. In the first place, making the diagnosis with certainty (and without the use of ultrasound) is difficult, and many babies of appropriate size for their gestational age will be included. The indiscriminate use of elective delivery would subject far too many women and babies to the small but real risks of this procedure. Frequently gestational dates and not fetal size are in error, and elective delivery would occasionally produce premature infants who are otherwise normal who, if left undisturbed in utero, would have grown to a more normal size and age. The proper use of amniocentesis, with the estimation of amniotic fluid creatinine, lecithin/sphingomyelin ratios, or the presence of fat-laden cells would undoubtedly reduce these errors in gestational dates to a minimum. We are not convinced that the ill-defined hazards of the latter weeks of pregnancy are threats sufficient to deny these infants the benefits of the last days in utero. Moreover, there is some evidence to suggest that with serial estriol determinations, amnioscopy, and oxytocin challenge tests, those infants in difficulty can be detected in ample time to be selectively delivered from the shadow of intrauterine danger. Studies have shown that mothers with estriols in the normal range and rising in the latter weeks of pregnancy will generally have healthy babies without intervention.[27,28,29] We have lost no infants in utero of our group with intrauterine growth retardation whose mothers' estriol levels have been within normal limits and rose on serial sampling. Abnormally low or falling estriol levels are more difficult to interpret. Not all such fetuses will die in utero, but the proportion of these patients whose babies are in danger is sufficiently high to consider elective delivery. Persistently low estriol values are commonly associated with pregnancies complicated by intrauterine growth retardation. The persistently low estriol titer, although worrisome, is not as ominous as the estriol value which decreases on serial sampling.

Our management of patients with suspected fetal growth retardation includes weekly sonography after 32 weeks' gestation, biweekly estriol determinations after 34 weeks' gestation, and weekly or biweekly amnioscopy as early after 35 weeks as the cervix will admit the amnioscope. Amniocentesis for creatinine and L/S ratio is performed at 37 to 38 weeks' gestation or earlier, if there is any evidence of fetal distress (consistently low or falling estriol values, or meconium staining of the amniotic fluid). In contrast to at least one other report,[30] we have found amniotic fluid creatinine concentration to be a highly reliable reflection of gestational age in patients with fetal growth retardation. Values in excess of 2.0 mg. per 100 ml. in patients whose serum creatinine concentration is not above 1.0

mg. per 100 ml. have consistently been associated with mature infants.[31] Other authors have reported the usefulness of establishing gestational dates with Nile blue sulfate staining of amniotic fluid cells in small for dates infants.[32] The oxytocin challenge test has recently been added to our management of these patients following the report of Ray and his co-workers.[33]

It is our feeling that unless there is definite evidence of fetal distress and well-established fetal maturity, the baby is better served by allowing pregnancy to continue until spontaneous labor occurs.

Therapeutic measures to improve fetal growth or prevent intrauterine growth retardation have not been well studied. Elliott has suggested that the use of folic acid in mothers who have previously had a small for dates baby is helpful in preventing the recurrence of this syndrome in these patients.[34] This work has not been confirmed by others. In reviewing a five year experience with twin pregnancies, we found that of those twins in whom the diagnosis was made by the thirtieth week of gestation, 50 per cent of the mothers were treated with bed rest in the hospital while the other 50 per cent were managed as outpatients, without a decrease in their ambulation. Bed rest did not decrease the incidence of prematurity or improve fetal or neonatal mortality rates, but there was an increase in weights of the twins born of mothers treated with bed rest for every gestational age, as compared to those whose mothers remained ambulatory. These data suggest that bed rest with its potential improvement in uterine blood flow may have a beneficial effect on intrauterine growth retardation.[35]

It has been demonstrated that labor is a time of particular risk for the small for gestational age fetus.[19] Whenever the syndrome is suspected before or during labor, the patient should be observed with continuous fetal heart and uterine contraction monitoring techniques. Early in labor, preparations for cesarean section should be made, so that if severe variable decelerations or late decelerations occur, uncorrected by changes in maternal position or the administration of oxygen, abdominal delivery can be performed without delay. If delivery is indicated because of decreasing estriol levels, the presence of meconium stained amniotic fluid, or for maternal indications (e.g., severe preeclampsia), induction of labor by amniotomy and the use of dilute intravenous solutions of oxytocin is not precluded, provided that continuous fetal heart monitoring techniques are available. Any evidence of fetal distress, demonstrated by changes in the fetal heart rate, is regarded as much more ominous in patients with intrauterine growth retardation than in otherwise normal babies. Consequently, cesarean sections tend to be done much earlier in patients with intrauterine growth retardation who demonstrate fetal bradycardia than in otherwise normal patients.

Small for gestational age babies are particularly susceptible to a number of immediate neonatal complications, including meconium aspiration, hypothermia, hypoglycemia, and hyperviscosity. It is imperative that, whenever possible, the pediatrician be notified of the impending delivery of a small for dates baby. If the syndrome is not discovered until the infant is born, the pediatric consultant should be notified at once. Careful surveillance of blood sugars, early feedings or intravenous therapy, meticulous care of temperature control, and thorough appraisal of the infant for congenital anomalies or congenital infections are all necessary in keeping the immediate and long-term morbidity and mortality rates for these infants at a minimum. It also would behoove obstetricians to become

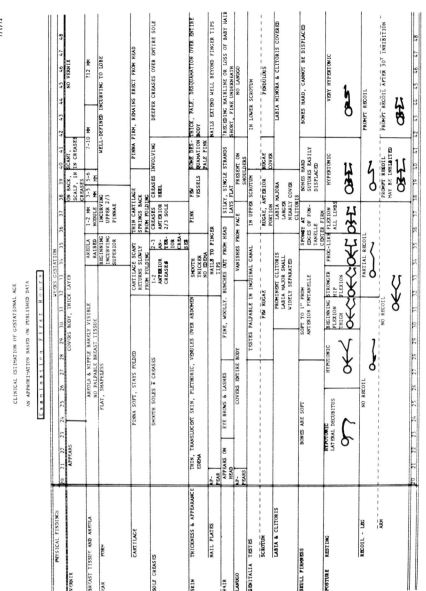

Figure 1-4. Chart used by physicians and nursing personnel in the University of Colorado Medical Center Nursery to estimate the approximate gestational age of the newborn during the first hours after delivery.

familiar with the physical characteristics of a newborn infant that help to establish its gestational age (Figure 1-4). In situations in which accurate menstrual dates are lacking and the patient has not been followed from the first trimester, these criteria will frequently aid the physician in determining if a low birth weight infant is in fact truly premature or simply small for its gestational age.

Summary

1. Intrauterine growth retardation is a term used to describe babies whose birth weights are below the tenth percentile for their gestational age.

2. Intrauterine growth retardation is commonly associated with multiple pregnancies, congenital abnormalities or congenital infections, and pregnancies complicated by renovascular disease. In over 50 per cent of cases, however, no specific maternal or fetal disease, apart from the growth retardation, can be identified.

3. Perinatal mortality and morbidity rates have been shown to be increased in this group of infants.

4. Intrauterine growth retardation can be correctly diagnosed prior to delivery in less than 75 per cent of cases.

5. There is no well-established treatment for intrauterine growth retardation, but fetal death and perinatal mortality and morbidity can probably be reduced by careful antepartum and intrapartum monitoring of the fetus, with prompt delivery if evidence of acute or chronic fetal distress is apparent.

REFERENCES

1. McBurney, R. D.: The undernourished full term infant. West. J. Surg. Obstet. Gynec. 55:363, 1947.
2. Lubchenco, L. O., Hansman, C., Dressler, M., and Boyd, E.: Intrauterine growth as estimated from live-born birth-weight data at 24 to 42 weeks of gestation. Pediatrics 32:793, 1963.
3. Gruenwald, P.: Chronic fetal distress and placental insufficiency. Biol. Neonat. 5:215, 1963.
4. Battaglia, F. C.: Intrauterine growth retardation. Am. J. Obstet. Gynec. 106:1103, 1970.
5. Usher, R. H.: Clinical and therapeutic aspects of fetal malnutrition. Ped. Clin. N. Amer. 17:169, 1970.
6. Bard, H.: Intrauterine growth retardation. Clin. Obstet. Gynec. 13:511, 1970.
7. Battaglia, F. C., and Lubchenco, L. O.: Practical classification of newborn infants by weight and gestational age. J. Pediat. 71:159, 1967.
8. Gruenwald, P.: Growth of the human fetus. I. Normal growth and its variation. Am. J. Obstet. Gynec. 94:1112, 1966.
9. Thomson, A. M., Billewicz, W. Z., and Hytten, F. E.: The assessment of fetal growth. J. Obstet. Gynaec. Brit. Comm. 75:903, 1968.
10. Babson, S. G., Behrman, R. E., and Lessel, R.: Live-born birth weights for gestational age of white middle class infants. Pediatrics 45:937, 1970.
11. Sterky, G.: Swedish standard curves for intrauterine growth. Pediatrics 46:7, 1970.
12. Tanner, J. M.: Standards for birth weight or intrauterine growth. Pediatrics 46:1, 1970.
13. Naeye, R. L.: Malnutrition, probable cause of fetal growth retardation. Arch. Path. 79:284, 1965.
14. Naeye, R. L.: Prenatal organ and cellular growth with various chromosomal disorders. Biol. Neonat. 11:248, 1967.
15. Ounsted, M.: Maternal constraint of foetal growth in man. Develop. Med. Child Neurol. 7:479, 1965.
16. Walker, J.: "Small for dates"—clinical aspects. Proc. Roy. Soc. Med. 60:877, 1967.
17. Butler, N. R., and Alberman, E. D. (eds.): Perinatal Problems: The second report of the 1958 British perinatal mortality survey. Edinburgh, E. & S. Livingstone, Ltd., 1963.
18. Lugo, G., and Cassady, G.: Intrauterine growth retardation; clinicopathologic findings in 233 consecutive infants. Am. J. Obstet. Gynec. 109:615, 1971.
19. Dawkins, M.: The "small for dates" baby in gestational age, size, and maturity. Clin. Develop. Med. 19:35, 1965.
20. Beargie, R. A., James, V. L., and Greene, J. W.: Growth and development of small-for-date newborns. Ped. Clin. N. Amer. 17:159, 1970.
21. Weiner, G.: The relationship of birth weight and length of gestation to intellectual development at ages 8 to 10 years. J. Pediat. 76:694, 1970.
22. Drillien, C. M.: The small-for-dates infant. Ped. Clin. N. Amer. 17:9, 1970.
23. Lubchenco, L. O.: Personal communication.
24. Beard, R. W., and Roberts, G. M.: A prospective approach to the diagnosis of intrauterine growth retardation. Proc. Roy. Soc. Med. 63:501, 1970.
25. Brush, M. G., Maxwell, R., Scherer, J., Taylor, R. W., and Tye, G.: Placental failure in the small-for-dates syndrome. Proc. Roy. Soc. Med. 63:1098, 1970.

26. Thompson, H. E., Holmes, J. H., Gottesfeld, K. R., and Taylor, E. S.: Fetal development as determined by ultrasonic pulse echo techniques. Am. J. Obstet. Gynec. 92:44, 1965.
27. Martin, J. C., Hähnel, R., Kean, B. P., and Troy, V. G.: Urinary oestrogen excretion in women with intrauterine fetal growth retardation. Aust. New Zeal. J. Obstet. Gynaec. 12:102, 1972.
28. Elliott, P. M.: Urinary oestriol excretion in retarded intrauterine growth. Aust. New Zeal. J. Obstet. Gynaec. 10:18, 1970.
29. Liggins, G. C., and Evans, M.: Patterns of oestriol excretion in abnormal pregnancy: a study of 234 cases. New Zeal. Med. J. 62:365, 1963.
30. Moore, W. M. O., Murphy, P. J., and Davis, J. A.: Creatinine content of amniotic fluid in cases of retarded fetal growth. Am. J. Obstet. Gynec. 110:908, 1971.
31. Droegemueller, W., Jackson, C., Makowski, E. L., and Battaglia, F. C.: Amniotic fluid for the assessment of gestational age. Am. J. Obstet. Gynec. 104:424, 1969.
32. Sharma, S. D., and Trussell, R. R.: The value of amniotic fluid examination in the assessment of fetal maturity. J. Obstet. Gynaec. Brit. Comm. 77:215, 1970.
33. Ray, M., Freeman, R., Pine, S., and Hesselgesser, R.: Clinical experience with the oxytocin challenge test. Am. J. Obstet. Gynec. 114:1, 1972.
34. Elliott, P.: Foetal salvage in retarded intrauterine growth of the foetus. Aust. New Zeal. J. Obstet. Gynaec. 7:13, 1967.
35. Jeffrey, R. L. J., Bowes, W. A., Jr., and Delaney, J. J.: The role of bed rest in twin gestation. (In press.)

Identification and Management of Intrauterine Growth Retardation

FREDRIC D. FRIGOLETTO, JR.
Harvard Medical School and Boston Hospital for Women

Introduction

Since the early 1950's there has been increasing concern over the significance of a discrepancy between the gestational age and the expected weight of the fetus at birth. Clifford[5] in 1954 described and classified in some detail the appearance of these infants and coined the term *placental dysfunction* to account for the observed changes in the skin and wasting of the subcutaneous tissue. The problem was highlighted in 1963 when Gruenwald[13] published his paper on chronic fetal distress and placental insufficiency. With the growing recognition that the newborn who has suffered from intrauterine deprivation with resultant growth retardation regardless of cause is vulnerable to metabolic, hematologic, and neurologic disorders, and has a higher perinatal mortality rate, obstetricians have become increasingly aware of this condition.[15]

The entity now has many synonyms—e.g., dysmaturity, placental insufficiency, small for dates baby, intrauterine growth retardation, and chronic fetal distress. Besides the characteristic appearance of the infant, the condition is considered to be present when by definition the neonate's weight falls in the lower tenth percentile of weight curves for infants of a given population at that particular gestational age.

Etiology

Many clinical states are associated with this syndrome; indeed, many of the conclusions which have been drawn from studies on the small for dates baby may be misleading or in error if they have been made without regard to particular underlying or associated conditions.[8] It is readily apparent that cases must be individualized and maternal, placental, and fetal factors critically assessed with respect to etiology, diagnosis, and eventual patient management. Thus, to advance

21

the identification and therapeutic management of such patients demands a multi-disciplinary approach.

Toxemia and hypertension, renal pathology, and collagen diseases have logically been associated with the etiology of this syndrome. It is assumed that in these conditions there is decreased uteroplacental perfusion, with resultant fetal malnutrition and fetal growth retardation. However, direct measurements of uteroplacental blood flow in these states have not been made. Nevertheless, it has been demonstrated in animals by Creasy[6] and others that following gradual occlusion of the uteroplacental vascular bed, there is a mean decrease of 30 per cent of fetal weight with a decrease in certain organ weights, especially in the brain-to-liver weight ratio. Chase[4] and colleagues recently have reported alterations in brain biochemistry in infants who had intrauterine growth retardation. Reductions in brain weight and cellularity seemed to be most marked in the cerebellum. The myelin lipids, cerebrosides, and sulfatides appeared to be reduced in concentration or total quantity to a greater extent than other lipids in such babies. However, in the human fetus, the size of the brain appears to be much less affected by growth retardation than any other part of the body, although little data exist pertaining to the eventual human brain development and mental status.[8]

Attempts to assess maternal malnutrition as a causal factor in low birth weight infants has and continues to be extensively studied, but currently the reported results are inconsistent and therefore inconclusive.[3] There is sufficient evidence to keep the question open that maternal nutrition affects birth weight. According to most studies, the mother's pregravid weight, weight gain during pregnancy, height, birth rank, and socioeconomic conditions are in varying degrees related to the infant's birth weight. However, many dietary survey studies have failed to find a significant relationship between maternal diet and birth weight. It must be pointed out that many of these studies suffer from one or more problems of experimental design—i.e., small numbers, inappropriate controls, and selection bias.[3] Nevertheless, certain observations made during unusual wartime conditions cannot be ignored. Studies of food deprivation during wartime indiciate that mean birth weights vary consistently with the level of nutrition in populations. However, severe and acute food shortage in the human female seems to result in failure to conceive and in an increase in early abortions rather than a decrease in birth weight of those fetuses who survive long enough to be viable.[8]

In addition to maternal factors, the placenta itself has been appraised to evaluate the influence of placental lesions on the small for dates baby. Most authorities agree that there is no single placental abnormality that is common to the low birth weight syndrome. There are certain lesions, however, which because of their relatively high frequency merit consideration. The associated morphological placental abnormalities vary greatly, from infarction, villous avascularity, fibrinosis, and premature aging, to nonspecific chronic villous inflammation, and many of these placentae are indistinguishable from those associated with normal, healthy babies.[2] In fact, Driscoll[2] found no clear evidence that placental infarction plays an important role in causation of dysmaturity. However, the placentas of dysmature infants tend to be lighter in weight for gestational age, the decrease in weight being roughly proportional to that of the infants themselves.[2]

Undoubtedly the inherent growth potential of the fetus is a significant determinant, which may help to explain the relatively large percentage of these cases in which no maternal or placental abnormality can be detected. Although the exact mechanism by which certain fetal abnormalities may result in intrauterine growth retardation is unknown, there is less controversy regarding the relationship between growth retardation and fetal viral infections, such as rubella, cytomegalic inclusion disease, toxoplasmosis, and chromosomal abnormalities. In summary, the etiology of this syndrome may include many factors, both maternal and fetal, and no single category will suffice.

Clinical Considerations

It is generally agreed that diagnosis of the syndrome is difficult and at times uncertain. However, when there are known predisposing factors, such as a previous history of a dysmature baby, unexplained intrauterine deaths, hypertension, and so forth, which could affect the fetus during gestation by the twenty-eighth week or earlier, careful and repeated observation should make the clinician suspicious of the presence of intrauterine growth retardation. Equally challenging and even more difficult to recognize and diagnose are the cases with a later onset, often referred to as a more acute form of the syndrome, in contrast to the more chronic form alluded to above. This may account for the infant who presumably has suffered from relatively acute weight loss, whose skin is loose or too large for its frame, but whose length may be normal or near normal, and who may be in a higher percentile than the tenth in weight. Although this infant may weigh seven pounds or more, he too has suffered from intrauterine "malnutrition" and possible asphyxia, but apparently of a much less chronic nature. Hence, for every parturient, close attention must be given to uterine size by whatever method of clinical measurement indicated—maternal weight, fetal activity, and estimation of quantity of amniotic fluid. Obviously, in many cases, even the most accurate observations will leave the clinician in doubt and he must turn to laboratory tests for assistance.

At amniocentesis a sample of clear amniotic fluid containing flecks of vernix caseosa is reassuring evidence that the syndrome is not present at the time to any significant degree. Meconium-stained fluid or only small amounts of fluid is highly suggestive of intrauterine malnutrition. However, these findings can be misleading; for example, there may be some meconium staining in an otherwise normal baby or a falsely dry tap. Likewise, a bloody tap may be defeating, although centrifuging the specimen will allow adequate inspection of the liquor. In addition to its appearance, the amniotic fluid should be evaluated for those components useful in determining fetal maturity.

With the increasing availability of estriol determinations and their use in assessing the high-risk pregnancy, 24 hour urinary estriol excretion rates and plasma levels have been studied in the intrauterine growth retardation syndrome. Many authors have demonstrated this fetal condition when maternal estriol excretion is diminished, but no absolute levels have been established. There is, however, a well documented group of normal patients who have consistently low estriol values for each particular period of gestation. Here the abnormal estriol excretion cannot be entirely explained. Although some of these babies may be compromised, many are healthy and vigorous, with no evidence of malnutrition. The other side of the coin likewise can be misleading: occasionally a mother with normal estriol values may give birth to a small for dates baby.[12] In other words, there is overlap in the distribution of the normal as well as the abnormal values of urinary estriols, with an up to 10 per cent chance of error. Nevertheless, with normal estriol excretion, the clinician can be reasonably confident that the fetus is not in immediate jeopardy.

Also, one must appreciate the day-to-day variation in urinary estriol determinations, perhaps as much as 40 per cent. However, there is no doubt that serial determinations can be of great help to the clinician in determining a trend and hence may assist in answering the plaguing question of whether or not to effect delivery at a given period in pregnancy.

More recently, ultrasonic fetal cephalometry has been studied with respect to the diagnosis of the dysmature syndrome. Willochs and Dunsmore,[20] in a relatively large series of cases, made a diagnosis of dysmaturity or intrauterine growth retardation if the weekly growth rate of the biparietal diameter was less than 0.17 cm. Using this criterion, it was found that 70 per cent of the dysmature cases could be identified and diagnosed correctly. Dewhurst[7] holds the view that the biparietal measurement provides the best method of intrauterine growth rate assessment currently available. An important point that has emerged from several investigators is that in intrauterine growth retardation normal fetal head growth is less rapid and more variable. The measurement of the biparietal diameter before 30 weeks correlates well with the gestational age and expected date of confinement, even when a single measurement is taken. Measurements taken after 30 weeks correlate less accurately with the due date but are nevertheless valid for rate of growth when serial determinations are obtained. It is reasonable to conclude that some skepticism is in order when determinations are done in late pregnancy, i.e., after the thirty-fourth week, because the overlap of dysmature and nondysmature fetal head measurements is too great.[9]

Although there are other hormonal and enzymatic assays which have been investigated in the diagnosis of the dysmature syndrome, none appear at this time to be more valid than those already discussed, and hence they will only be listed here: oxytocin challenge test; prematurely elevated amniotic fluid lecithin/sphingomyelin ratios; and placental alkaline phosphatase levels. Obviously what is needed is a relatively inexpensive, readily available, accurate diagnostic test that is specific in the identification of this syndrome of intrauterine growth retardation. Investigations continue in pursuit of such a technique or method. For example, Smith and Scanlon postulate that the dysmature fetus is undergoing increasing starvation.[19] The fetus thus begins to utilize his previously deposited fat stores, which results in hyperlipemia and hyperketonemia. If this occurs in the fetus, one might expect that the water-soluble ketone bodies would be present in amniotic fluid and hence aid in the antepartum diagnosis of the dysmature infant. The workers measured $D(-)\beta$-hydroxybutyrate in amniotic fluid in normal pregnancy and in those patients suspected of having the dysmature syndrome. Although there was overlap of the normal and affected infants, a value was established above which only dysmaturity was present.

The author and colleagues reported recently the finding of a maternal hypercoagulable state beyond that of normal pregnancy, which was associated with the dysmature syndrome.[10,17] In a few cases in which the syndrome was suspected clinically but the fetus was unaffected at birth, the coagulation factors were consistent with changes in a normal pregnancy. Hence, a periodic clotting profile in relation to a hypercoagulable state, especially a silicone clotting time, might prove helpful in identification of intrauterine growth retardation.[17] By analogy, the intravillous space may play some role in the early changes in blood clotting as observed in the Kasabach-Merritt (thrombopenia-hemangioma) syndrome. If so, this would reflect diminished intravillous blood flow and placental transport.

Treatment

Once the diagnosis is suspected and then confirmed, the major decision in patient management, currently at least, is to establish the optimal time to effect delivery, for the difficult question remains as to whether or not the fetus should be delivered as soon as studies for maturity indicate that it will not be afflicted with respiratory distress syndrome. In other words, is there less likelihood of irreversible damage to the fetus if it is delivered at 35 to 36 weeks than if it is permitted to continue to term and live in what is presumably an unfavorable intrauterine milieu, regardless of other considerations, such as a situation in which the pelvic findings are not conducive to successful induction of labor?

Indeed, when this syndrome is present prior to the thirty-fourth week of gestation, little is now available therapeutically except bed rest, which may enhance uteroplacental perfusion. However, in the realm of speculation, there are at least two approaches to the treatment of this perplexing problem which seemingly deserve consideration and investigation. On the basis of a long experience with the technique of transabdominal intrauterine fetal peritoneal transfusion for erythroblastosis fetalis, alimentation by fetal intraperitoneal nutritional supplements offers a possibility of combating the ravages of intrauterine malnutrition. Already reports have appeared describing the use of special diets or intravenous alimentation[11] in low birth weight infants in an attempt to provide optimal nutrition, otherwise not always possible, early in the postnatal course. This obviously presumes that the present complications of intravenous alimentation can be reduced to an acceptable level.[1]

Second, if the preliminary studies which indicate that a hypercoagulable state is associated with at least some of the cases of dysmature syndrome[10] are valid, then further investigations are necessary to evaluate the therapeutic role of long-term heparinization in the treatment of this disorder.

Conclusion

With rapidly increasing developments in the newborn intensive care unit, there has been a changing prognosis for the low birth weight infant.[16,18] It is therefore imperative that the obstetrician recognize the existence of the dysmature syndrome and effect delivery of such pregnancies when the chances of extrauterine survival are reasonable and before irreversible damage occurs to the fetus. Obviously this timing of delivery, which itself is controversial, is the crux of the matter in managing these pregnancies. Although the more sophisticated diagnostic tools are not available to all physicians caring for the parturient, a high index of suspicion and astute clinical acumen can suffice. Indeed, in the most subtle form of the syndrome—that which has its onset in the last few weeks of pregnancy—only meticulous attention to maternal weight, abdominal girth, and so forth, will warn of the presence of this syndrome in its subacute form. The suspicion of its presence, combined with determination of the status of fetal maturity, will then allow appropriately timed intervention in addition to thorough preparation for closely monitored labor in these high-risk fetuses.[14]

REFERENCES

1. Behrman, R. E.: Total intravenous alimentation: Foreword. J. Pediat. 81:127–182, 1972.
2. Benirschke, K., and Driscoll, S. G.: The Pathology of the Human Placenta. New York, Springer-Verlag, 1967.
3. Bergner, L., and Susser, M. W.: Low birth weight and prenatal nutrition: an interpretative review. Pediatrics 46:946–966, 1970.
4. Chase, H. P., Welch, N. N., Dabiere, C. S., Vasan, N. S., and Butterfield, L. J.: Alterations in human brain biochemistry following intrauterine growth retardation. Pediatrics 50:403–411, 1972.
5. Clifford, S. H.: Postmaturity with placental dysfunction. J. Pediat. 44:1, 1954.
6. Creasy, R. K., Barrett, C. T., De Swiet, M., Kahanpaa, K. V., and Rudolph, A.: Experimental intrauterine growth retardation in the sheep. Amer. J. Obstet. Gynec. 112: 566–573, 1972.
7. Dewhurst, C. J., Beagley, J. M., and Campbell, S.: Assessment of fetal maturity and dysmaturity. Amer. J. Obstet. Gynec. 113:141–149, 1972.
8. Drillien, C. M.: The small-for-date infant: etiology and prognosis. Pediat. Clin. N. Amer. 17:9–24, 1970.
9. Assessment of gestational age and prediction of dysmaturity by ultrasonic fetal cephalometry (editorial). Obstet. Gynec. Surv. 27:149, 1972.
10. Frigoletto, F. D., Tullis, J. L., Reid, D. E., and Hinman, J.: Hypercoagulability in the dysmature syndrome. Amer. J. Obstet. Gynec. 111:867–873, 1971.
11. Goldman, H. I., Leibman, O. B., Freudenthal, R., and Reuben, R.: Effects of early dietary protein intake on low-birth-weight infants: evaluation at 3 years of age. J. Pediat. 78:126–129, 1971.
12. Greene, J. W., and Beargie, R. A.: Use of urinary estriol excretion studies in the assessment of the high risk pregnancy. Pediat. Clin. N. Amer. 17:43–48, 1970.
13. Gruenwald, P.: Chronic fetal distress and placental insufficiency. Biol. Neonat. 5:215, 1963.
14. Low, J. A., Boston, R. W., and Pancham, S. R.: Fetal asphyxia during the intrapartum period in intrauterine growth-retarded infants. Amer. J. Obstet. Gynec. 113:351–357, 1972.
15. Lugo, G., and Cassady, G.: Intrauterine growth retardation. Amer. J. Obstet. Gynec. 109:615–622, 1971.
16. Rawlings, G., Reynolds, E. O. R., Stewart, A., and Strang, L. B.: Changing prognosis for infants of very low birth weight. Lancet 1:516–519, 1971.
17. Reid, D. E., Frigoletto, F. D., Tullis, J. L., and Hinman, J.: Hypercoagulable states in pregnancy. Amer. J. Obstet. Gynec. 111:493–504, 1971.
18. Robinson, R.: The small-for-dates baby—II. Brit. Med. J. 4:480–482, 1971.
19. Smith, A. L., and Scanlon, J. L.: Amniotic fluid D (−) β-hydroxybutyrate and the dysmature newborn infant. Amer. J. Obstet. Gynec. 115:569–574, 1973.
20. Willocks, J., and Dunsmore, I. R.: Assessment of gestational age and prediction of dysmaturity by ultrasonic fetal cephalometry. J. Obstet. Gynaec. Brit. Comm. 78:804–808, 1971.

Identification and Management
of Intrauterine Growth Retardation

Editorial Comment

As implied in the preface, greater emphasis is now being placed on assuring the new individual of being well born biologically. This is enhanced by the advances into the new frontier of intrauterine existence by amniocentesis and sonography. Undoubtedly, these represent the beginning of an extensive exploration of the biology of the normal and abnormal growth and development of the human fetus. Although discerning clinicians of previous eras were well aware that the fetus was in jeopardy in a variety of clinical states, their understanding of the onset and extent of this threat was based purely on clinical acumen and experience.

The various synonyms or terminologies for deviations in fetal growth patterns may well reflect the many unknowns that influence and control the intrauterine physiologic milieu. Perhaps no single term will suffice. This is suggested by the desire or recommendation to separate what might be regarded as intrauterine growth retardation involving the whole fetus and dysmaturity that may involve primarily the subcutaneous tissues of the fetus. However, this may be simply a matter of the degree of fetal malnutrition. Undoubtedly family standards or parent size should be given consideration in establishing normalcy for birth weight, but this would be of little value here, where rate of growth is the critical issue.

As indicated by the contributors, the clinical identification of the intrauterine growth retardation syndrome leaves much to be desired. However, in the laboratory, sonography has provided a reasonably accurate method of determining intrauterine growth retardation. It has been repeatedly demonstrated by several groups that in this syndrome the fetal biparietal diameter and thoracic measurements fail to increase in size in accordance with values established for normal rates of growth.

Hopefully, future advances will include more precise methods for early detection of failure of the fetus to grow in accordance with normal expectations. This is particularly pertinent during the critical period of 28 to 36 weeks' gestation, when the fetus must attain a state of maturity to insure its extrauterine survival. One of the basic questions at issue is whether the fetus suffering from intrauterine growth retardation should be delivered at an earlier period (32 to 35 weeks) in order to avoid irreversible central nervous system damage despite the increased risk of hyaline membrane disease. This raises an equally important query: namely, whether the effects of intrauterine malnutrition can be corrected after birth.

The treatment of intrauterine growth retardation currently is restricted to bed rest, which supposedly improves uteroplacental blood flow; possibly a regulation of nutritional factors, still to be defined, is also of value.

The rationale for bed rest currently is based on indirect evidence; the role of nutrition is truly speculative. The urinary estriol values often are found to rise with bed rest, indicating perhaps an increase in uteroplacental blood flow and an improvement, albeit temporary, in the fetal environment. With respect to nutrition, there has been a recent flurry of statements and publications contending that the fetal welfare is best served by what some might regard as uncontrolled maternal weight gain (but with little or no regard for the nutritional requirements of pregnancy) and this may have relevance here, especially to the idiopathic type of fetal growth retardation. The idiopathic type accounts for 50 per cent of the total in patients who give birth to infants that are growth retarded. Further, it has been noted that many of these mothers repeatedly produce infants so afflicted, after otherwise normal pregnancies.

It is evident that the original publications concerned in establishing the modifications of nutritional requirements for the pregnant state are unfamiliar or have been disregarded. Therefore, it seems appropriate to call attention to this void in lieu of the possibility that maternal nutrition may be an important factor in the possible prevention or management of fetal malnutrition. Hence, attention is directed to the careful and dedicated work of an outstanding nutritionist, the late Bertha S. Burke and her group of the Department of Maternal and Child Health, School of Public Health, Harvard University. To quote and slightly paraphrase these several papers ". . . (1) the old belief that the fetus is a nutritional parasite to the mother is false, but rather, if the mother is sufficiently depleted nutritionally, the fetus may suffer to spare the mother. . . . (2) The pregnant patient should be expected to gain 20 to 25 pounds above a desirable weight for her height and build. This implies that underweight women should gain more; the overweight woman may restrict her calories only when her protein, mineral, and vitamin needs are fully provided. . . . (3) As for all parturients, this includes approximately 80 grams of protein daily. If the latter is met, except for ascorbic acid, other supplements of vitamins, calcium, etc., are provided because of their natural association with protetin in food." In these studies, a relationship was established between a spectrum of diets ranging from very poor to excellent in protein content, and both the birth weight and—equally impressively—the birth length of the fetus.[1,2] Both were substantially decreased in diets poor in protein.

These findings are buttressed by observations in a recent paper on the caloric cost of pregnancy, in which the authors concluded that no increased requirements are needed if "adequate structural protein and other essential nutrients are provided."[3] This does not contradict the observation that the major source of maternal energy in pregnancy is carbohydrate, for the objective is to fulfill the fetal requirements. Moreover, maternal homeostasis involves, among many variables, a careful balance between placental lactogen and insulin activity. Placental lactogen levels have been observed to be low in many instances of intrauterine growth retardation, but the placenta may also be small. It will be of interest and presumably of some importance to note whether mothers, especially those who tend to have infants with intrauterine growth retardation after uncomplicated pregnancies, deviate nutritionally and metabolically from otherwise normal patients. That patients do differ in this regard is suggested by the fact that occasionally a parturient will gain very little weight during pregnancy despite the fact that her caloric intake may appear, and indeed is, in excess of the designated normal requirements for pregnancy.

All of this emphasizes the fallacy of basing conclusions on crude estimations of the relationship between the maternal weight gain and birth weight of the infant. The failure to consider certain variables mentioned here is to disregard totally the nutritional principles that influence the structural growth of the fetus. Moreover, to permit excessive maternal weight gain is to ignore the laws of health that will result in residual obesity for many women, to say nothing of the increased complications and hazards of pregnancy. In short, nutritional requirements and weight gain in pregnancy are not necessarily synonymous.

The day may be near when the fetus may be nourished directly by hyperalimentation, but this presupposes that it is sufficiently developed biochemically to utilize such supplements.

Granted that the sonogram, estriol estimations, and to a lesser degree placental lactogen determinations are invaluable, the precise regimen for assessment of fetal status still remains to be defined. In cases of growth retardation, in which the muscle mass is supposedly diminished, amniotic fluid creatinine values may be misleading in establishing fetal age. The sphingomyelin/lecithin ratio has provided the clinician with a nearly consistently accurate method in establishing the relative maturity of the fetus and the timing of delivery.

To generalize concerning the type of delivery to be preferred is hazardous, for in addition to the current clinical situation, the patient's history may well include past reproduction failures. Although pelvic delivery is safer for the mother despite the creditable reduction in the risk of cesarean section, the stress of labor on the growth retarded fetus cannot be minimized. Hence, the obstetrical management for each patient must be highly individualized as to both timing and method of delivery.

REFERENCES

1. Burke, B. S., Stevenson, S. S., Worcester, J., and Stuart, H. C.: Nutritional studies during pregnancy; relation of maternal nutrition to condition of infant birth; study of siblings. J. Nutrition 38:453, 1949.
2. Burke, B. S.: Nutritional needs of pregnancy—their importance to mother and fetus. Bulletin of Maternal Welfare, Sept.–Oct., 1956.
3. Emerson, K., Jr., Saxena, B. N., and Poindexter, E. L.: Caloric cost of normal pregnancy. Amer. Col. Obstr. Gynec. 40:6, 1972.

2

Treatment of Patients With Premature Rupture of the Fetal Membranes: (a) Prior to 32 Weeks; (b) After 32 Weeks

Alternative Points of View:

    By David Charles

    By Myron Gordon and Allan B. Weingold

    By Keith P. Russell and Joseph Cheung

    By William C. Scott

Editorial Comment

Treatment of Patients With Premature Rupture of the Fetal Membranes: (a) Prior to 32 Weeks; (b) After 32 Weeks

Management of Premature Rupture of the Membranes

DAVID CHARLES

Boston University School of Medicine and Boston City Hospital

Introduction

The management of premature rupture of the fetal membranes is of constant concern to the obstetrician, principally because of the complications that can arise from this entity. Interest in the problem is stimulated periodically by published or spoken pronouncements of various obstetric authorities, which often provoke a series of letters to medical journals, some agreeing with the experts, but most dissenting from the views expressed. Indeed, professional interest in this subject is perpetually simmering. Meanwhile, the problem remains unsolved and its incidence has not greatly declined during the past century, despite the sometimes acrimonious dissensions and proposals concerning etiology and treatment. Indeed, no single entity in obstetric practice is so surfeited with divergent views regarding causation and management as premature rupture of the membranes.

Although a cardinal feature of medicine is prevention, it would be utopian indeed to expect to eliminate entirely the premature rupturing of the membranes. At present we must modify our goals as far as the preventive aspects are concerned and concentrate upon minimizing or avoiding the development of the most serious complication, namely, sepsis. It is recognized that the likelihood of developing intrauterine sepsis increases as a function of time from the moment the fetal membranes rupture.

Etiology

Although certain entities, such as malpresentation and contracted pelvis, are commonly found in association with it, the etiology of premature rupture of

33

the membranes generally is unknown, and a number of hypotheses have been proposed in explanation.

Such factors as the incompetent cervix and increased intrauterine tension, resulting either from multiple pregnancy or from hydramnios, have been incriminated and undoubtedly account for some instances. Much has been written about defects in the tensile strength of the membranes as a possible cause, but this remains highly controversial. In truth, in the vast majority of cases, the exciting factor is unknown, and the reasons why some individuals repeat their obstetric history, with recurrent premature rupture of the membranes and premature labors, remain to be disclosed. Only now are we beginning to understand the role of the fetus in the initiation of labor. What effect the fetus itself may have on premature rupture of the membranes remains to be determined.

With the emancipation of civil laws and statutes concerning abortion, it would be well for us to remember that soon the Western hemisphere will meet the same problems that have been amply documented in Europe in patients who have had one or more therapeutic abortions. Premature rupture of the membranes and prematurity are common entities, presumably resulting from a compromised cervix, in countries where therapeutic abortion has been applied as a method of population control. It would be well for all obstetricians to take due cognizance of this fact.

Diagnosis

It is axiomatic that a definitive diagnosis of premature rupture of the membranes is necessary before therapy is begun. Although the diagnosis is evident when large quantities of amniotic fluid escape from the vagina, it is more difficult to distinguish if there is only a slight watery discharge. Urinary incontinence, increased cervical secretions, and leukorrhea must be differentiated. It is thought that a precise diagnosis can be obtained only by microscopic demonstration of fetal squames and other elements, such as hair, vernix caseosa, and cells which stain orange with Nile blue, in the discharge.

The importance of accurate diagnosis is obvious if the obstetrician is conversant with the seriousness of the entity and with the various morbid sequelae with which he may be confronted. All too frequently the physician has failed to adopt a prudent attitude towards the management of this problem.

Treatment

The definitive treatment of premature rupture of the fetal membranes requires the application of certain principles derived from our knowledge of what natural forces can accomplish and how, from a physiological and anatomical point of view, these forces can be aided and abetted. We must also remember our responsibility for the psychological, as well as the physical, health of our patients. This is especially pertinent in premature rupture of the membranes, since the unborn child is so frequently at risk from prematurity and infection. The obstetrician should endeavor to describe to his patient in general terms the nature of the condition and the course he is likely to adopt, as well as the objectives and probable effects of any of the measures he may recommend.

With respect to prevention, if a woman suffers from a severe vaginitis, the obstetrician immediately becomes aware of the dangers of infection should premature rupture of the membranes occur, but unfortunately the presence of virulent organisms is not always presaged by visible signs of an inflammatory process. It is safest to regard the vagina of every patient in labor as a source of potential intrauterine sepsis. Hence, it is highly important to avoid unnecessary pelvic examinations. Even when a vaginal examination is performed using strict aseptic precautions, chorioamnionitis can rapidly ensue, a fact that is well documented by Clark and Anderson,[1] who noted that in patients who became infected, 29.7 per cent had had a vaginal examination shortly before the infection developed and became clinically evident.

The majority of obstetricians recognize that once maximum maturity of a fetus has been attained, termination of the pregnancy is mandatory. Once rupture of the membranes has occurred, few would permit a woman at or beyond the thirty-seventh week of gestation to remain undelivered at home or in hospital. Here there should be no controversy as to management.

But what about pregnancy prior to the thirty-seventh week of gestation? Active attempts to prolong the pregnancy or the passive approach of "masterly inactivity" have been considered justifiable by some obstetricians when confronted with premature rupture of the membranes prior to weeks 35 to 37. It is frequently stated that spontaneous uterine activity occurs in over 80 per cent of individuals within 24 hours of rupture of the membranes.[1,2,3] In view of this, the question of what happens to the other patients must be raised. Are they allowed to languish in hospital or at home, exposed to the whole gamut of complications, which range from chorioamnionitis affecting the unborn child to maternal infection, with its implications regarding subsequent conception or even its threat to the mother's life itself? The medical literature contains many defenses of this attitude, which generally assert that complications are infrequent and rarely severe. This complacency perhaps is a logical result of an age in which maternal mortality is tabulated in deaths per 10,000 live births. However, it should be realized that Clark and Anderson[1] reported positive blood cultures in 13 per cent of their patients in whom infection was suspected. Maternal deaths from infection do occur, often in association with endotoxic shock and disseminated intravascular coagulation. Over a period of 13 years, Webster[2] reported 13 maternal deaths from sepsis in association with premature rupture of the membranes. Hence, there should be no disagreement that optimal therapy for the mother is prompt evacuation of the uterus, regardless of the duration of the gestation.

One may well ask, what about the infant's welfare? The obstetrician is indeed buffeted between Scylla and Charybdis. Active intervention means prematurity with its own specific risk to infant survival. On the other hand, even judicious neglect may foster infection and its sequelae, sometimes even death. Certainly it must be stated that every physician who practices obstetrics can cite an instance in which prolonged rupture of the membranes has existed for days or even weeks and eventually a healthy child has been delivered without subsequent difficulty. The physician, therefore, may be lulled into a false sense of security until his patient reappears in the office at a later date, complaining of secondary infertility that is found to result from tubal occlusion, a sequel to a low-grade postpartum infection. Such a sequence of events bespeaks the necessity of taking into account not only the life of the mother, but also her health and her subsequent reproductive prospects. One might also do well to inquire whether the child has developed normally and without any stigmata of central nervous system damage.

Regardless of the etiology, it is well recognized that a large number of infants weighing less than 2000 grams do not survive the neonatal period, even when they are presumably free of infection. However, it is reasonable to assume that the noninfected infant would have a better prognosis than one so afflicted. Moreover, spontaneous rupture of the membranes followed by labor prior to the thirty-fourth week of gestation is associated with a fetal loss that frequently is assigned to prematurity without considering other etiological factors. Clinically, the obstetrician is apt to be confronted by breech delivery with its inherent complications and risks, or with prolapse of the umbilical cord occurring independently or in association with breech presentation. The pathologist may report atelectasis and hyaline membrane disease as morphological conditions accounting for fetal demise. All too frequently, the major cause of death may be anoxia secondary to such complications of pregnancy as preeclampsia, hypertensive disease, or sundry other entities that are considered beyond control.

Furthermore, few infants in this predicament gain weight in utero even if a conservative, cautious attitude is adopted. Thus, it is germane to reiterate time and time again that the risk of lethal infection is always present, although sepsis in a fulminating form may not always ensue. Specifically, it would be well for all departments of obstetrics in their monthly staff conferences to present and discuss such cases in the presence of pathologists and pediatricians well versed in perinatal medicine. Surely we must realize that everyone is on the side of the angels!

From experience gleaned at Boston City Hospital, there is little doubt that an aggressive attitude towards the management of this condition, as advocated by Russell and Anderson in 1962, has minimized the risk of serious complications.[4] Hence, regardless of the length of the gestation, we feel that in cases of premature rupture of the membranes, the sooner the pregnancy is terminated, the better the maternal prognosis, and the better the child almost always fares.

Too many physicians have adopted the attitude that antibiotics should be administered routinely to all women with premature rupture of the membranes, to protect both mother and fetus against infection. The prophylactic use of these agents has resulted in the evolution of resistant strains of bacteria and compounded the ever-present risk of hospital infection. It must be remembered that infection is a continual hazard in the practice of obstetrics and, at the same time, the indiscriminate use of antibiotics can produce diagnostic and therapeutic dilemmas. A false sense of security is afforded to the physician who administers these agents in the absence of definite indications. They produce the optimal beneficial effect only when used at the right time, in the right place, in the right amounts, and for appropriate and specific infections.

Therefore, once a diagnosis of premature rupture has been attained, it is preferable to institute labor rather than run the risk of severe maternal or fetal infection. Surely, when premature rupture of the membranes occurs, the pregnancy itself is in jeopardy, and from a philosophical point of view, nature has attempted to take care of the situation. Indeed, obstetricians should consider premature rupture of the membranes as indicative of something remiss with the pregnancy.

In the past, there were many obstacles to the aggressive management of premature rupture of the membranes. Prior to the adoption of intravenous oxytocin, no method for the acceleration or accentuation of uterine activity existed, nor could we attenuate the interval between rupture of the membranes and initiation of labor. Even after therapeutic measures for induction of labor were accepted, delays still occurred, mainly because many physicians remained obdurate. Only when an overt or suspected maternal infection was present was vigorous therapy applied, and in such instances the septic process had already involved the fetus and placed it in jeopardy.

Active measures to initiate labor should be considered the rule and not the exception. As in all areas of obstetrics, when induction of labor is indicated, one must ever consider the possibility of abdominal delivery. It is true that whether it is necessary for maternal or for fetal reasons, the mere fact that induction is necessary should be considered as a possible indication for cesarean section, and this should always be foremost in the mind of the obstetrician, else he is practicing unpardonable obstetrics.

Present-day obstetrics has accepted the dictum that fulminating preeclampsia requires intervention, and all too frequently there is the risk of prematurity, but this is accepted in the interests of the mother and infant. If, therefore, we consider premature rupture of the membranes as an indication for delivery, the infant transferred to the pediatrician's care should, in the majority of instances, be capable of survival, since premature rupture of the membranes *per se* is not associated with uteroplacental insufficiency, such as occurs in the presence of preeclampsia, diabetes, and placental separation.

There are exceptions to every rule, and a conservative approach to premature rupture of the membranes can be judiciously adopted when the patient has had a series of obstetric disappointments or a history of infertility. Such a course of action applies only when the gestation is between the twenty-eighth and thirty-fourth week. The patient should be put to bed in the hospital, and once the diagnosis is substantiated, no further pelvic examinations should be performed. If fever occurs or the gestation has been judged to be of more than 34 weeks' duration, the pregnancy should be terminated.

It is now necessary to consider methods of inducing uterine action when nature has not taken care of its own—specifically, if the membranes have been ruptured for more than 12 hours and no uterine activity has occurred—since the risk to both mother and fetus increases exponentially. First and foremost, there is no justification for the subcutaneous or intramuscular administration of oxytocin to establish labor in individuals who have had premature rupture of the membranes. In fact, oxytocin should be administered only by the intravenous route and other methods considered to be as dead as the dodo. By the adoption of the intravenous route for administration, this pharmacologic agent can be infused with minute-to-minute control. Further precision has been achieved by the utilization of the Harvard pump, thereby circumventing the use of large volumes of fluid for oxytocin infusion. The latter is worthy of note, in view of the antidiuretic effects of the agent and the hazard of water intoxication. In fact, an infusion pump for oxytocin titration is now widely used for induction of labor.[5,6]

One must always realize that oxytocin administration, by whatever route, is not free from potential hazards. The response of the uterus to a specific dose varies enormously from patient to patient and even from hour to hour in the same individual. Any method that may be adopted to assess the therapeutic response to oxytocin, be it by an external or internal tokodynamometer, still requires the constant supervision of trained personnel. A major hazard is uterine hypertonicity, with potential fetal hypoxia owing to embarrassment of the uteroplacental circulation. Abnormal fetal heart rate patterns and alteration in acid balance, with decreased pH of the fetal blood may, therefore, be observed when an excessive dosage of oxytocin is administered.

Adequate monitoring of the fetal heart and uterine contractions is mandatory in conjunction with an aggressive approach to premature rupture of the membranes. Progress of labor should be measured by dilation of the cervix and not by the subjective reaction of the patient. It must be emphasized that such a policy can be conducted only when each patient is cared for individually. This means that a delivery unit is, in effect, a special care obstetric suite in which skilled nursing and medical staff are constantly in attendance. Similarly, to subordinate the rate of infusion of the oxytocin to the reaction of the patient is to allow her to dictate the course of labor.[7] In the absence of marked prematurity, analgesic drugs can be liberally prescribed. However, it is well worth recognizing the fact that when uterine action has been stimulated, the nature of the discomfort encountered by the patient changes, and the oxytocin infusion should be administered in conjunction with epidural anesthesia. The use of epidural anesthesia must be considered a significant advance in obstetric practice and not relegated only to the occasional patient with ruptured membranes. This form of management, with the improvements that have occurred in perinatal medicine, should be more liberally applied in obstetric practice.

In conclusion, it would be well to remember a comment by Oliver Wendell Holmes regarding puerperal infection, which also applies to premature rupture of the membranes—indeed, it pertains to the practice of medicine as a whole: "The duties of the practitioner to his profession should give way to his paramount obligations to society."

REFERENCES

1. Clark, D. M., and Anderson, G. V.: Perinatal mortality and amnionitis in a general hospital population. Obstet. Gynec. 31:714, 1968.
2. Webster, A.: Management of premature rupture of the fetal membranes. Obstet. Gynec. Surv. 24:485, 1969.
3. Gunn, G. C., Mishell, D. R., and Morton, D. G.: Premature rupture of the fetal membranes. Amer. J. Obstet. Gynec. 106:469, 1970.
4. Russell, K. P., and Anderson, G. V.: The aggressive management of ruptured membranes. Amer. J. Obstet. Gynec. 83:930, 1962.
5. Turnbull, A. C., and Anderson, A. B. M.: Induction of labour. Part III: Results with amniotomy and oxytocin titration. J. Obstet. Gynaec. Brit. Comm. 75:32, 1968.
6. MacVicar, J., and Howie, P. W.: Oxytocin titration on the outcome of labour following amniotomy. J. Obstet. Gynaec. Brit. Comm. 77:817, 1970.
7. O'Driscoll, K.: Impact of active management on delivery unit practice. Proc. Royal Soc. Med. 65:697, 1972.

Treatment of Patients With Premature Rupture of the Fetal Membranes: (a) Prior to 32 Weeks; (b) After 32 Weeks

Premature Rupture of the Membranes—A Rational Approach to Management

MYRON GORDON and ALLAN B. WEINGOLD

New York Medical College–Metropolitan Hospital Center

Premature rupture of the membranes is defined as spontaneous rupture of the amniochorionic membrane prior to the onset of uterine contractions (labor). It is a complication of pregnancy of unknown cause, of variably reported frequency, and of only partially satisfactory management. It is infrequently recognized before the middle of the second trimester, if it does occur at all in early pregnancy as a distinct entity, and usually it is not included in obstetrical reports before the twentieth to twenty-fourth weeks of gestation. We agree with Gunn *et al.*[1] that "most plans of management appear to be based upon personal experience rather than a careful analysis of large numbers of cases," and we would add that without prospective and controlled studies of various regimens, one must utilize all the data that can be made available in order to develop a rational therapeutic program. Thus, retrospective experience from large case studies can provide the broad background necessary for perspective, the detailed analysis of poor outcomes can demonstrate the pitfalls and deficiencies in management, and the personal institutional experience can provide characteristics of the local patient population and facilities which will modify the therapeutic program. In developing our own plan of management for premature rupture of the membranes, we have tried to draw upon all of the above experiences, with the anticipation that such a plan would be rational, practical, and reasonably successful.

Premature rupture of the fetal membranes occurs more frequently in patients of lower socioeconomic status, who have frequent pregnancies at short intervals, unstable home environments, and less than optimal health care. At the New York Medical College–Metropolitan Hospital Center, it complicates 2.0 per cent of the deliveries in private patients, 6.3 per cent of deliveries of ward patients, and 14.1 per cent of deliveries at Metropolitan Hospital Center (whose patients generally are lower socioeconomically). Following this complication, 23.2

39

TABLE 2-1. *Metropolitan Hospital Center Perinatal Mortality Rates for All Births, 1969–1971*

BY GESTATIONAL AGE	
Weeks	*Perinatal Mortality/1000 Single Births*
21–32	326
21–34	504
33–34	169
35–36	56
37–38	17
39–40	6
TOTAL	42

BY BIRTH WEIGHT	
Grams	*Perinatal Mortality/1000 Single Births*
500–999	961
1000–1499	586
1500–1999	218
2000–2499	35
2500–2999	15
3000–3999	9
TOTAL	42

per cent of the infants have low birth weights, and there is a 21 per cent perinatal mortality rate. It is another characteristic of the high-risk quality of pregnancy in disadvantaged patients, and as with other poor pregnancy outcomes, it tends to recur with subsequent pregnancies. The cause of premature rupture is unknown. Theories relating to etiological factors such as tensile strength, infection, and intercourse are unproved.

At Metropolitan Hospital Center, from January 1, 1969, to June 30, 1971, there were 5610 singleton deliveries. The perinatal mortality rates by weeks of gestation and by birth weight are shown in Table 2-1. Optimal survival rates are apparent at 39 to 40 weeks' gestation and when birth weights are in the range of 3000 to 3999 grams, although acceptable rates are seen for the immediately preceding values of both parameters.

Table 2-2 illustrates our experience with premature rupture of the membranes during this same period of time. From these data several points can be made:

1. In approximately one of every four patients with spontaneously ruptured membranes, the rupture occurred before the onset of labor.

2. The perinatal mortality rate increased as expected, particularly when the latent period exceeded 72 hours.

TABLE 2-2. *Premature Rupture of the Membranes, 1969–1971*

	Number of Cases	PERINATAL MORTALITIES		
		Number	*Rate/1000*	*Number of Immatures (<1000 gm.)*
Single births	5610	233	42	159
Spontaneous rupture of membranes	2937	145	49	52
No latent period	2141	96	44	38
Latent period ≤24 hrs.	637	26	41	7
25–72 hrs.	80	4	50	0
>72 hrs.	79	19	240	7
Total premature rupture of the membranes	796(14.1%)	49	61	14

TABLE 2-3. *Premature Rupture of Membranes With Infection, 1969–1971*

PREMATURE RUPTURE OF THE MEMBRANES (796 CASES)	PREMATURE RUPTURE OF THE MEMBRANES		PERINATAL MORTALITIES		
	Number	Per Cent of Cases	Number	Rate/1000	Number Immature
No Infection	719	90.4	31	40	6
Intrapartum Infection	77	9.6	18	230	8

3. Forty-eight per cent of the perinatal deaths (23/49) were accounted for by 20 per cent of the cases, and one third of these deaths were associated with immaturity.

4. Eighty per cent of the infants in cases of premature rupture were delivered within the first 24 hours.

Of the 796 cases of premature rupture of the fetal membranes, 77 or 9.6 per cent of the mothers became febrile during the intrapartum period. This complication increased the perinatal mortality rate sixfold (Table 2-3). Although representing only a small fraction (9.6 per cent) of the cases of premature rupture, intrapartum infection was associated with 36 per cent of the perinatal deaths and, of these, nearly 50 per cent of the infants were immature. Lastly, only four of the 233 perinatal deaths which occurred during this period were assigned a classification of infant or maternal infection as the primary cause of death, based upon clinicopathological findings.

From this, it is apparent that we are dealing with a problem in which the majority of cases reach a solution relatively early in the course of the disorder, and that, as with most high-risk obstetrical problems, it is the minority of cases for which the major therapeutic effort must be made in the hope of assuring the safest and most salutary outcome for mother and baby. Premature birth is probably responsible for the majority of cases of perinatal mortality, and, while clinical chorioamnionitis may be apparent in the mother, the diagnosis of infection in the infant may be quite difficult.

During the 15 year period of 1957 to 1971, there were seven maternal deaths associated with premature rupture of the membranes in a total of 50 maternal deaths (14.0 per cent) at the New York Medical College–Metropolitan Hospital Center. Relevant data concerning these seven mortalities are presented in Table 2-4. One maternal death occurred among the private patients (No. 5), and in only two cases (Nos. 2 and 3), both of which occurred more than 10 years ago, was there a direct relationship between management of premature rupture and the outcome. In one case (No. 6), one can only speculate as to any cause and effect relationship, and in case No. 7, the management of labor was probably the most relevant factor. Interestingly, there have not been any maternal deaths from clinical infection associated with premature rupture of the membranes since 1963.

For three cases in which clinical infection played a prominent role (Nos. 2, 4, and 5), there was a long delay on the part of the patient in presenting herself for medical care. In the series reported by Webster in 1969, all 13 of the maternal deaths at Cook County Hospital had similar delays of more than 12 hours before admission to the hospital. Thus, in our experience, chorioamnionitis and its attendant complications have not played a major role in recent maternal deaths. It is apparent that neglected cases or those infected at the time of admission require intensive care.

TABLE 2-4.   *Maternal Mortalities, 1957–1971*

CASE NO.	YEAR	AGE	PARITY	GESTA-TION	PREMATURE RUPTURE	DELIVERY	DEATH
1	1958	31	3-0-1-3	40	4 hr.	Normal spontaneous delivery; manual removal of placenta	Ruptured uterus
2	1959	32	1-0-6-1	33	1 week	Chorioamnionitis; spontaneous labor and delivery	Sepsis, acute renal failure
3	1961	33	6-0-0-6	36	Unknown	Failed induction 3 times; normal spontaneous delivery; stillborn	Postpartum hemorrhage, hysterectomy, hepatorenal failure
4	1962	23	4-0-0-4	25	3½ days	Heroin addict; in labor chorioamnionitis	Cardiac arrest, undelivered
5	1963	34	2-0-1-2	40	4 days	No care; in labor fever; disseminated intravascular coagulation; stillborn	Chorioamnionitis, disseminated intravascular coagulation
6	1964	38	4-1-3-5	37	4 hr.	Prophylactic antibiotics; normal spontaneous delivery 2 weeks later; normal postpartum	Cerebral hemorrhage 2 weeks post partum
7	1969	21	0-0-0-0	39	½ hr.	Spontaneous labor, supplemented; second stage, 3¾ hr.; low forceps delivery; saddle block anesthesia	Hypotension and cardiac arrest, no infection

To date, the only significant study of the effectiveness of prophylactic antibiotics in decreasing perinatal mortality rate was reported by Lebherz et al.[5] in 1961. This study showed that while the perinatal mortality rate was essentially the same for antibiotics-treated and placebo-treated cases, there was, however, a reduction in maternal morbidity, particularly in endometritis and puerperal pyelonephritis. The singular disadvantage of this study was that the agent selected had risks for both fetus and mother, demonstrated no selective placental transfer, and was not selectively effective against gram-negative organisms involved in chorioamnionitis.

In 1971–1972, we carried out a preliminary study utilizing a bactericidal, broad-spectrum antibiotic, ampicillin, which has been demonstrated to be selectively transferred across the placenta into the amniotic fluid, is not harmful to the fetus, and is effective against gram-negative organisms.

In brief, all patients with uncomplicated and confirmed premature rupture of the membranes were admitted to the hospital and an estimation of fetal maturity made from history, physical examination, ultrasound, and examination of the amniotic fluid for fetal squames. A single sterile speculum examination was carried out. Each case was classified as premature (less than 37 weeks' gestation) or term, and each case was placed in a treatment or nontreatment group on the arbitrary basis of the last digit of the admission number. The following groups were established:

1. Premature (Treat):   Ampicillin, 1 gram intramuscularly every 12 hours for 48 hours. Discharged with regimen of 500 mg. ampicillin orally every 8 hours for a total of 10 days.
2. Premature (Control):   Hospitalized, bed rest for 48 hours, discharged with cautions.
3. Term (Treat):   Same as Term (Control), plus infusion of 1 g. ampicillin in every 1000 cc. of 5 per cent dextrose in water until delivery.
4. Term (Control):   After a latent period of 12 hours, induction of labor begun and the infant was delivered within 24 hours.

Upon hospital admission after labor had begun, cultures were obtained of the amniotic fluid, and after delivery, of the cord blood and gastric aspirate. Specimens of the amnion, chorion, and umbilical cord were studied histologically.

For each group, the frequencies of clinical fetal morbidity and mortality, maternal morbidity, and bacteriological and histological evidence of infection have been recorded, and some of the data are summarized in Tables 2-5 to 2-7.

The frequency of positive cultures from various fetal sites (Table 2-5) shows significant differences for treated and control groups, depending on whether antibiotics were given to the premature or to term patients. Negative cultures from all sites occurred three times more frequently when antibiotics were given.

Bacteriologically, there were more than twice as many positive cultures of pathogenic organisms when antibiotics were withheld. This was most striking for *E. coli, Klebsiella*, and fermentative gram-negative rods (Table 2-6).

TABLE 2-5.   *Ampicillin Prophylaxis Study—Percentage of Positive Cultures by Site*

SITE OF CULTURE	PREMATURE		TERM	
	Treat (42)	*Control (38)*	*Treat (86)*	*Control (102)*
Amniotic Fluid	33.3	57.9	27.9	56.9
Gastric Aspirate	26.2	39.4	36.0	57.8
Cord Blood	11.9	18.4	12.8	11.8
Cord Section	47.6	68.4	27.9	40.2
All Negative	35.7	10.5	34.9	12.7
Positive Patients	64.3	89.5	65.1	87.3

TABLE 2-6.   *Ampicillin Prophylaxis Study—Organisms Cultured From All Sites*

	PREMATURE		TERM	
	Treat	*Control*	*Treat*	*Control*
Staphylococcus Coagulase Positive	0	0	1	5
Alpha *Streptococcus*	9	12	25	39
Beta *Streptococcus*	1	0	2	6
Streptococcus fecalis	2	4	3	12
Streptococcus zymogenes	1	2	1	6
Escherichia coli	7	13	18	33
Proteus mirabilis	1	3	3	4
Klebsiella aerogenes	5	11	5	12
Fermentative Gram-Negative Rods	5	14	6	18
Diplococcus pneumoniae	1	3	4	5
TOTALS	32	62	68	140

TABLE 2-7. *Ampicillin Prophylaxis Study—Maternal and Fetal Complications*

COMPLICATIONS	PRETERM		TERM	
	Treat	*Control*	*Treat*	*Control*
Maternal:				
Amnionitis	3(7.1%)	7(18.4%)	2(2.3%)	3(2.9%)
Other Fever (Prepartum)	0	1	3(3.4%)	3(2.9%)
Postpartum Morbidity	2(4.7%)	4(10.5%)	5(5.8%)	9(8.8%)
Fetal:				
Perinatal Deaths	12	10	1	2
Rate Per 100 Births	28.4	26.2	1.1	1.9

Clinically, prophylactic antibiotic therapy would seem to have been effective in decreasing the incidence of amnionitis or other causes of prepartum fever (pyelitis), as well as decreasing postpartum morbidity rates (Table 2-7). Antibiotics, given during delivery at term, would not be expected to decrease antepartum infection and would have only a marginal effect post partum. Most significantly, treatment seems to provide no advantage to the fetus for survival, the perinatal mortality rates being comparable for treated and control patients. The major cause of death was prematurity.

In summary, prophylactic antibiotics given prior to the onset of labor to those patients for whom induction is not contemplated will apparently have a salutary effect, which is measurable bacteriologically and clinically insofar as maternal and fetal infection is concerned. Perinatal mortality rates are not affected either for preterm or for term pregnancies.

From all of the foregoing we have reached the following conclusions:

1. The maternal risk of mortality can be mitigated by prompt and aggressive treatment of the clinically infected patient and of the patient who is neglectful of her own care and well-being.

2. The risk to the fetus increases with the duration of the latent period, and this risk is related primarily to immaturity and secondarily to infection.

3. Prematurity is the major cause of perinatal mortality, which in turn is significantly increased by amnionitis or intrapartum fever.

4. Positive bacteriological findings are more frequent than clinically apparent infections in newborns, and such infections are not a frequent finding at autopsy of infants that had been at risk.

5. The problem of management occurs mainly in the 20 per cent of the cases in which the latent period exceeds 24 hours, and more specifically, in the 10 per cent of cases in which the latent period exceeds three days. The latter group incorporates 40 per cent of the perinatal mortalities.

6. An acceptable perinatal mortality rate is attained when the gestational age reaches 37 weeks and the fetal weight approximates 2500 g.

7. If delay of delivery is not indicated, then delivery is best accomplished within the first 24 hours after rupture of the membranes.

8. Prophylactic antibiotics are effective in preventing maternal infection, clinical amniochorionitis, and postpartum morbidity. The antibiotic must be readily absorbed across the placenta and concentrate in the amniotic fluid.

With this as our basis, we have established a standard plan of management, which is summarized in the flow chart (Figure 2-1).

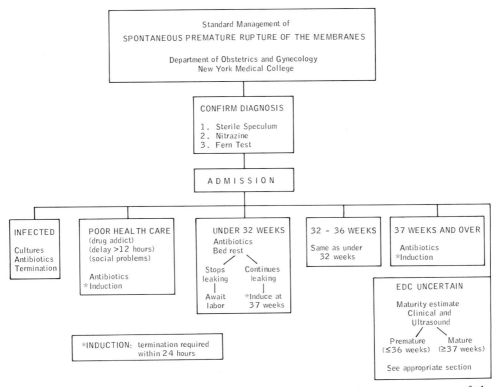

Figure 2-1. Flow chart summarizing plan of management of premature rupture of the fetal membranes.

Standard Management of Premature Rupture of Membranes

GENERAL PRINCIPLES

1. When the decision is made to terminate the pregnancy the infant will be delivered within 12 to 24 hours.

2. Antibiotic prophylaxis is ampicillin, 2 g. per day, in divided doses for 10 days. In labor, ampicillin is given directly intravenously in doses of 1 g. every 6 hours until delivery, and is continued orally for 48 hours post partum.

3. Pelvic examinations, which are to follow labor, are kept to a minimum; they are performed under sterile conditions and by the same individual for consistency of observation.

4. The pediatric staff is alerted to the case of premature rupture of the membranes in labor and takes necessary cultures from the infant.

SPECIFIC PRINCIPLES

Immediate efforts to terminate pregnancy will be initiated in the following instances:

1. When the fetus is judged to be mature, that is, having completed 259 days or 37 weeks of pregnancy and weighs approximately 2500 g.; or if the estimated date of confinement (E.D.C.) is in doubt, and there is evidence of matu-

rity obtained by clinical examination, ultrasound, amniotic fluid analysis, and X-ray study.

2. When there is clinical evidence of chorioamnionitis *or* when the potential for such infection is high—e.g., the patient delayed in presenting herself for care more than 12 hours after rupture of the membranes, she is a drug addict, there is history of poor health care.

3. Unsterile or repeated pelvic examinations have been done in confirmed case of premature rupture.

Observation and prophylactic antibiotic therapy will be initiated in the following instances: Gestation of less than 37 weeks; patient admitted to the hospital within 12 hours of the rupture, has had only a sterile speculum examination for confirmation of premature rupture, has a responsible attitude toward her own care, is afebrile, and has normal-appearing amniotic fluid upon examination.

The stage between 34 and 36 weeks' gestation is a "gray zone" where other factors may play a role in a decision:

a. Past obstetrical history: Repetitive perinatal loss, previous prematurity with abnormal neurological outcome, previous premature rupture with or without infection.

b. Complicating disease: Diabetes, chronic hypertensive disease, preeclampsia, heart disease.

c. Pregnancy at risk: Age, past obstetrical history.

Prior to 35 weeks, the perinatal mortality rate is unacceptable for induced delivery unless complications remove any options. In general, when in the course of "conservative" observation any untoward complication arises, i.e., change in character or odor of amniotic leakage, pyelonephritis, altered uterine activity (as in early labor), or if the patient signs out and is readmitted, steps to terminate the pregnancy should be initiated immediately.

If clinical chorioamnionitis supervenes, antibiotic therapy is intensified with the addition of aqueous penicillin (10 million units in each intravenous bottle) and kanamycin to the regimen. Ampicillin is increased to 12 g. per 24 hours. If the patient is not in labor and the cervix is very ripe (short labor anticipated) a 4 hour trial of induction is attempted. If the cervix is unripe or a long labor is anticipated, immediate cesarean section is selected. In labor, fetal monitoring is carried out with careful observation for fetal tachycardia, loss of beat-to-beat variability, or Type II dips. In any case, delay or arrest in progress of labor is indication for immediate termination.

While it will frequently seem that cesarean section is the method of delivery of choice for patients with these problems, it should be kept in mind that cesarean section in itself is not without risk to the patient in terms of anesthetic accidents, hemorrhage, wound disruption, infection, and embolization. Future cesarean sections have similar risks, with the addition of uterine rupture, prematurity, and an increased frequency of respiratory distress syndrome. The decision to perform a cesarean section cannot be undertaken lightly.

Cesarean hysterectomy is the procedure of choice in the presence of gross infection of the uterus, when sepsis is evident (shock, acute renal failure, hemolysis, or jaundice) for the multipara who desires sterilization, or in any circumstance in which leaving the uterus intact represents a significantly greater hazard to the patient than can be compensated for by retaining her ability to reproduce.

One question which we have not answered at all satisfactorily concerns proof of the value of the "conservative" approach in terms of significant prolongation of the pregnancy. Such proof can probably be gathered only by a prospective study of the random assignment of patients with premature rupture to an immediate termination group. In the absence of such a study, one must at present rely upon clinical experience and judgment. It does seem logical that, if prolongation of the pregnancy in premature cases does not in itself present an unacceptable risk to the mother or fetus, then it is preferable to immediate termination. With the regimen and qualifications outlined above, we believe that the risk is acceptable and that the conservative approach is preferable.

REFERENCES

1. Gunn, G. C., Mishell, Jr., D. R., Morton, D. G.: Premature rupture of the fetal membranes: a review. Amer. J. Obstet. Gynec. 106:469, 1970.
2. Hendricks, C. H.: Can we prevent premature membrane rupture? Hospital Practice 3:34, 1968.
3. Webster, A.: Management of premature rupture of the fetal membranes. Obstet. Gynec. Surv. 24:485, 1969.
4. Webb, G. A.: Maternal death associated with premature rupture of the membranes—an analysis of 54 cases. Amer. J. Obstet. Gynec. 98:594, 1967.
5. Lebherz, T. B., Hellman, L. P., Madding, R., Ametil, A., and Arje, S. L.: Double-blind study of premature rupture of the membranes. Amer. J. Obstet. Gynec. 87:218, 1963.

Treatment of Patients With Premature Rupture of the Fetal Membranes: (a) Prior to 32 Weeks; (b) After 32 Weeks

The Management of Premature Rupture of the Fetal Membranes—a Continuing Controversy

KEITH P. RUSSELL and JOSEPH CHEUNG

The Moore-White Medical Clinic

The clinical management of premature rupture of the fetal membranes has been a subject of continuing discussion and controversy by various investigators over the past decade, and it remains one of the most challenging clinical conditions which confronts the obstetrician. In 1961, we advocated the "aggressive" or active management of this condition. After 10 years it seems appropriate to take a second look at this advocacy.

The definition of premature rupture of the membranes has often varied from investigator to investigator. Technically, premature rupture is any rupture which results in loss of fluid before the onset of demonstrable labor. At or near term, this may occur with prodromal or preliminary uterine activity, leading rather soon into actual labor, so that it is not recorded as premature rupture of the membranes but is considered to be part and parcel of the onset of labor. For purposes of definition, it should be considered that premature rupture of the membranes has occurred if effective labor does not begin within one hour after rupture occurs. Since the rupture is sometimes difficult to time precisely, reports in the literature vary as to the incidence of the condition. In all series, however, spontaneous labor has usually been found to ensue within 12 hours. It is in that group in which this latter event does *not* occur that problems of management arise.

The original recommendations for the termination of those pregnancies complicated by rupture of the membranes occurring for long periods before labor begins were based upon a number of clinical observations, most of which still pertain:

1. It is well documented that there is an exceedingly high incidence of uterine infection the longer the period that elapses after fetal membrane rupture. The onset of such amnionitis in most cases occurs after 24 hours and usually within 48 hours. This infection may be minimal and localized, or it may be wide-

spread. An accurate prediction of the degree of infection that will occur cannot be made, but there are certain predisposing factors common to the more severe forms. Among these are vaginal invasion, such as repeated vaginal examinations or intercourse, and any form of instrumentation. Other predisposing factors include generally reduced resistance to infection associated with chronic anemia and malnutrition, and poor hygienic habits, such as unrestricted douching. Most of these occur in the lower socioeconomic population, but are not restricted to this group.

2. The incidence of amnionitis is not only high, but it is also certain to occur. This can be shown by following serial vaginal-cervical cultures. Such occurrence of infection is analogous to that which follows placement of an indwelling urethral catheter for a period of time. For obvious reasons, amnionitis is of much more ominous portent. After 24 hours without labor the incidence of infection exceeds 50 per cent, and is greatly increased and aggravated with the occurrence of prolonged labor.

3. Amnionitis under these circumstances most frequently results from enterobacillary organisms (gram-negative rods), including *E. coli, Pseudomonas* and *Proteus vulgaris*. This is significant because these bacteria are associated with a relatively high incidence of septic shock with all its ramifications—renal failure, disseminated intravascular coagulation (consumption coagulopathy), hypotension, and cardiac failure. In many series, the maternal mortality rate associated with septic shock has exceeded 60 per cent.

Anaerobic organisms also may cause amnionitis, and these require evacuation of infected tissues and enclosed spaces as a basic form of therapy.

4. Fetal and neonatal problems are a significant factor.
   a. The highest incidence of *unexplained* stillbirths has occurred in association with ruptured membranes. Approximately 60 per cent of stillbirths occur in the "cause unknown" category; that is, there may be no obvious explanation for fetal deaths, such as placental factors, (placenta previa, abruptio placentae), congenital malformations, intrauterine pneumonia, Rh incompatibilities. In this 60 per cent, the single most consistent associated finding has been membrane rupture.
   b. Perinatal morbidity and mortality rates show a three- to four-fold increase when membranes have been ruptured more than 48 hours before delivery. These figures correspond with those of Eastman previously published (Russell and Anderson[3]), and Freeman.[4]
   c. It has been demonstrated repeatedly that antibiotics given to the mother do not prevent a fatal outcome for the baby under these circumstances. The infant at birth is usually unable to metabolize and utilize properly many medications given, owing to the imperfect nature of his enzyme systems. Even the highly trained perinatologist finds his results are much better in the management of uninfected premature infants than in those who have been subjected to prolonged periods of intrauterine subclinical infection.

Although in all the above maternal and perinatal considerations premature rupture of the fetal membranes was the single common denominator, and despite much interest in this condition, the *etiology* of membrane rupture remains unknown. Contributing or predisposing factors include multiple pregnancy, hydramnios, vaginal infections, incompetent cervix, placenta previa, breech presentation, genetic abnormalities, and amnionitis. In early pregnancy, uterine instrumentation or attempts at termination of pregnancy must be considered. Danforth and others have shown that weakness in the tensile strength of the membranes themselves does not appear to be an etiologic factor. However, localized cervicovaginal infection spreading to the area of the endocervical os, over which the membranes lie, may predispose to breaks in the membranes.

The *diagnosis* of premature rupture of the membranes must be established by actual observation of pooling of the fluid in the vagina on speculum examination. Many patients complain of a "wetness" of vulvar and vaginal tissues, which they may interpret as fluid loss. However, such observation is insufficient for accurate diagnosis. In addition, some multiparous patients may suffer from urinary stress incontinence, which can be interpreted erroneously as premature rupture of the membranes unless proper evaluation is carried out.

Management

The active or aggressive management of premature rupture of the membranes calls for termination of the pregnancy by suitable means if labor does not ensue spontaneously within a reasonable period of time after rupture. This is generally held to be 24 hours, and in some cases the "reasonable period" should be 12 hours. Prolonged labor or extended attempts at induction should be avoided, and cesarean section instituted if induction fails. Cesarean hysterectomy should be considered if there is gross infection of the uterus.

Objections to the above course of management usually reside in the following categories:

1. "I've never had a problem." However, the incidence of premature rupture in which labor does not ensue within a short time is comparatively. The latent period is less than 24 hours in 90 per cent of cases. It takes large series to illustrate the problem.

2. "It will unnecessarily increase the incidence of cesarean sections to a high rate." In a large service (over 10,000 deliveries per year) cesarean section for ruptured membranes was utilized 43 times, increasing the overall cesarean section incidence by less than 0.5 per cent.

3. "The premature baby is better off in the uterus in these situations." This has been refuted by numerous studies (Breese; Freeman; Shubeck *et al.*); Freeman in particular has shown a marked reduction in perinatal morbidity rate with active management of premature rupture of the membranes. Also, most perinatologists have documented greater survival rates for noninfected premature infants as compared to infected ones, even though the latter may be more mature. Although all efforts to combat the causes of prematurity should be continued, newer techniques of management of the premature infant have greatly increased his chances of survival, particularly if these chances are not compromised by the presence of infection.

4. "The problem only exists in the indigent population." It is claimed that management problems with premature membrane rupture occur only in the patient population composed primarily of indigent and lower socioeconomic classes, and that active management is not warranted in private practice settings.

It is true that the incidence of maternal and perinatal morbidity and mortality is higher in the indigent groups, with their poorer nutrition, anemia, increased susceptibility to infection, and poorer standards of hygiene. It is likewise true that practically all obstetrical complications and morbidity rates are higher in this group. This fact has led to greater attention to efforts to improve the management of all facets of obstetrical care for these patients, including active management of premature rupture of the membranes. However, maternal mortality studies in California and elsewhere have repeatedly recorded deaths in private practice as well, when the presence of prematurely ruptured membranes was ignored or mismanaged.

If one elects to follow the conservative course of management of premature membrane rupture, a rigid protocol must be followed. This includes:

1. Prohibition of all sexual activity and douching by the patient.
2. Amniotic fluid must remain clear at all times.
3. There must be no uterine contractions.
4. The patient must remain afebrile.
5. No vaginal examinations should be performed (after initial establishment of the diagnosis).

It is obvious that, of these five rules of management, only one, the fifth, is under direct control of the physician. Patients often do not follow specific instructions, or are forgetful. Any bacteriostatic activity the amniotic fluid might possess is rendered ineffectual by the admixture of blood or meconium, and of course neither the physician nor the patient can foresee exactly when such might occur, or to what degree. Uterine contractions are difficult to evaluate subjectively, and and it is known that the uterus undergoes mild contractions throughout the third trimester. Finally, leukocytosis may precede temperature elevation as a beginning of infection. The appearance of fever means that the optimum time for delivery has already passed.

For these and other reasons cited we do not recommend watchful waiting or "wait and call back" as the management of choice for premature rupture of the membranes.

Typical case histories taken from maternal mortality files in our community follow. (Cases from the maternal mortality studies of the California Medical Association Committee on Maternal and Child Care. Dr. Russell is immediate past chairman of the committee.)

CASE I

A 22 year old woman, para 0, was admitted to a hospital in the forty-second week of pregnancy with a 3 hour history of ruptured membranes. Five hours later, spontaneous labor began. In the fourteenth hour of labor, her temperature rose to 105° F.; in the eighteenth hour of labor (26 hours after membrane rupture), because of documented cephalopelvic disproportion, she was delivered of a depressed infant by low cervical section. The placenta showed microscopic evidence of severe amnionitis.

Twenty-four hours later, her temperature, which had fallen after delivery, rose to 102° F. Intravenous antibiotics were started. On the third postoperative day there was severe ileus, and on the fourth postoperative day jaundice was noted.

On the fifth postoperative day, her urinary output fell and the blood urea nitrogen rose to 88 mg./100 ml. Shortly afterward, she became irrational and required restraints. In a few hours she died.

Autopsy showed endometritis, parametritis, and generalized peritonitis. Cultures of the blood, uterus, and peritoneal cavity yielded *E. coli* and *Proteus*.

Comment. The presence of ruptured membranes should have weighted the decision for cesarean section much earlier. In addition, the condition called for early and massive antibiotic therapy.

CASE II

A 31 year old woman, para 1, was admitted to the hospital in the thirty-sixth week of pregnancy, a "few hours" after spontaneous rupture of the membranes. Her cervix was unripe. Four days and four vaginal examinations later, the cervix was still unripe. Her temperature rose to 101.3° F. and she experienced a shaking chill. Subsequently *Pseudomonas* was cultured from her blood. Tetracycline therapy and intravenous oxytocin administration were begun.

Five hours later, a moribund 5 lb. 13 oz. infant was born precipitously under saddle block anesthesia. An adherent purulent placenta was removed piecemeal. Within 15 minutes of delivery, the patient's blood pressure fell to shock levels. The total blood loss was 400 cc. Administrations of aramine, chloramphenicol, hydrocortisone, streptomycin, blood, and Levophed proved ineffectual. Over the next 30 hours, the patient remained in septic shock, exhibiting increasing oliguria and respiratory distress. Shortly before her death, her white blood cell count was 56,000 per cubic millimeter.

Autopsy showed marked pulmonary edema, myocarditis, adrenal hemorrhage, and severe endoparametritis.

Comment. Aggressive management of ruptured membranes would have been far preferable.

CASE III

A 31 year old woman, gravida 6, para 4, ab 1, at 35 weeks' gestation was admitted to a hospital 12 hours after spontaneous rupture of her membranes, with a temperature of 100° F. Urinalysis was negative. Forty hours after admission, induction of labor with intravenous oxytocin was begun. Four hours later, chloramphenicol was added to the oxytocin infusion because her temperature had risen to 102.6° F. Two hours later, a 5 lb. 13 oz. healthy infant was born under pudendal block anesthesia.

In the next hour, uterine atony failed to respond to multiple oxytocin infusions and continuous uterine massage. The blood pressure fell to 0/0 despite administration of oxygen and one unit of plasma. Blood loss was severe. Subsequent treatment included 2500 cc. of blood, 8 g. fibrinogen, 250 mg. hydrocortisone, and a desperation hysterectomy under oxygen. The uterus never did contract and the patient expired.

Comment. This is a frequently found chain of events with neglected ruptured membranes. Overwhelming infection interferes with all organ systems. Greater attention to the "membrane factor" might have been life-saving.

CASE IV

A 30 year old woman, para 3, cesarean section 3, entered a hospital in the twenty-fifth week of pregnancy with a two day history of ruptured membranes and a temperature of 101.4° F. Immediate treatment included intravenous fluids and chloramphenicol. Five hours after admission, an intravenous oxytocin infusion was begun. Following a 3 hour labor, a stillborn, foul smelling infant was born in bed.

A postpartum clotting deficiency was corrected by 7 g. fibrinogen along with 1500 cc. of blood. Chloramphenicol was continued.

Twelve hours after delivery, the patient complained of epigastric distress. In the next few hours, she became dyspneic and her blood pressure dropped to 70/64. Eighteen hours after delivery, an abdominal tap demonstrated a hemoperitoneum.

At laparotomy, the uterus was found to be intact. A 2 to 2½ inch laceration of the caudate lobe of the liver was bleeding freely and the abdominal cavity contained an estimated 3000 cc. of blood. By this point the patient was in an irreversible shock and did not respond to a total of 7000 cc. of blood replacement or to a thoracotomy.

Autopsy confirmed the diagnosis of amnionitis and endoparametritis, as well as the previously noted ruptured liver.

Comment. Proper management of ruptured membranes includes warning all pregnant patients to report promptly any loss of fluid. This patient did not report until fever had been established. Clotting deficiencies occur in a significant number of patients with severe amnionitis. The preoperative diagnosis was uterine rupture of previous cesarean section scar, secondary to oxytocin administration. However, intra-abdominal hemorrhage was due to a ruptured liver, a rare entity.

CASE V

A 22 year old multipara was delivered at term of a 7 lb. 4 oz. infant by low cervical cesarean section under spinal anesthesia. The membranes had been ruptured for 42 hours and her temperature had spiked to 105° F. during 8 hours of active labor.

Twenty-four hours later, when her temperature reached 102° F., therapy with tetracycline was begun. Cultures of her urine at this time showed *E. coli* sensitive to chloramphenicol and kanamycin.

By the next day, her abdomen was moderately distended and her urine output had fallen to 25 cc. per hour despite an intravenous input of 160 cc. per hour.

During the next 3 days, her ileus became increasingly severe and she remained febrile, with a temperature of up to 102° F. and a urinary output of 5 to 10 cc. per hour. Tetracycline therapy was continued, along with intravenous fluids, supplemental potassium, and one infusion of 250 cc. of plasma.

On the fifth postoperative day she was clinically jaundiced and irrational. With the onset of a hypotensive episode, penicillin (5 million units), hydrocortisone (500 mg.), and sodium bicarbonate were given. Shortly thereafter she expired.

The principal autopsy finding was generalized peritonitis, with 1000 cc. of purulent peritoneal fluid. *Escherichia coli* was cultured from the blood, peritoneal fluid, and uterine cavity.

Comment. Induction of labor before 42 hours elapsed after rupture of the membranes and earlier cesarean section would probably have led to a happier outcome.

Conclusion

After further experience with the management of prematurely ruptured membranes, we find no substantive reasons for changing our recommendation for the active or aggressive treatment of this condition. Premature rupture of the membranes is a *complication* of pregnancy and must be managed as such; to regard it as a "natural course of events" or a nontreatable condition is to invite disaster in the long run. We must accept the fact that premature rupture of the membranes is a serious and potentially lethal threat to both mother and infant. The fact that 90 to 95 per cent of these occurrences present no problem should not deny concerned management to the other 5 to 10 per cent, in whom life itself or future reproductive potential may be seriously threatened.

REFERENCES

1. Breese, M. W.: Spontaneous premature rupture of the membranes; a clinical study. Amer. J. Obstet. Gynec. 88:251, 1964.
2. Freeman, M.: Unpublished data.
3. Russell, K. P., and Anderson, G. V.: The aggressive management of ruptured membranes. Amer. J. Obstet. Gynec. 83:930, 1962.
4. Shubeck, F., Benson, R. C., Clark, W. W., Jr., *et al.*: Fetal hazard after rupture of the membranes; a report from the collaborative project. Obstet. Gynec. 28:22, 1966.
5. Webb, G. A.: Maternal death associated with premature rupture of the membranes. Amer. J. Obstet. Gynec. 98:594, 1967.
6. Webster, A.: Management of premature rupture of the fetal membranes. Obstet. Gynec. Surv. 24:485, 1970.

Treatment of Patients With Premature Rupture of the Fetal Membranes: (a) Prior to 32 Weeks; (b) After 32 Weeks

WILLIAM C. SCOTT, M.D.

University of Arizona School of Medicine and Arizona Medical Center

Among the more perplexing problems of our specialty of obstetrics and gynecology is the unabating incidence of premature rupture of the membranes. The application of our burgeoning knowledge within the field of perinatology is steadily reducing mortality within the live-born infant class. However, prematurity is still responsible for roughly half of all infant deaths, with 40 per cent of these being brought about following spontaneous or induced labor after premature rupture of the membranes. The removal of nature's normal barrier to intrauterine infection surprisingly is of little consequence to the mature infant, but many times is disastrous to the younger fetus. This discussion will outline the present status of knowledge of premature rupture of the membranes and will discuss the application of our newer diagnostic procedures to the improvement of results in the immature infant.

TABLE 2-8.   *Incidence of Spontaneous Premature Rupture of the Membranes*

	TOTAL DELIVERIES	PREMATURE RUPTURE OF THE MEMBRANES	PER CENT
Sacks and Baker[68]	6269	415	6.6
Lanier et al.[39]	7637	473	6.2
Breese[5]	44,723	2887	6.4
Clark and Anderson[11]	32,022	1009	3.1
Gunn *et al.*[24]	17,562	1884	10.7
Rovinsky and Shapiro[66]	30,336	3800	12.5
	138,549	10,468	7.5

A compilation of the large reported series to date, Table 2-8, reveals some variation in incidence, undoubtedly resulting from known difficulties in establishing exact time of rupture in relation to onset of labor. The majority of reports accept a one hour latent period as proper definition. Eastman[19] included all cases of rupture before labor, disregarding the latent period, and reported a 13 per cent incidence, compared to the lower figures in Table 2-8.

No satisfactory solution to the etiology of this condition has yet been presented. Taylor and associates[72] have shown that many of these patients display markedly increased uterine irritability throughout pregnancy. Polishuk and his colleagues[56] claim to show an ethnic predisposition in women of European origin based on decreased membrane tensile strength, while Danforth and his co-workers[16] demonstrated tensile strength far above normal intra-amniotic pressures. Of unknown relation to the above are the findings of Wideman and colleagues,[78] who found the incidence of premature rupture of the membranes to be 15 per cent in patients with severe ascorbic acid deficiency, compared with only 1 per cent for patients with normal levels of this vitamin. Speculations of the relationships of infection, congenital defects, maternal age, parity, trauma, and numerous other possibilities seem to be of declining importance as suggested etiological factors. Like toxemia, preventive treatment awaits further elucidation of an etiology not yet understood but of vital importance for reducing our present perinatal mortality rate.

Diagnosis

The diagnosis of premature rupture of the membranes is in most instances obvious from the sudden release of clear amniotic fluid from the vagina and its continued dribbling after. Confirmation is needed and is most important, since management depends on positive knowledge. Differentiation between amniotic fluid and urine or endocervical mucus is most practically made by the tests in Table 2-9.

TABLE 2-9.   *Diagnosis of Ruptured Membranes*

TEST	REPORTED ACCURACY
Nitrazine	94–97%
Amniotic fluid crystallization	75–98%
Nile blue	98%

The manner of diagnosis is of utmost importance, most particularly as the time from estimated date of confinement increases. All of these diagnostic maneuvers should be carried out in such a fashion as to keep the introduction of pathogenic organisms into the vagina and cervix—or through the cervix and into the uterus—to a minimum. That it is amniotic fluid exuding from the vagina can be confirmed by the nitrazine test or ferning, or possibly by obtaining enough fluid to demonstrate fetal squames at the vaginal orifice. When the vagina needs to be examined, only a sterile speculum under aseptic conditions should be used. Here the cervix may be visualized, the presenting part displaced, and the presence of fluid released confirmed and tested. Introducing gloved fingers into the vagina and cervix adds nothing to the diagnosis, rarely affects management, and may markedly alter the risk of infection. Furthermore, attempts to sterilize the vagina with antibiotics and thus prevent ascending infection, such as those of Brelje and Kaltreider,[6] have proved futile.

After the diagnosis of amniorrhexis is established, certain immediate and delayed complications may be anticipated. Prolapse of the umbilical cord surprisingly is infrequent, with an average incidence of 0.3 to 0.6 per cent, rising to

2 to 3 per cent in the more premature infants.[24,67,68] Fetal mortality in these few cases, however, especially with vertex presentation, is horrendous, reaching 60 per cent.[5] With breech presentation, as might be expected, occult prolapse during

TABLE 2-10.   *Fetal Mortality by Presentation*

	BREECH	VERTEX
2000–2500 grams	17.8%	13.1%
1500–1999 grams	60 %	32.3%
1000–1499 grams	86.2%	45.7%
500– 999 grams	89 %	100 %

labor is a constant concern. Breech presentation in itself is of ominous significance when the membranes rupture early. Occurring in about 6.3 per cent of all cases of premature rupture of the membranes, with a perinatal mortality rate of about 25 per cent, the incidence of breech is much higher (16 to 18 per cent) in the fetus under 2500 g., and these cases have a mortality rate of 36 to 40 per cent.[24] The perinatal mortality risk for the fetus under 1500 g. is almost double when a breech rather than vertex presentation exists.

Risks to Fetus and Mother

Perhaps the greatest immediate risk to the fetus is prematurity itself. Two reviews of 4771 cases of premature rupture of the membranes reported 786 babies weighing less than 2500 g., an incidence of 18 per cent.[5,24] This is approximately three times the incidence of prematures in the total newborn population. Since perinatal mortality rate rises sharply as fetal weight declines, obviously this factor alone weighs heavily in infant loss. When the latent period between rupture of membranes and onset of labor is considered, it will be seen that the addition of infection to prematurity is often the coup de grâce leading to fetal demise.

The invasion of the uterus by pathogens not only causes amnionitis and deciduitis, but may also present as endometritis and parametritis. Wilson and his colleagues[80] found maternal infection associated with one in two infected infants. Other studies[11,24,59,66,68,70] indicate an overall maternal morbidity rate of up to 18 per cent, either intrapartum or postpartum. Maternal mortality, on the other hand, is exceedingly rare but exists in sufficient numbers to warrant serious con-

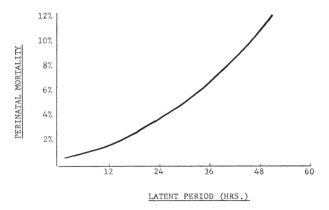

Figure 2-2. Relationship of perinatal mortality to duration of latent period. (From Gunn, G. C., Mishell, D. R., Jr., and Morton, D. G.: Amer. J. Obstet. Gynec. *106*:477, 1970.)

sideration. Webb,[74] analyzing California statistics, calculated maternal deaths secondary to rupture of the membranes as 1 in 5551, but Webster,[75] in reporting Cook County Hospital 10 year statistics of 226,878 deliveries, found 13 maternal deaths from sepsis associated with premature rupture of the membranes. Using the same method of calculation as Webb, this gives an incidence of 2.4 per 5000. Thus, even though the risk to the fetus is far greater, we cannot disregard the mother in the management decision.

The Latent Period

Numerous studies[2,28,24,59] have repeatedly stressed the importance of the latent period in the development of ascending infection and the increasing hazards with time to both mother and baby. The mature fetus enjoys a significantly lesser risk, for while the latent period totals less than 24 hours in 50 to 54 per cent, in the term pregnancy it varies from 81 to 95 per cent.[5] Howard and Bauer[28] report perinatal mortalities of 0.28 to 0.5 per cent in the term pregnancy in which the infant is delivered within 24 hours of rupture of the membranes. Spontaneous onset of labor in these cases will nearly always solve the problem in the last four weeks of pregnancy and, when necessary and not obstetrically contraindicated, pitocin induction is now almost universally standard procedure for the few not in labor at the end of 12 to 24 hours. Hellman and Pritchard[26] recommend cesarean section for the occasional patient not in labor in 12 hours. The aggressive management of Russell and Anderson,[67] using cesarean section to insure termination of all pregnancies within 24 hours after rupture of the membranes, raised their rate of cesarean sections from 4.5 to 12 per cent but reduced fetal deaths by two-thirds.

Since it is obvious that the neonatal death rate rises in a linear fashion with the length of the latent period, the percentage associated with premature rupture of the membranes doubles from 14 to 30 between 24 and 48 hours,[24,39] and therefore the controversy over management between the conservatives and activists has involved primarily the premature infant. Not being able to accurately assess the fetal size or ability to survive extrauterine existence, the clinician was always tempted to believe that additional intrauterine time was worth the risk of infection. Indeed, Pryles and his associates[59] found that 59 per cent of infants born to mothers whose latent periods over 24 hours were premature, and all authors agree that there is an inverse relationship between length of gestation and latent period.

After a 24 hour latent period, the incidence of amnionitis rises to involve from 10 to 30 per cent of pregnancies. Breese,[5] in addition, has graphed the rising mortality rate with both diminishing fetal size and increasing latent period.

TABLE 2-11. *Perinatal Mortality by Weight and Latent Period*

Weight	LATENT PERIOD	
	Under 48 Hr.	Over 48 Hr.
2000–2500 grams	9.6%	20.6%
1500–1999 grams	31.2%	42.8%
1000–1499 grams	60.8%	63.1%
500– 999 grams	55 %	100 %

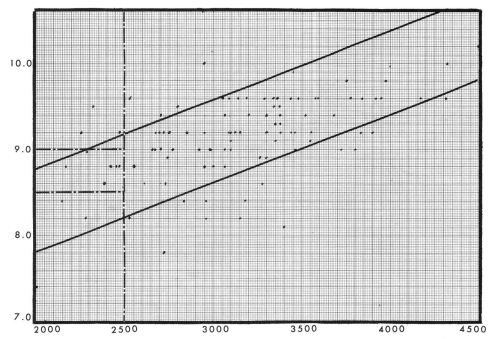

Figure 2-3. Weight of infant estimated by biparietal diameter alone. (From Thompson, H. E., *et al.*: Fetal development as determined by ultrasonic pulse echo techniques. Amer. J. Obstet. Gynec. 92:44–52, 1965.)

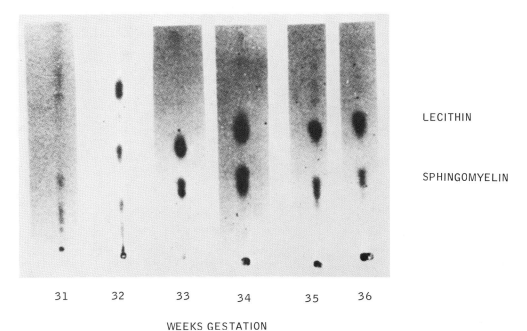

LECITHIN

SPHINGOMYELIN

31   32   33   34   35   36

WEEKS GESTATION

Figure 2-4. Thin-layer chromatography of phospholipids in amniotic fluid. (From: Clinical diagnosis and natural history of the idiopathic respiratory distress syndrome of the newborn. An invitational symposium. J. Reprod. Med. 8:243, 1972.)

Bryans (Lanier *et al.*[39]) also shows a marked rise from 8 per cent to 46.19 per cent infant mortality when maternal infection coexists. These figures have led to the conclusion that the infant over 2000 g. is best treated similarly to the mature infant, with prompt delivery. Estimates as to fetal size through clinical examination have always been grossly inaccurate, and many decisions made on that basis are later regretted.

Ultrasonography has now changed this to a degree, for Thompson[73] has calculated a formula by which he has been able to determine fetal size within 300 g., using the B scan and chest circumference. The biparietal diameter of the fetal head may also be measured to within a 2 mm. accuracy, adding a second dimension for the assessment of fetal growth. The experiences of our ultrasound laboratory support the view that the combined results of these two measurements are indeed correlating well with gestational age and fetal size. Ultrasonography is a standard procedure prior to the planned induction of any labor and is extremely valuable when infant size is borderline or questionable.

Postnatal Risks

The major threat to extrauterine existence of the premature infant is the respiratory distress syndrome, or hyaline membrane disease. The pioneering work of Gluck and his associates[23] has given us a means of accurately assessing fetal lung maturity. Adequate amounts of surfactant in the alveolar lining insure alveolar stability during respiration and thus are necessary for normal respiratory function. This surfactant, produced by the type II epithelial cells of the alveoli, is a complex lipoprotein containing 90 per cent dipalmital lecithin.[36,48] This substance is synthesized from phosphatidyl ethanolamine by transmethylation via the enzyme N-methyl-transferase.[52] Concentrations of this enzyme are high in the microsomal fractions of lung extract. Brumley[7] has shown a markedly lowered pulmonary synthesis of phosphatidyl choline, with low fetal Po_2 and acidosis, especially in the premature.

There is a rapid increase in amniotic fluid lecithin after weeks 32 to 34 and

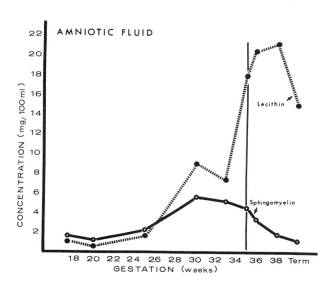

Figure 2-5. Mean concentrations of amniotic fluid of sphingomyelin and lecithin during gestation. The acute rise in lecithin at 35 weeks marks pulmonary maturity. (From Gluck, L., et al.: Diagnosis of the respiratory distress syndrome by amniocentesis. Amer. J. Obstet. Gynec. *109*:441, 1971.)

by amniocentesis, measurements of lecithin phosphate directly or comparatively, as the lecithin/sphingomyelin (L/S) ratio, have proved to be of great value in predicting lung maturity.[3,77] The lecithin/sphingomyelin ratio technique was developed to avoid potential errors caused by variation in amniotic fluid volumes affecting lecithin concentration. Recent reports[25,63] have challenged the value of Gluck and his group's initial work, but in each instance the original technique had been altered to be less complex and to produce faster results, to the detriment of accuracy. Those institutions using the original method, including ours, continue to find the test of great value. In borderline cases, in which it is feasible to obtain uncontaminated amniotic fluid following rupture of the membranes, an L/S ratio over 2 or lecithin levels over 3.5 mg. would rapidly dispose toward quick delivery.[3]

Additional evidence of fetal liver maturity may easily be obtained, using the same specimen, by determining the creatinine level. Zwirek and Pitkin[55] in 1968 showed a progressive rise in creatinine concentration in late gestation, and a level of 2 mg. per 100 ml. or over is comforting corroborating evidence of viability in extrauterine existence.[18] In the small for gestational age infant, however, the creatinine concentration does not correlate well and lecithin levels are a better guide.[50,51]

The original work of Kittrich[32] recognized the fetal squames in amniotic fluid when stained by Nile blue sulfate. Husian and Sinclair[29] developed a method yielding equally good results with hematoxylin and eosin or Papanicolaou staining techniques. The predictions of fetal maturity with this method, however, are considered by some to be less reliable than the methods using creatinine and lecithin concentrations.[18]

When ultrasound confirms the size and creatinine and lecithin levels indicate maturity, there is no difficulty in deciding management if the membranes are ruptured. In the smaller infant, not yet mature and subject to respiratory distress

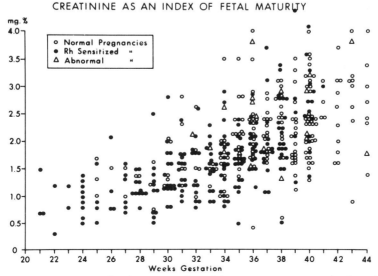

Figure 2-6. Creatinine levels as an index of fetal maturity. (From: Clinical diagnosis and natural history of the idiopathic respiratory distress syndrome of the newborn. An invitational symposium. J. Reprod. Med. 8:243, 1972.)

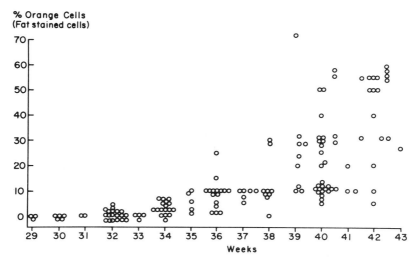

Figure 2-7. Nile blue sulfate stain of amniotic cells as an index of fetal maturity. (From: Clinical diagnosis and natural history of the idiopathic respiratory distress syndrome of the newborn. An invitational symposium. J. Reprod. Med. 8:243, 1972.

syndrome, perinatal mortality rates can be improved only by attempts to produce maturity before deadly infection ensues. Kotas and Avery,[37] using rabbits, and Knelson,[36] working with lambs, have been able to accelerate lung surfactant synthesis by the administration of hydrocortisone and prednisolone. Ewerbeck and Helwig[20] in Germany treated 10 premature infants who had respiratory distress syndrome with prednisolone. Five of these infants died, but none as a result of hyaline membrane disease. Provenzano[58] reported preliminary beneficial results without side-effects in similar work between 1950 and 1953. At the present time, such work is still regarded as experimental as far as its effectiveness and overall safety to the infant are concerned,[17] particularly, as Reynolds[62] points out, because the lag time between steroid administration and the induction of the enzyme system may not be rapid enough to be of clinical benefit. In the light of our abysmal ignorance of the etiology of premature rupture of the membranes, with consequent inability to control its incidence, such developments as we have just described appear at the moment to be our only hope for saving more of these infants.

Effects of Antibiotics

Rovinsky and Shapiro,[66] Lebherz and associates,[40] and Russell and Anderson[67] have all demonstrated the lack of effectiveness of prophylactic antibiotic therapy following rupture of the membranes in decreasing perinatal mortality rate. Maternal morbidity rates for endometritis, parametritis, and pyelitis are all reduced by antibiotic treatment during labor and the postpartum period, for with labor there may be hematogenous spread mediated by the contractile forces of the uterus. Breese[5] reports a lowering of the fetal mortality rate from 37 to 29 per cent with antibiotics administered in labor.

All antibiotics in use today rapidly cross the placental barrier, and the obstetrician must therefore consider the effect upon the fetus whenever medication is given to the mother during pregnancy, labor, or lactation.[4,10,31,33,43,53] That these agents may have hidden effects not immediately recognized is demonstrated by the nine year lag between Scott and Taylor's[69] advocating chloramphenicol in obstetric infections to Kent and Wideman's[30] reporting of its toxicity, and Burns and his colleagues' description of the "gray syndrome."[8]

TABLE 2-12.   *Effect of Drugs on Fetus and Neonate*

Streptomycin	Deafness
Tetracyclines	Bone Anomalies Dental Staining
Nitrofurantoin	Hemolysis
Novobiocin	Hyperbilirubinemia
Chloramphenicol	Cardiovascular Collapse "Gray Syndrome"
Sulfonamides	Kernicterus
Kanamycin	Possible Neurotoxicity
Gentamicin	Possible Ototoxicity

The fetal liver has a marked deficiency of oxidative enzymes necessary for detoxification of drugs in utero. The principal metabolic pathway is either acetylation or conjugation with uridine diphosphoglucuronic acid by the enzyme glucuronyl transferase.[1] The practical implications are impaired acetylation of sulfonamides and decreased conjugation of other antibiotics.[39,42,49] The sulfonamides reduce binding of proteins, resulting in an increased fraction of diffusible bilirubin, and when they are administered near the time of birth, the fetus may be delivered before the placenta can aid in clearance, resulting in neonatal kernicterus.[42]

Penicillin and streptomycin become highly concentrated in the fetus, owing to the low clearance capacity of the kidney for organic acids.[1] So far no tolerance limits for penicillin have been exhibited, but Conway and Birt[14] report fetal deafness associated with administration of streptomycin to the mother.[49,64] The tetracyclines pose special problems, owing to deposition of analogues in the tooth crown when fetal teeth are undergoing mineralization during late pregnancy, as well as deposition of tetracycline phosphors in the skeleton and resulting growth retardation.[13,33,38,61] The "gray syndrome" of chloramphenicol toxicity is secondary to the high fetal concentration of this agent and develops from the resulting inhibition of protein synthesis. This inhibition, an interference with the attachment of RNA to ribosomes, precludes the synthesis of enzymes so necessary for extrauterine existence—an effect which continues after birth.[49,76] Novobiocin also is implicated in competitive interference with bilirubin conjugation, while the cephalosporins so far have not been shown to be toxic.[1,9,41,71]

Dailey[15] has recently shown the increasing antibiotic resistance of coliform organisms in neonatal infections. Thirty-eight per cent of the species or strains were resistant to ampicillin, streptomycin, and the tetracyclines, but fewer were resistant to cephalothin and kanamycin. Our preferred mode of maternal therapy in infection is large doses of penicillin (30 to 60 million units per day intravenously) in the nonallergic patient, or Keflin in doses of 1 to 2 g. every 4 hours in cases in which sensitive organisms are resistant to penicillin. Kanamycin has a wider spectrum of effectiveness, but its fetal nephrotoxicity and neurotoxicity are unproved.[46] Gentamicin has potential ototoxicity but is effective when *Proteus* and *Pseudomonas* infections are superimposed.[34,47] The drugs mentioned are effective primarily against the major pathogenic organisms which may invade the uterus following premature rupture of the membranes. Selection of the drug with maximum effectiveness and minimum fetal risk can therefore be made intelligently. Other modalities of therapy may be added in severe maternal infections, such as septic shock.

Preserving the immature fetus within the uterus following premature rupture of the membranes deserves not only the careful sterile diagnostic handling previously described but also isolation from the hospital environment with its virulent pathogens. Most would prefer to maintain the patient at home, without intravaginal manipulations, recording the temperature twice daily, and restricting activity. As long as the patient is afebrile and without purulent vaginal discharge, this management is continued, with weekly sonograms being taken, until fetal size reaches 2000 g., at which time labor is induced or cesarean section performed.

Diagnosing Intrauterine Infections

The diagnosis of intrauterine infection is fraught with potential danger.[21] To make sense out of the bacteriological findings in the vagina is nearly impossible for, as Prystowsky[60] says, the microbiologic findings in the cervix, placenta, and vagina are "a big sea of ignorance." Prevedourakis and his co-workers[57] found 7.8 per cent positive amniotic fluid cultures without fetal or maternal morbidity, and identical organisms in both the fetal throat and urine as in the vagina and cervix, even without rupture of the membranes. Barbaro[2] found pathogens in 45 of 96 patients, 77 per cent of which were anaerobic *Streptococcus* or gram-negative organisms. Even the initial cultures following rupture of the membranes were positive in 33 per cent, but in only 3 per cent was actual infection established. Wilson and his co-workers[80] found the cord to show inflammation in 39 per cent, with only 8 per cent of infants actually infected. Mandsley and associates,[45] analyzing 3000 samples from 494 cases of premature rupture of the membranes, found maternal deciduitis in 89 per cent and chorioamnionitis in 27 per cent, yet 50 per cent of the uterine cultures were negative. Hosmer and Sprunt[27] found cord blood, gastric aspirate, and infant blood cultures 50 to 80 per cent negative or misleading. Pryles and his colleagues[59] concluded after examining 358 cases that 80 per cent of infants with umbilical cord vasculitis did well without treatment, therefore antibiotic therapy needed additional justification.

The febrile patient, particularly with purulent or foul-smelling amniotic fluid and uterine tenderness, presents a much more ominous picture, as well as a much more positive diagnostic conclusion. When amnionitis is present, Bryans and Lanier have reported 50 per cent fetal loss.[39] Pryles and his co-workers[59] found 57 per cent of babies to be ill when maternal fever was present, and Clark and Anderson[12] report 17 per cent of stillbirths and 14.4 per cent of all neonatal deaths occurring in the presence of amnionitis. The presence of infection may be difficult to document bacteriologically, but when clinically present demands immediate uterine evacuation, despite the size of the infant. Procrastination at this point could well lead to severely prejudicing the mother's health while not improving fetal chances of survival. The choice of obstetrical delivery is that which is most expedient.[54] Willson and colleagues[79] justify cesarean section if effective labor cannot be induced and delivery expected within 24 hours. Cesarean hysterectomy often should be the choice where induction fails and gross infection exists, particularly when further childbearing is not a factor.

Summary

Since at the present time the obstetrician is unable to effectively prevent spontaneous rupture of the membranes, his management of the patient with this condition must be impeccable. Prompt confirmation of the diagnosis by sterile speculum examination and analysis of the leaking fluid should be followed by evaluation of fetal size and corroboration by sonogram if necessary. Induction of labor when not obstetrically contraindicated should be initiated within 12 to 24 hours in the fetus weighing 2000 g. or more, with cesarean section or cesarean hysterectomy when induction fails. The immature fetus may be allowed to remain in the uterus until it reaches this degree of maturity or until clinical infection supervenes, at which time rapid delivery with antibiotic coverage in labor is indicated. At delivery, aerobic and anaerobic cultures of infant blood from two different sites should be obtained for intelligent neonatal and postpartum therapy. Such management hopefully will result in maintaining as low a perinatal loss as is possible at the present state of our knowledge of this perplexing obstetrical problem.

REFERENCES

1. Adamson, K., Jr., and Joelsson, I.: The effects of pharmacologic agents upon the fetus and newborn. Amer. J. Obstet. Gynec. 96:437, 1966.
2. Barbaro, C. A.: Foetal prognosis after spontaneous premature rupture of the membranes. Med. J. Australia 2:57, 1967.
3. Bhagwanani, S. G., Fahmy, D., and Turnbull, A. C.: Prediction of neonatal respiratory distress by estimation of amniotic fluid lecithin. Lancet 1:159–635, 1972.
4. Bray, R. E.: Transfer of ampicillin into fetus and amniotic fluid from maternal plasma in late pregnancy. Amer. J. Obstet. Gynec. 96:938, 1966.
5. Breese, M. W.: Spontaneous premature rupture of the membranes. Amer. J. Obstet. Gynec. 81:1086, 1961.
6. Brelje, M. D., and Kaltreider, D. F.:The use of vaginal antibiotics in premature rupture of the membranes. Amer. J. Obstet. Gynec. 94:889, 1966.
7. Brumley, G. W.: Lung development and lecithin metabolism. Arch. Int. Med. 127:413, 1971.
8. Burns, L. E., Hodgman, J., and Cass, A. B.: Fatal circulatory collapse in premature infants receiving chloramphenicol. New Eng. J. Med. 261:1318, 1959.
9. Burland, W. L., Simpson, K., and Samuel, P. D.: Combining cephaloride and streptomycin for the treatment and prophylaxis of neonatal infections. Postgrad. Med. J. (Suppl.) 46:85, 1970.
10. Charles, D. J.: Placental transmission of antibiotics. J. Obstet. Gynec. Brit. Emp. 61:750, 1954.
11. Clark, D. M., and Anderson, G. V.: Perinatal mortality and amnionitis in a general hospital population. Obstet. Gynec. 31:714, 1968.
12. Clark, D. M., Anderson, G. V., and Burchell, R. C.: Premature spontaneous rupture of the membranes. Amer. J. Obstet. Gynec. 88:251, 1964.

13. Cohlan, S. P., Bevelander, G., and Tiamsic, T.: Growth inhibitions of prematures receiving tetracycline. Amer. J. Dis. Child. *105*:453, 1963.
14. Conway, N., and Birt, B. D.: Streptomycin in pregnancy: effect on the foetal ear. Brit. Med. J. *2*:260, 1965.
15. Dailey, K. M.: Incidence of antibiotic resistance and R factors among gram negative bacteria isolated from the neonatal intestine. J. Pediat. *80*:198, Feb. 1972.
16. Danforth, D. N., McElin, T. W., and Stites, M. N.: Studies on fetal membranes: I. Bursting tension. Amer. J. Obstet. Gynec. *65*:480, 1953.
17. Delamos, R. A., Shermeta, D. W., Knelson, J. H., Kotas, R. J., and Avery, M. E.: The induction of the pulmonary surfactant in the fetal lamb by the administration of corticosteroids. Pediat. Res. *3*:505, 1969.
18. Droegemueller, W., Jackson, C., Makowski, E. L., and Battaglia, F. C.: Amniotic fluid examination as an aid in the assessment of gestational age. Amer. J. Obstet. Gynec. *104*:424, 1967.
19. Eastman, N. J.: Editorial discussion of Roth, N. E.: Early rupture of the membranes: significance, etiology and prognosis. Obstet. Gynec. Surv. *10*:14, 1955.
20. Ewerbeck, H., and Helwig, H.: Treatment of idiopathic respiratory distress with large doses of corticoids. Pediatrics *49*:467, 1972.
21. Franciosi, R. A.: Fetal infection via the amniotic fluid. Rocky Mountain Med. J. *67*:32, 1970.
22. Freidman, M. L., and McElin, T. W.: Diagnosis of ruptured fetal membranes. Amer. J. Obstet. Gynec. *104*:544, 1969.
23. Gluck, L., Kulovich, M. V., Borer, R. C., Jr., Brenner, P. H., Anderson, G. G., and Spellacy, W. N.: Diagnosis of the respiratory distress syndrome by amniocentesis. Amer. J. Obstet. Gynec. *109*:440, 1971.
24. Gunn, G. C., Mishell, D. R., Jr., and Morton, D. G.: Premature rupture of the fetal membranes. Amer. J. Obstet. Gynec. *106*:469, 1970.
25. Gusdon, J. P., and Waite, B. M.: A colorimetric method for amniotic fluid phospholipids and their relationship to the respiratory distress syndrome. Amer. J. Obstet. Gynec. *112*:62, 1972.
26. Hellman, L. M., and Pritchard, J. A.: Williams Obstetrics. 14th Ed. New York, Appleton-Century-Crofts, 1971.
27. Hosmer, M. E., and Sprunt, K.: Screening method for identification of infected infant following premature rupture of maternal membranes. Pediatrics *49*:283, 1972.
28. Howard, P. J., and Bauer, A. R.: Infection in the newborn infant and its association with prolonged rupture of the amniotic membranes. Henry Ford Hosp. Med. J. *15*:161, 1967.
29. Husain, O. A. N., and Sinclair, L.: Studies on the cytology of amniotic fluid and of the newborn infant's skin in relation to maturity of the infant. Proc. Roy. Soc. Med. *64*:1213, 1971.
30. Kent, S. P., and Wideman, G. L.: Prophylactic antibiotic therapy in infants born after premature rupture of membranes. J.A.M.A. *171*:1199, 1959.
31. Kiefer, L.: The placental transfer of erythromycin. Amer. J. Obstet. Gynec. *69*:174, 1955.
32. Kittrich, M.: Editorial. Lancet *1*:132, 1972 (Geburtsh. Frauenheilkd. *26*:156, 1963).
33. Klein, J. O., and Marcy, S. M.: Infection in the newborn. Clin. Obstet. Gynec. *13*:321, 1970.
34. Klein, J. O., Herschel, M., Therakan, R. M., and Ingall, D.: Gentamycin in serious neonatal infections: absorption, excretion, and clinical results in 25 cases. J. Infect. Dis. (Suppl.) *124*:224, 1971.
35. Kline, A. H., Blattner, R. J., and Zunin, M.: Transplacental effect of tetracyclines on teeth. J.A.M.A. *188*:178, 1964.
36. Knelson, J. H.: Environmental influence on intrauterine lung development. Arch. Int. Med. *127*:421, 1971.
37. Kotas, R. V., and Avery, M. D.: Accelerated appearance of pulmonary surfactant in the fetal rabbit. J. Appl. Physiol. *30*:358, 1971.
38. Kutscher, A. H., Zegarelli, E. V., Tovell, A. M., Hochberg, B., and Hauptman, J.: Discoloration of deciduous teeth inducted by administration of tetracycline ante partum. Amer. J. Obstet. Gynec. *96*:291, 1966.
39. Lanier, L. R., Jr., Scarbrough, R. W., Jr., Fillingim, O. W., and Baker, R. E., Jr.: Incidence of maternal and fetal complications associated with rupture of the membranes before onset of labor. Amer. J. Obstet. Gynec. *93*:398, 1965.
40. Lebherz, J. B., Hellman, L. M., Madding, R., Anctil, A., and Arje, S. L.: Double-blind study of premature rupture of the membranes. Amer. J. Obstet. Gynec. *87*:218, 1963.
41. Lokietz, H., Dowben, R. M., and Hsia, D. Y-Y.: Studies on the effect of novobiocin on glycuronyl transferase. Pediatrics *32*:47, 1963.

42. Lucey, J. F., and Driscoll, T. J.: Hazard to newborn infants of administration of long-acting sulfonamides to pregnant women (letter to Editor). Pediatrics 24:498, 1959.

43. MacAulay, M. A., Abou-Sabe, M., and Charles, D.: Placental transfer of ampicillin. Amer. J. Obstet. Gynec. 96:943, 1966.

44. MacDonald, H. N., and Isherwood, D. M.: Assessment of gestational age from amniotic fluid. Lancet 1:321, 1972.

45. Mandsley, R. F., Brix, G. A., Hinton, N. A., Robertson, E. M., Bryans, A. M., and Haust, M. D.: Placental inflammation and infection. Amer. J. Obstet. Gynec. 95:648, 1966.

46. McCracken, G. H., Jr.: Changing pattern of the antimicrobial susceptibilities of *Escherichia coli* in neonatal infections. Pediatrics 78:942, 1971.

47. McCracken, G. H., Jr., and Jones, L. G.: Gentamicin in the neonatal period. Amer. J. Dis. Child. 120:524, 1970.

48. Menzel, D. B.: Perspective and conclusions: symposium on pollution and lung biochemistry. Arch. Int. Med. 127:375, 1971.

49. Mirkin, B. L.: Effects of drugs on the fetus and neonate. Postgrad. Med. 47:91, 1970.

50. Moore, W. M. O.: Assessment of gestational age from amniotic fluid. Lancet 1:493, 1972.

51. Moore, W. M. O., Murphy, P. J., and Davis, J. A.: Creatinine content of amniotic fluid in cases of retarded fetal growth. Amer. J. Obstet. Gynec. 110:908, 1971.

52. Morgan, T. E.: Biosynthesis of pulmonary surface-active lipid. Arch. Int. Med. 127:401, 1971.

53. Morrow, S. J., Jr., Palmisano, P., and Cassady, G.: The placental transfer of cephalothin. Pediatrics 73:262, 1968.

54. Overstreet, E. W., and Romney, S. L.: Premature rupture of the membranes—consultation. Amer. J. Obstet. Gynec. 96:1037, 1966.

55. Zwirek, S. J., and Pitkin, R. M.: Direct spectrophotometric estimation of amniotic fluid volume. Amer. J. Obstet. Gynec. 101:934, 1968.

56. Polishuk, W. Z., Kohane, S., and Wiznitzer, N.: Premature rupture of membranes in different ethnic groups. Israel J. Med. Sci. 1:450, 1965.

57. Prevedourakis, C. N., Strigou-Charalambis, E., St. Michalas and Alvanou-Iakovakis, M. Intrauterine bacterial growth during labor. Amer. J. Obstet. Gynec. 113:33, 1972.

58. Provenzano, R. W.: Editorial comment on Ewerbeck, H., and Helwig, H.: Treatment of idiopathic respiratory distress with large doses of corticoids. Pediatrics 49:468, 1972.

59. Pryles, C. V., Steg, N. L., Nari, S., Gellis, S. S., and Tenney, B.: A controlled study of the influence on the newborn of prolonged premature rupture of the amniotic membranes and/or infection in the mother. Pediatrics 31:608, 1963.

60. Prystowsky, H.: Management of premature rupture of membranes. Northwest Med. 64:124, 1965.

61. Rendle-Short, T. J.: Tetracycline in teeth and bone. Lancet 1:1188, 1962.

62. Reynolds, J. W.: Comment on H. Ewerbeck's letter to Editor on treatment of idiopathic respiratory distress with large doses of corticoids. Pediatrics 49:467, 1972.

63. Rivkind, J., and Pisani, B. J.: Premature rupture of fetal membranes. Postgrad. Med. 42:52, 1967.

64. Robinson, G. C., and Cambon, K. G.: Hearing loss in infants of tuberculous mothers treated with streptomycin during pregnancy. New England J. Med. 271:949, 1964.

65. Roux, J. F., Nakamura, J., Brown, E., and Sweet, A. Y.: The lecithin-sphingomyelin ratio of amniotic fluid: an index of fetal lung maturity? (letter to Editor). Pediatrics 49:464, 1972.

66. Rovinsky, J. J., and Shapiro, W. J.: Management of premature rupture of membranes: I. Near term. Obstet. Gynec. 32:855, 1968.

67. Russell, K. P., and Anderson, G. V.: The aggressive management of ruptured membranes. Amer. J. Obstet. Gynec. 83:930, 1962.

68. Sacks, M., and Baker, T. H.: Spontaneous premature rupture of the membranes. Amer. J. Obstet. Gynec. 97:888, 1967.

69. Scott, W. C., and Taylor, E. S.: The use of chloramphenicol in obstetric infections. West. J. Surg. Obstet. Gynec. 60:36.

70. Shubeck, F., Benson, R., Clark, W. W., Berendes, H., Weiss, W., and Duetschberger, J.: Fetal hazard after rupture of the membranes. Obstet. Gynec. 28:22, 1966.

71. Sutherland, J. M., and Keller, W. H.: Novobiocin and neonatal hyperbilirubinemia. An investigation of the relationship in an epidemic of neonatal hyperbilirubinemia. Amer. J. Dis. Child. 101:447, 1961.

72. Taylor, E. S., Morgan, R. L., Bruns, P. D., and Drose, V. E.: Spontaneous premature rupture of the fetal membranes. Amer. J. Obstet. Gynec. 82:1341, 1961.

73. Thompson, H. E.: Diagnostic Ultrasound. New York, Plenum Press, 1966.

74. Webb, G. A.: Maternal death associated with premature rupture of the membranes. Amer. J. Obstet. Gynec. 98:594, 1967.

75. Webster, A.: Management of premature rupture of the fetal membranes. Obstet. Gynec. Surv. 24:485, 1969.
76. Weiss, C. F.: Chloramphenicol in the newborn infant. New Eng. J. Med. 262:787, 1962.
77. Whitfield, C. R., and Sproule, W. B.: Prediction of neonatal respiratory distress. Lancet 1:382, 1972.
78. Wideman, G. L., Baird, G. H., and Balding, O. T.: Ascorbic acid deficiency and premature rupture of fetal membranes. Amer. J. Obstet. Gynec. 88:592, 1964.
79. Willson, J. R., Beecham, C. T., and Carrington, E. D.: Obstetrics and Gynecology. 4th Ed. St. Louis, C. V. Mosby Co., 1971.
80. Wilson, M. D., Armstrong, D. H., Nelson, R. C., and Boak, R. A.: Prolonged rupture of fetal membranes. Amer. J. Dis. Child. 107:138, 1964.

Treatment of Patients With Premature Rupture of the Fetal Membranes: (a) Prior to 32 Weeks; (b) After 32 Weeks

Editorial Comment

It has long been appreciated that spontaneous rupture of the fetal membranes prior to the onset of labor is a potential hazard for both the mother and the fetus. Prior to the introduction of chemotherapeutic and antibiotic agents, many maternity clinics pursued the policy that "the sun should never set more than once on the parturient with rupture of the fetal membranes in the undelivered state." The emphasis was placed on the maternal outcome, for intrauterine infection at that time could only be treated supportively and all too often ineffectively.

Now the emphasis is being placed on the fetal welfare, and here the subtleness of intrauterine infection comes to the fore. Certainly, fetal infection may occur when the maternal vital signs are normal, a fact that should be considered also when abdominal delivery is being contemplated. Moreover, the question of the long-term sequelae in the newborn to prolonged exposure to intrauterine infection must still be answered. In fact, this angle has never been investigated except in a preliminary way. Granted the evidence is still meager, there *is* some to indicate that severe damage to the central nervous system in the newborn may manifest itself several months after birth, when there was a latent period of several days or weeks after rupture of the fetal membranes. The hospital course of such infants was unremarkable and infection was not of clinical concern. However, the placental vessels contained extensive inflammatory exudate.[1] This situation might well contribute to a decrease in fetoplacental blood flow and result in a chronic state of hypoxia. When the expectant or conservative treatment is pursued, weekly sonograms of the fetus might afford an index of its growth rate. Should intrauterine growth retardation be demonstrated, a possibility that has been mentioned by one of the contributors, the fetus is best delivered to avoid hypoxic damage. This is a further illustration of the fact that fetal and neonatal results should not be gauged by perinatal mortality rates alone, but rather should include the ultimate outcome of the infant some months or a year or more following birth.

The incidence of premature rupture of the membranes appears to be closely related to the socioeconomic status of the patients, and this may account somewhat for the attitude and differences in opinion held by physicians regarding management of this complication. Whatever else, good medical practice requires that the physician be aware of and take steps to protect the patient against possible adverse influences in her environment.

For example, it is commonplace to recommend that the patient with prematurely ruptured membranes be discharged and sent home after a short period of observation rather than continue to be hospitalized until delivery. The maternal deaths cited by the contributors makes one question the wisdom of such a policy. It must be emphasized that the patient often comes initially or returns to the hospital already suffering from serious and possibly lethal intrauterine infection. Surely we must not leave it to the patient to decide whether or not she is developing an intrauterine infection. It would appear that we are again confronted with a possible compromise in patient care as a result of the costliness of hospitalization. Certainly the reliability of the patient to follow instructions closely and the limitations imposed by her environment must be given consideration in her overall management. Again, we must ask whether the nonprivate patient is being subjected to a different quality of care than the private patient. Are these women being properly and adequately instructed, for example, about not indulging in intercourse or at least in only a modified form—i.e., avoidance of deep penetration—during the last 8 to 10 weeks of gestation? Are they having repeated vaginal examinations, and by several examiners, without the taking of proper sterile precautions? What indeed are the factors accounting for the incidence, recorded by Drs. Gordon and Weingold, of premature rupture of the fetal membranes occurring in 2 per cent in private patients and in 14 per cent of the socioeconomically deprived? How can we ignore these findings, for they are common to the majority if not all of the nonprivate obstetric services in this country? Although the etiology of this condition is not entirely clear, it certainly appears that there is an element of preventability.

Besides prevention, what then can be done to manage intrauterine infection conservatively? First, avoid anything that might infect the patient with rupture of the fetal membranes. If a pelvic examination must be performed, it should be done under the most rigid sterile conditions. Second, antibiotics have been advocated and cautiously condemned; apparently they do not influence intrauterine fetal loss but appear to decrease postpartum maternal morbidity, according to one contributor's study. However, as mentioned, there is the possibility that the fetus is unable to manage antibiotics biochemically, and hence these agents may adversely affect the neonate in the long run. Third, despite the apparently favorable effect in controlling morbidity in the mother, the same authors caution that if abdominal delivery is required, cesarean hysterectomy should be considered.

There is general agreement that, whatever the policy to be pursued, an infant weighing 2000 to 2500 g. or more fares better in the pediatric intensive care unit than in the mother's uterus. Also, the fetal mortality rate rises precipitously when intrauterine infection becomes evident, and prompt termination of the pregnancy appears to be indicated.

When the fetus weighs less than 2000 g., conservative management of the patient is usually advocated. However, if the incidence of central nervous system damage in the neonate exposed to intrauterine infection following premature rupture of the fetal membranes proves to be similar to that seen in the fetus of 1500 g. or thereabouts in patients managed conservatively for placenta previa, the remarks made in the Editorial Comment in Chapter Four might apply here (see page 137). One must therefore raise the question of whether the conservative or expectant treatment of premature rupture of the fetal membranes in the more premature infants is the correct move. It must be stated, however, that there appear to be fewer unavoidable fetal deaths than in placenta previa, while the sequelae of irreversible central nervous system damage are still to be determined or indeed proved in the fetus delivered after prolonged rupture of the fetal membranes. As one of the contributors has written in a letter which accompanied his manuscript, "I don't think that the right study of premature rupture of the fetal membranes has been done yet."

REFERENCES

1. Reid, D. E.: The right and the responsibility. Amer. J. Obstet. Gynec. *108*:828, 1970. Preliminary data on severe central nervous system damage in the neonate exposed to prolonged rupture of the fetal membranes.

3

The Management of Impending Labor Prior to the Thirty-Fifth Week

Alternative Points of View:

By Tom P. Barden

By Luis A. Cibils

By Robert Landesman

Editorial Comment

The Management of
Impending Labor Prior to the Thirty-Fifth Week

Tom P. Barden

University of Cincinnati Medical Center

Prematurity is the major contributing factor to neonatal morbidity and mortality, associated with approximately two-thirds of neonatal deaths in the United States. Premature birth weights of 500 to 2499 g. occur in nearly 10 per cent of the approximately four million births each year in the United States. It is well established that population segments which are socioeconomically deprived have a high frequency of prematurity and high neonatal morbidity and mortality rates. Infants weighing less than 1500 g. at birth in particular show a significantly increased incidence of epilepsy, cerebral palsy, and mental retardation. Long-term hospitalization of these infants places a tremendous burden on hospital facilities, as well as an overwhelming financial obligation on the responsible parties. Although the reduction of maternal mortality rates has been dramatic in recent decades, the decline in neonatal deaths with advancing medical knowledge has been much more gradual. These statistics, plus our improving knowledge of uterine physiology and labor, have stimulated interest in developing a treatment for premature labor that is successful regardless of etiology—which at any rate is unknown—and yet is safe for both fetus and mother. Our incomplete knowledge of the physiology of labor at term, as well as prior to term, contributes to the obvious confusion over when to attempt inhibition of premature labor, as well as the choice of method. The following discussion will review the rapidly growing literature relating to labor physiology, define premature labor, consider indications and contraindications to therapy, and review both the available methods of therapy and those under investigation.

Physiology of Labor

During recent years, research has produced several major hypotheses regarding the onset and control of human labor. The first, proposed by the studies of Csapo,[26,27] states that placental production of progesterone during pregnancy produces a local "progesterone block" on the motility of the underlying uterine site. At the onset of labor, the concentration of progesterone in the myometrium adjacent to the placenta is decreased, and the resulting organized or "symmetrical" uterine contractions produce progressive labor. In support of this theory, the work of Kumar and associates[45] indicated that a higher concentration of progesterone is present in the myometrium overlying the placental site than elsewhere in the uterus. On the other hand, Brenner and Hendricks[14] reported that oral administration of medroxyprogesterone, 80 mg. daily, had no effect on duration of pregnancy or labor. In contrast, Bengtsson[10] found that by injecting 150 to 400 mg. of medroxyprogesterone into the anterior wall of the uterus, uterine activity was suppressed in 9 of 10 patients in early premature labor. Wood and co-workers[71] subsequently studied a series of term patients given intravenous and intramuscular 17-hydroxyprogesterone, and intra-amniotic and intramyometrial medroxyprogesterone. They concluded that administration of large doses of progestogens in late pregnancy sometimes produces a partial suppression of uterine activity. Wood and Pinkerton[72] found a discrepancy in uterine motility in a case of uterine duplication in which the fetus occupied one side, concluding that the pregnancy inhibited uterine motility in the occupied side. Also in support of the theory was the more recent report of Csapo and associates[28] reporting laboratory evidence of plasma progesterone withdrawal prior to abortion following intra-amniotic instillation of hypertonic saline. Scommegna and co-workers[60] found that intravenous infusion of pregnenolone sulfate, the immediate precursor of progesterone, significantly inhibited term labor. From recent studies[77,78] Csapo has suggested that prostaglandin $F_{2\alpha}$ is the intrinsic myometrial stretching. The level of intrinsic or extrinsic stimulant activity to the threshold of progesterone block of cyclic uterine activity may determine the onset of progressive labor. Csapo and co-workers[79] reported that labor in rats may be delayed or interrupted by the administration of naproxen, a known inhibitor of prostaglandin synthesis. Although the progesterone block theory is widely accepted, there are no reports establishing the efficacy of progesterone therapy to inhibit premature labor in humans.

A second hypothesis, introduced by Caldeyro-Barcia and Sereno,[23] states that human myometrium becomes progressively more sensitive to a relatively constant level of circulating oxytocin during pregnancy, until a critical level is attained, producing clinical labor. Further, the work of Fuchs[33] indicated that in rabbits, the infusion of ethanol blocked the hypothalamohypophyseal release of oxytocin, as well as of antidiuretic hormone. Fuchs and associates[34] reported that the administration of ethanol markedly reduced uterine activity in nonpregnant women. A sequel to this work is found in the recent study by Zlatnik and Fuchs[73] in which 42 patients in threatened premature labor participated in a controlled study using intravenous ethanol versus 5 per cent glucose in water. Delivery was delayed for at least three days in 81 per cent of the ethanol group, and in only 38 per cent of the glucose-in-water group, a significant difference. A possible fetal source of oxytocin triggering labor was suggested by the studies of Chard and associates,[24] who used a specific radioimmunoassay for oxytocin to confirm that maternal blood levels of oxytocin were not detectable in 81 per cent of a series of patients in labor; however, oxytocin levels were detectable in 76 per cent of umbilical arterial plasma samples collected at the time of delivery. In paired umbilical vessel samples, the concentrations were lower in venous than in arterial samples, suggesting a fetal source of oxytocin. Evidence that appears contrary to this hypothesis of labor control was presented by Karim and Sharma,[42] who studied a series of women with fetal death in the third trimester to demonstrate that intravenous ethanol inhibited uterine activity produced by intravenous infusion of prostaglandins, but it failed to modify the effect in other cases, in which uterine activity was stimulated by intravenous oxytocin. Further evidence for the possible role of prostaglandins in the initiation of labor was presented by Karim[43] when he reported the appearance of prostaglandin $F_{2\alpha}$ in the blood of pregnant women at the onset of labor.

Another hypothesis of the etiology of labor evolved from the work of Ahlquist,[2] who postulated that the action of sympathomimetic hormones on smooth muscle is mediated through two sets of receptors, the alpha and beta adrenergic receptors. In the human in late pregnancy, norepinephrine produces myometrial stimulation via the alpha receptors, and epinephrine produces uterine relaxation through stimulation of the beta receptors.[62,63] The studies of Sutherland[65] have established that stimulation of beta adrenergic receptors, producing myometrial relaxation, is associated with increased intracellular amounts of cyclic 3,'5'-adenosine monophosphate (cyclic AMP). Most of the agents currently being investigated for uterine inhibitory properties are beta adrenergic sympathomimetic amines, structurally related to epinephrine. Further evidence to support the rationale of using these compounds to inhibit unwanted uterine activity is offered by the work of Coutinho and Vieira Lopes,[25] who found a uniform inhibition of uterine activity by aminophylline. Aminophylline is a methylxanthine which blocks the action of phosphodiesterase, the enzyme which normally destroys cyclic AMP.[67]

A common denominator among some of these hypotheses of labor etiology is afforded by the work of Brotánek and his colleagues[16] who, by using a thermistor probe placed in the anterior lip of the cervix to register uterine blood flow,[17] observed a decrease of uterine blood flow with maneuvers for induction of labor, and improved uterine blood supply associated with decreased uterine activity. Other studies, of Brotánek and Hodr,[18,19] indicated a decrease of uterine blood flow shortly after the initiation of oxytocin infusion, and demonstrated that intravenous infusion of isoxsuprine produced an increase of uterine blood flow as it inhibited uterine motility. Brotánek and his associates[20] also reported that in spontaneous labor, uterine blood flow decreases for about 30 seconds before the onset of contractions. From a clinical perspective, it is well known that the incidence of premature labor is increased in conditions associated with compromised uterine blood flow, such as heavy smoking, maternal cardiac disease, chronic hypertension, uterine anomalies, multiple pregnancy, and hyponutritive states. In contrast, the mechanism of action of ethanol or various beta adrenergic sympathomimetic amines in inhibition of labor may well be mediated in part through improved uterine blood flow.

Thus we are presented with a variety of likely mechanisms of labor initiation, which are probably functioning simultaneously. It is not surprising that a variety of agents have been studied for possible use in inhibition of unwanted uterine activity.

Premature Labor

There is no consensus on a standard definition of premature labor as determined by a prospective clinical judgment. Regardless of criteria that we may establish, in a certain number of patients labor-like activity in time will cease spontaneously. Gestational histories are notoriously inaccurate, uterine size varies in pregnancies of comparable duration, and clinical estimation of fetal weight may be significantly in error. It is apparent that almost all patients in labor have relatively regular uterine contractions at intervals of less than 10 minutes, associated with progressive changes of the cervix and fetal descent. True labor contractions tend to become more regular and to increase in frequency, intensity, and painfulness as labor progresses; however, it is apparent from virtually all studies of uterine inhibiting agents that early treatment tends to be more successful than attempts at inhibition when labor is advanced. Thus in approaching the management of premature labor, either clinically or in study of an experimental agent, it is unwise to await significant evidence of advancing dilation, fetal descent, or increasing subjective evidence of labor before initiating therapy. Generally, the estimation of fetal weight tends to be more accurate than an estimation of gestation based on menstrual history. Premature labor might then be defined as the development of relatively regular contractions of less than 10 minute intervals, associated with concomitant changes of cervical effacement or dilatation, or both, and fetal descent in a patient between 20 and approximately 36 weeks' gestation, with fetal weight of 500 to 2499 g.

In approximately 50 per cent of premature labors, the pathogenesis is uncertain. Low socioeconomic status is the most frequent identifiable factor and may variously involve nutrition, hygiene, bacterial flora, susceptibility to infection, genetic factors, pregnancy in the younger and older age groups, higher incidence of multiple pregnancy, greater frequency of multiparity, coital frequency, and inadequate prenatal care. Numerous reports on prematurity describe a 10 to 15 per cent incidence related to elective obstetric procedures. Prematurity occurs more frequently in patients who live at high altitudes, who smoke, or who have asymptomatic bacteruria.[1] Providing prenatal care with the best available treatment for any obstetric complications that may occur, such as toxemia, placenta previa, incompetent cervix, and Rh isoimmunization, may decrease the frequency of premature labor somewhat, but there is no convincing evidence that care as it now exists, if extended to all, will significantly reduce prematurity rates. An effective and safe treatment of premature labor is needed which can be initiated in the labor room when the diagnosis is established and no apparent contraindications to inhibition of labor are present.

MANAGEMENT OF PREMATURE LABOR

Once a clinical diagnosis of premature labor has been made, a decision as to the course of further management must be forthcoming. There is no doubt that certain conditions may prevail in pregnancy that promote premature labor to the advantage of the yet immature fetus, when further intrauterine existence offers nothing but serious compromise. In contrast, certain maternal conditions that trigger premature labor are self-limiting, or correctable with proper management. In these situations, it is clear that vigorous therapy to stop the premature labor and resolve the maternal disease state is indicated to afford a better outcome for the fetus. In some clinical circumstances, the decision of whether to attempt inhibition or to permit premature delivery becomes a delicate judgment problem.

At present, it is generally agreed that the following conditions are contraindications to active treatment directed toward inhibiting premature labor:

Maternal

       Chronic hypertensive cardiovascular disease

       Other maternal heart disease

       Uterine anomaly or tumor

       Intrauterine infection

       Advanced labor

Fetoplacental

       Placental separation

       Placental insufficiency

          Diabetes mellitus

          Chronic hypertension

          Advanced toxemia

       Ruptured membranes

       Fetal anomaly

       Fetal distress (chronic)

       Fetal death

Chronic hypertension is generally aggravated by superimposed pregnancy, and is not amenable to most forms of therapy during pregnancy. It is thought to promote premature labor by the associated compromising of uterine blood supply and presence of placental insufficiency. Many of the agents in current use for inhibition of premature labor also produce maternal tachycardia and potential danger if there is preexisting cardiac disease. A compromise of intrauterine space by an anomaly or tumor is considered too strong a stimulus to premature labor to be inhibited by existing drugs. It is not possible at present to adequately treat intrauterine infections, and thus there is nearly unanimous agreement that this diagnosis contraindicates active inhibition, and generally indicates a need for induction of labor. A consensus prevails that if cervical dilation has advanced to 4 cm. or more, active intervention is fruitless. A diagnosis of placental separation or placental insufficiency indicates potential fetal jeopardy and is considered a contraindication to therapy. Presence of ruptured membranes associated with premature labor is generally considered a contraindication to pharmacologic inhibition of labor owing to the high incidence of intrauterine infection with continued pregnancy. If there are known fetal anomalies, evidence of chronic fetal distress, or a diagnosis of fetal death in utero, active intervention in premature labor is not indicated.

METHODS CURRENTLY AVAILABLE

From the preceding discussion it becomes apparent that a diagnosis of premature labor is often very tentative, awaiting evidence of progressive labor. We also understand that virtually all treatment modes will fail if labor becomes too advanced. The result is that a significant number of cases of premature labor may appear to be successfully treated, by whatever management schemes are used, when in fact they would have been diagnosed "false labor" had there been no treatment.

There are relatively few studies of the influence of bed rest upon uterine activity, and yet the practice of advising bed rest for threatened premature labor is obviously widespread. It is of interest that in well controlled studies of specific medicaments in treatment of premature labor,[70,73] which will be discussed in detail below, there were significant delays of labor by bed rest alone in 38 per cent and 48 per cent, respectively. There is no doubt that bed rest should be an adjunct to any pharmacologic treatment of premature labor.

The influence of psychic factors on uterine motility is poorly understood. There is some evidence that catecholamines are elevated during stressful situations.[31,68] It is established that intravenous infusion of epinephrine in low dosages will inhibit contractions, whereas norepinephrine promotes an increase of uterine activity.[7,75] It is not clear if sedatives, so widely accepted as an integral part of the therapy of threatened premature labor, are beneficial by influencing levels of catecholamines or only by helping enforce bed rest.

At the present, in the United States, there is no consensus on treatment of premature labor. The two most widely employed agents for inhibiting uterine motility are ethanol and isoxsuprine hydrochloride. It is clear that neither of these agents is ideal, for both produce undesirable side effects, are not uniformly effective, and involve complicated dosage schedules for optimal results. The results of quantitative studies of these, plus other available agents for the treatment of premature labor, follow.

ETHANOL.   Ethanol is thought to inhibit labor by blocking the release of fetal or maternal oxytocin, and possibly by improving uterine blood flow.[33,34,58] The treatment regimen most often utilized consists of 7.5 to 15 ml. of a 9.5 per cent ethanol solution per kilogram of body weight per hour for two hours as a loading dose, and then 1.5 ml. per kg. body weight per hour as a maintenance dose for an additional 6 to 10 hours.[76] The infusion is stopped if labor continues despite the loading dose. At least one group has recommended continuing maintenance with oral whiskey containing 45 per cent ethanol per volume in doses of 60 ml. every eight hours.[54] Most simply stop ethanol therapy after the conclusion of the intravenous maintenance dose, continuing the bed rest for an additional 24 to 48 hours. As previously described, the most thorough study of the success of ethanol in threatened premature labor was reported by Zlatnik and Fuchs,[73] who found that delivery was delayed for at least three days in 81 per cent of the ethanol-treated group and 38 per cent of the glucose-in-water group. In another study of ethanol treatment of 20 threatened cases of premature labors, Graff[38] was unable to delay delivery significantly; however, he continued the maintenance dose for only one hour after cessation of contractions. During the intravenous infusion of ethanol, patients often experience nausea, vomiting, restlessness, depression, and attacks of crying. Although no evidence of fetal distress is apparent from fetal heart rate monitoring performed in most of the human studies, it is of interest that studies of ethanol effects in the rhesus monkey[66] indicate that the fetuses become progressively asphyxiated. In contrast, the studies of Dilts[30] on pregnant ewes indicated that the infusion of ethanol did not alter the fetal acid-base state, although there was a decrease in uterine blood flow. Wagner and associates[69] reported that intravenous infusion of ethanol to six low birth weight infants produced no significant changes of alertness, motor activity, circulation, respiration, or acid-base status.

ISOXSUPRINE.   In 1956, Brucke and his co-workers[21] introduced isoxsuprine, a synthetic phenethanolamine. Later Lish and his associates[53] reported on the myometrial inhibitory effects of isoxsuprine hydrochloride in experimental ani-

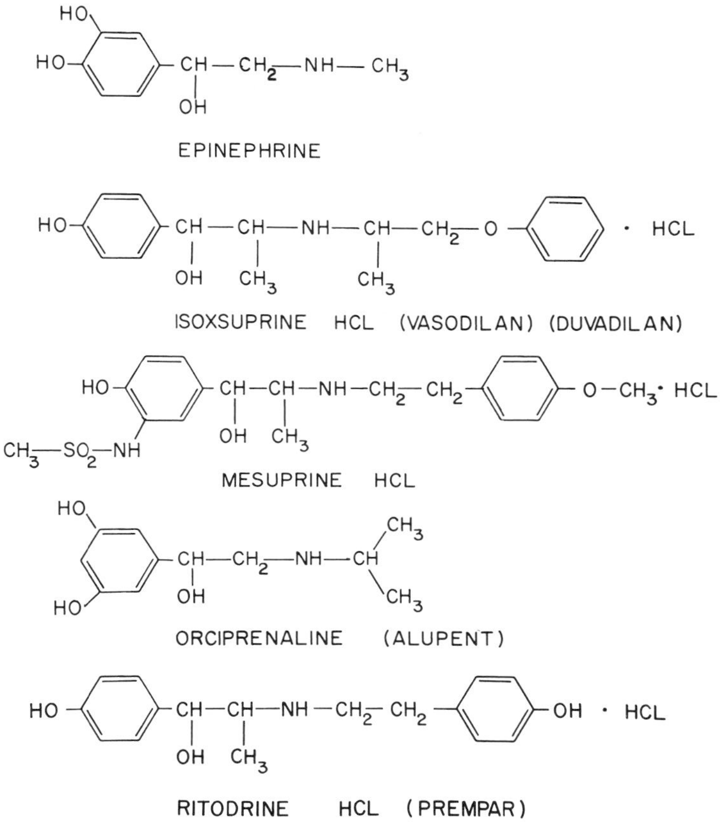

Figure 3-1.   Epinephrine and related compounds.

mals. They suggested that the mechanism of action of this compound was predominantly sympathomimetic and mediated through the uterine beta adrenergic receptors. This contention was supported by studies of Barden and Stander[8] reporting complete blocking of uterine inhibitory and cardiovascular effects of isoxsuprine by pretreatment of patients with propranolol, a beta adrenergic blocking agent. The studies of Bishop and Woutersz[12] and of Hendricks and associates[39] established the ability of isoxsuprine to decrease motility of the intact human gravid uterus. The similarity in structural formulas of epinephrine, isoxsuprine, and other compounds to be discussed is illustrated in Figure 3-1.

In treatment of premature labor, the efficacy of isoxsuprine hydrochloride (Vasodilan) has been in part established by the report of Bishop and Woutersz,[12] who treated 156 patients in premature labor, finding brief or no response in 36 per cent of cases, but significant delay in 64 per cent, with 42 per cent of cases having been delayed long enough to produce infants weighing 2500 g. or more. Hendricks and associates[39] reported that in 6 of 9 patients in premature labor with intact membranes, there was significant delay of labor following treatment with isoxsuprine. They observed that labor was not significantly delayed when membranes were ruptured or labor advanced. Zobel[74] reported that in using isoxsuprine treatment of premature labor, only 52 per cent of patients had significant delay and 37 per cent reached fetal weight of 2500 g. prior to delivery. Das[29] reported on treatment of 25 cases of premature labor with isoxsuprine and compared them to a control group of 25 cases treated with rest, sedatives, and antispasmolytics. Labor in 72 per cent of the isoxsuprine group was postponed by 1 to 12 weeks, in contrast to the situation in the control group, in which 75 per cent were delivered of their babies within 24 hours.

Other reports are concerned with the prophylactic use of isoxsuprine for delaying premature labor in patients at risk. Mathews and associates[57] treated 103 patients who had a history of premature delivery or were carrying twins in the current pregnancy with 120 mg. of oral isoxsuprine daily. Eight of 12 deliveries occurring before 36 weeks were in the isoxsuprine group. Briscoe[15] tested oral isoxsuprine, 40 mg. daily, against a placebo as prophylaxis of premature labor in 1165 patients, and found no significant difference in the incidence of prematurity.

Although isoxsuprine hydrochloride is not yet officially approved for treatment of premature labor, it is quite apparent that it is being used by a significant number of obstetricians for the treatment of this pregnancy complication. At the present time, the "routine" management of unwanted clinical premature labor in many hospitals consists of bed rest, avoidance of pelvic examinations, sedation with barbiturates or phenothiazines, and the administration of isoxsuprine hydrochloride. The usual dosage is 0.5 mg. per minute intravenously for 40 to 60 minutes. In most patients, uterine contractions gradually subside and cease during the isoxsuprine infusion. All patients develop a maternal tachycardia of 30 to 50 beats per minute over preinfusion heart rate, fetal heart rate occasionally increases slightly, and approximately 10 per cent of the patients develop significant hypotension, at times associated with fetal distress, as manifested by the development of late decelerations, tachycardia, and loss of baseline irregularity. During the infusion of isoxsuprine, patients occasionally complain of palpitations or nervousness, which may require decreasing the dosage. Depending on the degree of tolerance to the intravenous infusion of isoxsuprine, an intramuscular dosage of from 5 to 20 mg. every 3 to 6 hours is started at the conclusion of the intravenous infusion. If evidence of labor recurs, the intravenous infusion may be repeated. Generally, the intramuscular dosage is most effective if it is adjusted to maintain a moderate maternal tachycardia. After 24 hours, oral isoxsuprine may be started at the same dosage as for the intramuscular route, and this is continued for 3 to 10 days, while the patient gradually resumes ambulation.

The side-effects of isoxsuprine therapy are generally tolerable; however, it is imperative for fetal safety that in the event of maternal hypotension or fetal distress, the isoxsuprine infusion be stopped immediately. The effects of the drug subside rapidly, and there is usually no need for further specific therapy to counter the maternal hypotension.[12, 44, 64] It is strongly advised that patients receiving isoxsuprine, or any of the related compounds to be discussed, remain in the lateral decubitus position during the therapy in order to avoid supine hypotension as the uterus relaxes. There have been no reports of neonatal complications that might be attributable to this drug in pregnancy, but there have been no properly designed studies to adequately gather such data.

OTHER DRUGS.   There are numerous other compounds which enjoy a reputation as uterine relaxants, but generally they are ineffective or produce undesirable side-effects. Succinylcholine was found to have no significant inhibitory effect on uterine activity in term labor.[40] Intravenous magnesium sulfate will only partially inhibit labor.[46] Amyl nitrite inhalation will produce brief uterine relaxation in about 50 per cent of cases of term labor.[47] Intravenous epinephrine will inhibit uterine activity but also produces significant cardiovascular effects and is associated with a post-infusion "rebound" of uterine activity.[36,41] Lutrexan, an aqueous extract of sow corpus luteum, is widely used in treatment of threatened premature labor. Majewski and Jennings[55,56] reported a 68.4 per cent success rate in treating 79 patients in presumed premature labor. However, their study failed to utilize controls, and there have been no additional reports of studies of Lutrexan to establish its efficacy or safety in treating premature labor.

DRUGS UNDER INVESTIGATION.   Orciprenaline (Alupent), or metaproterenol (Figure 3-1), is a derivative of isoproterenol that is available in Europe and South America, but has not been made available for clinical investigation in the United States. It presumably acts via sympathomimetic beta adrenergic stimulation. Baillie and associates[3] recently reported on a series of 30 patients in premature labor treated with diazepam plus orciprenaline in doses of 12 to 80 μg. per minute, intravenously, for 20 minutes. The treatment was repeated as needed to maintain uterine inhibition. Labor in approximately two-thirds of the patients was delayed to beyond 36 weeks' gestation. The treatment was associated with moderate maternal tachycardia and moderate diastolic hypotension. Fetal tachycardia occurred with higher infusion rates. Caldeyro-Barcia and co-workers[22] reported on the successful use of orciprenaline to inhibit uterine contractions associated with fetal distress, followed by resolution of fetal acidosis prior to delivery by cesarean section. Favier and Helfferich[32] treated 77 patients in premature labor with orciprenaline and found little success when membranes were ruptured, but in 43 cases with intact membranes, labor was delayed for more than 24 hours in 35 patients and for more than 7 days in 25 women.

Mesuprine hydrochloride (Figure 3-1) is a methanesulfonamide derivative of isoxsuprine that was introduced by Larsen and Lish[52] in 1964. Subsequently a series of studies[6,11,48] revealed that this compound, compared to isoxsuprine, was a more potent uterine relaxant with fewer cardiovascular effects. Initial studies of mesuprine in human premature labor[5,48] revealed moderate effectiveness. Before further trials using adequate controls could be initiated, all studies of mesuprine were stopped in late 1970 because of the finding of leiomyomas in the ovaries of some rats fed large doses for a year or more. The drug remains unavailable for clinical investigation.

Ritodrine hydrochloride (Prempar) (Figure 3-1) is another sympathomimetic amine which was synthesized in the continuing search for new compounds with potent inhibitory effects upon the uterus. Initial studies[9,35,49] revealed that ritodrine was capable of producing uterine relaxation with minimal beta mimetic cardiovascular responses. Subsequently, in the United States, Barden[4] studied the effects of ritodrine on uterine and cardiovascular responses in term pregnancy and in the early postpartum period, to find effective uterine relaxation with maternal tachycardia, but very minimal alterations of maternal blood pressure. Thus, ritodrine appeared to have a distinct advantage over the other sympathomimetic amines. Wesselius-de Casparis and associates[70] have recently reported on a double-blind placebo-controlled collaborative study of 91 patients in premature labor. Premature labor was arrested and delivery significantly postponed in 80 per cent of the patients receiving ritodrine and in 48 per cent of the placebo group. In these studies, the treatment consisted of 200 μg. per minute of

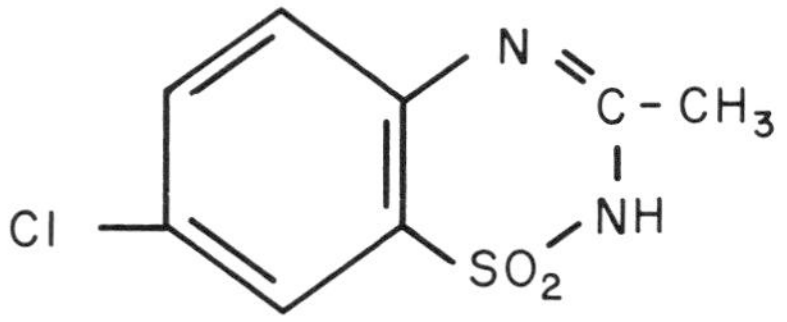

Figure 3-2.   Diazoxide.

ritodrine intravenously for 24 to 48 hours, followed by a course of 10 mg. of oral ritodrine four times daily for 5 to 7 days. Patients continued bed rest for 4 days and then gradually resumed ambulation. Similar trials of ritodrine for premature labor are now in progress in the United States.

Diazoxide (Hyperstat) (Figure 3-2), is an antidiuretic benzothiadiazine introduced as an antihypertensive compound, but found to possess smooth muscle relaxing properties.[13] Landesman and co-workers have reported on the efficacy of diazoxide in relaxing isolated human myometrium,[50] as well as in relaxing uterine activity in human term labor.[51] In the latter study, administration of diazoxide consistently reduced the spontaneous uterine activity of patients in labor, while concomitantly producing a moderate decrease in maternal blood pressure and an increase in maternal, but not fetal, heart rate. Its similarity in action to the previously discussed phenylethylamines is possibly due to a depression of the degradation of intracellular cyclic adenosine monophosphate.[61] Diazoxide has been shown to suppress insulin secretion and elevate blood sugar.[13] These actions prompted studies exploring its usefulness in the hypoglycemia associated with islet cell carcinoma[37] and idiopathic infantile and leucine-sensitive hypoglycemia.[59] In an unreported series of 15 term and 10 premature human labors we studied the effects of administration of diazoxide in doses of 60 mg. intravenously, repeated four times at 15 minute intervals. In term labors there was minimal uterine inhibition, moderate increase in maternal heart rate, and no significant change in maternal blood pressure or fetal heart rate. In the premature labor series, there was more apparent inhibition of uterine activity, but labor was delayed in only 5 of the 10 patients. Dosage studies of diazoxide are needed, for an effective dosage regimen utilizing a brief series of intravenous injections over a brief period would certainly be more convenient than the long intravenous infusions that are necessary with some of the other investigational drugs. Diazoxide may well be useful also in treating hypertensive toxemia associated with threatened premature labor, or in treating precipitate labor.

Summary

Premature birth is the principal cause of neonatal mortality and morbidity. To date, an ideal management of premature labor has not been identified, and most of the management schemes have been based on rather tentative grounds. At present, efforts are being made to identify and correct prenatal factors responsible for prematurity; however, there is little evidence that dramatic breakthroughs in this area of research are likely. Therefore, a search is in progress for an agent that will safely inhibit unwanted uterine activity without endangering the health of mother or fetus/neonate. Bed rest and sedation, plus intravenous infusion of either ethanol or isoxsuprine hydrochloride, are the most widely used treatment schemes for premature labor that are utilized in the United States at present. Other compounds, which may prove to be more efficacious than existing treatments, are still under investigation. In conjunction with the effort to develop a treatment for premature labor, it is imperative that simultaneous progress be made in developing methods for more accurately assessing the status of the fetal environment prior to stopping the process of labor.

REFERENCES

1. Abramowicz, M., and Kass, E. H.: Pathogenesis and prognosis of prematurity. New Eng. J. Med. 275:878, 1966.
2. Ahlquist, R. P.: A study of the adrenotropic receptors. Amer. J. Physiol. 153:586, 1948.
3. Baillie, P., Meehan, F. P., and Tyack, A. J.: Treatment of premature labour with orciprenaline. Brit. Med. J. 4:154, 1970.
4. Barden, T. P.: Effect of ritodrine on human uterine motility and cardiovascular responses in term labor and the early postpartum state. Amer. J. Obstet. Gynec. 112:645, 1972.
5. Barden, T. P.: Inhibition of human premature labor by mesuprine hydrochloride. Obstet. Gynec. 37:98, 1971.
6. Barden, T. P., and Stander, R. W.: Myometrial and cardiovascular effects of two methane-sulfonamido-phenethanolamines. Amer. J. Obstet. Gynec. 96:1069, 1966.
7. Barden, T. P., and Stander, R. W.: Effects of adrenergic blocking agents and catecholamines in human pregnancy. Amer. J. Obstet. Gynec. 102:226, 1968.
8. Barden, T. P., and Stander, R. W.: Myometrial and cardiovascular effects of an adrenergic blocking drug in human pregnancy. Amer. J. Obstet. Gynec. 101:91, 1968.
9. Baumgarten, K., Frohlich, I., Seidl, A., Lim-Rachmat, F., and Sokol, K.: Uber einen neuen intravenös anwendbaren Wehenhemmer ohne Kreislaufwirkung. Wien. Klin. Wchnschr. 81:102, 1969.
10. Bengtsson, L. P.: Experiments on the suppressive effect of a synthetic gestogen on the activity of the pregnant human uterus. Acta Obstet. Gynec. Scand. 41:124, 1962.
11. Bishop, E. H., Bolognese, R. J., and Piver, U. S.: Effect of methanesulfonamide on uterine contractions. Obstet. Gynec. 28:784, 1966.
12. Bishop, E. H., and Woutersz, T. B.: Arrest of premature labor. J.A.M.A. 178:812, 1961.
13. Blackard, W. G., and Aprill, C. N.: Mechanism of action of diazoxide J. Lab. Clin. Med. 69:960, 1967.
14. Brenner, W. E., and Hendricks, C. H.: Effect of medroxyprogesterone acetate upon the duration and characteristics of human gestation and labor. Amer. J. Obstet. Gynec. 83:1094, 1962.
15. Briscoe, C. C.: Failure of oral isoxsuprine to prevent prematurity. Amer. J. Obstet. Gynec. 95:885, 1966.
16. Brotánek, V., Hendricks, C. H., and Yoshida, T.: Importance of changes in uterine blood flow in initiation of labor. Amer. J. Obstet. Gynec. 105:535, 1969.
17. Brotánek, V., Kazda, S., and Roth, L.: A method for studying uterine blood flow in pregnant women. Physiol. Bohemoslov. 11:358, 1962.
18. Brotánek, V., and Hodr, J.: Dangers to the foetus during induction of labour by oxytocin. In Horský, J., and Štembera, Z. K., eds.: Intrauterine Dangers to the Fetus. New York, Excerpta Medica Foundation, 1967.
19. Brotánek, V., and Hodr, J.: The effect of isoxsuprine on uteroplacental circulation. In Horský, J., and Štembera, Z. K., eds: Intrauterine Dangers to the Fetus. New York, Excerpta Medica Foundation, 1967.
20. Brotánek, V., Hendricks, C. H., and Yoshida, T.: Changes in uterine blood flow during uterine contractions. Amer. J. Obstet. Gynec. 103:1108, 1969.
21. Brucke, F., Hertting, G., Lindner, A., and Loudon, M.: Zur Pharmakologie einer neuen gefässerweiternden Substanz aus der p-Oxy-Ephedrin-Reihe. Wien. Klin. Wchnschr. 68:183, 1956.
22. Caldeyro-Barcia, R., Magaña, J. M., Castillo, J. B., Poseiro, J. J., Méndez-Bauer, C., Pose, S. V., Escarcena, L., Casacuberta, C., Bustos, J. R., and Giussi, G.: A new approach to the treatment of acute intrapartum fetal distress. In Perinatal Factors Affecting Human Development, Washington, Pan American Health Organization, 1969, p. 248.

23. Caldeyro-Barcia, R., and Sereno, J. A.: The response of the human uterus to oxytocin throughout pregnancy. *In* Caldeyro-Barcia, R., and Heller, H., eds.: Oxytocin. New York, Pergamon Press, 1961, p. 177.

24. Chard, T., Hudson, C. N., Edwards, C. R. W., and Boyd, N. R. H.: Release of oxytocin and vasopressin by the human foetus during labor. Nature 234:352, 1971.

25. Coutinho, E. M., and Vieira Lopes, A. C.: Inhibition of uterine motility by aminophylline. Amer. J. Obstet. Gynec. 110:726, 1971.

26. Csapo, A.: Progesterone "block." Amer. J. Anat. 98:273, 1956.

27. Csapo, A.: Defence mechanism of pregnancy. *In* Ciba Foundation Study Groups: Progesterone and the Defense Mechanism of Pregnancy. Boston, Little, Brown and Co., 1961.

28. Csapo, A. I., Kuobil, E., Pulkkinen, M., Van der Molen, H. J., Sommerville, I. F., and Wiest, W. G.: Progesterone withdrawal during hypertonic saline-induced abortions, Amer. J. Obstet. Gynec. 105:1132, 1969.

29. Das, R. K.: Isoxsuprine in premature labor. J. Obstet. Gynaec. India 19:566, 1969.

30. Dilts, P. V., Jr.: Effect of ethanol on uterine and umbilical hemodynamics and oxygen transfer. Amer. J. Obstet. Gynec. 108:221, 1970.

31. Elmadjian, F., Hope, J. M., and Lamson, E. T.: Excretion of epinephrine and norepinephrine under stress. J. Clin. Endocr. 17:608, 1957.

32. Favier, J., and Helfferich, M.: Experiences with the use of orciprenaline (Alupent) in cases of threatened premature delivery. Ned. T. Geneesk. 114:2120, 1970.

33. Fuchs, A. R.: The inhibitory effect of ethanol on the release of oxytocin during parturition in the rabbit. J. Endocr. 35:125, 1966.

34. Fuchs, A., Coutinho, E. M., Xavier, R., Bates, P. E., and Fuchs, F.: Effect of ethanol on the activity of the nonpregnant human uterus and its reactivity to neurohypophyseal hormones. Amer. J. Obstet. Gynec. 101:997, 1968.

35. Gamissaus, O., Esteban-Altirriba, J., and Maiques, V.: Inhibition of human myometrial activity by a new B-adrenergic drug (DU-21220). J. Obstet, Gynaec. Brit. Comm. 76:656, 1969.

36. Garrett, W. J.: The effects of adrenaline and noradrenaline on the intact human uterus in late pregnancy and labour. Obstet. Gynaec. Brit. Comm. 61:586, 1954.

37. Graber, A. L., Porte, D., and Williams, R. H.: Clinical use of diazoxide and mechanism for its hyperglycemic effects. Diabetes 15:143, 1966.

38. Graff, G.: Failure to prevent premature labor with ethanol. Amer. J. Obstet. Gynec. 110:878, 1971.

39. Hendricks, C. H., Cibils, L. A., Pose, S. V., and Eskes, T. K. A. B.: The pharmacologic control of excessive uterine activity with isoxsuprine. Amer. J. Obstet. Gynec. 82:1064, 1961.

40. Iuppa, J. B., Smith, G. A., Colella, J. J., and Gibson, J. L.: Succinylcholine effect on human myometrial activity. Obstet. Gynec. 37:591, 1971.

41. Kaiser, I. H.: The effect of epinephrine and norepinephrine on the contractions of the human uterus in labor. Surg. Gynec. Obstet. 90:649, 1950.

42. Karim, S. M. M., and Sharma, S. D.: The effect of ethyl alcohol on prostaglandin E_2 and $E_{2\alpha}$ induced uterine activity in pregnant women. J. Obstet. Gynaec. Brit. Comm. 78:251, 1971.

43. Karim, S. M. M.: Appearance of prostaglandin $F_{2\alpha}$ in human blood during labor. Brit. Med. J. 4:618, 1968.

44. Karim, M.: Isoxsuprine and the human parturient uterus. J. Obstet. Gynaec. Brit. Comm. 70:992, 1963.

45. Kumar, D., Goodno, J. A., and Barnes, A. C.: Isolation of progesterone from human pregnant myometrium. Nature (Lond.) 195:1204, 1962.

46. Kumar, D., Zourlas, P. A., and Barnes, A. C.: In vitro and in vivo effects of magnesium sulfate on human uterine contractility. Amer. J. Obstet. Gynec. 86:1036, 1963.

47. Kumar, D., Zourlas, P. A., and Barnes, A. C.: In vivo effect of amyl nitrite on human pregnant uterine contractility. Amer. J. Obstet. Gynec. 91:1066, 1965.

48. Landesman, R., Wilson, K., and Zlatnik, F. J.: The myometrial relaxant properties of isoxsuprine and 2 methanesulfonamide derivatives. Obstet. Gynec. 28:775, 1966.

49. Landesman, R., Wilson, K. H., Coutinho, E. M., Klima, I. M., and Marcus, R. S.: The relaxant action of ritodrine, a sympathomimetic amine, on the uterus during term labor. Amer. J. Obstet. Gynec. 110:111, 1971.

50. Landesman, R., and Wilson, K. H.: The relaxant effect of diazoxide on isolated gravid and nongravid human myometrium. Amer. J. Obstet. Gynec. 101:120, 1968.

51. Laudesman, R., de Souza F., J. A., Coutinho, E. M., Wilson, K. H., and de Sousa F., M. B.: The inhibitory effect of diazoxide in normal term labor. Amer. J. Obstet. Gynec. 103:430, 1969.

52. Larsen, A. A., and Lish, P. M.: A new bio-isostere: Alkylsulphonamidophenethanolamines. Nature (Lond.) 203:1283, 1964.
53. Lish, P. M., Hillyard, I. W., and Dungan, K. W.: The uterine relaxant properties of isoxsuprine. J. Pharmacol. Exp. Ther. 129:438, 1960.
54. Luukkainen, T. Väistö, L., and Järvinen, P. A.: The effect of oral intake of ethyl alcohol on the activity of the pregnant human uterus. Acta Obstet. Gynec. Scand. 46:486, 1967.
55. Majewski, J. T., and Jennings, T.: A uterine relaxing factor for premature labor. Obstet. Gynec. 5:649, 1955.
56. Majewski, J. T., and Jennings, T.: Experiences with a uterine relaxing hormone in premature labor. Obstet. Gynec. 9:322, 1957.
57. Mathews, D. D., Friend, J. B., and Michael, C. A.: A double-blind trial of oral isoxsuprine in the prevention of premature labour. J. Obstet. Gynaec. Brit. Comm. 74:68, 1967.
58. McDonald, R. L., and Lanford, C. F.: Effects of smoking on selected clinical obstetric factors. Obstet. Gynec. 26:470, 1965.
59. Merev, T. R., Kassoff, A., and Goodman, A. D.: Diazoxide in the treatment of infantile hypoglycemia. New Eng. J. Med. 275:1455, 1966.
60. Scommegna, A., Burd, L., Goodman, C., and Bieniarz, J.: The effect of pregnenolone sulfate on uterine contractility. Amer. J. Obstet. Gynec. 108:1023, 1970.
61. Schultz, G., Senft, G., Losert, W., and Sitt, R.: Biochemische Grundlagen der Diazoxid-Hyperglykämie. Arch. Exper. Path. u. Pharmakol. 253:372, 1966.
62. Stander, R. W., and Barden, T. P.: Adrenergic receptor activity of catecholamines in human gestational myometrium. Obstet. Gynec. 28:768, 1966.
63. Stander, R. W., and Barden, T. P.: Adrenergic mechanisms in human myometrial control. In Mack, H. C., ed.: Prenatal Life. Detroit, Wayne State University Press, 1970.
64. Stander, R. W., Barden, T. P., Thompson, J. F., Pugh, W. R., and Werts, C. E.: Fetal cardiac effects of maternal isoxsuprine infusion. Amer. J. Obstet. Gynec. 89:792, 1964.
65. Sutherland, E. W., and Rall, T. W.: The relation of adenosine-3'5'-phosphate and phosphorylase to the actions of catecholamines and other hormones. Pharmacol. Rev. 12:265, 1960.
66. Terusada, H., Kotaro, S., Comas-Urrutia, A. C., Mueller-Henbach, E., Moyer-Milic, A. M., Baratz, R. A., Morishima, H. O., James, L. S., and Adamsons, K.: Effect of ethanol upon uterine activity and fetal acid-base state of the rhesus monkey. Amer. J. Obstet. Gynec. 109:910, 1971.
67. Triner, L., Overweg, N. I. A., and Nahas, G. G.: Cyclic 3,5'-AMP and uterine contractility. Nature (Lond.) 225:282, 1970.
68. Euler, U. S., and Lundberg, V.: Effect of flying on the epinephrine excretion in Air Force personnel. J. Appl. Physiol. 6:551, 1953.
69. Wagner, L., Wagner, G., and Guerrero, J.: Effect of alcohol on premature newborn infants. Amer. J. Obstet. Gynec. 108:308, 1970.
70. Wesselius-de Casparis, A., Thiery, M., Yo le Sian, A., Baumgarten, K., Bosens, I., Gamissans, O., Stolk, J. G., and Vivier, W.: Results of double-blind multicentre study with ritodrine in premature labor. Brit. Med. J. 3:144, 1971.
71. Wood, C., Elstein, M., and Pinkerton, J. H. M.: The effect of progestogens upon uterine activity. J. Obstet. Gynaec. Brit. Comm. 70:839, 1963.
72. Wood, C., and Pinkerton, J. H. M.: A comparison of the myometrial activity in the pregnant and non-pregnant side of a septate uterus. J. Obstet. Gynaec. Brit. Comm. 70:669, 1963.
73. Zlatnik, F. J., and Fuchs, F.: A Controlled study of ethanol in threatened premature labor. Amer. J. Obstet. Gynec. 112:610, 1972.
74. Zobel, G. J.: The use of isoxsuprine in premature labor. J. Amer. Osteopath. Ass. 66:1276, 1967.
75. Zuspan, F. P., Cibils, L. A., and Pose, S. V.: Myometrial and cardiovascular responses to alterations in plasma epinephrine and norepinephrine. Amer. J. Obstet. Gynec. 84:841, 1962.
76. Zuspan, F. P., Barden, T. P., Bieniarz, J., Cibils, L. A., Fuchs, F., Landesman, R., Mercer, J. P., Moawad, A. H., and Paverstein, C. J.: Premature labor: its management and therapy. J. Reprod. Med. 9:93, 1972.
77. Csapo, A. I.: On the mechanism of the abortifacient action of prostaglandin F$_{2\alpha}$. J. Reprod. Med. 9:400, 1972.
78. Csapo, A. I.: The prospects of PGs in postconceptional therapy. Prostaglandins 3:245, 1973.
79. Csapo, A. I., Csapo, E. F., Fay, E., Henzl, M. R. and Salau, G.: The delay of spontaneous labor by naproxen in the rat model. Prostaglandins 3:827, 1973.

The Management of
Impending Labor Prior to the Thirty-Fifth Week

Luis A. Cibils

The University of Chicago and The Chicago Lying-In Hospital

A rational management of undesirable preterm labor must be based on a clear understanding of the physiologic phenomena involved. The difficulties in applying this obvious principle reside in our incomplete knowledge of the physiology of normal labor and of the factors governing it. Some of the therapeutic approaches for arresting premature labor are based upon the acceptance of hypotheses explaining the initiation of normal labor, whereas others are based on observations of pharmacologic responses of the uterus to specific preparations.

THE PROGESTERONE HYPOTHESIS

From studies carried out in animals, mainly in rabbits, Csapo elaborated the hypothesis that progesterone is the hormone responsible for the maintenance of pregnancy. Its high circulating levels during pregnancy would keep the myometrium resting membrane potential very high and thereby incapable of a uniform, coordinated contraction.[30,52] To explain the observations in humans, Csapo postulated a refinement of that hypothesis, indicating that progesterone synthesis by the placenta creates an extremely high concentration of the hormone in the myometrium overlying it, while the rest of the uterus is exposed to significantly lesser concentrations and, therefore, the contractions of the uterus are asymmetric, meaning that they are irregular, incoordinated, and unable to affect the lower segment and cervix. As term approaches, according to this hypothesis, the steady increase in uterine volume and rapid decrement of progesterone synthesis by the placenta tend to facilitate a lower, and now uniform, resting membrane potential and thereby make possible a complete, "symmetric" uterine contraction.[10,26,28,29,76] Premature labor would be the consequence of diminished progesterone synthesis by the placenta, loss of asymmetry, and prematurely effective contractions to efface and dilate the cervix.

THE OXYTOCIN SENSITIVITY HYPOTHESIS

It is known that the nonpregnant human uterus has a very poor response to oxytocin stimulation, while the term uterus is extremely sensitive to it.[18,19,34,73,74] Caldeyro-Barcia postulated, based on his observations of human subjects, that the sensitivity of the uterus increased steadily throughout pregnancy, until the thirty-fourth week of gestation, when it plateaus.[18,19] According to Theobald, the sensitivity of the uterus to oxytocin reaches its maximum very suddenly in the hours preceding labor,[34,74] the normally circulating oxytocin being then sufficient to trigger labor. When the maximum sensitivity to oxytocin is reached prematurely, labor would start likewise.

PHARMACOLOGIC OBSERVATIONS

Although there is no formally structured hypothesis to this effect, suggestions have been made that catecholamines play a major role in the labor triggering process.[2,7,65,66,67] Observations that epinephrine and norepinephrine have a very marked effect upon the myometrium at minimal circulating concentrations have been made over the past 25 years,[23,49,50,59,63,77] indicating the possibility that adrenergic receptors may, indeed, play part in the normal mechanism of labor. It has been shown that estrogens and progesterone alter the norepinephrine content of uterine and paracervical adrenergic neurons.[33,57,58,70] Likewise, the catecholamine content of the pregnant uterus seems to be significantly less than that of the nonpregnant uterus.[40,64,70]

The above-mentioned empirical clinical observations, tied to the biological findings later described, constituted the rationale for a number of studies aimed at finding a sympathomimetic drug which would selectively inhibit uterine contractions without significantly affecting other sympathetically innervated organs or systems.

Lately, some workers have attempted a "multitarget" approach,[12,14] attacking through more than one of the described mechanisms.

Progesterone

This so-called "hormone of pregnancy" is secreted at a high rate by the corpus luteum and later by the placenta. In some animal species, it has a clearly quiescing effect upon the myometrium. In humans, in an attempt to reach the uterus with the highest possible concentrations or for the most prolonged action, progesterone has been given orally, injected directly into the myometrium or the amniotic cavity, or administered intravenously or intramuscularly.

ORAL. Brenner and Hendricks[16] conducted a double-blind study in a group of normal patients in the last four weeks of pregnancy, one half of the group receiving 20 mg. of medroxyprogesterone per day. The course of pregnancy and all parameters of labor and delivery were indistinguishable in both groups of patients, suggesting that prolonged ingestion of a potent progestogen neither delayed the expected onset of labor nor influenced the normal duration of labor or its contraction pattern.

INTRAMUSCULAR. Progesterone was administered in what are considered large doses (400 mg. every 6 hours) to near-term patients or to patients in labor, who were then observed for the onset of spontaneous uterine activity, the extent of cervical dilation, the duration of labor, and the response of the uterus to the administration of oxytocin.[60,61] These patients reacted no differently than did the untreated or control group studied under the same experimental conditions. The possibility that the amount of progesterone administered may have been insufficient, even despite the large doses, remained as a plausible explanation for the lack of effect.

Another series of observations carried out by Csapo and his associates,[27] using very high doses of intramuscular medroxyprogesterone during early labor, did not reveal a significantly depressing effect upon uterine activity. Labors progressed undisturbed to normal deliveries. Moller and Fuchs were unable to demonstrate, in a double-blind study, the effect of acetoxyprogesterone given in threatened abortions in early or midpregnancy.[56]

INTRA-AMNIOTIC.   Hendricks and his colleagues[47] injected large quantities of progesterone in the amniotic cavity of a series of patients in early or late prelabor. From those observations it could only be concluded that there was no clear quiescent effect, the results being equivocal, at best. The response to infusion of physiologic doses of oxytocin was unchanged.

INTRAVENOUS.   Since it is a liposoluble hormone, progesterone presumably would not reach the myometrium at a concentration comparable to those being secreted by a normally functioning placenta. Kumar and his associates[51] decided to dissolve the hormone in 50 per cent ethyl alcohol, thereby facilitating the intravenous administration. In a small series of cases, the infusion of large amounts of progesterone in a relatively short period of time produced only a transient diminution in uterine activity, and the labors progressed to completion without incident. These effects occurred even though the progesterone blood levels were "15 to 20 times higher than those found normally at this stage of gestation," and twice as high as values for the intervillous space.[68] Very high concentrations of circulating progesterone were measured in peripheral blood over one hour after the infusions had been discontinued, when the uterine activity had fully recovered and the labors were progressing rapidly. Scommegna and colleagues[69] administered large doses of pregnenolone, a progesterone precursor, intravenously, and produced only transient diminution of the uterine contractions of spontaneous labor.

INTRAMYOMETRIAL.   Bengtsson[9] used the direct injection of medroxyprogesterone into several spots of the myometrial wall to arrest premature labor in a selected number of patients. This progestogen preparation is claimed to be 10 to 20 times more potent than progesterone, on a weight-for-weight basis. In a number of cases in early phase of premature labor, uterine activity was suppressed, whereas in more advanced stages of labor, progress was not arrested with a dosage of 250 to 400 mg. Theoretically, this treatment should create a classical "asymmetric" condition of the uterus.

The experience would indicate the progesterone, or more potent progestogens, administered either on a long-term basis or for acute situations, is unable to suppress, significantly or at all, uterine contractions of the pregnant human uterus in either early or late pregnancy. This assessment seems valid for normal as well as abnormal uterine activity, regardless of the route of administration and would strongly suggest that progesterone is not the ideal preparation to arrest premature labor.

Oxytocin Suppressants

The reports that an aminopeptidase ("oxytocinase") was present in the plasma of pregnant patients and that its concentration increased with the progress of pregnancy created hopes that it could be used to control undesired uterine contractions. Attention was turned toward methods of suppressing the release of oxytocin, assuming that it plays a paramount role in premature and normal spontaneous labor.

The rapid intravenous infusion of isotonic electrolyte-free solutions creates a "volume expansion" in the intravascular space and, hopefully, slows down the release of ADH and oxytocin by the hypothalamus-pituitary. This effect has been shown to be present, but very transiently, in studies carried out in early spontaneous labors,[12,14] and seems to be of no practical value when attempting to arrest premature labor.

Ethanol

In a very elegant series of experiments in rabbits, A. R. Fuchs and G. Wagner demonstrated the primary role of oxytocin in the process of labor, and the possibility of blocking its release by administration of ethyl alcohol.[35,36,39] Use of ethanol infusion as an analgesic in labor had resulted in a decrease in uterine activity[8,31] but the mode of action remained obscure. It was F. Fuchs who postulated that administration of ethanol in premature labor should decrease uterine contractions by interfering with oxytocin release by the hypothalamus. His first series of experiments[37,38] clearly demonstrated that, indeed, infusion of ethanol at the proper doses, maintained for a sufficient period of time, could arrest premature labors in a significant number of treated patients. The fact that maintenance of the infusion is necessary to obtain significant prolongation of pregnancy was demonstrated by the consistent failures reported by Graff,[42] who discontinued ethanol infusion only one hour after contractions were controlled. A subsequent randomized series by Zlatnik and Fuchs[78] demonstrated by sequential statistical analysis that ethanol infusion given in clinical premature labor will prolong the pregnancy significantly more often than infusion of glucose in water. Following Fuchs' first reports,[37,38] several individuals have used the same method in clinically diagnosed premature labor with acceptable success. Our own experience has been very satisfactory, a case in point being shown in Figures 3-3 and 3-4. This somewhat unorthodox case illustrates the dilemmas the clinician must face when treating the individual patient:

S.M. was a G-4, P-3, 26 year old class C diabetic patient who had her three children born by cesarean section at 37 weeks. Only the first one lives, the other two dying neonatally. When she approached 35 weeks of her fourth gestation her insulin requirements dropped (from 70 units neutral protamine Hagedorn and 30 units of regular insulin per day), while the 24 hour urinary estriol excretion was 22 mg. and an oxytocin challenge test was negative. The lecithin/sphingomyelin ratio was 1.2. She went into premature labor (Figure 3-3), and it was decided to attempt to prolong her pregnancy until a more satisfactory test of pulmonary maturity could be obtained. Uterine contractions ceased and ethanol was discontinued after 10 hours, but activity resumed 22 hours later and another ethanol course was started (Figure 3-4). The infusion was maintained

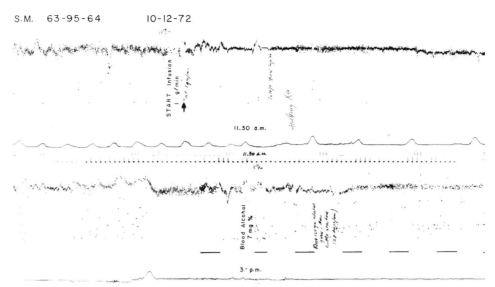

Figure 3-3. Continuous uterine contractility and fetal heart rate monitoring. Tracing at top left represents premature labor contractility. Ethanol infusion (1 g./min.) was begun at the arrow. The bottom tracing reproduces the pattern recorded 3 hours later, with blood level of 7 mg./100 ml. The infusion rate was then 0.1 g./min. The uterus is almost quiescent, while the fetal heart rate remains unchanged, with good rapid baseline fluctuations. There was good estriol excretion, but very low lecithin/sphingomyelin (L/S) ratio. Alcohol infusion was discontinued 6 hours after last part of record shown.

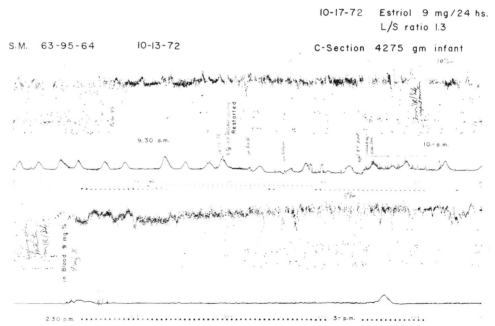

Figure 3-4. Same case, one day later, when uterine activity had resumed (top left). Ethanol was restarted on the same schedule (middle of upper record) and produced rapidly satisfactory effects. Four hours later, lower tracing, the contractility was very low, with a blood level of 9 mg./100 ml. of alcohol. The fetal heart rate continued to indicate good fetal condition. The maintenance dose was continued for 4½ days, with urinary estriol level falling steadily. Cesarean section produced a typically diabetic infant in heart failure, who recovered well in spite of a very low L/S ratio.

for 4½ days, during which time daily estriol determinations were performed. When these fell, and despite a low L/S ratio of 1.3, the cesarean section was performed and a large infant delivered. Although revealing findings consistent with heart failure, the infant was in good condition at 24 hours. Both infant and mother were discharged in good condition on the seventh postoperative day. The mother's insulin requirements returned to prepregnancy values (40 units of N.P.H. insulin daily).

In our experience, there are few maternal side-effects, mainly nausea, vomiting, and restlessness. There seems to be no appreciable effect upon the fetus, even when the maternal blood levels reach 15 mg. The fetal heart rate maintains its baseline values as well as the physiologic fluctuations. Those infants who were born shortly after an alcohol infusion was discontinued were in good condition, with a blood ethanol concentration equivalent to the mother's.[38] The oral administration of ethanol has been suggested by some investigators,[55] but, although it may be more pleasant for some patients, it has the inconveniences of unpredictable absorption rate and the need to drink very large quantities in a short time.

Adrenergic Preparations

Studies of the effects of epinephrine and norepinephrine upon the human uterus in advanced pregnancy were published by Kaiser and Harris in 1950,[49,50] following earlier studies by Woodbury and Abreu.[77]

What at first seemed confusing results were later better understood with the acceptance of Ahlquist's concept of the existence of alpha and beta adrenergic receptors,[1] as well as the recognition that some organs or systems have varying numbers of these receptors, and, probably, changing degrees of receptivity.[21]

Further studies confirmed these observations and clearly established that epinephrine works predominantly as a beta receptor agent upon the human uterus in late pregnancy,[6,59] whereas norepinephrine seems to be exclusively an alpha receptor substance.[2,6,23] The fact that epinephrine is only "predominantly" a beta receptor agent was shown by recovery of uterine activity under continuous infusion and a marked "rebound" when it was discontinued.[23,49,50] In addition to this, the marked cardiovascular effects made an epinephrine a very impractical drug to be used as an uterine relaxant. More specific beta receptor substances were subsequently synthesized.

IsoxSUPRINE. This synthetic "epinephrine-like" or beta mimetic preparation was predicted to produce less tachycardia than epinephrine and to be effective when administered orally. When assayed in animals, it was found to have excellent uterine relaxant properties. The first observations on humans confirmed that this drug is an excellent uterine relaxant.[22,48] Unfortunately, the cardiovascular effects are still very significant, producing tachycardia and hypotension in a large proportion of cases.[6,20,22,48] In Figure 3-5 is illustrated a case of a patient with premature labor who was given large doses of isoxsuprine to control the excessive uterine activity. This was brought under control only after infusing the drug at a rather high rate and dosage. The effects upon blood pressure and pulse rate, showing moderate hypotension and tachycardia, are also illustrated. Some recovery was documented in the recording obtained the next day, these side-effects did not recur with oral administration of the drug (Figure 3-6), and labor

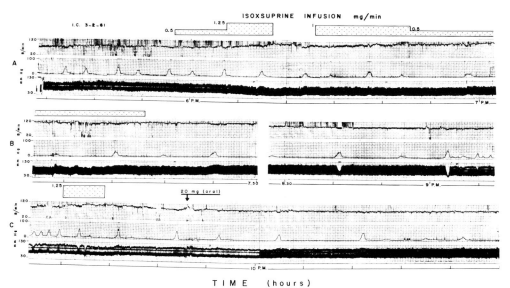

TIME   (hours)

Figure 3-5. Premature labor at 29 weeks gestation in a G-4, P-3 patient. The top part of each tracing records the maternal pulse rate, the middle the intrauterine pressure by trans-abdominal catheter, and the lower part the arterial pressure recorded by intrafemoral catheter. The scales are shown on the left. Tracing A and the left half of B represent 2 hours 20 minutes of continuous recording; the right half of B and C represent another period of continuous recording, but an intervening 40 minutes is not shown on this record. The isoxsuprine infusion and dose is indicated by the dotted area over the respective tracings. The labor-like uterine activity was only modestly diminished by 500 μg./min. infusion; this was increased to 1250 μg./min., then 1000 μg./min., after which the excessive activity was controlled. Subsequently, the infusion was lowered to 500 μg./min. and finally discontinued. It had to be restarted (bottom left) when a burst of contractions indicated renewed activity; this and 20 mg. given by mouth controlled the contractions. It is very important to note that the pulse rate rises as the drug is given, while there is only a moderate hypotension, reaching lowest values, at the time of highest infusion rate. (From Hendricks, C. H., *et al.*: The pharmacologic control of excessive uterine activity with isoxsuprine. Amer. J. Obstet. Gynec. 82:1064–1075, 1961.)

was successfully postponed. Another patient, in more advanced pregnancy, who required a lower infusion rate to arrest uterine contractions, is described in Figure 3-7. She also had moderate hypotension and tachycardia. These two cases demonstrate some of the difficulties in predicting the degree of response to a given dose. Each uterus seems to have different threshold of sensitivity to the drug, and this is not necessarily dependent on the state of pregnancy.

The dose most frequently found to be effective has been 500 micrograms (μg.) per minute. With this infusion rate, one generally obtains a good uterine response (Figures 3-7 and 3-8) within 10 minutes, but if the effect is not satisfactory, one should not hesitate to increase the infusion rate up to 1000 or 1250 μg. per minute, provided that the cardiovascular system tolerates that dose (Figure 3-5). Once the desired level of uterine activity has been reached, the drug infusion must be maintained for at least 90 minutes before being discontinued. In most cases, 10 mg. of isoxsuprine was given intramuscularly every 4 to 6 hours for 2 days before switching to the oral form of the preparation, prescribed at 80 mg. per day in divided doses. This maintenance dose will produce only a moderate degree of tachycardia.

The cardiovascular effects of the drug also differ markedly from patient to patient, the most extreme example of low tolerance being illustrated in Figure

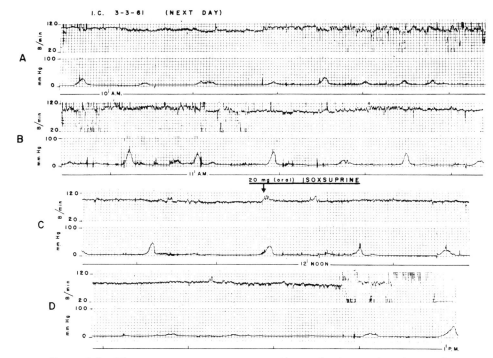

Figure 3-6. The same patient as in Figure 3-5, one day later. Three hours of continuous recording of intrauterine pressure and maternal pulse rate are shown. The very low activity (*A*) started to increase (*B*), and an oral dose of 20 mg. isoxsuprine (*C*) seemed to have succeeded in reducing the activity. Note the moderate tachycardia present throughout. This patient was discharged on oral medication and readmitted 11 days later with premature rupture of membranes. Allowed to go into labor without interference, she delivered a 1950 gm. infant (the largest of her four), who did well. (From Hendricks, C. H., *et al.*: The pharmacologic control of excessive uterine activity with isoxsuprine. Amer. J. Obstet. Gynec. 82:1064–1075, 1961.)

3-8. A very marked difference in the tolerance of patients to isoxsuprine infusion is obvious on comparing the blood pressure responses for the cases shown in Figures 3-5 and 3-7 with Figure 3-8. Among the controllable factors influencing this response, the clinician must remember that borderline hypovolemic states predispose to severe hypotension when sympathetic compensatory actions are interfered with by infusing beta receptor agents. Proper hydration is a safeguard against this possibility. Hypotension owing to vena cava compression can easily be corrected by turning the patient on her side. The use of vasoconstrictors is usually ineffective, as shown in Figure 3-8. In addition, some have a selective action on the uteroplacental vessels and, therefore, further jeopardize the condition of the infant.[43,44,45,46]

Isoxsuprine infusion side-effects upon the fetus do not seem very significant. We were unable to detect any, but Stander and his associates[71] recorded a very moderate increase in the baseline fetal heart rate.

Because of the undesirable cardiovascular side-effects of isoxsuprine, the search has continued for a beta receptor agent with more specific effect upon the myometrium, and other drugs have been tested in late human pregnancy.

HYDROXYPHENYLISOPROPYLARTERENOL (CC-25). This agent was used in a small series by Stolte and his co-workers,[72] with good uterine relaxing effects but

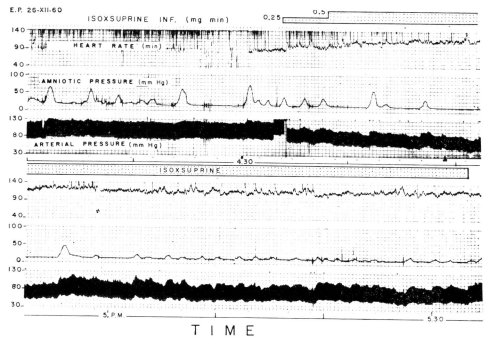

Figure 3-7. Multipara at 34 weeks in premature labor, cervix 4 cm. dilated and 50 per cent effaced. One hour 25 minutes of continuous recording. The high uterine activity did not respond well to a 250 μg./min. (0.25 mg./min.) infusion rate, but diminished dramatically after this was increased to 500 μg./min. (dotted area). Note that the heart rate started to rise right after the infusion was begun, and that the blood pressure dropped likewise. They stabilized after one-half hour of infusion. This patient was discharged on oral medication and readmitted 20 days later, when she was allowed to continue labor, and delivered a 2350 gm. infant who did well. (From Cibils, L. A., and Zuspan, F. P.: Pharmacology of the uterus. Clin. Obstet. Gynec. 11:34–68, 1968.)

also with a marked cardiovascular response. Eskes and his colleagues[32] attempted to block the undesirable cardiovascular response by infusing a beta blocking agent, propranolol. Unfortunately, however, this agent also blocks the uterine response to the drug.

METAPROTERENOL. This is another derivative of isoproterenol, and has been used extensively in Latin America and Europe, where its uterorelaxing properties in term pregnancies have been clearly demonstrated.[17,62] The experience with premature labor is more limited, but the results look promising at the present time.[3] As a potent beta receptor agent it produces a very marked tachycardia in the mother, with more moderate but still significant hypotension, which is dose-related. In this respect, the effect upon the blood pressure seems to be equivalent to or more marked than that of isoxsuprine. An additional side-effect is the marked fetal tachycardia triggered by the drug infusion,[3,17,62] although it has not been reported in all series studies. One disadvantage of this particular preparation is that uterine activity may recover, or "escape," during a steady infusion rate, necessitating further increase in order to maintain a good effect.[17] In this respect, this drug is similar to epinephrine.[50,59,63]

MESUPRINE. A derivative of isoxsuprine, mesuprine was synthesized with the hope that it would have fewer cardiovascular effects than the parent product. A limited number of studies have been carried out to evaluate its uterine relaxing

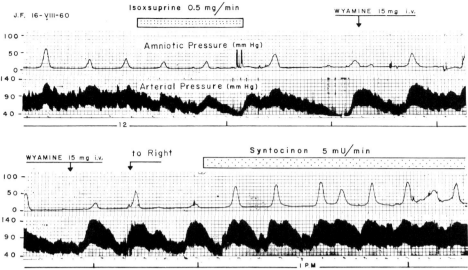

Figure 3-8.   Term pregnancy in early spontaneous labor. One hour 25 minutes of continuous intrauterine and arterial pressure recording. The dramatic effect of 500 μg./min. isoxsuprine (4.5 mg. total dose) (dotted area) is clearly illustrated. In less than 4 minutes, the blood pressure began to drop, and the systolic was 50 at 8 minutes. Discontinuing the infusion did not immediately improve the picture, nor did two intravenous injections of 15 mg. Wyamine each. Turning the patient helped somewhat (bottom), but by then the drug had already been discontinued 30 minutes, and the patient had been receiving rapid intravenous fluids. This patient's cardiovascular system has exhibited the most marked sensitivity in our experience. (From Cibils, L. A.: Inhibitory effects of isoxsuprine on uterine contractility. Amer. J. Obstet. Gynec. *94*:762–764, 1966.)

properties. It is effective in the nonpregnant uterus, but the cardiovascular response is still significant.[21,53] The same effect is observed in advanced pregnancy, either at term[5] or in cases of premature labor,[15] although the hypotensive effects do not seem too severe. Unfortunately, subsequent studies with this drug have been halted by decision of the manufacturers.

RITODRINE.   This is another derivative of isoxsuprine, which has had extensive clinical trials in Europe[41,75] but is still in early stages of clinical investigation in the United States. It has been shown to have uterine relaxing properties in the nonpregnant uterus.[25] Although it produces no significant hypotension, there is an associated tachycardia. Landesman and his colleagues[54] and Barden[4] have shown that the drug is an effective uterine relaxant for the term pregnant uterus. Furthermore, their reports concur that ritodrine causes a moderate tachycardia, with a negligible effect upon the blood pressure.

In the presence of preterm uterine contractions, the drug appears to have the same uterine relaxing effect. Wesselius-de Casparis and associates[75] report a cooperative study carried out in Europe, and Bieniarz and colleagues[13] have confirmed these findings in a small series studied in the United States.

The side-effects produced by therapeutic doses of ritodrine in premature labor are a moderate to marked and consistent tachycardia, with a minimal effect, if any, upon the blood pressure. If blood pressure decreases, it consists of a moderate drop of diastolic pressure only, with resultant increase in the pulse pressure (Figures 3-9 and 3-10). This effect, coupled with a significant tachycardia, would suggest that the cardiac output is increased. Bieniarz[11] has been

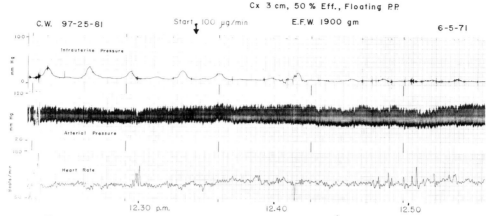

Figure 3-9. Premature labor in a G-6, P-2 patient at 32 weeks gestation. The high uterine activity began to diminish shortly after ritodrine was started at 100 μg./min. (arrow). Note the progressive widening of the pulse-pressure without hypotension, and the steady increase of the pulse rate.

able to prove this fact by direct measurement (dye dilution technique); the cardiac output increment is, furthermore, in direct proportion to the infusion rate of the drug.

Our own observations support the above-mentioned effects of ritodrine. Figures 3-9 and 3-10 illustrate the uterine contractions of a patient in premature labor who received the drug at a rate of 100 μg. per minute, with rapid and satisfactory uterine relaxation. Her systolic blood pressure was minimally increased, while the diastolic pressure dropped and, as a consequence, the pulse pressure is increased. Diminished peripheral resistance and vasodilatation are suggested by the absence of the dicrotic notch after the drug affected the cardiovascular system. The significantly increased pulse rate and pulse pressure would suggest that the cardiac output is also increased. We have observed a significant hypotension in only one case when using intravenous ritodrine.

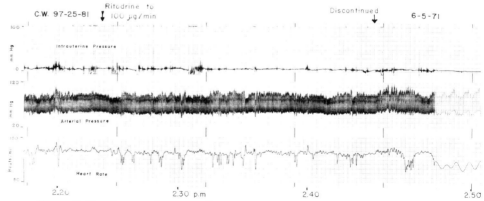

Figure 3-10. Same patient as in Figure 3-9, two hours later. Ritodrine was discontinued at the arrow, and there were no uterine contractions recorded. The blood pressure, unchanged, maintained the increased pulse-pressure. Note at the end of the arterial pressure tracing (taken at high paper speed) the absence of the dicrotic notch. The pulse rate remains increased and stable. The patient was discharged on oral medication. Readmitted 32 days later, with premature rupture of membranes, she delivered a 2675 gm. infant who did well.

An adequate and effective infusion rate may start at 50 μg. per minute, with the upper limit being 400 μg. per minute. The uterine activity diminishes within five minutes, and when the infusion rate is adequate will continue until almost complete quiescence has occurred (Figure 3-10). As with isoxsuprine, we maintain the drug infusions for two hours after the desired level has been reached. Intramuscular injections of 5 mg. of ritodrine every 4 to 6 hours should be sufficient to maintain the effect during the first postinfusion day, oral medication of 10 mg. every 4 to 6 hours being satisfactory in subsequent days.

The effects upon the fetus are manifested by moderate tachycardia, not exceeding 170 beats per minute.[62,75] A limited number of fetal acid base studies indicate that this parameter is not adversely affected by drug infusion.[75]

COMBINATION. Bieniarz and associates[14] studied the control of excessive uterine activity by what they called "multitarget" approach, utilizing simultaneous administration of a large fluid volume, ethanol, pregnenolone, and ritodrine. Apparently they were able to suppress uterine activity, but not necessarily beyond that of single-target medication methods. However, from a theoretical standpoint, and until a clear explanation is found regarding the factors controlling the onset and progression of labor, this approach deserves further trial.

Summary

From the foregoing facts, it appears that, at the present time, there are two acceptable means of arresting premature labor: infusion of ethanol or administration of a beta adrenergic drug (ritodrine) with minimal effect upon the blood pressure. The requirements of administration, as well as the theoretical basis for their clinical use, have been outlined briefly. When the fetal membranes are intact and the cervical dilatation is minimal, these methods have produced encouraging results. Excluding those cases in which a known mechanical factor is triggering the process, as in abruptio placentae or premature rupture of the membranes, there should be a high success rate in averting premature labor by these methods.

REFERENCES

1. Ahlquist, R. P.: A study of the adrenotropic receptors. Amer. J. Physiol. 153:586-600, 1948.
2. Althabe, O., Schwarcz, R. L., Sala, N. L., and Fisch, L.: Effect of phentolamine methanesulfonate upon uterine contractility induced by l-norepinephrine in pregnancy. Amer. J. Obstet. Gynec. 101:1083-1088, 1968.
3. Baillie, P., Meehan, F. P., and Tyack, A. J.: Treatment of premature labor with orciprenaline. Brit. Med. J. 4:154-155, 1970.
4. Barden, T. P.: Effect of ritodrine on human uterine motility and cardiovascular responses in term labor and the early postpartum state. Amer. J. Obstet. Gynec. 112:645-652, 1972.
5. Barden, T. P., Stander, R. W.: Myometrial and cardiovascular effects of two methanesulfonamidophenethanolamines. Amer. J. Obstet. Gynec. 96:1069-1077, 1966.
6. Barden, T. P., and Stander, R. W.: Myometrial and cardiovascular effects of an adrenergic blocking drug in human pregnancy. Amer. J. Obstet. Gynec. 101:91-96, 1968.
7. Barden, T. P., and Stander, R. W.: The effects of propranolol upon uterine activity in term human pregnancy. J. Reprod. Med. 2:188-195, 1969.
8. Belinkoff, S., and Hall, J.: Intravenous alcohol during labor. Amer. J. Obstet. Gynec. 59:429-432, 1950.

9. Bengtsson, L. P.: Experiments on the suppressive effect of a synthetic gestagen on the activity of the pregnant human uterus. Acta Obstet. Gynec. Scand. 41:124-142, 1962.
10. Bengtsson, L. P., and Csapo, A. I.: Oxytocin response, withdrawal, and reinforcement of defense mechanism of the human uterus at midpregnancy. Amer. J. Obstet. Gynec. 83:1083-1093, 1962.
11. Bieniarz, J.: Personal communication.
12. Bieniarz, J., Burd, L., Motew, M., and Scommegna, A.: Inhibition of uterine contractility in labor. Amer. J. Obstet. Gynec. 111:874-885, 1971.
13. Bieniarz, J., Motew, M., and Scommegna, A.: Uterine and cardiovascular effects of ritodrine in premature labor. Obstet. Gynec. 40:65-73, 1972.
14. Bieniarz, J., Burd, L., and Scommegna, A.: Multitarget approach to prevention of prematurity. Obstet. Gynec. 37:632-633, 1971.
15. Bishop, E. H., Bolognese, R. J., and Piver, M. S.: Effect of methanesulfonamide on uterine contractions. Obstet. Gynec. 28:784-786, 1966.
16. Brenner, W. E., and Hendricks, C. H.: Effect of medroxyprogesterone acetate upon the duration and characteristics of human gestation and labor. Amer. J. Obstet. Gynec. 83:1094-1098, 1962.
17. Caldeyro-Barcia, R., Magana, J. M., Castillo, J. B., Poseiro, J. J., Mendez-Bauer, C., Pose, S. V., Escarcena, L., Casacuberta C., Bustos, J. R., and Giussi, G.: A new approach to the treatment of acute intrapartum fetal distress. In Perinatal Factors Affecting Human Development. Washington, D.C., Pan American Health Organization, 1969.
18. Caldeyro-Barcia, R., and Poseiro, J. J.: Oxytocin and contractility of the human uterus. Ann. N. Y. Acad. Sci. 75:813-830, 1959.
19. Caldeyro-Barcia, R., and Sereno, J. A.: The response of the human uterus to oxytocin throughout pregnancy. In Caldeyro-Barcia, R., and Heller, H., eds.: Oxytocin. New York, Pergamon Press, 1961.
20. Cibils, L. A.: Inhibitory effects of isoxsuprine on uterine contractility. Amer. J. Obstet. Gynec. 94:762-764, 1966.
21. Cibils, L. A.: Effect of mesuprine hydrochloride upon non-pregnant uterine contractility and the cardiovascular system. Amer. J. Obstet. Gynec. 111:187-196, 1971.
22. Cibils, L. A., and Hendricks, C. H.: Effecto de la isoxsuprina sobre la contractilidad del utero humano gravido. Mem. X Reun. Gin. Obstet. (Mexico) 1:418-437, 1961.
23. Cibils, L. A., Pose, S. V., and Zuspan, F. P.: Effect of l-norepinephrine infusion on uterine contractility and cardiovascular system. Amer. J. Obstet. Gynec. 84:307-317, 1962.
24. Cibils, L. A., and Zuspan, F. P. Pharmacology of the uterus. Clin. Obstet. Gynec. 11:34-68, 1968.
25. Coutinho, E. M., de Sousa, B. M. B., Wilson, K. H., and Landesman, R.: The inhibitory action of a new sympathomimetic amine (DU-21220) on the nongravid uterus. Amer. J. Obstet. Gynec. 104:1053-1056, 1969.
26. Csapo, A. I.: The onset of labor. Lancet 2:277-280, 1961.
27. Csapo, A., de Sousa-Filho, M. B., de Souza, J. C., and de Souza, O.: Effect of massive progestational hormone treatment on the parturient human uterus. Fertil. Steril. 17:621-636, 1966.
28. Csapo, A. I., Jaffin, H., Kerenyi, T., Lipmen, J. I., and Wood, C.: Volume and activity of the pregnant human uterus. Amer. J. Obstet. Gynec. 85:819-835, 1963.
29. Csapo, A. I., and Lloyd-Jacob, M. A.: Effect of uterine volume on parturition. Amer. J. Obstet. Gynec. 85:806-812, 1963.
30. Csapo, A. I., and Takeda, H.: Effect of progesterone on the electric activity and intrauterine pressure of pregnant and parturient rabbits. Amer. J. Obstet. Gynec. 91:221-231, 1965.
31. Chapmen, E. R., and Williams, P. T.: Intravenous alcohol as an obstetrical analgesic. Amer. J. Obstet. Gynec. 61:676-679, 1951.
32. Eskes, T., Stolte, L., Seelen, J., Moed, H. D., and Vogelsang, C.: Epinephrine derivatives and the activity of the human uterus. II. Amer. J. Obstet. Gynec. 92:871-881, 1965.
33. Falck, B., Owman, C., Rosengren, E., and Sjoberg, N. O.: Reduction by progesterone of the estrogen-induced increase in transmitter level of the short adrenergic neurons innervating the uterus. Endocrinology. 84:958-959, 1969.
34. Farr, C. J., Robards, M. F., and Theobald, G. W.: Changes in myometrial sensitivity to oxytocin in man during the last six weeks of pregnancy. J. Physiol. 196:58-59, 1968.
35. Fuchs, A. R.: Oxytocin and the onset of labor in rabbits. J. Endocr. 31:217-224, 1964.
36. Fuchs, A. R.: The inhibitory effect of ethanol on the release of oxytocin during parturition in the rabbit. J. Endocr. 35:125-134, 1966.

37. Fuchs, F.: Treatment of threatened premature labour with alcohol. J. Obstet. Gynaec. Brit. Comm. 72:1011-1013, 1965.
38. Fuchs, F., Fuchs, A. R., Poblete, V. F., and Risk, A.: Effect of alcohol on threatened premature labor. Amer. J. Obstet. Gynec. 99:627-637, 1967.
39. Fuchs, A. R., and Wagner, G.: The effect of ethyl alcohol on the release of oxytocin in rabbits. Acta Endocr. 44:593-605, 1963.
40. Gaffney, T. E., Burket, R. L., and Woronkow, S.: Catecholamine content of the pregnant and non-pregnant human uterus. Obstet. Gynec. 99:627-637, 1967.
41. Gamissans, O., Esteban-Altirriba, J., and Marquis, V.: Inhibition of human myometrial activity by a new beta adrenergic drug, DU-21220. J. Obstet. Gynaec. Brit. Comm. 76:656, 1969.
42. Graff, G.: Failure to prevent premature labor with ethanol. Amer. J. Obstet. Gynec. 110:878-880, 1971.
43. Greiss, F. C.: The uterine vascular bed: adrenergic receptors. Obstet. Gynec. 23:209-213, 1964.
44. Greiss, F. C.: Differential reactivity of the myoendometrial and placental vasculatures: vasodilatation. Amer. J. Obstet. Gynec. 111:611-622, 1971.
45. Greiss, F. C., Gobble, F. L., Anderson, S. G., and McGuirt, W. F.: Effect of sympathetic nerve stimulation on the uterine vascular bed. Amer. J. Obstet. Gynec. 97:962-967, 1967.
46. Greiss, F. C., Gobble, F. L., Anderson, S. G., and McGuirt, W. F.: Effect of parasympathetic stimulation on the uterine vascular bed. Amer. J. Obstet. Gynec. 99:1067-1072, 1967.
47. Hendricks, C. H., Brenner, W. E., Gabel, R. A., and Kerenyi, T.: The effect of progesterone administered intra-amniotically in late human pregnancy. In A. C. Barnes, Ed.: Progesterone. Augusta, Michigan, Brook Lodge Press, 1961.
48. Hendricks, C. H., Cibils, L. A., Pose, S. V., and Eskes, T. K. A. B.: The pharmacologic control of excessive uterine activity with isoxsuprine. Amer. J. Obstet. Gynec. 82:1064-1075, 1961.
49. Kaiser, I. H.: The effect of epinephrine and norepinephrine on the contractions of the human uterus in labor. Surg. Gynec. Obstet. 90:649, 1950.
50. Kaiser, I. H., Harris, J. S.: The effect of adrenalin on the pregnant human uterus. Amer. J. Obstet. Gynec. 59:775, 1950.
51. Kumar, C., Goodno, J. A., Barnes, A. C.: In vivo effects of intravenous progesterone infusion on human gravid uterine contractility. Bull. Johns Hopkins Hosp. 113:53-56, 1963.
52. Kuriyama, H., and Csapo, A.: Placental and myometrial block. Amer. J. Obstet. Gynec. 82:592-599, 1961.
53. Landesman, R., Coutinho, E. R., and Wilson, K.: The effect of oxytocin and 2-methanesulfonamide derivatives of isoxsuprine on the human nongravid uterus. Amer. J. Obstet. Gynec. 102:212-218, 1968.
54. Landesman, R., Wilson, K., Coutinho, E. M., Klima, A. M., and Marcus, R. S.: The relaxant action of ritodrine, a sympathomimetic amine on the uterus during term labor. Amer. J. Obstet. Gynec. 110:111-114, 1971.
55. Luukkainen, T., Vaisto, L., and Jarvinen, P. A.: The effect of oral intake of ethyl alcohol on the activity of the pregnant human uterus. Acta Obstet. Gynec. Scand. 46:486-493, 1967.
56. Moller, K. J. A., and Fuchs, F.: Double-blind controlled trial of 6-methyl,17-acetoxyprogesterone in threatened abortion. J. Obstet. Gynaec. Brit. Comm. 72:1042-1044, 1965.
57. Owman, C., Rosengren, E., and Sjoberg, N. O.: Origin of the adrenergic innervation to the female genital tract of the rabbit. Life Scien. 5:1389-1396, 1966.
58. Owman, C., and Sjoberg, N. O.: Difference in rate of depletion and recovery of noradrenaline in long and short sympathetic nerves after reserpine treatment. Life Scien. 6:2549-2556, 1967.
59. Pose, S. V., Cibils, L. A., and Zuspan, F. P.: Effect of l-epinephrine infusion on uterine contractility and cardiovascular system. Amer. J. Obstet. Gynec. 84:297-306, 1962.
60. Pose, S. V., and Fielitz, C.: The effects of progesterone on the response of the pregnant human uterus to oxytocin. In Caldeyro-Barcia, R., and Heller, H., eds.: Oxytocin. New York, Pergamon Press, 1961.
61. Pose, S. V., Fielitz, C., Alvarez, H., Sica Blanco, Y., and Cibils, L. A.: Effect of progesterone on the contractility of the human uterus. Proc. XXI Internat. Congr. Physiol. Scien. (Buenos Aires) 281, 1959.
62. Poseiro, J. J., Guevara-Rubio, G., Magana, J. M., and Caldeyro-Barcia, R.: Accion de la orciprenalina (Alupent) sobre la contractilidad del utero humano gravido, el

sistema cardiovascular materno y la frecuencia cardiaca fetal. Arch. Ginec. Obst. (Uruguay) 23:99, 1968.

63. Reynolds, S. R. M., Harris, J. S., and Kaiser, I. H.: Clinical Measurement of Uterine Forces in Pregnancy and Labor. Springfield, Ill., Charles C Thomas, 1954.

64. Rosengren, E., and Sjoberg, N. O.: Changes in the amount of adrenergic transmitter in the female genital tract of rabbit during pregnancy. Acta Physiol. Scand. 72:412-424, 1968.

65. Sala, N. L., Fisch, L., and Schwarcz, R. L.: Effect of cervical dilatation upon milk ejection in humans and its relation to oxytocin secretion. Amer. J. Obstet. Gynec. 91:1090-1094, 1965.

66. Sala, N. L., Schwarcz, R. L., Althabe, O., Fisch, L., and Fuentes, O.: Effect of epidural anesthesia upon uterine contractility induced by artificial cervical dilatation in human pregnancy. Amer. J. Obstet. Gynec. 106:26-29, 1970.

67. Schwarcz, R. L., Sala, N. L., Althabe, O., and Fish, L.: Effect of atropine upon uterine contractility induced by artificial cervical dilatation. Amer. J. Obstet. Gynec. 98: 577-580, 1967.

68. Scommegna, A., Burd, L., and Bieniarz, J.: Progesterone and pregnenolone sulfate in pregnancy plasma. Amer. J. Obstet. Gynec. 113:60-65, 1972.

69. Scommegna, A., Burd, L., Goodman, C., and Bieniarz, J.: The effect of pregnenolone sulfate on uterine contractility. Amer. J. Obstet. Gynec. 108:1023-1029, 1970.

70. Sjoberg, N. O.: Increase in transmitter content of adrenergic nerves in the reproductive tract of female rabbits after estrogen treatment. Acta Endocr. 57:405-413, 1968.

71. Stander, R. W., Barden, T. P., Thompson, J. F., Pugh, W. R., and Werts, C. E.: Fetal cardiac effects of maternal isoxsuprine infusion. Amer. J. Obstet. Gynec. 89:792-800, 1964.

72. Stolte, L., Eskes, T., Seelen, J. Moed, H. D., and Vogelsang, C.: Epinephrine derivatives and the activity of the human uterus. I. Amer. J. Obstet. Gynec. 92:865-870, 1965.

73. Theobald, G. W.: Oxytocin reassessed. Obstet. Gynec. Surv. 23:109-131, 1968.

74. Theobald, G. W., Robards, M. F., Suter, P. E. N.: Changes in myometrial sensitivity to oxytocin in man during the last six weeks of pregnancy. J. Obstet. Gynaec. Brit. Comm. 76:385-393, 1969.

75. Wesselius-de Casparis, A., Thiery, M., Yo le Sian, A., Baumgarten, K., Brosens, I., Gamissans, O., Stolk, J. G., and Vivier, W.: Results of a double-blind study with ritodrine in premature labour. Brit. Med. J. 3:144-147 1971.

76. Wood, C., and Pinkerton, J. H. M.: A comparison of the myometrial activity in the pregnant and non-pregnant side of a septate uterus. J. Obstet. Gynaec. Brit. Comm. 70:669-671, 1963.

77. Woodbury, R. A., and Abreu, B. F.: Influence of epinephrine upon the human gravid uterus. Amer. J. Obstet. Gynec. 48:706, 1944.

78. Zlatnik, F., and Fuchs, F.: A controlled study of ethanol in threatened premature labor. Amer. J. Obstet. Gynec. 112:610-612, 1972.

The Management of
Impending Labor Prior to the Thirty-Fifth Week

ROBERT LANDESMAN

*Cornell University Medical School, New York Hospital,
and Jewish Memorial Hospital*

Labor is premature when it occurs between the twentieth and the thirty-fifth weeks of pregnancy. The accurate determination of the duration of pregnancy provides the basis for the critical timing of drug therapy in premature labor. It is our goal to prevent the onset of the labor until the thirty-eighth week. Maintaining intravenous therapy for many days requires the intensive use of medical personnel and produces an emotional crisis for the gravid patient requiring confined activities in the hospital. Dating the pregnancy from the onset of the last menstrual period has frequently been inaccurate. The technique of sonography, along with direct measurement of fetal skull diameters, has provided evidence of maturity that is accurate to within two weeks. This technique usually confirms the estimated duration of pregnancy calculated by other means. If the recalled last menstrual date differs widely from the sonographic measurements, the latter is usually considered more reliable. However, reduced rates of growth of the fetus, such as may occur in toxemia or in certain congenital states, diminish the value of sonographic estimates. Nevertheless, the entire clinical picture will always provide some final estimate of the degree of maturation.

During the maturation and development of the fetus, uterine contractions may ensue at any time. These may gradually increase in intensity, developing into true labor. The earlier the onset of labor, the higher the percentage of fetal loss. The fetal mortality rate ranges as high as 90 per cent to 100 per cent from 20 to 25 weeks' gestation, and as low as 5 to 10 per cent from 33 to 35 weeks'. Premature labor may be an indication of abnormalities in fetal development: congenital anomalies of the fetus may be associated with early delivery. In certain instances, these congenital aberrations may be ascertained by obtaining fetal cells via amniotomy. Cell cultures and chromosomal analysis may require weeks for completion and final diagnosis. During the time required for genetic study, efforts to block uterine activity may be advisable. The selection of patients for chromosomal analysis at this time requires careful consideration of clinical factors, since there are not enough genetic laboratories available to study all the fetal specimens associated with the premature onset of labor. In patients in whom previous congenital abnormalities have occurred and the chance of recurrences is high— such as in Down's syndrome or hemophilia—chromosomal studies should receive the highest priority. Anencephaly or hydrocephaly may be accurately diagnosed by radiopaque dye injected in the amniotic sac. Recent efforts to postpone labor in one patient continued successfully for four weeks. Pregnancy finally terminated in delivery of a premature infant weighing 700 g. who did not survive. The autopsy, showing bilateral agenesis of the kidneys, provided the full diagnosis which unfortunately was unknown at the time of the onset of premature labor. Although the exact number of serious anomalies at various stages of pregnancy is unknown, term infants may have a 0.5 per cent incidence of abnormalities. During the seventh and eighth months of pregnancy, this may be several times higher.

Management

At the present time, two methods of controlling uterine contractions are possible. The first is via the adrenergic pathways and the second is through the use of parenteral ethyl alcohol. Both techniques may inhibit uterine contractions in early labor and have been shown to postpone delivery in premature labor. Each of these agents produces side-effects, which to some extent limits their use. Further controlled studies comparing the efficiency and side-effects of both methods are in progress. Randomized control investigations with ritodrine and ethyl alcohol studied separately have demonstrated that both groups had a greater success rate in stopping premature labor than the controls.

RITODRINE HYDROCHLORIDE

The most promising beta adrenergic stimulating drug (beta receptor agent) for blocking uterine contractions is ritodrine hydrochloride.[1] Isoxsuprine was initially tried at a number of centers and appeared to be potentially effective. However, no evidence was presented to indicate it had a greater degree of effectiveness than occurred in control groups. Ritodrine is over five times more effective than isoxsuprine in controlling uterine contractions, and it does not have isoxsuprine's toxicity. Orciprenaline or metaproterenol[2] has also been extensively used to control uterine contractility. Orciprenaline does not have the sustained action of ritodrine and not infrequently results in hypotension. Since ritodrine, from our experience, has the most promising qualities, the technique for its administration will be outlined.

Ritodrine therapy is begun intravenously, usually for six hours, and is continued for at least two hours following cessation of uterine activity. This is followed by oral treatment until 38 weeks' gestation or until delivery. Ritodrine is readily dissolved in 5 per cent glucose and water and initially administered at 50 μg. per minute. The rate of infusion may be gradually increased 50 μg. per minute every 10 minutes until adequate uterine relaxation appears or unacceptable side-effects occur. In these latter instances, the dose may be reducd until an acceptable level is achieved. Although we have had no criteria suggesting indications for its use, propranolol hydrochloride, a specific cardiovascular antagonist, should be available during the administration. One milligram of propranolol given intravenously will counteract the cardiovascular effects of ritodrine. The maximum intravenous dose of ritodrine is 500 μg. per minute. Thirty minutes before expected discontinuance of intravenous therapy, oral medication is begun at a dosage rate of 5 to 20 mg. of ritodrine every 4 to 6 hours. Patients who require and tolerate high intravenous doses usually tolerate higher oral doses, which may be as high as 20 mg. every 4 hours. Tablets should be taken 20 minutes before meals when possible. After several days of hospital maintenance, the patient may return home on oral ritodrine. Two visits each week for evaluation are mandatory to monitor dosage and to assess cardiovascular status.

ETHANOL

Ethanol,[3] the other important agent for the control of premature labor, is to be continued intravenously for at least 6 hours following the cessation of uterine activity. Repeated intravenous ethanol may be required, but no oral treatment is recommended. Two ampules containing 50 ml. of 95 per cent ethanol are mixed with 900 ml. of 5 per cent dextrose and water. This stock solution contains 9.5 per cent (volume for volume) of ethanol or 75.4 g./liter. The initial loading dose is 7.5 ml. per kg. body weight per hour for two hours. The maintenance dose is continued for 10 hours at 1.5 ml. per body weight per hour. If labor stops during treatment but begins again after discontinuation, the treatment is resumed at a proportionately lower secondary loading dose. If uterine activity resumes after 10 hours have elapsed, the control loading dose is readministered. Tachycardia, flushing, nausea, and vomiting are not infrequent. Central nervous system effects, characterized by stupor, sleepiness, and occasional agitation, with extreme restlessness, may be part of the generalized alcohol toxicity. Constant nursing care is mandatory during the loading phase of this therapy.

Comparisons

Comparisons of ritodrine and ethyl alcohol afford strong indications for the use of either one. However, neither may be considered the perfect therapy for the problem of premature labor. In three instances, we have administered both ethyl alcohol and ritodrine to a patient after one of the agents proved unsuccessful. An additional delay of labor of at least one week was obtained when the second therapy was administered. At the present time, because of the diversity of toxicity of these two agents, the use of both simultaneously should be used only as a last resort.

Bieniarz and his associates[4] recently described the use of ritodrine for the therapy of early premature labor. In Figure 3-11 is illustrated the case of a 33 week multipara who commenced labor with the cervix 1 cm. dilated and 50 per cent effaced. Ritodrine inhibited contractions only incompletely, after a delay of 80 minutes. The initial dosage of ritodrine was 100 μg. per minute, increased to 380 μg. per minute, unsuccessfully. The addition of ethanol to the treatment regimen relaxed the uterus rapidly and completely. Six weeks later, the patient gave birth to a near term infant.

Diazoxide, a benzothiadiazine structurally related to the thiazide diuretics, has no diuretic action. Its primary action is related to its profound effect on

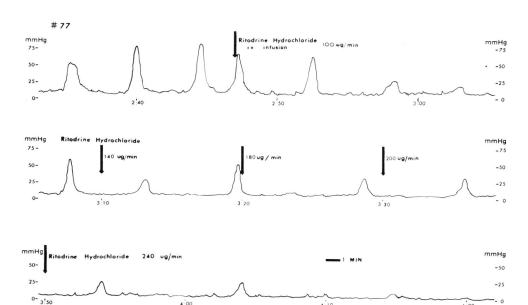

Figure 3-11. Ritodrine is unsuccessfully administered to control premature labor. The addition of ethanol results in a successful delay of labor. Intra-amniotic direct recordings indicate their results. (From Bieniarz, J., *et al.*: Uterine and cardiovascular effects of ritodrine in premature labor. Obstet. Gynec. *40*:65, 1972.)

smooth muscle relaxation and its antihypertensive properties.[5] Finnerty used diazoxide as an antihypertensive agent in toxemia of pregnancy. He noted that the drug frequently stopped labor and reduced uterine contractility. Diazoxide was administered intravenously in 18 nongravid patients in a dose range of 150 to 337 mg.[6] Profound uterine relaxation resulted in all patients. Testing was extended to the contracting uterus during term labor. Relaxation again resulted, but not in as intensive a degree as in the nongravid uterus. On occasion there was an extensive blood pressure drop, which promptly reversed spontaneously. This pressure drop appeared to be related to individual sensitivity. Diazoxide is not effective orally and is most effective intravenously when administered rapidly (in less than 30 seconds).

J.D. was a 27 year old para 3, gravida 7, abortions 3, living children 2. All deliveries were premature. She was admitted August 2, 1968, 31 weeks gravid. Figure 3-12 shows the external monitoring of uterine contractions. Initial dose of 402 mg. diazoxide successfully controlled contractions for 5 days. On August 7, a dose of 306 mg. was required. On August 9, 318 mg. and three days later, 396 mg., were required to control contractility. On August 13, a total dose of 530 mg. was unsuccessful. A standard ethanol infusion was then administered and completely controlled contractility. Patient was readmitted 4 weeks later and was delivered of a well, 2200 g. infant, the largest and most mature. Diazoxide was administered in five instances in a patient with premature labor. Over a period of 11 days, 1.95 g. of intravenous diazoxide were given, which checked the contractions. However, when ethanol was added, it postponed delivery for an additional 4 weeks.

Use of Labor-Inhibiting Agents

What is the potential applicability of labor-inhibiting agents to the various clinical categories of premature labor prior to the thirty-fifth week? Zlatnik[7] has

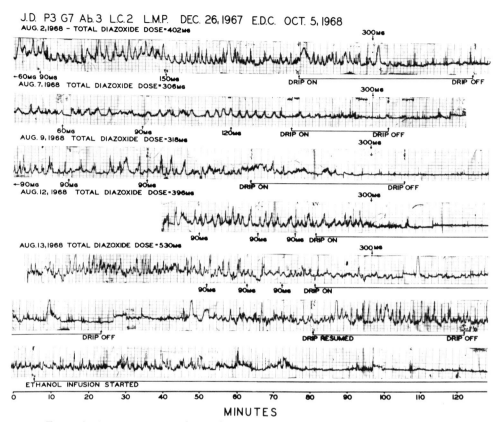

Figure 3-12. Intravenous diazoxide was administered on occasions in eleven days. Ethanol was then successfully added. External recordings indicate the combined results.

recently analyzed some of these subgroups. From March 1, 1970, to July 12, 1971, there were 2287 deliveries at The New York Hospital clinical service, of which 8.4 per cent, or 191, were premature. Only 42 mothers, or only 25 per cent of the premature infants born during this period, satisfied Zlatnik's requirements for inclusion in a study evaluating the effects of ethanol in preventing premature labor. His strict criteria for admission to the ethanol study included only cervical dilatation under 4 cm., with intact membranes and without bleeding. The largest category excluded were 49 infants, or 31 per cent, who were estimated to weigh over 2500 g. Only 8 of these infants had a gestational age of 37 weeks and obviously, although their weights were premature, these represented the larger, borderline infants, almost all of whom would survive without the inhibition of labor.

The second largest category, comprising 45 patients or 28 per cent, was excluded from ethanol therapy because of ruptured membranes. Wesselius-de Casparis and her colleagues,[8] studying a small group of patients with ruptured membranes, showed that ritodrine, a beta adrenergic agent, delayed the onset of labor, as compared to results obtained with a small control group. A study is now in progress to determine the value of ritodrine in cases of ruptured membranes.[9] The reduction of motility may be an important factor in preventing intrauterine infection. In the future, new organ-specific beta blockers, associated with higher potency beta adrenergic compounds and antibiotics, may successfully delay labor for weeks, providing additional maturation time sufficient for infant survival.

A third group of 28 patients, or 18 per cent, were excluded from the ethanol study because of imminent delivery. These patients had a cervix dilated beyond 4 cm. and were in the middle of a driving terminal labor. Coutinho,[10] using available inhibitory agents, has delayed delivery for many hours, even when the cervix was 7 to 8 cm. dilated. The new organ-specific blocking agents may provide more effective dose therapy when used with available agents. Improved education of pregnant women concerning the earliest manifestations of labor, more frequent prenatal visits, and external uterine monitoring may reduce the number of patients in this category and permit early therapy in the course of labor. In addition, patients with a history of previous premature delivery may be singled out for early selected care.

Multiple gestations, representing 8 cases or 5 per cent in the studied series, were also excluded. Because of widespread use of ovulatory agents, in some clinics multiple births have more than doubled. Multiple gestations were excluded from the ethanol series for statistical reasons and because they present a special problem. The diagnosis of multiple gestation has improved as a result of the additional use of electronic fetal heart monitors and sonography. X-ray diagnosis, multiple fetal heart tones, and a uterine size which is greater than expected for the duration of pregnancy are the main criteria for diagnosis. The earlier recognition of a multiple gestation before the onset of premature labor, made possible by these methods, permits the institution of prophylactic measures to delay labor until maturity. Common techniques to further delay the onset of labor include reduced physical activity, sedation, prolonged period of bed rest, and prohibition of regular work. Oral ritodrine has been administered prophylactically in several multiple pregnancies over a period of weeks. Braxton-Hicks contractions were markedly curtailed. A randomized study is in progress to determine whether ritodrine delays labor in the presence of multiple gestation. In addition, Flynn[9] has obtained suggestive evidence that ritodrine produces increased fetal rates of growth by improving the fetal blood supply. The final decision concerning possible prophylactic use of a beta adrenergic compound for delaying labor and possibly increasing the rate of growth of the fetus must await clinical randomized trial. Such therapy for the prevention of premature labor in multiple pregnancies appears to be extremely promising.

Intrauterine growth retardation involved a small group of 7 patients, or 4 per cent. This may not occur if uterine blood flow is increased by beta adrenergic compounds and at the same time, if labor is delayed, a two-edged sword may be available for therapy. Trials of this type are essential in order to determine if drug therapy will be of any benefit. Augmentation of blood supply may be beneficial in preeclampsia (present in 5 patients, or 3 per cent of this series), but there is no evidence that labor-inhibiting agents are effective in reversing the toxemia syndrome. Erythroblastotic infants constituted an additional 3 per cent (5 patients) of the premature group. The severity of the disease determines when the delivery is indicated. During intrauterine transfusions or other manipulations, labor-inhibiting drugs may prevent uterine contractions. A seriously compromised erythroblastotic infant fares better in the premature nursery than in utero. The only category which contraindicates labor inhibitors is profuse third trimester bleeding, found in 4 per cent, or 7 patients. The increased uterine tone and contractility frequently reduces blood loss.

Summary

The management of impending labor prior to the thirty-fifth week has improved somewhat during the past decade. The early clinical recognition of an overactive uterus and a dilating cervix may permit the successful management of the uterine contractility with our available drug therapy. The additional recognition of cases in which serious congenital anomalies exist in utero will contraindicate the use of drug therapy. Although these techniques of therapy may provide some glimmer of hope for the occasional salvage of infants who would have died as a result of prematurity, maximum salvage of premature infants will be provided by better maternal nutrition and more intensive prenatal care. Special attention given to patients with multiple pregnancies, repeat prematurity, toxemia, and familial congenital anomalies will provide the early clues for further successes in the management of prematurity associated with labor prior to 35 weeks of gestation.

REFERENCES

1. Landesman, R., Wilson, K. H., Coutinho, E. M., Klima, I. M., and Marcus, R. S.: The relaxant action of ritodrine, a sympathomimetic amine, on the uterus during term labor. Amer. J. Obstet. Gynec. *110*:111, 1971.
2. Zilianti, M., and Aller, J., Action of orciprenalime on uterine contractility during labor. Amer. J. Obstet. Gynec. *109*:1073, 1971.
3. Fuchs, F., Fuchs, A. R., Poblete, V. F., Jr., and Risk, A.: Effect of alcohol on threatened premature labor. Amer. J. Obstet. Gynec. *99*:627, 1967.
4. Bieniarz, J., Motew, M., and Scommegma, A.: Uterine and cardiovascular effects of ritodrine in premature labor. Obstet. Gynec. *40*:65, 1972.
5. Finnerty, F. A., Jr., Kakviatos, N., Tuckman, J., and Magill, J.: Clinical evaluation of diazoxide, a new treatment for acute hypertension. Circulation *28*:203, 1963.
6. Landesman, R., de Souza, J. A., Coutinho, E. M., Wilson, K. H., and de Sousa, M. B.: The inhibitory effect of diazoxide in normal term labor. Amer. J. Obstet. Gynec. *103*:430, 1969.
7. Zlatnik, F. J.: The applicability of labor inhibition to the problem of prematurity. Amer. J. Obstet. Gynec. *113*:704, 1972.
8. Wesselius-de Casparis, A., Thiery, M., Yo Le Sian, A., Baumgarten, K., Brosens, I., Gamissans, O., Stolk, J. G., and Vivier, W.: Results of a double-blind multicentre study with ritodrine in premature labor. Brit. Med. J. 3:144, 1971.
9. Flynn, M.: Personal communication (1972).
10. Coutinho, E. M.: Personal communication (1972).

The Management of
Impending Labor Prior to the Thirty-Fifth Week

Editorial Comment

Despite notable advances in recent years, several made by the contributors to this chapter, the factors precipitating labor continue to remain elusive.

Theories of the etiology of labor have now broadened to include the possibilities that labor may be initiated either systemically or locally, and by a single agent or several acting synergistically—for example, prostaglandin together with oxytocin. Whatever the substance or substances involved, they may be either maternal or fetal in origin.

The possible participation of the sex steroids in myometrial motor activity has been of continuing interest and investigation. Although the value for progesterone and estrogen changes little prior to the expulsion of the placenta, this is not to say that these placental hormones do not exert a local effect on the uterus. These hormones may be concerned more with providing for uterine accommodation and a favorable milieu for fetal growth than with influencing myometrial motor activity. Moreover, the progesterone output by the placenta for the various periods of pregnancy is so variable that previous indications for adjunctive progesterone therapy in pregnancy complications are no longer valid (see Chapter 22).

That labor may be initiated locally is supported by the observation that in the double uterus, each side containing a fetus of a twin pregnancy, one fetus may be delivered while the other uterine horn may remain quiescent and its fetus may be delivered several weeks later.

The local initiation of labor and methods to inhibit labor have acquired increased attention, stimulated by the possible influence of the sympathomimetic catecholamines and the recent observations on the prostaglandins. Norepinephrine activates the alpha adrenoceptors, causing the myometrium to contract. Activation of beta adrenoceptors inhibits myometrial motor activity. Thus, a dual approach is presented for the inhibition of labor—namely, the blockade of alpha adrenoceptors or the activation of beta adrenoceptors. An inhibition of beta adrenoceptors would permit the unopposed action of norepinephrine, resulting in myometrial contractions.

It is interesting to note that the cervix, especially at the uterovaginal junction, is unusually rich in adrenergic nerves, and would thus provide a storage site for norepinephrine. To speculate further, any factor that might cause the cervix to change its initial configuration or relationship through myometrial motor activ-

110

ity, resulting from administration of oxytocin, or the presence of a laminaria or bougie, might release norepinephrine and thus initiate or accentuate labor. An example of this possibility is the observation that myometrial motor activity commonly ceases following cerclage that may restore the cervix to normal; the adrenergic nerve endings are no longer exposed and norepinephrine ceases to be released. Finally, it should be noted that monoamine oxidase destroys catecholamines, and the placenta is rich in this enzyme. If perhaps, then, a balanced state exists in pregnancy, and if this is upset by placental aging, by changes within the placenta, or by a reduction in uteroplacental blood flow, as in toxemia of pregnancy, norepinephrine would no longer be inactivated adequately by the enzyme.

4

The Value and Dangers in the Conservative Management of Placenta Previa

Alternative Points of View:

By Edward H. Bishop

By Russell Ramon de Alvarez and Jon Michael Passmore

By Abe Mickal and Phillip H. Rye

By Kenneth R. Niswander and Frederick W. Hanson

Editorial Comment

The Value and Dangers in the Conservative Management of Placenta Previa

EDWARD H. BISHOP

University of North Carolina

A clarification of the meaning of "conservative management" is appropriate before entering into a detailed discussion of our subject. At one time it was considered that, once a diagnosis of placenta previa had been made, not only was prompt and active treatment indicated, but also any temporization whatever was totally unjustified. Subsequently the reports of Johnson[1] and later those of MacAfee and his colleagues[2] suggested that frequently, depending on certain circumstances, delay of delivery for an interval after the initial symptoms leading to a diagnosis of placenta previa appeared not only was justifiable but also helped to reduce the high neonatal mortality rate resulting from premature delivery. This concept was supported by the observation that the initial hemorrhage was rarely, if ever, fatal and that subsequent hemorrhages were rarely lethal if the maternal hemoglobin was kept at acceptable levels. It is this scheme of deferment of delivery until the fetus has attained more favorable maturity that is considered "conservative management." If this concept is justified, the advantage is obvious, but whether or not this course actually results in an improved neonatal survival has been questioned by some. Even if we accept the possibility of improved neonatal survival rates, associated disadvantages may complicate the conservative approach. Prolonged and costly hospitalization, multiple blood transfusions, and the increased fetal risk associated with secondary hemorrhages are among the potential hazards associated with a conservative approach. Additionally, we have too often observed that, because of these undesirable factors, a compromise type of management has been instituted under the guise of conservative therapy. As a result of the pressure instigated by the financial, emotional, or personal stresses of prolonged hospitalization, the patient with placenta previa in a temporarily quiescent stage frequently has been allowed to leave the hospital while awaiting "more optimal" gestational age. Too often, in spite of explicit instructions and supposedly adequate precautions, a subsequent serious hemorrhage has occurred under less than acceptable circumstances where therapy is concerned. Although often a tempting "solution," we feel that the use of such compromise methods is not tenable with good practice.

Possibly the best method of discussing the management of placenta previa is by outlining our present and usual plan.

All patients with bleeding judged to be more than "show" or "spotting" must be admitted at once to the hospital for further evaluation. A rough method of evaluating the amount of bleeding is to determine if it has been sufficient to require the use of a perineal pad. This represents sufficient indication for admission and evaluation, even though the actual amount of blood loss deemed by the patient to be sufficient for the use of this sort of protection varies according to personal idiosyncrasies.

Because placenta previa is almost exclusively a complication of multiparity, particular attention must be given to *any* bleeding among this group of patients during the last half of pregnancy.

Following admission, evaluations of the amount of blood loss, of the vital signs of both the mother and the fetus, and of the laboratory findings will indicate when there is the need for immediate therapy. Obviously, when either the mother or the fetus is in jeopardy from blood loss, prompt treatment of actual or impending shock is indicated, followed by, or simultaneous with, prompt delivery by the most expeditious method. Although the original hemorrhage sometimes may abate reasonably promptly and the status of both the patient and the fetus improve after appropriate therapy, including blood replacement, it has been our firm conviction that little can be gained and much can be lost by temporizing and delaying definitive therapy if the original hemorrhage has been severe. Under such circumstances, we believe that conservative therapy has many more disadvantages than advantages.

Most often the patient is admitted with only a moderate amount of bleeding, without evidence of any immediate threat to either maternal or fetal life. These happily favorable circumstances permit a more deliberate management of the problem. First, we have the opportunity to confirm or eliminate the provisional diagnosis of placenta previa by:

1. X-ray placental localization.
2. Ultrasonic examination.
3. Isotope localization of the placenta.
4. Amniography.

Second, once the diagnosis has been confirmed, time is available for determining the best method of subsequent therapy. This decision can be made only after combined evaluation of several factors, listed here:

FETAL GESTATIONAL AGE.   If the gestational age is reliably estimated to be 36 weeks or more, and if the estimated fetal weight is in excess of 2500 g., little can be gained by conservative therapy and much can be lost by procrastination. Under such favorable circumstances, once the presumptive diagnosis has been confirmed, termination of pregnancy is indicated. If the stage of fetal development is questionable, it is sometimes necessary to perform special test for fetal maturity before a definite conclusion can be attained. Among these evaluations are x-ray determination of fetal bone development, cytologic and histochemical examinations of the amniotic fluid, measurement of the amniotic fluid creatinine levels, the lecithin/sphingomyelin demonstration of the presence or absence of favorable amounts of amniotic surfactant. Only when the fetus is unquestionably immature is conservative therapy and continuation of pregnancy justifiable.

TYPE OF PLACENTA PREVIA.   Although this is often determined by the same methods used for making the diagnosis, occasionally final determination of the type can be made only by vaginal examination. However, it is essential to stipulate that such an examination should be performed *only* under proper circumstances—in the operating room, with preparation for immediate surgical intervention if necessary, and with adequate equipment for blood replacement and necessary personnel immediately available. It is our conviction that there is little place for procrastination when a diagnosis of a central placenta previa has been made. Although it is not ideal to deliver an infant with a decreased chance of survival owing to prematurity, delay in the presence of a central placenta previa not only seldom succeeds but also increases the peril for both the mother and the fetus. This risk is less for the placenta previa with lesser degree of encroachment on the area of the internal os. Therefore, for these more moderate situations, conservative therapy may be indicated if the other circumstances listed above are favorable.

VAGINAL BLEEDING.   The choice between aggressive and conservative therapy is dependent upon the amount of vaginal bleeding and the number of bleeding episodes. As mentioned earlier, a life-threatening hemorrhage is an absolute indication for prompt and active therapy, but we believe that a second serious hemorrhage is an equally important indication for prompt termination of pregnancy. When a second serious hemorrhage occurs, any subsequent episodes of bleeding may terminate in fetal loss.

PRESENCE OF LABOR.   The symptoms of placenta previa occasionally occur during early labor. When this occurs, obviously there is neither justification nor opportunity for conservative therapy.

Once the decision has been made to terminate the pregnancy, the actual method is determined by consideration of numerous factors. Among these are:

1. Type of placenta previa.
2. Severity of bleeding.
3. Parity.
4. Condition of the cervix.
5. Presence or absence of labor.
6. Fetal presentation.
7. Condition of the patient and the fetus.

At one extreme are patients with a central placenta previa, those with a series of hemorrhages, and nulliparous patients with unfavorable cervices, all of whom are usually best managed by delivery via cesarean section. At the other extreme are the multiparous patients at or near term, in early labor, with a partially dilated cervix and a marginal placenta previa. This group may be safely and successfully managed by amniotomy followed by either induction or stimulation of labor. Between these two extremes are many situations for which the decision regarding the method of delivery can be made only by an evaluation of the relative importance of all the factors listed above.

Abnormal fetal presentations are a frequent problem in the pregnancy already complicated by placenta previa, and must be considered when deciding upon the optimal method of delivery. There is little justification for attempting vaginal delivery in a pregnancy complicated by a placenta previa and additionally by the presence of an abnormal fetal presentation.

In summary, it is our conclusion that "conservative management of placenta previa" is indicated and justified only when:

1. The fetus weighs less than 2500 g. or is of less than 36 weeks' gestational age.

2. The vaginal bleeding is not excessive or repetitive.

3. The placenta previa is *not* centrally located.

4. The statuses of the fetus and the mother are not in immediate jeopardy.

5. The circumstances and the physical facilities permit continuous hospitalization until the optimal time for delivery has been attained.

When conservative therapy is indicated or elected, no compromise can be made. The patient must be kept in the hospital, after the initial hemorrhage, from the time of admission to the time of delivery. During this period, adequate blood for replacement and adequate personnel and physical facilities for immediate treatment must be available at all hours should a change in circumstances require a sudden alteration in the planned method of therapy. Obviously, then, conservative therapy will be elected for only a small number of patients, since the first bleeding episode occurs most often when the fetus is of an age at which it can survive outside the uterus. When the original episode of bleeding occurs earlier than this, it is frequently associated with the more serious forms of placenta previa, which are less amenable to conservative management. Conservative therapy is therefore justified only when it does not threaten the life of either the mother or her fetus.

It must be recognized that except under the most ideal circumstances —circumstances which are difficult to achieve—it is difficult to document an improvement in perinatal mortality rate resulting from conservative therapy. In electing conservative therapy, one must consider the relative frequencies of not only perinatal mortality but also neonatal morbidity. The fetus who has survived multiple hypoxic episodes resulting from repeated hemorrhages may have also suffered neurologic and developmental abnormalities. Conservative management of placenta previa is justified only when the risk of prematurity is so great that an alternative method of management offers little hope for the survival of a healthy neonate.

REFERENCES

1. Johnson, H. A.: The conservative management of some varieties of placenta previa. Amer. J. Obstet. Gynec. 50:248, 1945.
2. MacAfee, C. H. G., Millar, W. G., and Harley, G.: Maternal and fetal mortality in placenta previa. J. Obstet. Gynaec. Brit. Comm. 69:203, 1962.

The Value and Dangers in the Conservative Management of Placenta Previa

Russell Ramon de Alvarez and Jon M. Passmore
Temple University School of Medicine

Bleeding in the late second trimester and third trimester of pregnancy should always arouse the suspicion that placenta previa is present. The differential diagnosis should include special attention to abruptio placentae, marginal sinus rupture, rupture of the uterus, carcinoma of the cervix, polyps (cervical, decidual, or vaginal), candidiasis and other chronic infections, granulomas, associated hydatidiform mole, and trauma. A careful history and record of the findings at the initial antepartum examination are most helpful in arriving at the diagnosis of chronic cervical or vaginal lesions.

Because a close etiologic correlation exists among uterine pathology, endometrial trauma (including previous uterine surgery), and pathologic changes in the placenta, a careful and detailed history of previous obstetric and operative procedures will bring into focus the possibility of placenta previa.

The use of portable scintillation detectors to identify the distribution of radioisotopes through the placental circulation offers the most practical and economic means of determining the location of the placenta. We have achieved an accuracy of 90 to 95 per cent, as have other examiners.[1] The administration of radioiodinated human serum albumin to the pregnant patient provides an important aid in diagnosing placenta previa. The technique of scanning the abdomen to localize the placenta is quite accurate after the twenty-eighth week of pregnancy but is almost useless prior to that time. Although it approaches the same degree of accuracy in localizing the placenta, B scan ultrasonography needs costly apparatus and the numbers of qualified personnel to operate the equipment are limited. The reluctance of health administrators to place or encourage the use of this desirable equipment in obstetric areas where it would be most frequently used also imposes limitations on the assessment of this valuable diagnostic tool. Automatic scintillation counting is definitely superior to the portable detectors, but the methods and equipment currently available are not practical for use in obstetric suites. The high degree of inaccuracy of the Doppler ultrasonograph and soft tissue radiography in localizing the placenta does not justify their use as

119

routine methods for investigating the bleeding of late pregnancy. Nevertheless, the radiograph does serve a great and important function in determining the position of the fetus, the number of fetuses present, the type of pelvis, the existence of obstruction, and other features commonly associated with low implantation of the placenta.

Amniography, while more accurate, is reputed to be a cause of premature labor. Thermography has received some study; however, the results, when we have used it, were inconclusive. Vaginal or rectal examination prior to delivery are both dangerous and deceptive and, because the possibility of hemorrhage is so great, the physician is likely to restrict his palpation, sacrificing thoroughness for safety of the patient and the fetus. A vaginal examination is warranted only in an obstetric operating room situation, where immediate delivery is an alternative. Recently, an increase in urinary human chorionic gonadotropin excretion has been reported not only to be diagnostic of placenta previa but has even been suggested to indicate the diagnosis before the onset of hemorrhage.[2] Unfortunately, no one has been able to substantiate these claims.

When bleeding owing to placenta previa begins in the second trimester, there is a high probability that placenta previa is partially or completely covering the internal os. Even so, in the interests of the fetus, conservative management of the bleeding is advisable and desirable whenever the placenta is found to be located in the lower uterine segment.

Conservative Management

Once the diagnosis of placenta previa is likely or certain, care is directed to the prevention of bleeding, the control of hemorrhage, and the replacement of blood lost. Although the purpose of conservative therapy during mid-trimester or early third trimester is to allow a longer period time for the intrauterine development of the premature fetus, there is no good reason to delay active diagnostic investigation and treatment of placenta previa if the fetus is at or near term or if labor has begun.

Labor commonly precipitates hemorrhage in cases of placenta previa. In the near future, it may be possible to arrest labor with considerable success with the use of beta adrenergic blocking agents, such as ritodrine hydrochloride.[3] With the drugs now available, the conservative management of placenta previa may be more successful.

When the fetus is judged to be capable of surviving (37 weeks' gestation and 2500 g. minimum weight), further attempt to prolong the pregnancy serves no good purpose and may, in fact, be detrimental to fetal survival.

If placental localization is reasonably certain, amniocentesis through an area not covered by the placenta, and study of the amniotic fluid creatinine, bilirubin, fetal cells, and lecithin/sphingomyelin ratio are helpful. Recently a rapid and reliable test for determination of surfactant, as an index of fetal maturity, has become available.[4]

When conservative treatment of placenta previa is elected, the patient should be hospitalized immediately; women who experience early bleeding may require as much as 12 weeks' hospitalization before viability of the fetus is attained. Although the characteristically recurrent, small hemorrhages are rarely fatal in the absence of vaginal manipulation, uncontrollable hemorrhage demands prompt termination of pregnancy. As a general rule, hospitalization is vital to successful conservative expectant therapy.

Prohibitive hospital costs may force the home management of these patients. In the follow-up of these patients, repeated hemoglobin determinations are made. In the hospital or at home, bed rest is mandatory and perineal pad counts are helpful to assess blood loss. Semmons has advised termination of pregnancy when a single episode of hemorrhage results in a blood loss greater than 600 ml.[5] Of course vaginal examination, intercourse and any other vaginal manipulative procedures, tampons, douches, or inserts are contraindicated. It is helpful to place these patients on stool softeners in an effort to avoid straining at defecation that may increase bleeding as a result of increased intra-abdominal pressure; of course, enemas are not to be used.

Emergency Treatment

To provide for emergency treatment of hemorrhage, 1000 ml. or 2 units of blood properly typed and cross-matched must always be available in the hospital blood bank for each patient with placenta previa. Following admission, immediate replacement of lost blood is essential, and transfusion will also be necessary if values from the weekly determinations of hemoglobin level fall below 11.0 g./100 ml. Because of the availability of modern blood typing and blood replacement methods, some authors advocate bed rest at home to spare the patient today's soaring hospital costs. This approach is not recommended but, when economic considerations demand observation at home, a minimum of 2000 ml. of blood should be available continuously for possible immediate replacement if and when necessary upon admission to the hospital.

If the gestation progresses without a provocative event, or when the fetus is judged to be of a size sufficient to be without risk of developing the respiratory distress syndrome, a "double set-up" examination may be performed. Such an examination may be necessary at an earlier gestational age or because of recurrent hemorrhage. Hemorrhage during labor is also grounds for the "double set-up" examination. For this examination, an anesthetist must be present, as well as two obstetricians, one to perform the diagnostic investigation and the other, standing by gowned and gloved, fully prepared to deliver the infant abdominally should severe hemorrhage be precipitated. To this end, full preparation for cesarean section must have been made; scrub nurses and equipment should be present and consents to the procedure signed. It is essential that blood for replacement be at hand, but at times hemorrhage may force definitive examination before cross-match is complete. The use of type O rhesus negative blood should be considered in these circumstances.

At the time of examination one of four types of low-lying placenta may be found: (1) the placenta previa centralis (total), wherein the entire internal os is occluded; (2) the placenta previa partialis, in which the internal os is partially occluded by the placenta; (3) the placenta previa marginalis, in which the placenta lies at the borders of the internal os; and (4) the simple low-lying placenta attached to the lower uterine segment but without encroachment on the area of the internal os.

Total placenta previa absolutely requires abdominal delivery. When total placenta previa is diagnosed, there is no alternative to cesarean section as the means of delivering both the infant and the placenta. Transplacentation version or any other manipulation of total placenta previa is emphatically contraindicated.

When partial placenta previa is present and covers a quarter or less of the internal os, it may be treated by artifical rupture of the fetal membranes plus carefully monitored oxytocin stimulation. A cesarean section set-up should be at hand if the necessity arises to cope with recurrent hemorrhage or fetal distress. The partial placenta previa does not strictly preclude vaginal delivery, since the presenting part may tamponade the abnormally situated placenta with minimization of blood loss. However, as with placenta previa marginalis and variously positioned low-lying placentas, such tamponade occasionally may result in fetal distress, characterized as late decelerations. In such cases, fetal distress should require prompt abdominal delivery. In partial placenta previa, hemorrhage will dictate cesarean delivery more frequently than will fetal distress.

Placenta previa marginalis and low-lying placentas are to be regarded with respect and suspicion, because the edge of the placenta may become exposed during further dilatation of the cervix, with conversion of the original diagnosis to partial placenta previa, with all the risks attendant on this condition.

Should dangerous hemorrhage occur at any time during labor after the manual determination of the location of the placenta, cesarean section is immediately performed in order to arrest the bleeding and avoid fetal hypoxia.

Postpartally, hemorrhage may occur from the placental implantation site in the lower uterine segment as a result of relatively poor contraction of the lower segment, and may necessitate surgical intervention. Uterine packing is mentioned here only to be condemned. Placenta accreta, more commonly encountered in placenta previa cases, may demand immediate hysterectomy.

Even with attentive care, however, conservative management is not 100 per cent effective. Treatment is termed successful, of course, only when both mother and fetus survive without undue morbidity. Although in our experience, conservative therapy has markedly increased the number of live births, it is not always possible to assure significantly decreased neonatal mortality. Profuse hemorrhage, which must be controlled and can only be stopped by delivery, often precludes conservative therapy. Consequently, fetal or perinatal death attributable to hypoxia or prematurity ensues. An inaccurate assessment of fetal weight prompting delivery of low birth weight babies further increases mortality. Fetal growth itself is in no way retarded by the presence of placenta previa.

In actual practice, one may be forced to act in behalf of the mother rather than the fetus by choosing an early delivery. This is not an arbitrary decision, but should be tempered by considerations of the quality of neonatal care available and the possibility of transporting the small and feeble infant to a major neonatal care center. The presence of such centers has certainly reduced the mortality and morbidity rates of these neonates.

Cyclopropane anesthesia, usually preferred when there is hypovolemic shock, often produces an immediate depressing effect, which is thought to be detrimental to fetal survival. The possibility of fetal blood loss occurring during maternal hemorrhage is also receiving increased attention. While the mother's life should never be jeopardized, delivery should be considered only after conservative therapy has been proved clearly inadequate.

With attentive care, the maternal mortality rate in placenta previa is low. Postpartum and postoperative morbidity rates still offer problems, however, particularly as a result of infection. The type of placenta previa present appears to be unrelated to total blood loss, frequency of bleeding, or fetal outcome, although hypovolemic shock is usually associated with placenta previa centralis.

Because multiparity is an especially notable etiologic feature of this condition, most parous women who have experienced placenta previa prefer to eliminate the possibility of pregnancy and the hazards of a similar future complication undergoing tubal sterilization at the time of cesarean section or later at laparoscopy.

Although conservative management has become more practicable with newer technology, it has created significant new problems of its own. There are few satisfactory answers in a situation in which preservation of the fetus endangers the life of the mother; yet, technological advances in placental localization, in the determination of the likelihood of fetal survival, and in availability of emergency neonatal transport and care have given the physician a greater armamentarium in the management of these cases. Even with new and sophisticated technology and advances in the delivery of health care, there is no substitute for alertness, discretion, and sound clinical judgment based upon extensive obstetrical experience.

REFERENCES

1. Hibbard, L. T.: Placenta previa. Amer. J. Obstet. Gynec. *104*:172-184, 1969.
2. Maeder, H. P., and Lippert, T. H.: Placenta previa increta and increased chorionic-gonadotropin excretion. Lancet 2:604-605, 1971.
3. Bieniarz, J., Motew, M., and Scommegna, A.: Uterine and cardiovascular effects of ritodrine in premature labor. Obstet. Gynec. *40*:65-73, 1972.
4. Clements, J. A., Platzker, A. C. G., Tierney, D. F., Hobel, C. J., Creasy, R. K., Margolis, A. J., Thibeault, D. W., Tooley, W. H., and Oh, W.: Assessment of the risk of the respiratory distress syndrome by a rapid test for surfactant in amniotic fluid. New Eng. J. Med. *286*:1077–1081, 1972.
5. Semmons, J. P.: A second look at expectant management of placenta previa. Postgrad. Med. *44*:207-212, 1968.

The Value and Dangers in the
Conservative Management of Placenta Previa

ABE MICKAL and PHILLIP H. RYE

Louisiana State University Medical Center

The incidence of placenta previa in the Louisiana State University Services at the Charity Hospitals of Louisiana averages 0.38 per cent, or 1 in 261 deliveries. Conservative management is our procedure of choice, provided that the condition does not demand emergency or immediate care.

The basic concept of conservative management is to increase fetal salvage rate without jeopardizing the well-being of the mother. This attitude has gained support over the past years because of the improvements in obstetrical techniques, anesthesia, blood banks, prenatal care, and monitoring of labor. Of equal importance are the improved facilities for care of newborns, especially premature and high-risk infants.

Before the use of cesarean section, vaginal delivery was associated with a maternal mortality rate of 10 per cent and a perinatal infant mortality rate ranging from 60 to 80 per cent. In addition to the high mortality rates were increased morbidity rates and longer recovery periods. The judicious and expert use of cesarean section has dramatically reduced the maternal mortality rate to less than 1 per cent and the perinatal infant mortality to about 10 to 15 per cent.

Etiology

The exact etiology of placenta previa is unknown. It is presumably a complication of multiparity, as the ratio is approximately 7:1 for women who have borne children versus primiparous patients. Multiparity and previous intrauterine surgical procedures tend to result in a decreased vascular supply to the lower uterine segment. The placenta of a low implanted zygote, therefore, must fan out over a greater area of the lower uterine segment to secure adequate blood, with subsequent encroachment on the cervical os. This placental involvement of the cervical os has been statistically reported to be marginal in 37 per cent of patients, partial in 33 per cent (with less than 30 per cent of cervical os in-

124

volved), and total in 30 per cent of cases. The partial and total placenta previas are our areas of most concern and it is principally in these two situations that the clinician must make the decision between immediate and conservative management of the case.

There are certain conditions which demand immediate care, and in which the conservative method cannot or should not be exercised, namely:

1. Serious and progressive bleeding.
2. Presence of active labor with or without fetal demise.
3. Gestations of 37 weeks or more, with term sized infants and active bleeding.
4. Positive evidence of fetal distress.

Cases of placenta previa not falling into any of the above categories can be managed by the conservative approach and delivered electively, at the most opportune time for both baby and mother. One must remember that no deaths have been reported resulting from the initial spontaneous hemorrhage in placenta previa. The deaths that do occur have been from recurrent bleeding or following examinations when placenta previa was not suspected or adequately provided for.

All painless vaginal bleeding of significance must be presumed to result from placenta previa until proved otherwise. A high index of suspicion is mandatory. Hospitalization and a thorough evaluation is a small price to pay for the ultimate well-being of mother and child. The earlier placenta previa is diagnosed, the better the prognosis. Close cooperation between the patient and doctor is essential to avoid the many pitfalls and thus insure safe continuation of the pregnancy, with improved fetal maturity and salvage rate.

Management

In the Louisiana State University Service all patients suspected of having placenta previa are admitted to the hospital and managed according to the following protocol, outlined in brief:

1. Obstetrical and general history and physical examination.
2. Blood examination, to include complete blood count, Rh determination, fibrinogen level, typing and cross-matching of 1000 ml. or 2 units of blood, and so forth.
3. Abdominal palpation to outline the fetus. Localize the fetal heart tones and placental souffle.
4. X-ray for placental localization.
5. Pelvic examination with "double set-up" technique.
   a. Inspection of external genitalia.
   b. Speculum evaluation of vagina and cervix for bleeding sites.
   c. Gentle digital palpation of the lower uterine segment and cervix to detect presence of interposing structures between uterine wall and fetal parts. An engaged fetal vertex usually denotes the likely absence of partial placenta previa and certainly of central or total placenta previa.
   d. Gentle exploration of cervix, if permissible (no forcing). Blood clots cannot be differentiated from placenta and no forceful attempt

should be made to do this. The presence of clots as well as placenta over the cervical os is sufficient to justify treatment as placenta previa.

6. Bed rest with limited privileges paralleling the clinical course and progress.

7. Delivery, elective if possible, at the most opportune time (fetal maturity determined by amniotic fluid studies).

8. At time of cesarean section, the bladder flap is reflected and the lower uterine segment is exposed and inspected. A low transverse incision is carried out if conditions permit, otherwise a low longitudinal or classical incision is made. One must carefully inspect the endometrial cavity after removing the placenta. A few needed sutures at bleeding areas of the placental site at this time can be most rewarding in preventing postpartum hemorrhage.

As already stated, the ultimate goal is a mature, healthy baby and a healthy mother, otherwise the need for conservative management would not exist. In appropriate cases, Morgan[1] and Semmens[2] have both reported a perinatal infant mortality rate of 9.6 per cent by this method of management. Pedowitz[5] reported a perinatal infant mortality rate of 13 per cent in 77 cases of placenta previa managed conservatively.

There are, however, dangers to this method of management, and one must weigh the values as well as the dangers in each case, for certainly no uniform, "across the board" philosophy can apply in placenta previa. We must acknowledge that the resultant increase in fetal salvage far outweighs the dangers.

The outline below denotes the values as well as the dangers in the conservative management of placenta previa:

Values:
1. *Increased fetal salvage.*
2. Avoids unnecessary intervention when other causes of vaginal bleeding are present, i.e., marginal sinus rupture, low-lying placenta.
3. Reduces complications of lower uterine segment and cervix because elective cesarean section is performed.
Dangers:
1. Intrauterine fetal demise, possible hypoxic episodes.
2. Overtreatment of suspected but not confirmed placenta previa.
3. Misdiagnosis of situations requiring immediate care, such as abruptio placentae, and so forth.
4. Increased maternal morbidity and mortality rates as a result of procrastination.

Case History

R.S., case no. L62-9343, gravida 4, para 3, previous cesarean section for cephalo pelvic disproportion, last menstrual period 2/5/72, estimated date of confinement 11/11/72

8/14/72   Admitted with history of painless vaginal bleeding. 24–26 weeks' gestation. Workup and examination confirmed previable pregnancy with central placenta previa (positive placental scan). Hematocrit,

36 ml./100 ml. Recommendation: conservative management in hospital.

9/15/72   Moderately active bleeding. Hematocrit, 32 ml./100 ml. Given 2 units packed cells. Continue hospitalization and observation.

9/26/72   Moderately active bleeding. No labor. Hematocrit, 32 ml./100 ml. Given 2 units packed cells. Continue hospitalization and observation.

10/1/72   Early labor. Active bleeding. Repeat cesarean section with delivery of viable 3 lb 5 oz female with Apgar score 7/8. Bilateral tubal ligation was done. Discharged on fifth post section day with hematocrit 36 ml./100 ml. and in good clinical condition. Baby is doing well.

CONCLUSION.   This case illustrates the possibility that exists in some cases of placenta previa, in which the conservative management allows the baby to grow and mature. Care must be exercised in making the proper diagnosis and in developing good rapport with the patient. Good team work can produce similar results. The risk to the mother can be justified and minimized if the necessary precautions are taken.

REFERENCES

1. Morgan, J.: Placenta previa: report of a series of 538 cases (1938–1962). J. Obstet. Gynaec. Brit. Comm. 72:700, 1965.
2. Semmens, J. P.: A second look at expectant management of placenta previa. Postgrad. Med. 44:207, 1968.
3. Hellman, L., and Pritchard, J.: Williams Obstetrics. 14th Ed. New York, Appleton-Century-Crofts, 1971.
4. Taylor, E. S.: Beck's Obstetrical Practice. 9th Ed. Baltimore, Williams & Wilkins Co., 1971.
5. Pedowitz, P.: Placenta previa: an evaluation of expectant management and the factors responsible for fetal wastage. Am. J. Obstet. Gynec. 93:16, 1965.

The Value and Dangers in the Conservative Management of Placenta Previa

Kenneth R. Niswander and Frederick W. Hanson
University of California at Davis School of Medicine

Five to six per cent of pregnant patients will have bleeding during the third trimester of pregnancy. Placenta previa accounts for approximately one-third of the cases of third trimester bleeding.[1] The last 25 years have seen little or no improvement in perinatal infant mortality rate associated with placenta previa. The recent reports of Hibbard,[2] Nesbitt and associates,[3] and Niswander and co-workers[4] clearly illustrate this lack of improvement.

Early in the twentieth century, perinatal mortality rates with placenta previa were variously reported as between 40 and 75 per cent. Maternal mortality rates in the range of 10 per cent were experienced frequently. In 1927, Bill[5] reported that maternal mortality rates improved dramatically, to a rate of 1 per 100, apparently as a result of the more aggressive therapeutic approach to the patient. Earlier hospitalization, transfusion, and increased use of cesarean section were the chief weapons employed. Despite the improved statistics, hemorrhage remains a leading cause of maternal mortality in the United States. Unfortunately, the aggressive approach to the management of placenta previa did not consider the fetus.

The dictum of aggressive management spread and remained preeminent until 1945, when Macafee[6] and Johnson[7] advocated a more conservative approach in selected cases of placenta previa. Williams[8] and, more recently, Semmens[9] have supported conservative management.

Macafee, in his classic article,[6] clearly established the objectives of expectant management:

1. The reduction of foetal mortality without unfavourably affecting the maternal death rate.
2. The preservation of an open mind with regard to the appropriate treatment of a particular case, i.e., that each case should be treated, not necessarily on any standard lives, but in accordance with the conditions found.

Hypoxia and prematurity have accounted for most of the perinatal deaths, and these two risks tend to "squeeze" the fetus from opposite directions. Although

128

conservative management is continued in an effort to gain fetal maturity, the fetus remains constantly at risk because of the likelihood of a subsequent major maternal hemorrhage. Should such hemorrhage occur, the resultant shock and intrauterine hypoxia may be fatal or cause irreparable damage to the fetus. On the other hand, while delivery of the fetus shortly after a relatively minor bleeding earlier in pregnancy may avert the risk of a later and serious intrauterine hypoxic episode, this can be accomplished only at the cost of an essential degree of fetal maturity. The finest obstetric judgment is needed if we are to avoid either of these undesirable extremes.

Nesbitt and his associates[3] studied the perinatal losses among gravidas of upstate New York giving birth between 1942 and 1958, on whom a diagnosis of placenta previa had been recorded on the birth record. Their studies indicated that a rising cesarean section rate could decrease the stillborn loss, but this gain was likely to be cancelled by an increased neonatal loss. Record and McKeown,[10] reporting on 1023 cases of placenta previa from Birmingham, England, concluded that an increased use of cesarean section accounted for about one-third of the drop in perinatal death rate recorded between 1942–1943 and 1950–1952, whereas one-half of the improvement was attributable to prolongation of gestation.

In the United States, many are understandably distressed by the relatively high infant perinatal loss in this country, compared to rates in other industralized countries.[11] It seems most appropriate to continue seeking ways of decreasing perinatal loss in the United States. With this objective in mind, we have studied the perinatal deaths associated with placenta previa occurring in an obstetric population available to us for study. Hoping to determine that some of these deaths might have been avoided, we have assumed that such a review would also suggest measures that would decrease the loss associated with placenta previa.

Materials and Methods

We have reviewed all cases of placenta previa managed between the years 1960 and 1967 at the Buffalo General Hospital and the Buffalo Children's Hospital, as well as the previously reported cases from a collaborative project.[4] The review included 78 cases of placenta previa among 16,132 deliveries (5:1000) at the Buffalo General Hospital, 83 from 24,872 deliveries (3:1000) at the Buffalo Children's Hospital, and 238 in 40,262 deliveries (6:1000) from other hospitals reporting to the collaborative project.

Results

Table 4-1 relates the degree of placenta previa to the perinatal death rate per 1000 total births. The perinatal death rate with the lesser degrees of placenta previa is only slightly lower than that associated with the more severe degrees of low implantation. Table 4-2 shows a diminishing cesarean section rate as the degree of placenta previa decreases from total to low-lying, with an overall cesarean section rate for the entire group of 58.0 per cent. Table 4-3 illustrates the well-known relationship between placenta previa and prematurity. Nearly 50 per cent of the infants in the cases reviewed weighed less than 2500 g. at birth.

TABLE 4-1.   *Perinatal Mortality Rate by Degree of Placenta Previa**

	CASES		DEATHS			DEATH RATE
DEGREE	No.	Per Cent	Fetal	Neonatal	Total	PER 1000
Total	104	26.4	5	14	19	183
Partial	71	17.8	7	10	17	239
Marginal	72	18.1	7	7	14	194
Low-lying	142	35.4	6	13	19	134
Unknown	9	2.3	1	0	1	—
Total	398	100.0	26	44	70	176

* From Niswander, K. R., and Ray, M.: Management of second and third trimester bleeding. *In* D. E. Reid and T. C. Barton, eds.: Controversy in Obstetrics and Gynecology I. Philadelphia, W. B. Saunders Co., 1969, p. 70.

TABLE 4-2.   *Cesarean Section Rate by Degree of Placenta Previa**

		SECTIONS	
DEGREE	No.	No.	Per Cent
Total	104	99	95.2
Partial	71	52	73.2
Marginal	72†	31	43.1
Low-lying	142	40	28.2
Unknown	9	9	—
Total	398	231	58.0

* From Niswander, K. R., and Ray, M.: Management of second and third trimester bleeding. *In* D. E. Reid and T. C. Barton, eds.: Controversy of Obstetrics and Gynecology I. Philadelphia, W. B. Saunders Co., 1969, p. 70.
† One case unknown if delivery was cesarean.

TABLE 4-3.   *Relationship of Perinatal Mortality Rate to Infant Weight**

BIRTHWEIGHT		DEATHS			DEATH RATE
(GRAMS)	No.	Per Cent	Fetal	Neonatal	PER 1000
<1500	55	13.8	16	23	709
1500–1999	45	11.3	3	7	222
2000–2499	79	19.8	3	9	152
≥2500	218	54.8	4	5	41
Unknown	1	0.3	0	0	—
Total	398	100.0	26	44	176

* From Niswander, K. R., and Ray, M.: Management of second and third trimester bleeding. *In* D. E. Reid and T. C. Barton, eds.: Controversy in Obstetrics and Gynecology I. Philadelphia, W. B. Saunders Co., 1969, p. 70.

Our perinatal mortality rate is similar to those reported by other investigators, though not as low as was reported recently by Semmens.[9] To determine if our perinatal loss could have been lowered by more perceptive management, the neonatal deaths and fetal deaths have been analyzed separately, in an effort to recognize the basis for a choice between continuation of conservative treatment in order to avoid deaths from prematurity versus earlier delivery in an effort to avoid the results of severe intrauterine hypoxia.

It seemed evident that certain situations reduced the desirability of continuing conservative management or, indeed, made such treatment impossible. When labor or excessive bleeding could not be disregarded, the perinatal loss was accepted as unavoidable (Table 4–4). However, four neonatal deaths might have been avoided by a delay of intervention. Table 4–5 lists the clinical details of these cases.

Infant 1 was delivered by cesarean section because the mother was bleeding "moderately" and because the 37 week gestational length was thought to be adequate for extrauterine survival; prematurity was the primary cause of fetal death. Infant 2 was delivered under almost identical circumstances. These

TABLE 4-4. *Unavoidable Neonatal Deaths**

REASON	NO.
Labor	15
Premature rupture of membranes	3
Shock or two or more transfusions	16
Congenital anomaly	1
Birthweight > 2500 grams Gestation > 37 weeks	2
Erythroblastosis fetalis	1
Prolapse of cord	2
	40
Avoidable?	4

* From Niswander, K. R., and Ray, M.: Management of second and third trimester bleeding. *In* D. E. Reid and T. C. Barton, eds.: Controversy in Obstetrics and Gynecology I. Philadelphia, W. B. Saunders Co., 1969, p. 70.

TABLE 4-5. *Avoidable Neonatal Deaths**

NO.	WEEKS OF GESTA- TION	BIRTH WEIGHT	DEGREE OF PREVIA	CAUSE OF DEATH	DELIVERY	PRESENTA- TION	REMARKS
1	37	2268	Low	Prematurity	Section	Vertex	"Moderate" bleeding
2	37	2098	Marginal	Prematurity	Section	Vertex	"Moderate" bleeding
3	32	1474	Total	Prematurity	Section	Transverse	3 separate "moderate" bleedings
4	33	2098	Total	Prematurity; Hyaline membrane disease	Section	Transverse	"Moderate" bleeding

* From Niswander, K. R., and Ray, M.: Management of second and third trimester bleeding. *In* D. E. Reid and T. C. Barton, eds.: Controversy in Obstetrics and Gynecology I. Philadelphia, W. B. Saunders Co., 1969, p. 70.

cases indicate that the most careful clinical estimations of fetal weight are notoriously inaccurate and such errors contribute to the perinatal loss that is likely to be charged to placenta previa.

Infant 3 was delivered at 32 weeks' gestation after three separate and distinct but "moderate" bleeding episodes. It seems quite possible that a continuation of conservative management might have permitted the necessary degree of fetal maturation to be reached.

Infant 4 was delivered at 33 weeks' gestation. Cesarean section was considered to be indicated because of a transverse lie and x-ray evidence of a total placenta previa. Vaginal bleeding had been only moderate. In this instance, too, deferment of aggressive management might have assured the necessary degree of fetal maturity.

TABLE 4-6.   *Unavoidable Fetal Deaths**

REASON	NO.
Fetal weight < 1500 grams	15
Gestation < 32 weeks	3
Congenital anomaly	1
Section for maternal shock	2
Macerated fetus due to severe preeclampsia	1
	22
Avoidable?	4

* From Niswander, K. R., and Ray, M.: Management of second and third trimester bleeding. *In* D. E. Reid and T. C. Barton, eds.: Controversy in Obstetrics and Gynecology I. Philadelphia, W. B. Saunders Co., 1969, p. 70.

Some of the 26 fetal deaths seemed unavoidable (Table 4-6). However, details of the management of these patients is indicated in Table 4-7.

Infant 5 was delivered unnecessarily early. The patient had experienced only minimal bleeding until a pelvic examination precipitated such severe bleeding that labor was induced in order to "stop the bleeding."

Infants 6 and 7 both suffered the consequences of 50 per cent abruptio placentae, in which the placenta was implanted low in the uterus. Although one patient underwent cesarean section and the other was delivered vaginally following an induction of labor, both infants died of hypoxia. Since cesarean section is usually regarded as the "radical" management and vaginal delivery following induction of labor as the "conservative" therapy for abruptio placentae, here we note the failure of both approaches in an attempt to avoid perinatal loss under almost identical circumstances.

Since infant 8 died of hypoxia during a labor induced to control moderate bleeding, one can conclude that cesarean section in this instance might have provided a healthy infant who would have survived.

Discussion

It has been established without doubt that a certain percentage of patients with placenta previa will benefit from the application of a course of conservative management as originally described by Macafee. We are not aware of any recent literature to the contrary. The only real controversy concerns proper selection of patients who will benefit from conservative management. In most cases, the fetus alone stands to benefit from conservatism, and indeed this may be the only way to lower the perinatal mortality rate associated with placenta previa. Evidence indicates that improper selection of patients will increase maternal risks by exposing the mother to the hazard of severe hemorrhage and its attendant morbidity and mortality dangers. The sole purpose of conservative management is the reduction of fetal prematurity. Patients who are in labor or are considered to be at term clearly are not candidates.

What amount of bleeding precludes the application of conservative management? Semmens has suggested that a "point of no return" in the conservative management of placenta previa has been reached when a single episode

TABLE 4-7.   *Avoidable Fetal Deaths*[*]

NO.	GESTATION (WEEKS)	BIRTH WEIGHT (GRAMS)	DEGREE OF PREVIA	TIME OF DEATH	CAUSE	DELIVERY	CLINICAL SEVERITY OF DISEASE	SHOCK	REMARKS
5	38	907	Total	<24 before delivery	Unknown	Vaginal	Moderate	No	Severe bleeding followed by pelvic exam. Induced to "stop bleeding."
6	35	2155	Low + 50% abruptio	At delivery	Hypoxia	Section	Moderate	No	FHS heard just before section.
7	40	3402	Marginal + 50% abruptio	During labor	Hypoxia	Vaginal	Moderate	No	Induced for abruptio.
8	36	2665	Marginal + 50% abruptio	During labor	Hypoxia	Vaginal	Moderate	No	Induced when bleeding was "moderate."

* From Niswander, K. R., and Ray, M.: Management of second and third trimester bleeding. *In* D. E. Reid and T. C. Barton, eds.: Controversy in in Obstetrics and Gynecology I. Philadelphia, W. B. Saunders Co., 1969, p. 70.

of bleeding has resulted in blood loss exceding 600 ml. We agree with this warning, and when labor ensues or excessive bleeding occurs, the choice of management is relatively easy. A more difficult problem presents when a gravida with
x-ray confirmed central or partial placenta previa approaches term without
having developed a severe bleeding episode. Since cesarean section is certain
to be contemplated for the delivery, an early elective section before an expectedly
severe bleed seems likely to avoid a preventable fetal death. Only the risk of
neonatal death owing to prematurity stays the hand of the surgeon for too long
on some occasions. Categoric resolution of this dilemma is not possible, and the
art of medicine continues to supersede science.

A final point, which has received scant attention in the literature and
which requires serious consideration, is the question of fetal growth associated
with placenta previa. Does it proceed at a normal rate? Conservative management is based on the premise that fetal growth and maturity proceed normally.
A recent publication by Gabert would appear to support the idea that placenta
previa does not retard or in any way impede fetal growth.[12] Our experience supports this point of view (Figure 4-1). It should be noted, however, that both
our data and Gabert's are plotted on a birthweight–gestation graph which is
foreign to our own populations and which may not be precisely applicable to
our own populations because of differences in race, sex of infant, nutritional
status of the mother, and many other factors.

"Good" therapy requires an astute clinical appraisal of all pertinent factors
plus utilization of such supplemental tools as blood transfusion and radiography.
However, a critical analysis of the management of pregnancies in which perinatal
death was associated with placenta previa only occasionally suggests that better
therapy would have avoided a perinatal mortality. In only two of the 44 neonatal
deaths we have reviewed would conservative management have been of value
and possibly have prevented a fetal death. One of the 26 fetal deaths might have
been avoided if vaginal examination had been delayed. A second infant delivered

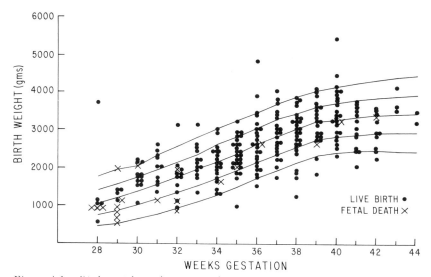

Figure 4-1.   Birth weight and gestation data on a series of patients with placenta previa
plotted on graph prepared from data of Gruenwald[13] of an unselected population.

vaginally who died of hypoxia might have survived if cesarean section had been employed. Even if all post hoc appraisals have been correct (a highly questionable assumption), more astute clinical judgment could have lowered the perinatal mortality rate in this series only from 176 to 166.

In conclusion, we have found no basis upon which to offer more than agreement with Pedowitz when he suggests that "further reduction in fetal wastage must await developments that will control or prevent [uncontrolled hemorrhage, the onset of labor, or intrauterine death] in order to permit the pregnancies to continue until the fetus is of adequate size."[14] If the obstetrician will appreciate the value of conservative management but exercise his best "clinical judgment" while continuing to anticipate the risk of a fetal life-threatening maternal bleeding episode, the lowest possible perinatal mortality rate will result. In this study, however, we have found little reason to believe we can substantially reduce the related fetal loss until the etiology of placenta previa is known and low implantations of the placenta can be avoided.

REFERENCES

1. Reid, D. E., Ryan, K. J., and Benirschke, K., Ed.: Principles and Management of Human Reproduction. Philadelphia, W. B. Saunders Co., 1972.
2. Hibbard, L. T.: Placenta previa. Amer. J. Obstet. Gynec. 104:172–184,1969.
3. Nesbitt, R., Yankauer, A., Schlesinger, E., and Allaway, N.: Investigation of perinatal mortality rates associated with placenta previa in upstate New York, 1942–1958. New Eng. J. Med. 267:381–386, 1962.
4. Niswander, K. R., Friedman, E. A., Hoover, D. B., Pietrowski, H., and Westphal, M. C.: Fetal morbidity following potentially anoxigenic obstetric conditions. II. Placenta previa. Amer. J. Obstet. Gynec. 95:846–852, 1966.
5. Bill, A. H.: Treatment of placenta previa by prophylactic blood transfusion and cesarean section. Amer. J. Obstet. Gynec. 14:523–529, 1927.
6. Macafee, C. H. G.: Placenta praevia–a study of 174 cases. J. Obstet. Gynaec. Brit. Emp. 52:313, 1945.
7. Johnson, H. W.: The conservative management of some varieties of placenta previa. Amer. J. Obstet. Gynec. 50:248, 1945.
8. Williams, T. J.: The expectant management of placenta previa. Amer. J. Obstet. Gynec. 55:169, 1948.
9. Semmens, J. P.: A second look at expectant management of placenta previa. Postgrad. Med. 44:207–212, 1968.
10. Record, R. G., and McKeown, T.: Investigation of foetal mortality associated with placenta praevia. Brit. J. Prev. Soc. Med. 10:25–31, 1956.
11. Chase, H.: International comparison of perinatal and infant mortality. Public Health Service Publications, No. 1000—Series 3—No. 6.
12. Gabert, H. A.: Placenta previa and fetal growth. Obstet. Gynec. 38:403–406, 1971.
13. Gruenwald, P.: Growth of the human fetus; normal growth and its variations. Amer. J. Obstet. Gynec. 94:1112–1119, 1966.
14. Pedowitz, P.: Placenta previa: an evaluation of expectant management and the factors responsible for fetal wastage. Amer. J. Obstet. Gynec. 93:16–25, 1965.

The Value and Dangers in the
Conservative Management of Placenta Previa

Editorial Comment

In the late 1930's and early 1940's, with the advent of blood banks, many North American clinics began to consider delaying the delivery of patients suspected of having a placenta previa in cases in which the fetus was considered too premature to survive and the extent of the bleeding was not life threatening. The idea was also expressed that fetal survival was enhanced if the mother's condition could be stabilized and the rate of intravillous blood flow was restored to normal for at least a period of time prior to delivery. As cited by the contributors to this chapter, Macafee and Johnson in their writings described this approach to the management of patients with placenta previa and offered evidence that fetal wastage could be reduced from 30 to 15 per cent.

However, we no longer can assess results on the basis of perinatal and neonatal mortality rates alone, but must be constantly aware of the presence of morbidity and what it signifies. As might be anticipated, the neonatal morbidity rate appears to be greatest in the two most trying obstetrical conditions to manage: namely, premature rupture of the fetal membranes and late pregnancy bleeding prior to the thirty-fifth or thirty-sixth week of gestation. The incidence of neurological damage to the fetus in instances of late pregnancy bleeding is some eight times (50:1000 to 60:1000) or more than the average frequency in the general population (7:1000) and it is higher than that of the premature group (40:1000), which contains many of the infants from the above obstetrical complications. For example, in the collaborative study referred to by Drs. Niswander and Hanson, the baseline incidence of cerebral palsy was 7:1000 for all pregnancies, but rose sharply to 40:1000 in the premature group. Still required is an assessment of the time in pregnancy the initial bleeding occurred, the amount of the bleeding, and the number of bleeding episodes. All of these obviously must play a role in influencing the incidence of permanent damage to the central nervous system of the newborn from hypoxia through a disturbance in the intravillous circulation either directly or through a fall in maternal blood pressure. Similar to renal blood flow, a systolic blood pressure of 70 to 80 mm. Hg may affect the rate of intravillous blood flow and placental transport.

The diagnosis of placenta previa by placental localization and the determination of fetal age has permitted a more rational approach to the management of patients with late pregnancy bleeding. Certainly, placental localization by methods such as ultrasound avoids the necessity for vaginal examination. Unless the pregnancy is of 36 weeks' duration or longer, vaginal examination is contra-indicated, for it may cause recurrent bleeding that may reach proportions that demand an immediate delivery.

It must be recognized that the accuracy of the various methods of placental localization is still open to controversy. All the methods are reliable in the last five weeks of pregnancy, but in these circumstances one might proceed to examine the patient under "double set-up" precautions and establish the diagnosis without the aid of placental localization. What is not entirely known is how accurate the various methods are at earlier stages of pregnancy, the time when the clinician is most desirous of establishing or excluding the diagnosis without recourse to vaginal examination. Hence, the question is posed: what is the accuracy of these methods at 26, 30, and 34 weeks of pregnancy? Ultrasound scan appears to qualify best in this regard. Also, it is well to determine whether the placenta is implanted on the anterior or posterior uterine wall. There is some question about the ability of methods other than ultrasound to identify the placenta when implanted on the posterior uterine wall. Since the posterior wall is anatomically shorter than the anterior uterine wall by a few centimeters, a posterior implant is more likely to be a placenta previa and the degree of previa is apt to be greater. Also, as Stallworthy[1] has emphasized, when the placenta is implanted on the posterior wall of the lower uterine segment, the vertex is less likely to enter the pelvis, having to bypass the sacral promontory and placenta simultaneously. This is a consideration when rupture of the membranes may be contemplated as the preferred method of treatment. In fact when the placenta previa is posteriorly located, elective cesarean section is undoubtedly indicated even in type II of the British nomenclature (marginal type). The risk is more especially to the fetus, and the selection of the method of delivery is dictated in large measure by the extent of placental encroachment on the lower uterine segment. Again, ultrasound scan appears to be more accurate than other methods in determining the degree of placenta previa.

When the placenta is found by placental localization to be in the upper uterine segment, the patient may safely be discharged from the hospital after a 24 to 48 hour observation period. A 48 hour stay is recommended, for some patients have been discharged immediately when the scan proved to be negative for placenta previa, only to return shortly with extensive placental separation and absence of fetal heart tones.

The presence of the placenta in the lower segment calls for a definite plan of management. We hold the view that basically the patient with placenta previa should remain in the hospital for however long, until delivery. Perhaps there is no better illustration of the compromises that are now being made in overall patient care because of the current prohibitive cost of hospitalization than is seen in the conservative treatment of a patient with placenta previa.

As Niswander and Hanson's data indicate, any further reduction in the prenatal mortality rate in placenta previa will occur mainly in patients who qualify for conservative treatment. However, in their series of patients so treated, the number of infants salvaged was surprisingly small. With the high toll of unavoidable fetal deaths, whether expectant treatment is justified remains to be seen. This would apply especially to patients who bleed prior to the thirty-third week of pregnancy, since, as previously stated, the central nervous system damage in this group is substantial. In patients of 33 to 35 weeks' gestation or in cases in which the fetus weighs 2000 g., it would appear reasonable to pursue conservative treatment to avoid hyaline membrane disease, when hypoxic damage is less of a threat. Before the contemplated delivery at 36 to 37 weeks' gestation is carried out, it is mandatory that the fetal age and size be established by lecithin/sphingomyelin ratio and sonography determinations of the biparietal diameter of the fetal head, respectively.

However, prior to the thirty-third week, and in the belief that hyaline membrane disease does not contribute per se to central nervous system damage, the question is posed whether pregnancy should be terminated forthwith rather than pursuing a policy of conservative treatment. It is readily granted that the death rate from hyaline membrane disease in this earlier period will be high, but, as shown by Niswander and Hanson, unavoidable fetal loss is 50 to 60 per cent in patients being treated conservatively. The infants who do escape hyaline membrane disease and survive by such a policy presumably would be free of permanent hypoxic damage.

In any event, these patients should be in a hospital environment which includes an intensive infant care unit. All the facilities, including ultrasound, must be available and the operating room prepared so that abdominal delivery may be carried out within minutes if there is recurrent bleeding. The anesthetic should be administered by a Board certified anesthesiologist.

It has been recommended that centers be established regionally to care for patients with all forms of high-risk pregnancy. These centers, with medical specialists—i.e., perinatologists, and so forth—undoubtedly would need to be supported by national and state funds so that these cases are not financially burdensome to the hospital, and the patient may enter without economic constraints.

Finally, it is our belief that the fetus should be transported in utero rather than after delivery to an intensive pediatric care unit from those hospitals without such facilities. Until these centers come into being, the patient and her concerned physician will somehow muddle through at the risk that the newborn may be the victim of irreversible nervous system damage and a recipient of a totally blighted life. If some four million of our citizens are so victimized, and with some evidence that the numbers can be reduced by at least two million with proper facilities and care, we would inquire what is truly meant by medical priorities.

REFERENCES

1. Stallworthy, J.: The dangerous placenta. Amer. J. Obstet. Gynec. 61:720, 1951.

5

The Status of
Fetal Monitoring
in Decision Making
in Patient Management

Alternative Points of View:

By L. S. James, Edward T. Bowe, and Henry R. Rey

By E. J. Quilligan and Roger K. Freeman

By Robert A. Stookey and Mortimer G. Rosen

Editorial Comment

The Status of Fetal Monitoring in Decision Making in Patient Management

L. S. James, Edward T. Bowe, and Henry R. Rey

Columbia University College of Physicians and Surgeons and Babies Hospital

Fetal Monitoring

In the past 15 years, advances in instrumentation have led to the introduction of biophysical and biochemical monitoring techniques in many areas of medicine. For a number of reasons, acceptance of these techniques as useful adjuncts to the practice of obstetrics has been quite limited. Arguments to oppose their use are many and at times vociferous. "There is no evidence to show that it will reduce mortality and morbidity." "The cost would be prohibitive." "Serious heart rate changes can be detected clinically." "It is unnecessary meddling which interferes with the normal physiological process of labor and upsets delivery room routine."

Such arguments only serve to maintain the status quo and will not help to resolve the controversy. They miss the fact that the principal contribution of monitoring is to provide the physician with more precise information not available by standard clinical methods. This should permit earlier detection of fetal difficulty and thus provide a means for lowering both mortality and morbidity rates. The arguments ignore the contributions from clinical investigations which have confirmed a significant relationship between abnormal fetal heart rate patterns and fetal acidosis, hypoxia, and poor condition at birth. They ignore the animal experiments which have provided new information on the mechanisms of various fetal heart rate patterns.

Technical difficulties

Mistrust of instrumentation has undoubtedly contributed to the lack of acceptance. Earlier models were complex, difficult to use, and not designed to

This investigation was supported by United States Public Health Service Grants GMO9069 and HLI4218.

141

withstand the wear and tear of rough usage by inexperienced personnel in a busy obstetric unit. Machine failure and breakdown has not been infrequent. Clipping an electrode to the scalp of the fetus and incising the scalp to obtain a capillary sample of blood has been regarded as unduly traumatic, and the wires were inconvenient for the physician and uncomfortable for the patient.

Reliable instrumentation which is relatively easy to use is now available. With greater demands for monitors, continued improvement in design can be anticipated. The introduction of ultrasonic detectors has facilitated the external recording of the fetal heart rate and enabled monitoring to be introduced earlier in labor, without the need of rupturing the membranes or placing scalp electrodes. The electrode design itself has been greatly improved, and records can be obtained free from extraneous interference. Advances in design of the blood gas meters, which are now more stable, simple to use, and automated, have simplified the measurements of pH, Pco_2 and Po_2.

RECOGNITION AND INTERPRETATION OF HEART RATE PATTERNS

Inability to recognize the various heart rate patterns and a general lack of understanding of the mechanisms involved have also contributed to the lack of acceptance.

There is now both well-documented experimental evidence and a wealth of clinical observation to indicate that the three major heart rate patterns (early deceleration or Type I dip, late deceleration or Type II dip, and variable deceleration) all result from specific mechanisms. Difficulty in recognizing these patterns has been in part an effect of a too rapid or too slow paper speed, lack of instrumentation sensitivity, and extraneous interference producing artifacts. Standardization and improvements in instrumentation should alleviate these problems.

Early deceleration is primarily caused by vagal stimulation, which may occur as a result of head molding or pressure (reflex from the meninges), pressure on the fontanelle, carotid sinus, or eyeball, and some forms of cord occlusion. Usually it is not of serious consequence, but it should alert the physician to possible serious difficulties.

Late deceleration or Type II dip reflects fetal bradycardia which commences during a uterine contraction and persists for 30 to 60 seconds after the contraction is over. The fetus who exhibits this pattern of bradycardia is usually severely asphyxiated and depressed at birth. As a consequence, late deceleration has been termed hypoxic bradycardia and is related to placental insufficiency. It has been correlated in humans with fetal hypoxia, from results of both a tissue Po_2 electrode and sampling of fetal capillary blood. It has also been produced in an experimental model in the pregnant subhuman primate in which cardiovascular and acid-base state can be monitored directly. In those fetuses which become acidotic, hypoxic, and hypotensive as labor advanced, there is an increase in baseline heart rate and late deceleration of the fetal heart rate following each uterine contraction. The late deceleration appears as a marked transient bradycardia and is accompanied by a further decrease in fetal oxygen levels. In those fetuses which remain well oxygenated, there is no change in heart rate or in the level of oxygenation during uterine contractions of similar intensity. Late deceleration is abolished or suppressed when the level of fetal oxygenation is increased by administering a high concentration of oxygen to the mother. Since the fetal acidosis and hypotension remain, it is concluded that fetal hypoxia is the essential component producing late deceleration of the heart rate.

Variable deceleration has been clinically correlated with occlusion of the umbilical cord, and this pattern of change has also been reproduced experimentally by interfering with blood flow in the umbilical arteries or vein. It is usually innocuous but again its presence should alert the physician to possible difficulties later.

Finally, there is now a substantial body of literature on the relationship between loss of baseline irregularity or beat to beat variation and poor fetal outcome.

It should be emphasized that neither the fetal heart rate patterns nor the beat to beat variation can be detected solely by listening. Listening alone is comparable to attempting the diagnosis of various cardiac disorders with a stethoscope while ignoring the EKG. A written record is essential. Not only are many of the heart rate changes inaudible during uterine contractions, but also their exact relationship to the contraction needs to be determined. In addition, there are details of changes in the fetal electrocardiograph, ectopic beats, conduction abnormalities, S-T changes, and so forth, which can be recognized only if recorded. Of equal importance is the educational value of the written record; abnormalities or trends missed by intermittent listening are available, and there is no question as to the events and the exact sequence of events.

MEANING AND VALIDITY OF FETAL CAPILLARY SAMPLES

The development of a respiratory and metabolic acidosis during an asphyxial episode is reflected by a fall in pH. Thus, the determination of fetal acid-base state by measurement of pH and Pco_2 gives a measure of an asphyxial or hypoxic insult to the fetus.

The question as to whether a fetal capillary sample is representative of circulating arterial blood or is a reliable index of fetal acid-base state has set another obstacle in the path of acceptance of monitoring.

The validity of fetal capillary blood as an index has been verified in several ways. A positive correlation exists between the values for pH in the latest scalp sample and those of the umbilical artery and vein. This positive correlation is also found for hematocrit values. Although the slightly higher fetal capillary hematocrit levels observed probably do imply some mild degree of stasis in the regional blood flow from which the samples are taken, these observed differences in hematocrit values are not statistically significant. Again, there is evidence to support the contention that the presence of caput succedaneum rarely causes erroneous values was found when the pH values obtained from the fetuses of a group of multiparous patients were compared to those of fetuses of nulliparous patients at the end of labor. Other evidence that fetal capillary blood obtained from the presenting part during labor is an accurate reflection of fetal arterial and venous acid-base state has been obtained using catheters implanted in monkey fetuses during labor. A positive correlation was found when the pH of the fetal capillary blood was compared with that obtained in simultaneous samples of blood from the carotid artery and jugular vein. The agreement between samples extended over a pH range of 7.3 to 6.8.

The value of a single measurement of pH as a predictor of the infant's condition at birth has, in our experience, been found to be misleading in approximately 18 per cent of cases. These have been subdivided into two main groups, designated "false normal" and "false abnormal." Those instances in which the fetus is minimally acidotic during labor, with a pH of 7.2 or higher, and yet is depressed at birth have been termed false normals. Those instances in which the fetus is observed to be acidotic, with a pH below 7.2, but is nevertheless vigorous at birth have been termed false abnormals.

Asphyxia, while an important cause of depression at birth, is only one of a number of factors that can lead to depression of the central nervous system. Other factors include sedative drugs or anesthetics, infection, airway obstruction, congenital anomalies, precipitous delivery, and asphyxial episode between the time of fetal blood sampling and delivery of the infant. Maternal medication or anesthesia probably accounts for more false normal values than any other cause in the above list. The major contributing factor in the false abnormal group is maternal acidosis, which occurs if labor is unduly long or associated with excessive muscular effort. It also occurs when the mother receives inadequate fluid or calories, as a result of starvation and dehydration. If maternal acidosis is of sufficient duration, it will be reflected in the fetus. Infants in this group can be distinguished by evaluating the maternal acid-base state. A maternal venous sample from the antecubital vein obtained without stasis, or a capillary sample, is quite satisfactory for this purpose.

From the foregoing discussion it may be seen that correlation between fetal pH and the condition of the infant at birth is not a simple direct relationship. Many factors must be taken into account; the proportion of infants in the false normal category or false abnormal category will be influenced by the practice of both obstetrics and obstetrical anesthesia, and may therefore vary from clinic to clinic. If no attention is paid to maternal hydration and caloric requirements, the proportion of infants in the false abnormal group will be increased. If, on the other hand, heavy maternal sedation is employed, or if the infants are delivered under potent inhalation anesthetic agents, the proportion of infants in the false normal group will be quite high. In our own experience, the proportions of false abnormals and false normals are 7.6 per cent and 10.4 per cent, respectively. It would seem important for the physician to make an attempt to establish in his own practice what proportion of infants are included in these two particular groups. With this knowledge he will have a better chance of predicting the outcome for an individual patient.

From our own experience the introduction of fetal blood sampling has resulted in a fivefold improvement in the predictability of outcome of labor over the clinical observation of both heart rate irregularities and the presence of meconium.

COMBINED HEART RATE AND ACID-BASE MONITORING

Cardiovascular status and acid-base state are not independent variables. Therefore, the monitoring of heart rate is not an alternative to acid-base monitoring; instead, the two methods should be considered as complementary. Although interrelated, each one provides information of a different order. A less than optimal or deteriorating environment might first be revealed by heart rate changes during the stress of a uterine contraction. The severity of the deterioration can be assessed by the fetal acid-base state.

As in other areas of medicine, such as surgical or medical intensive care, biophysical and biochemical monitoring are both important for continued assessment and evaluation of the patient.

RISKS, EDUCATION, AND TRAINING

As with every procedure, there are definite risks associated with monitoring, particularly if a catheter is introduced into the uterus for measuring the intensity of uterine contractions. There are two reports of uterine perforation, and fetal bleeding may follow scalp sampling. Abscess formation has occurred following both placement of scalp electrodes and scalp sampling. The risk is undoubtedly greater for those with little experience or for those who have been poorly instructed. In our own clinic, we have had less than a 1 per cent incidence of fetal complications and no maternal complications in nearly 1500 monitored patients.

When there has been careful instruction of physicians in the correct techniques, and when due attention is paid to all precautions and safeguards, the risks of monitoring are minimal, perhaps of comparable order to a venipuncture or a low forceps delivery. Education in the operation, use, and care of fetal monitors should be extended to nurses as well as physicians. Interpretation of the heart rate patterns should also be taught to both nurses and physicians. In the future, this will become simpler with the application of computer technology; automatic pattern recognition systems will be tied in with alarm systems.

The development of educational programs for obstetrical monitoring is probably one of the foremost needs to assure the implementation of these techniques into clinical practice. In our own experience, once a physician is knowledgeable about the physiology of labor and acid-base balance, has confidence in handling the instrument, and is familiar with the various heart rate patterns and the mechanisms involved, he becomes unwilling to conduct a delivery without the benefit of additional information. Too often in the past a monitor has been bought or lent, minimal instruction has been given by a salesman, and the instrument is left to be "tried out" by a junior physician. Such a trial is doomed to failure.

Education of the nursing staff is an essential component of a monitoring program. It is important both from the point of view of care and use of equipment, as well as for its value in alerting the physicians to abnormalities. It will also help free the nursing staff from the burden of individually observing and recording data from each patient.

The mother must also be educated during the antepartum period. In this modern age of television, intensive care units, and computer technology, the general public is already prepared to accept new instrumentation for better diagnosis and treatment. If the mother is educated during her antenatal visits, there will be no reason for alarm over instruments when she comes into labor.

The lack of adequate education of both physicians and patients has undoubtedly led to many misconceptions and is probably responsible for the view expressed by some obstetricians that the electronic equipment is alarming to the patient, and that the whole operation of monitoring is a potentially danger-ous interference, likely to impede the normal physiological progress of labor.

CONTROL STUDY

The possibility of conducting a controlled study to determine the benefit of fetal monitoring has been raised. Such a study would require a monitored group for which information was available to the physician, a monitored group for which information was not available, and a nonmonitored group which would be followed only by standard clinical methods. Because of the experimental infor-mation on the mechanisms of various heart rate patterns and the clinical correla-tions between loss of baseline irregularity, late deceleration, and fetal hypoxia, and because of the demonstrated relationships between fetal hypoxia, acidosis, and brain damage, it would not be morally defensible to gather such information and withhold it from the physician or patient. Furthermore, to conduct such a study in an institution in which the physicians were not aware of the significance of the findings would not resolve this ethical dilemma.

Monitoring is not a treatment but a means of gathering more information. A controlled study would be warranted should there be significant risks associ-ated with the techniques. As already discussed, the risk is minimal and these techniques even in relatively inexperienced hands have been shown to be safe. It should be pointed out that monitoring of heart rate, electrocardiogram, blood pressure, or acid-base state were all introduced into operating rooms, surgical recovery rooms, and intensive care units without there ever being a demand for a controlled trial.

The value of monitoring depends upon an understanding and an interpre-tation of the findings by the physician, who then takes appropriate action. Moni-toring without appropriate action will not change the outcome, nor will it provide an answer as to the value of monitoring.

WHOM TO MONITOR

Ideally some level of monitoring should be available to every patient. Unanticipated complications may occur even in the most normal pregnancies.

For those at lowest risk, external monitoring of heart rate and uterine pressure will be sufficient to detect any potential problem. Should untoward dif-ficulties arise, and more precise information be deemed necessary, the mem-branes can be ruptured, a scalp sample taken, and a clip electrode applied directly. For those at high risk, the same sequence may be followed, but the physician should be aware of the present limitations of the indirect external system.

MONITORING AND CESAREAN SECTION RATE

The cesarean section rate has been reported to decrease rather than increase with the introduction of monitoring. There are probably several reasons for this. Intermittent compression of the umbilical cord can produce marked irregularity of the fetal heart without seriously jeopardizing the fetus. It is likely that many cesarean sections have been performed unnecessarily for this very reason. Monitoring, particularly of the fetal acid-base state, allows the obstetrician to follow these patients with confidence, and many can proceed to deliver normally.

Cost

The cost of introducing monitoring into an obstetric unit is not insignificant. However, the same argument has been raised in the past in relation to other new diagnostic techniques. The cost of an initial outlay is between $15,000 and $40,000, depending on the number of deliveries to be monitored. This cost has to be weighed against that of maintaining a brain-damaged individual, which has been estimated to be approximately $20,000 per year. This does not take into account the untold mental suffering of the parents and family of the brain-damaged child.

It has been claimed that a large number of additional personnel would be needed, which would greatly increase the cost. Such an argument is erroneous, since the present delivery room personnel can be taught to use the equipment and interpret the results. Monitoring of every patient has been successfully introduced even in a small community hospital with no resident house staff. For larger hospitals, some additional staff is desirable, particularly a bioengineer or the equivalent and a laboratory technician.

Historical perspective

Similar resistance has been encountered in the past, when new diagnostic techniques were first introduced into clinical practice. X-ray pelvimetery is a good example. Initially, this was a research technique, limited to a few university centers. Now it is available in nearly every hospital with a sizable obstetrical service. Analysis of blood for acid-base state and electrolyte composition was also purely a research investigation less than 20 years ago. Advances in instrumentation technology and education of physicians now make these investigations mandatory for the management of such conditions as diabetic acidosis, severe hydration, or diarrhea.

Summary

It now seems that we have reached a point in time when new diagnostic technology should be introduced into obstetrics as it has been into medicine, surgery, and pediatrics. Monitoring of the mother and fetus will provide the physician with additional and more precise information. Improvement in mortality and morbidity rates will depend on the physician's interpretation and action. Monitoring without acting on the results will not change the outcome. The successful introduction of monitoring into the practice of obstetrics requires not only new instrumentation but also education of doctors, nurses, and patients: For doctors and nurses, education in the care and operation of the equipment and interpretation of the results; for patients, education to increase confidence and reduce fear. Finally, a monitoring program will not be successful without strong support and leadership from the senior obstetricians and a well organized team approach.

With presently available technology, continuous intrapartum surveillance of the fetal heart rate, and intermittent capillary blood sampling, we have the ability to detect earlier potentially damaging hypoxia, upon which the obstetrician can make a decision for early intervention and expedient delivery. The important questions to ask are, "Is fetal monitoring going to provide more information upon which meaningful decisions can be made and is it going to increase the safety of the fetus during labor?" To both of these questions, the answer most certainly is "Yes."

REFERENCES

1. James, L. S., Morishima, H. O., Daniel, S. S., Bowe, E. T., Cohen, H., and Niemann, W. H.: Mechanism of late deceleration of the fetal heart rate. Am. J. Obstet. Gynec. *113*:578–582, 1972.
2. Bowe, E. T., Beard, R. W., Finster, M., Poppers, P. J., Adamsons, K., James, L. S.: Reliability of fetal blood sampling. Am. J. Obstet. Gynec. *107*:279–287, 1970.

The Status of Fetal Monitoring in Decision Making in Patient Management

Monitoring the High-Risk Fetus

E. J. QUILLIGAN
University of Southern California School of Medicine

ROGER K. FREEMAN
*University of Southern California School of Medicine
and Los Angeles County Hospital*

The ability to gauge precisely the intrauterine status of the fetus is a goal sought by physicians since antiquity and one that is not yet fully realized. The physician caring for a pregnant mother is interested primarily in whether or not the fetus is undergoing growth and maturation in utero. He also has the ultimate objective of assuring that the fetus at delivery has the potential to fulfill its entire genetic endowment. For purposes of discussion we will attempt to define efforts to judge intrauterine growth and maturation and ability to tolerate uterine activity as separate entities.

EVALUATION OF INTRAUTERINE GROWTH

Perhaps one of the oldest facets to be monitored and the least well done today is intrauterine growth. About the only functions the physician or midwife of antiquity had to monitor were whether or not the uterus was increasing in size and whether or not the fetus was active. Many myths developed correlating the amount of fetal activity and sex of the infant. Hippocrates thought that if movements are first felt in the third month the fetus is female and if first felt in the fourth month the fetus is male.

The monitoring of fetal growth was only slightly better until very recently. The conscientious obstetrician measures the height of the uterine fundus above the symphysis pubis at each visit; however, a recent study by Beazley and Underhill[1] demonstrated that there is wide variation in fundal heights both from patient to patient and within the same patient. They felt that the variability was wide enough to rule out the usefulness of fundal height measurements for either gestational age or intrauterine growth.

149

The relatively recent use of ultrasonic A scanning to measure the fetal biparietal diameter and to follow that diameter as an index of fetal growth does show great promise.[2]

FETAL MATURITY

Recent advances have greatly enhanced the obstetrician's ability to monitor fetal maturity. Until the advent of amniotic fluid analysis for creatinine and lecithin/sphingomyelin ratio, the physician was forced to utilize last menstrual period dates, onset of fetal activity, timing of first hearing of fetal heart tones, and epiphysial X-rays to determine fetal maturity in utero. All the latter are subject to wide variation in relationship to the gestational age of a particular fetus. Thus, in many instances, the physician's estimate of fetal age was in error by as much as 4 weeks. Tragic consequences could and did occur as a result of these mistakes, the most common error being the delivery of a premature child by elective repeat cesarean section.

In 1967, Pitkin and Zwerek[3] found a good correlation between amniotic fluid creatinine and fetal age; specifically, they found that any fetus with an amniotic fluid creatinine greater than 2 mg./100 ml. was probably of 36 weeks' gestation or more. Since their original article was published, other investigators have confirmed their work. There are, however, both false positives and false negatives with this test. The false positives that we have observed often occur in mothers with hypertensive vascular disease, many of whom have elevated blood creatinine levels. However, if one uses the test only when the maternal blood creatinine level is normal, this will eliminate the majority of this type of error (false positives). The false positive error is potentially the most serious for the fetus; however, the false negative value can also direct the obstetrician toward placing the fetus in jeopardy by indicating that the fetus should remain in a potentially hostile environment when in reality it is mature. The false predictions described may not in reality be "mispredictions." Amniotic fluid creatinine is probably a measure of either fetal muscle mass or fetal renal maturity or both, and thus these parameters may be quite accurately reflected by this test.

Since most premature fetuses die of respiratory distress, a more accurate assessment of the intrauterine fetal potential for external survival should involve evaluation of fetal pulmonary maturity. It has been known since 1961 that the principal surface active material in the lung is a dipalmitoyl lecithin.[4] This led Gluck and co-workers[5] to examine amniotic fluid for lecithin, determine the lecithin/sphingomyelin ratio and relate it to fetal pulmonary maturity. The correlation appears to be quite good. The majority of reports to date state an incidence of false positive values which is very low. In general, those infants who have developed respiratory distress and have ratios greater than 2 have been severely depressed at birth. It is possible that severe hypoxia and acidosis may adversely affect the ability of an otherwise normal lung to produce surfactant. The incidence of false negative values in our study is higher than that reported by Gluck and associates. If the lecithin/sphingomyelin ratio was between 1.7 and 1.9, 8.7 per cent of the infants died with respiratory distress. With ratios between 1.4 and 1.6, 25 per cent died with respiratory distress; with ratios between 1.1 and 1.3, 33 per cent died, and with ratios of less than 1.0, 100 per cent died with respiratory distress. Thus the test seems highly valuable if the ratio is above 2 and slightly less valuable when ratios are lower.

EVALUATION OF FETAL WELL-BEING DURING THE THIRD TRIMESTER

Two tests that we have found of great value are the determination of 24-hour urinary estriol levels and the oxytocin challenge test.

The use of urinary estriol to follow high-risk fetuses during the third trimester of pregnancy has been used since 1963, when Greene and Touchstone[6] reported on 279 pregnancies that were followed with 24-hour urinary estriol determinations. Since that time, the relative contributions of fetus, placenta, and mother to the total urinary estriol have been well studied. The real value of using estriol as a guideline for fetal well-being has been subject to considerable discussion. Originally Greene felt the test was most valuable in assessing the status of a fetus of a diabetic mother, but he now feels this is not the case.[7] He does feel the test is helpful in the management of hypertensive pregnant patients. Our own view is that 24-hour urinary estriol determinations can be helpful in many types of high-risk pregnancy, including diabetes, hypertension, and postmaturity. To obtain reliable test results one must follow certain guidelines:

1. The laboratory must do recovery studies with each determination.

2. The test must be available on a daily basis.

3. While simultaneous determination of creatinine in the urine will help to detect incomplete collections, the day-to-day fluctuations in creatinine excretion are about as great as those of estriol, thus making changes in estriol/creatinine ratio less valuable than the true estriol excretion determination from accurately collected specimens.

Recovery studies help to reduce the wide variations obtained in estriol determinations that result from the laboratory procedure itself. For example, investigators using acid hydrolysis may find marked differences in the yield of estriol on the same patient's urine sampled two days apart, and since each step in the determination has potentials for fluctuation, recovery procedures using labeled estriol as an internal standard will help to minimize these problems.

Performing the test daily helps minimize the chances of missing a significant decrease in estriol value. In a recent study of 60 pregnant diabetic patients, Goebelsmann and associates[8] found that 60 per cent of the significant drops in estriol would have been missed had the test been performed on a biweekly basis. Using a daily determination also gives the obstetrician the opportunity to follow a pattern of excretion, which is most important, since a diagnosis of fetal jeopardy can seldom be made on the basis of a single determination. In our laboratory, a fall of 40 per cent from the mean of the three days preceding the fall is considered significant. Using this technique, we have had only one unexpected fetal death in over 300 high-risk pregnancies. Since we have, in general, interrupted the pregnancy when the fall was 50 per cent or greater, we cannot honestly state how many fetuses would have been lost had we not acted. In some instances, the estriol values may start at very low levels and remain so. This is particularly true in the hypertensive diseases of pregnancy, making the calculation of a significant fall particularly difficult.

It is very important that the patient's drug ingestion history be known when evaluating urinary estriol excretion. Maternal exogenous corticosteroid administration will depress fetal pituitary activity and consequently fetal adrenal activity, as well as those of the mother, thus lowering the fetal androgenic precursors available to the placenta and reducing estriol secretion. Ampicillin appears to lower estriol excretion, while Mandelamine and glucose interfere with the determination.

A second test which may assist in the antepartum evaluation of the fetus is the oxytocin challenge test. This test is based on the response of the fetal heart to uterine contractions. The test is performed by stimulating uterine activity with an oxytocin infusion given by pump while recording both fetal heart rate and uterine activity. The uterine activity is recorded by an external tocodynamometer and the fetal heart rate by either an ultrasonic transducer or a microphone. The oxytocin infusion is started at 0.5 milliunits per minute and increased until there is regular uterine activity until a late deceleration of the fetal heart rate occurs. If there is no late deceleration of the fetal heart rate after 30 minutes of uterine activity, the test is said to be negative. In our own experience we have had only one infant die in utero within one week of a negative test, this in the face of several hundred tests on high-risk fetuses. This would seem to indicate that a negative test can, in general, give the obstetrician confidence that the fetus will tolerate its environment for at least another week. What of a positive test? In a recent study,[9] we performed the test but did not give the managing obstetrician our results. These fetuses died in utero after a positive test. There were also more low Apgar scores in the fetuses with positive tests than in those with negative test results. The oxytocin challenge test appears to become positive before the estriol level falls. However, this is not to say that all fetuses with a positive test will either have a low Apgar score or die in utero. We have had cases in which the fetus tolerated labor without difficulty after obtaining a positive oxytocin challenge test. The test is, therefore, most helpful when results are negative, which reassures the obstetrician that the fetus is not in jeopardy. In the face of both a positive oxytocin challenge test and falling estriol values, however, we feel the fetus should be delivered.

EVALUATION OF THE FETUS DURING LABOR

The time-honored method of fetal evaluation during labor is observation of changes in the fetal heart rate. The introduction of better transducers (scalp electrodes and ultrasonic and phonocardiographic transducers) plus good electronic design has enabled Hon and Quilligan[10] and others to classify patterns of fetal heart rate change in response to uterine contractions. These patterns are the well known early, late, and variable decelerations (Figure 5-1). All types of late deceleration (mild, moderate, and severe) and the more severe variable deceleration are associated with a higher incidence of fetal compromise. Since some fetuses are not in jeopardy with the above-mentioned patterns, other criteria must be utilized to further define the specific fetus at risk. Two areas of the fetal heart rate tracing are worth noting. Both involve the baseline fetal heart rate, in contrast to the periodic changes mentioned above. Normally there is a baseline irregularity of about 3 to 5 cycles per second. This represents an interplay between the sympathetic and parasympathetic control of the heart rate and seems

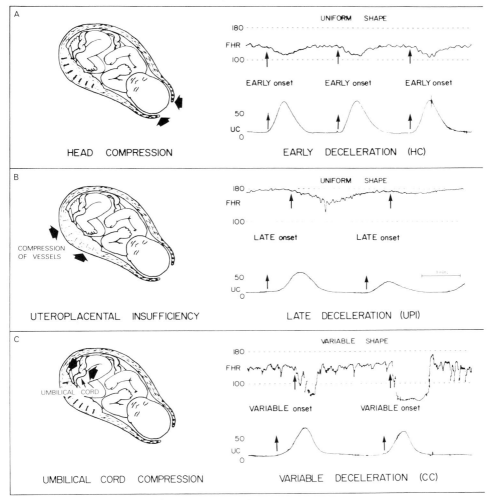

Figure 5-1.   Patterns of fetal heart rate change in response to uterine contractions.

to disappear in the compromised fetus.[11] Also, in general, the severely compromised fetus will have a baseline tachycardia; however, this tachycardia is not always present in the distressed fetus and may be present when the fetus is perfectly healthy, as in cases of maternal fever.

A second method of evaluating the fetus during labor is to observe its acid-base status. The technique for this was developed by Dr. Erich Saling,[12] who found that it was possible to collect blood from the fetal scalp during labor simply by making a 2 to 3 mm. wide and 2 mm. deep incision in the fetal scalp through a partially dilated cervix. The blood, collected in heparinized glass capillaries, can then be analyzed for pH, Pco_2, and base defict. If the proper instruments are used and the physician is absolutely certain the scalp bleeding has stopped before ceasing observation of the puncture site, complications are minimal. It is one thing to state a test is relatively easy and harmless, but we must also ask "Of what benefit is it?" Of fundamental importance to the maintenance of fetal neuronal integrity is a proper oxygen supply to those neurons. If the fetus is deprived of its oxygen supply, it can exist for a short period using anaerobic metabolism. Anaerobic metabolism is accompanied by a buildup of lactic acid in the blood, and the fetus therefore develops a metabolic acidosis. This fetal hypoxia is usually the result of a decreased maternal blood flow through the intervillous space or severe constriction of the umbilical vessels. In either instance, carbon dioxide is not adequately transferred from the fetus to mother; thus a respiratory acidosis also develops in the fetus. If only the pH is obtained from the fetus, the physician cannot know whether a metabolic or respiratory acidosis or combination of the two is present. For this reason, simultaneous measurements of carbon dioxide tension or base deficit, or both, should be made. Since the fetus can to some extent reflect the acid-base status of the mother, it is important to know her status as well. This can easily be determined by using capillary blood or nonstatic venous blood. The acid-base values obtained from scalp usually are slightly above the umbilical artery values and coincide well with carotid artery values[13]; thus they would seem to be an accurate reflection of fetal values. An exception to this statement is seen with severe fetal caput succedaneum. Owing to the marked edema and stasis, the scalp pH values may be significantly lower than those of the umbilical artery.

In our view, continuous fetal heart rate monitoring and fetal scalp blood sampling are complementary procedures. If the fetal heart rate shows no periodic decelerations (other than the benign early or mild variable), and there is normal baseline variability, scalp sampling need not be utilized. However, if there are moderate or marked variable decelerations, any degree of late decelerations, or loss of baseline variability, a scalp sample should be taken. If the pH is greater than 7.25, and in the absence of maternal alkalosis, one may withhold sampling unless periodic changes continue, in which case the fetus should be sampled in 15 to 20 minutes. Assuming there is no decrease in the fetal pH, no further sampling is needed unless the character of the periodic decelerations becomes more severe. If the initial pH is less than 7.25, one should sample again in 5 to 10 minutes, and if it is less than 7.20, sample again immediately. A decreasing pH or a pH which stays below 7.20 indicates fetal jeopardy.

Summary and Conclusions

All the previously described tests give the physician a better insight into the status of the fetus in its intrauterine environment. No single test is 100 per cent accurate, nor should a single test constitute the sole basis for management of a specific pregnancy. All factors concerning that pregnancy must be evaluated when arriving at a judgment concerning the fetus. Was the pregnancy complicated by maternal disease? What is the past reproductive history? The answers to these questions, plus many others, must fit into the equation before arriving at a final answer.

We have found the use of these techniques very helpful in managing high-risk pregnancies. In 1970 the stillbirth rate for our patients, as well as the neonatal mortality rate, was as good for the monitored high-risk mother as it was for the unmonitored normal mother.[14] This statement to us implies two things: (1) It is possible to significantly lower perinatal mortality rates in the high-risk pregnancy, and (2) if all patients were monitored the perinatal mortality rate in the low-risk pregnancy could perhaps also be lowered.

The change in perinatal mortality is probably only the tip of the iceberg. There are undoubtedly many brain-damaged children who could have been normal and healthy if they were properly monitored during pregnancy. This statement is much harder to prove, owing to a lack of longitudinal studies on monitored fetuses. Only indirect inferences can be made. We know the monitored fetuses have better 5 minute Apgar scores than unmonitored fetuses, and since there is a correlation between 5 minute Apgar scores and subsequent brain damage, one might predict that the monitored infant is less likely to be brain damaged. This is not to say that well designed longitudinal studies are not needed; every facet of present techniques needs continual testing and continual improvement. In addition, new techniques must be developed.

REFERENCES

1. Beazley, J. M., and Underhill, R. A.: Fallacy of the fundal height. Brit. Med. J. 4:404, 1970.
2. Willocks, J., Donald, I., Campbell, S., and Dunsmore, I. R.: Intrauterine growth assessed by ultrasonic fetal cephalometry. J. Obstet. Gynec. Brit. Comm. 74:639, 1967.
3. Pitkin, R., and Zwirek, S.: Amniotic fluid creatinine. Amer. J. Obstet. Gynec. 98:1135, 1967.
4. Klaus, M. H., Clements, J. A., and Havel, R. J.: Composition of surface-active material isolated from beef lung. Proc. Nat. Acad. Sci. U.S.A. 47:1858, 1961.
5. Gluck, L., Kulovich, M., Borer, R., Jr., Brenner, P., Anderson, G., and Spellacy, W.: Diagnosis of the respiratory distress syndrome by amniocentesis. Amer. J. Obstet. Gynec. 109:440, 1971.
6. Greene, J. W., Jr. and Touchstone, J. C.: Urinary estriol as an index of placental function. Amer. J. Obstet. Gynec. 85:1, 1963.
7. Greene, J. W., Jr.: Personal communication.
8. Goebelsmann, U. T., Freeman, R. K., Mestman, J. H., Nakamura, R. M., and Woodling, B.: Estriol in pregnancy. II. Daily urinary estriol assays in the management of the pregnant diabetic. Amer. J. Obstet. Gynec. 115:795, 1973.
9. Ray, M., Freeman, R. K., Pine, S. and Hesselgesser, R.: Clinical experience with the oxytocin challenge test. Amer. J. Obstet. Gynec. 114:1, 1972.
10. Hon, E. H., and Quilligan, E. J.: Classification of fetal heart rate. II. A working classification. Conn. Med. 33:779, 1967.
11. Kubli, F. W., Kaeser, O., and Hinselmann, M.: Diagnostic management of chronic placental insufficiency. In Pecile, A., and Finzi, C. (Eds.): The Feto-Placental Unit. Amsterdam, Excerpta Medica Foundation, 1969.
12. Saling, E.: Neues Vorgehen zur Untersuchung des Kindes unter Geburt. Arch. Gynäk. 197:108, 1962.
13. Adamsons, K., Beard, R. W., and Myers, K. E.: Comparison of the composition of arterial, venous, and capillary blood of the fetal monkey during labor. Amer. J. Obstet. Gynec. 107:435, 1970.
14. Paul, R. H.: Clinical fetal monitoring: Experience on a large clinical service. Amer. J. Obstet. Gynec. 113:573, 1972.

The Status of Fetal Monitoring in Decision Making in Patient Management

Fetal Monitoring: During Labor

ROBERT A. STOOKEY and MORTIMER G. ROSEN

The University of Rochester School of Medicine and Dentistry

Introduction

As with all other laboratory tests, the interpretation and relative importance of monitoring data must be considered in light of the clinical status of the patients (mother and fetus) at that moment in time. Monitoring information often is not so clear-cut that it alone will allow the physician to predict with certainty the condition of the fetus at delivery. With these limitations in mind, we will proceed to discuss fetal monitoring as it is used by physicians in our monitoring unit. No attempt will be made to cover the entire subject of monitoring, which rates a textbook of its own. Rather, representative monitored cases of labor will be presented as examples for discussion of our overall approach to this subject.

Types of Monitoring

The general categories of fetal monitoring systems now in clinical use include biochemical studies on maternal and fetal blood samples, and continuous external or internal uterine pressure and fetal heart rate recordings. It has been our experience that fetal scalp blood sampling is helpful in patient management; however, many of the hospitals using electronic monitoring may find scalp blood sampling inconvenient, both because the technique demands the presence of additional personnel, and because more time and effort is required of the physi-

---

This study was supported by United States Public Health Service Training Grant HD-00015-11A1. Also supported by the Grant Foundation, Inc., and the John A. Hartford Foundation, Inc.

Appreciation is expressed to Mrs. Margaret Steinbrecher and Mrs. Linda Bachelder for their continuing assistance in the fetal monitoring program.

cian in obtaining and interpreting the samples. This attitude toward scalp blood sampling has been described previously.[1]

The examples to be discussed will be derived from continuous recordings of uterine pressure and fetal heart rate as obtained from in utero sensors, since this is the fetomaternal monitoring system most frequently used at present. To some extent, similar inferences can be accorded to extra-abdominal monitoring techniques, with allowances made for some loss of precision—for example, in intrauterine pressure measurement.

Intrauterine Pressure Monitoring

Direct recording of intrauterine pressure (IUP) provides information not easily obtained by palpation of the uterine fundus through the abdominal wall. Abnormalities or changes in uterine tone and contraction patterns can be more precisely evaluated by direct intrauterine pressure measurements than by manual or external recording techniques. The IUP tracings have defined uterine contraction patterns which were previously unrecognized.

SYNTOCIN STIMULATED LABOR.   One of the more clear-cut improvements in patient care related to monitoring consists of objective observations of artificially stimulated uterine contractions. These observations allow us to determine the optimal rate of syntocin infusion and to observe disorders in contraction patterns which often are otherwise unrecognized.

Figure 5-2 illustrates normal-appearing contractions of fairly consistent rate, amplitude, and shape, with good relaxation between contractions. When this situation is present, we may be relatively sure that the stimulation of uterine contractions is adequate. The level of stimulation should be maintained unless the contraction pattern deteriorates, the fetal heart rate becomes abnormal, or the clinical circumstances (failure of progressive dilatation of the cervix and descent of the presenting part) suggest that the fetus will not accommodate to the pelvis despite apparently adequate forces of labor.

In Figure 5-3, A and B, we note infrequent uterine contractions of low amplitude seen during the early stages of a syntocin induction. Since no progression of cervical dilatation was observed, the rate of the syntocin induction was increased in accordance with our usual procedure in managing induced or stimulated labor. Following this increase in syntocin infusion rate, more frequent contractions were observed with poor uterine relaxation and almost no resting interval between the contractions. The fetal heart rate began to fall, showing both baseline bradycardia (Figure 5-3, C and D) and delayed deceleration (Figure 5-3, E and F). Therapeutic measures were instituted: the syntocin infusion was stopped, oxygen was administered, and the patient was turned on her side. The fetal heart rate and intrauterine pressure recordings returned to a more

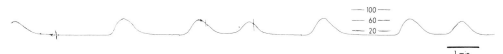

1 min.

Figure 5-2.   Induction of labor with intravenous syntocin: normal contraction pattern. Intrauterine pressure is measured in millimeters of mercury.

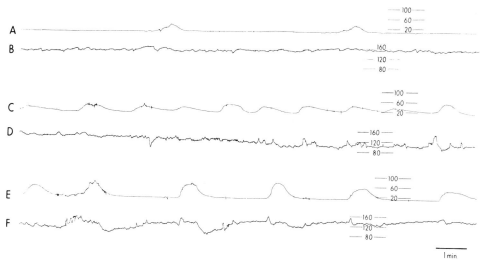

Figure 5-3. *A,B,* Induction of labor with intravenous syntocin. Soon after beginning of induction, infrequent contractions of low amplitude are seen. *C,D,* Same patient after increased infusion rate of syntocin; frequent contractions with poor relaxation and baseline fetal brady-cardia are noted. *E,F,* Delayed decelerations ensue. Because of these, therapeutic measures were instituted (see text). (*A,C,E:* intrauterine pressure in millimeters of mercury; *B,D,F:* fetal heart rate in beats per minute.)

normal pattern. Then, with careful resumption of syntocin stimulation, the spon-taneous delivery of a healthy infant was effected. No further abnormalities of the fetal heart rate or IUP recordings were noted. If continuous monitoring had not been used, the initial evidence of fetal distress might not have been recognized early enough to be adequately corrected by conservative measures. After the episode of fetal distress, the reinstitution of syntocin infusion would not have been carried out without continuous recordings of the resulting uterine contrac-tions and fetal response.

During syntocin stimulation of labor in another patient (Figure 5-4) the

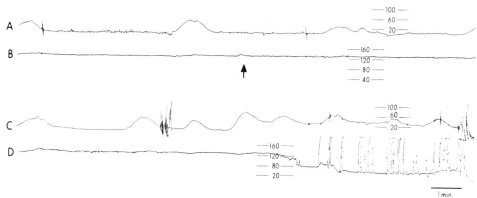

Figure 5-4. Induction of labor with intravenous syntocin. Syntocin infusion rate was increased at arrow, and this was followed by increased contraction frequency, incomplete uterine relaxation, and severe fetal bradycardia which did not respond to therapeutic measures. Emergency cesarean section was performed (see text). (*A,C,* Intrauterine pressure in milli-meters of mercury; *B,D,* fetal heart rate in beats per minute.)

infusion rate of syntocin was increased (at the arrow, Figure 5-4, A and B), followed by a dramatic increase in contraction frequency and intrauterine pressure baseline (Figure 5-4, C and D), and then by a marked fetal bradycardia. The syntocin was discontinued, oxygen was given, and the fetal vertex was elevated. At the same time the operating room was being readied for cesarean section. The bradycardia persisted while the patient was transferred to the operating room. An emergency cesarean section was performed, with the delivery of an Apgar 7 infant. The cord venous blood pH was 7.08, with a respiratory acidosis combined with a more severe metabolic acidosis. The elevated uterine pressure recorded by monitor was the only abnormality noted to explain the fetal bradycardia and acidosis. The persistent bradycardia (circa 60 beats per minute for several minutes in this instance) negated any less definitive measures. Had the heart rate returned to normal, delivery by cesarean section under emergency conditions might not have been necessary at that time. Continuous monitoring made it possible for this critical decision to be made, or changed, up to the moment of surgery.

OTHER ABNORMAL UTERINE CONTRACTION PATTERNS. As noted earlier, many varieties of contraction patterns are seen during fetal monitoring and as yet not all are clearly understood. These patterns are usually not detected by clinical methods of observation. For example, not all contractions are symmetrical in shape. Paired and even triplet patterns of contractions (Figure 5-5, A) are seen. At times, the spacing of contractions is too close to permit return of intrauterine pressure to resting levels. These contraction abnormalities often antedate fetal heart rate abnormalities. In specific situations (after placenta previa has been ruled out) spontaneous labor with evidence of antepartum bleeding warrants observation for increased uterine tonus which in its early stages can be most easily documented by intrauterine pressure monitoring. Finally, the patient who fails to progress in labor can be more accurately evaluated if contraction patterns are recorded by monitor (Figure 5-5, B). While the presence of atypical labor patterns is more frequently perceived with these techniques, the clinical management of the patient is still dictated by her progress toward delivery in the presence of these circumstances and the response of the fetal heart rate to these atypical patterns.

SUMMARY. It is apparent that measurement of intrauterine pressure may be of considerable value in management of the patient in labor, particularly in conjunction with fetal heart rate recordings. It provides precise, continuous infor-

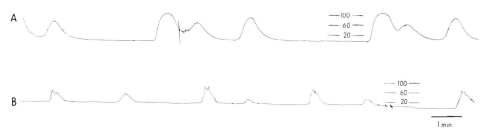

Figure 5-5. A, Induction of labor with intravenous syntocin: abnormal contraction pattern, with new contractions occurring during the relaxation phase of the previous contraction, is seen. B, Induction of labor with intravenous syntocin: abnormal contraction pattern with contractions of low and variable amplitude, seen in a patient who was making little clinical progress in labor. Increased infusion rate was followed by a normal contraction pattern and uncomplicated labor and delivery. (Intrauterine pressure measured in millimeters of mercury.)

mation, often essential to appropriate patient management. Syntocin induction of labor is in itself one of the more frequent indications for monitoring. In the examples cited previously, plans for emergency delivery were instituted while conservative therapeutic measures were being implemented. In both these instances, similar measures were undertaken initially with each patient, but very different subsequent management was required because of the difference in fetal responses to these measures as recorded by the monitors. Precise monitoring observations aided the physicians in deciding upon the clinical management appropriate to the individual situation.

Fetal Heart Rate Assessment

Among the original reasons for exploring electronic monitoring techniques were problems relating to fetal heart rate variation. In 1940, Lund,[2] using clinical fetal heart auscultation, stated that "The rate and rhythm of the fetal heart constitute the most satisfactory if not the only method for constant study of the fetus during pregnancy and labor. Accurate interpretations are as yet incomplete. . . ." These statements, made more than 30 years ago, are still appropriate. Although accurate methods of recording fetal heart rate are now available, interpretation of the data obtained remains incomplete.

Fetal heart rate variations have been described in terms of decelerations, with variations in pattern and time of onset of these decelerations with respect to in utero pressure changes.[3,4] These definitions will not be repeated here. According to various authors, the classical patterns, when present, correlate well with Apgar scores after birth,[4,5] and with fetal acid-base values during[3,5,6] and after labor.[7,8] It is not uncommon, however, for combinations of different patterns to occur during the same labor, as well as fetal heart rate decelerations which do not fit the described criteria. Several examples are presented below in the clinical settings which are essential to their interprtation.

DECELERATION PATTERNS EARLY IN LABOR. Clinical decisions must be influenced by the time at which abnormalities in monitoring information are seen as well as by the supposed predictive value of this information. In Figure 5-6 we see combinations of different decelerative patterns and the clinical course of one such labor. At first, early in labor (Figure 5-6, A and B), we see regular contractions of normal amplitude and shape, associated with fetal heart rate decelerations that were interpreted by the obstetrician as early decelerations. Labor continued, and one hour later (Figure 5-6, C and D), we note a combination of deceleration patterns, some of which are similar to those seen earlier, but these are now associated with an increase in irregularity of the fetal heart rate tracing and finally a U-shaped deceleration (at the arrow), which suggested fetal distress and the possibility of umbilical cord compression. The patient was turned onto her side, given oxygen and atropine, and watched. Decelerations varying in shape persisted. One hour later (Figure 5-6, E and F), we see pronounced and prolonged bradycardia. The obstetrician felt that termination of labor was indicated, and as the fetus was undeliverable vaginally, he elected to perform a cesarean section. An Apgar 9 infant was delivered in the presence of a large amount of fresh meconium. A prolapsed umbilical cord was noted to be present

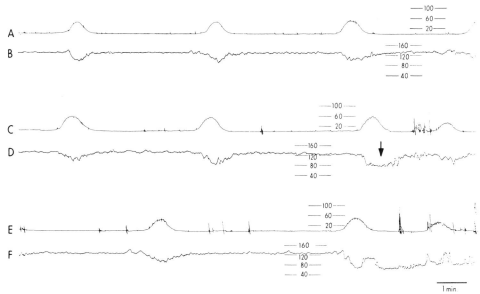

Figure 5-6.   A,B, Early spontaneous labor, with a normal contraction pattern and early
fetal heart rate deceleration. C,D, Same patient, one hour later. Early decelerations persist and
a "U"-shaped deceleration occurs (at arrow). E,F, One hour later, after therapeutic measures
were instituted. Decelerations persist and a prolonged bradycardia is noted. Cesarean section
was performed (see text). (A,C,E: intrauterine pressure in millimeters of mercury; B,D,F:
fetal heart rate in beats per minute.)

alongside the vertex, compressed against the maternal pelvis. The mode of delivery in this instance depended upon the stage of labor and the persistence and
severity of the deceleration patterns. Scalp micro-blood examinations might have
been helpful in reaching a decision at an earlier stage. Had the obstetrician felt
that vaginal delivery would soon be possible, he might well have elected to continue close observation as long as the fetal heart rate returned to normal. However, as conservative measures failed to alleviate the profound bradycardia,
delivery was thought to be the treatment of choice.

DECELERATIONS DURING THE SECOND STAGE OF LABOR.   Frequently when
the vertex is well applied in the pelvis, and again later, in the second stage of
labor, associated with maternal "bearing down," high uterine pressures are
recorded and pronounced fetal heart rate changes may be observed. In Figure
5-7, A and B, we see the onset of maternal "bearing down," with contractions
and the associated fetal heart rate decelerations. Between contractions, the heart

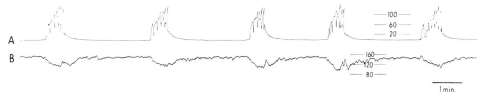

Figure 5-7.   Fetal heart rate decelerations occurring with maternal "bearing down" just
prior to spontaneous delivery of a healthy infant with an Apgar score of 9. (A, Intrauterine
pressure in millimeters of mercury; B, fetal heart rate in beats per minute.)

rate returned to normal, progress in labor continued, and shortly thereafter an Apgar 9 term infant was delivered spontaneously. This type of "bradycardia" when heard by auscultation has frequently provoked hasty forceps interventions in late labor. Through monitoring we have noted that transient bradycardia with "bearing down" is a not uncommon occurrence, apparently having no association with overt fetal morbidity. Continuous monitoring under these circumstances provides the most accurate means of assessing fetal condition until delivery is effected, with minimal trauma to mother and infant.

OTHER HEART RATE AND RHYTHM CHANGES. Persistent abnormalities of the baseline fetal heart rate (outside the normal range of 120 to 160 beats per minute are occasionally noted. In some instances these changes can be explained —for instance, fetal tachycardia in the presence of maternal fever is not an uncommon finding. It is our experience that tachycardia does not always denote fetal distress. At other times, the significance of these various abnormalities remains obscure and must be considered in light of any of the more specific changes which may ensue.

The loss of normal *baseline irregularity* of the fetal heart rate is also of interest,[4,9] but its clinical significance and prognostic value appear to be somewhat limited. Occasionally, baseline irregularity disappears transiently for unknown reasons. This phenomenon is also seen following drug administration to the mother (Figure 5-8, *A* and *B*), apparently being unassociated with fetal distress. At other times this phenomenon is associated with severely depressed infants.

SUMMARY. Many questions regarding the interpretation of fetal heart recordings remain. When patterns of deceleration are seen which are suggestive of a compromised fetus, management decisions rest upon the definition of additional parameters, including the stage and quality of the patient's labor, the adequacy of her pelvis, her present and past obstetrical history, and the response of the fetus to therapeutic measures. Fetal acid-base values as determined by scalp micro-blood examinations, when available, can also be very useful in confirming or questioning the interpretations of recordings made in monitoring. It is in this context that the data provided by a monitoring system contribute to improved patient care.

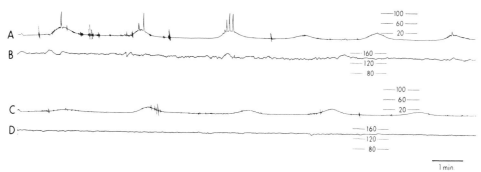

Figure 5-8. *A,B,* Normal baseline fetal heart rate irregularity during spontaneous labor. *C,D,* Same patient after caudal anesthesia. Contractions are somewhat diminished in amplitude and frequency, and baseline fetal heart rate irregularity is nearly eliminated, although the rate is normal. Irregularity of the fetal heart rate resumes as the anesthetic effects wear off. (*A,C,* Intrauterine pressure in millimeters of mercury; *B,D,* fetal heart rate in beats per minute.)

When Should Fetal Monitoring Be Used?

In the continuing effort to reduce unexpected and unexplained fetal morbidity and mortality incurred during labor, the time may come when nearly all patients in labor are monitored. At present, monitoring facilities on most obstetrical services are not sufficient to serve all patients' needs, nor are all patients or indeed all physicians prepared to make routine use of the technique unless specific indications exist. In general, we feel that any patient in whom it is demonstrated that the fetus is at increased risk over the "normal" obstetrical population is a candidate for monitoring. Included in this category are patients with antepartum abnormalities, such as preexisting medical illness, toxemia, small for gestational age fetuses, postmaturity, and previous fetal death, to mention only a few. In addition to these candidates for monitoring are patients identified during labor with "fetal distress," as indicated by presence of meconium, fetal bradycardia or arrhythmia, and, as noted earlier, any patient in whom labor is artificially induced, for whatever reason.

In our experience, the use of monitoring in a high-risk antepartum and intrapartum group has been associated with a cesarean section rate of 17 per cent, which is higher than that of our obstetrical population as a whole (7.4 per cent).[10] Similar findings have been reported by others.[11] It does not surprise us that on occasion we deliver babies with high Apgar scores, although the tracings suggested fetal distress. Conversely—and less frequently—we deliver infants who are severely depressed for no apparent reason, after obtaining tracings in which no abnormality was seen. These instances serve only to indicate both the limitations of the technique—of which we are already aware—and the need for further study.

Conclusion

It is clear that monitoring provides us with useful information. Because of the still unsolved problems of data interpretation, this technique may fail at times to eliminate our uncertainty entirely. The predictive value of monitoring is to some extent limited to a short period of time following the observed episode. Fetal prognosis and outcome may be altered, for example, by supportive measures instituted at the bedside or by a subsequent traumatic delivery. Progressively deteriorating clinical situations requiring rapid intervention must be separated from those which are stable and can be observed. Appropriate interpretation may prevent unnecessary procedures as well as indicate when emergency procedures are necessary. The value of electronic monitoring can be augmented by the use of fetal scalp blood examinations when indicated by abnormal fetal heart rate patterns.

It must be appreciated that our ability to evaluate fetal outcome with respect to clinical management in labor and delivery is diminished by our limited ability to assess the infant's immature neurophysiology and intellectual function in the neonatal period. Because of inconsistencies in results, judgment based on the first few moments of life is of limited predictive value with regard to the infant's later development. Most clearly deficient are our ability to accurately define subtle abnormalities in the developmental status of the infant and our ability to assess how these abnormalities may relate to our clinical management of labor. Until these questions are answered, the relative value of monitoring cannot be completely assessed.

REFERENCES

1. Tatelbaum, R. C., and Rosen, M. G.: Applicability and acceptability of fetal scalp blood sampling technique. Obstet. Gynec. 32:290–292, 1968.
2. Lund, C. J.: The recognition and treatment of fetal heart arrhythmias due to anoxia. Am. J. Obstet. Gynec. 40:946–957, 1940.
3. Kubli, F. W., Hon, E. M., Khazin, A. F., and Takemura, M.: Observations on heart rate and pH in the human fetus during labor. Am. J. Obstet. Gynec. 104:1190, 1969.
4. Caldeyro-Barcia, R., Mendez-Bauer, R., Poseiro, J. J., Escarcena, L. A., Pose, C. V., Bieniarz, J., et al.: Control of human fetal heart rate during labor. In Donald E. Cassels, Ed.: The Heart and Circulation in the Newborn and Infant. International Symposium on the Heart and Circulation in the Newborn and Infant, Chicago, 1965. New York, Grune and Stratton, 1966.
5. Wood, C., Newman, W., Lumley, J., and Hammond, J.: Classification of fetal heart rate in relation to fetal scalp blood measurements and Apgar score. Am. J. Obstet. Gynec. 105:942–948, 1969.
6. Hon, E. M., Khazin, A. F., and Paul, R. H.: Biochemical studies of the fetus. II. Fetal pH and Apgar scores. Obstet. Gynec. 33:237, 1969.
7. Quilligan, E. J., Katigbak, E., Nowacek, C., and Czarnecki, N.: Correlation of fetal heart rate patterns and blood gas values. 1. Normal heart rate values. Am. J. Obstet. Gynec. 90:1343, 1964.
8. Mendez-Bauer, C., Arnt, I. C., Gulin, L., Escarcena, L., and Caldeyro-Barcia, R.: Relationship between blood pH and heart rate in the human fetus during labor. Am. J. Obstet. Gynec. 97:530–545, 1967.
9. Hon, E. M., and Yeh, S.-Y. Electronic evaluation of the fetal heart rate. X. The fetal arrhythmia index. Med. Res. Eng. 8:14, 1969.
10. Strong Memorial Hospital: Unpublished data.
11. Paul, R. H.: Clinical fetal monitoring. Am. J. Obstet. Gynec. 113:573, 1972.

The Status of Fetal Monitoring
in Decision Making in Patient Management

Editorial Comment

The contributors to this chapter have made major contributions to the technique of fetal monitoring. Drs. Quilligan and Freeman chose to consider the subject of monitoring the fetus during pregnancy and labor. Dr. James and his associates discuss in some detail the interrelationship of the biochemical determinations of the fetus and how these values may relate to deviations in the fetal heart rate during the course of labor. Drs. Stookey and Rosen place emphasis on factors that influence the fetal heart rate in labor and consider what to do about correcting pathological states. All of these authors recognize the requirements for and limitations of satisfactory monitoring. As one of the contributors to this chapter has commented, "I have finally come to realize that a successful monitoring program cannot be instituted without strong support of the obstetrical chief and his staff and the addition of the electronics engineer." Undoubtedly, the presence of the electronics engineer is a requirement in programs geared to research and the acquisition of new knowledge.

Clinicians have long known that changes in the fetal heart rate are meaningful and subject to interpretation. They were aware that a degree of fetal bradycardia is a component of normal labor and that pathologic bradycardia is often preceded by a period of fetal tachycardia. Also, it was appreciated that a delay in recovery from a bradycardia some time after the contraction ceased (now referred to as dip II) was more ominous than a mere drop in fetal rate early on during the contraction, followed by rapid return to normal rate. However, only as a result of monitoring is it now realized that the deviations in baseline fetal heart rate may be pathologic.

Therefore, in the broadest sense, monitoring of the fetus in utero and especially in labor may be said to embody the entire philosophy of modern obstetrics—namely, to provide the necessary safeguards that will ensure that the new individual will be born without biological handicaps. In order to attain this objective it is necessary to continue to challenge current attitudes and practice. For example, the idea of prolonged labor as a means of patient management should be discarded. Certainly, hypoxic fetal distress is commonly observed in patients who experience excessively long labors, resulting in a substantial fetal loss and leaving its scars on an undetermined number of neonates. As demonstrated by Dr. Rosen, fetal monitoring is essential in the augmentation of labor to identify the onset of fetal distress should it occur and to take steps to correct it.

Moreover, it is generally accepted that in all high risk pregnancies, the fetus should be monitored through labor or until delivered by whatever is the appropriate method necessary to meet the problem.

Several questions remain unanswered, which undoubtedly will be resolved in time. An example in support of this statement is cited here. The question has frequently been asked whether a pathologic disturbance in fetal heart rate is consistent with fetal oxygen deficit and to what degree, if any. Both Dr. James and his associates and Drs. Quilligan and Freeman submit evidence that the pH of a scalp sample of fetal blood correlates rather closely with the extent of pathologic bradycardia in somewhat over 80 per cent of cases, truly an important observation. A criticism is also made to the charge that the cesarean section incidence increases inordinately whenever fetal heart monitoring is introduced. But again, this is difficult to assess unless all the patients are being monitored, not simply those at high risk. The most pressing question is whether monitoring assists in reducing neonatal morbidity—more specifically, regarding cerebral palsy and other devastating damage to the central nervous system. As indicated by Drs. Quilligan and Freeman, the data are meager, but if the concept is valid that a lowering of perinatal mortality rate is accompanied by reduction in the neonatal morbidity rate, one would expect the answer to be affirmative.

To have a permanent record of the behavior of fetal heart with each uterine contraction is a basic requirement not only in patient care but also in the investigation of fetal distress and possible long-term effects on the newborn. Instrument monitoring is obviously required if every patient is to be benefited, for it is unrealistic to expect that this can be achieved by a single individual on the nursing staff. For total effectiveness the instruments for routine clinical usage should be subject to ready application by the nursing staff. They should be externally located and operate without the need for intrauterine invasion. They should announce to a central board at the nursing station any deviations in fetal heart rate and the caliber of the uterine contractions. All of this does not remove the ultimate responsibility of the nursing staff or the obstetrician-gynecologist, for both must be immediately available to meet any contingency in the event that the recording indicates the fetus is in jeopardy.

6

Preferable Methods of Pain Relief in Labor, Delivery, and Late Pregnancy Complications

Alternative Points of View:

By Otto C. Phillips

By Bradley E. Smith

By Jess B. Weiss

Editorial Comment

Preferable Methods of Pain Relief in Labor, Delivery, and Late Pregnancy Complications

OTTO C. PHILLIPS

Western Pennsylvania Hospital and
University of Pittsburgh School of Medicine

It is now possible to offer agents and techniques to relieve all parturients of all pain. American women are well aware of this; most of them, therefore, expect some type of relief during labor and delivery. Some demand not only this, but total oblivion. Others have been taught, and insist, that the birth process is a natural phenomenon; as such, it should not be associated with pain, and artificial means of pain relief should not be necessary. Between these two extremes lies a broad spectrum, a variety of opinions and approaches—and actual needs.

If parturition is truly a natural phenomenon, what is the place for unnatural drugs and techniques? Since most therapeutic measures are assessed by weighing the benefits against the side-effects, how do we appraise obstetric analgesia and anesthesia? Are these adjuncts really necessary parts of modern practice or are they unnatural and hazardous luxuries?

Obstetrics in the United States is a hospital practice, and in this practice it is an established fact that the vast majority of our obstetric patients do receive some chemical means of pain relief for delivery. Furthermore, most attendants feel that analgesia and anesthesia during labor and delivery have earned an integral place in modern obstetric practice. This stand is based on the conviction that pain relief offers more than personal comfort to the mother, that a thoughtfully chosen analgesic regime, properly administered and at the right time, can improve the process of labor. In addition, it seems well documented that an adequate anesthesia makes possible the accomplishment of difficult or otherwise impossible pelvic deliveries.

Volumes have been published on the physiology, pharmacology, and techniques of obstetric anesthesia. It is therefore no great problem to assimilate the necessary information and skills simply to render a parturient pain-free or unconscious. Dr. Robert MacIntosh, the eminent British anesthesiologist, has pointed out, however, that any fool can offer admirable operating conditions by simply giving more anesthesia. Sound medical judgment of the physician should offer something in addition—safety. The obstetric patient is a special challenge; she is different from any other patient receiving anesthesia. Many anatomical and physiological changes occur during pregnancy which would be considered signs of a diseased state in the nonpregnant patient. In addition, most drugs given the mother have a direct or indirect effect on the fetus. These factors need to be taken into account by the obstetric anesthetist.

In addition to the above considerations, the obstetric patient comes to the physician for relief of pain from what is usually a self-limiting and self-resolving condition. At times there may also be disagreement between the physician and the patient regarding her *wishes* as compared to her *needs*. With the wide range of demands by patients (and all-too-frequent acquiescence by physicians), however, we might take another look at this natural phenomenon—labor—and at the basic role of analgesia and anesthesia in obstetric practice. This is the purpose of the present discussion, which will encompass three broad aspects: the need, the risk, and the personnel required.

The Need for Anesthesia

"Really normal labor is not a painful process. The use of anesthetics in such labor can afford no advantage and can even work an injury to the patient. In all cases of normal parturition the employment of anesthetics is as undesirable as would be the use of opiates during the period of normal menstruation."[16] The author of this quotation, writing in 1881, went on to point out that in civilized society the majority of mankind are living under abnormal conditions. He inferred, therefore, that most women did not experience normal labor, and that therefore it is usually associated with discomfort and pain. This discussion of labor and modern society was written by Henry Lyman in a textbook on anesthesia. Much published then, as now, was concerned with what was normal and abnormal, natural and unnatural. Webster defines "natural" as "conforming to the customary sequence or character of things and events." Normal may be considered a synonym; abnormal and unnatural are antonyms to both. What, therefore, is normal and natural; what is abnormal and unnatural?

Labor and delivery are usually painful, and this phenomenon is characteristic not only of modern but also of past societies. When Euffame MacAlyne of Edinburgh sought relief from her labor pains in 1591, she was buried alive for this felony. The years ahead brought a little more compassion, but available means of pain relief suggested negligible benefits. In 1677 a Massachusetts colonist proposed a prescription that included, among other things, a lock of virgin's hair and 12 ant eggs.[12] By 1800, more physiological efforts had been made. Dr. Benjamin Rush, a medical student at the University of Pennsylvania, wrote "An Essay on the Means of Lessening the Pains of Parturition." He proposed a method that worked—copious bloodletting, which obtunded the sensorium and achieved profound muscular relaxation. This effective but hazardous approach was expounded in a number of medical articles during the ensuing years. These and many other references to early efforts to relieve pain in labor suggest that in those days it was a common problem. Pain, then as now, was thus natural, or normal.[4]

Anthropological studies, in addition, fail to confirm the proposal that the pain of labor has arisen only with our advanced civilization.[7] While childbirth itself is universally looked upon as a natural event, almost all cultures make some attempt to aid the parturient in the hope that the delivery will proceed smoothly. During pregnancy, the mother is often subjected to an extensive set of taboos and rituals that relate to her diet, physical activities, social life, and sexual contacts. With the onset of labor, preparations for birth may be minimal or quite elaborate. Most frequently, attendants simply massage the abdomen and thus manipulate the fetus, but the mother may also be given ointments to make her supple, drugs to ease her pain, and amulets accompanied by ritual and prayer to help her and the child.

It has been alleged that primitive people are in general less sensitive to pain than their civilized counterparts. It is difficult to compare pain in a "raw" form from one culture to another. It is a subjective phenomenon, conditioned by culture and environment.[11] In some societies, stoicism in the presence of pain is highly valued. It is therefore praiseworthy and a matter of honor to respond with minimal expression, and indifference and hostility may be the response to a request for help. Most mothers in primitive societies have become aware that few if any techniques are likely to relieve their pain and that overt complaints will elicit criticism—with few benefits being obtained. Among the Navaho Indians, for instance, a woman who does not cry out is highly praised, and it is usual for a mother to go through the entire labor process with little more than a few groans. Suffice it to say that despite variations in responses from one society to another, evidence suggests that no society exists in which women do not experience pain in childbirth.

We can safely conclude, therefore, that throughout the world, and probably throughout history, the process of human parturition has been painful. This is "the customary sequence or character of things"; natural childbirth can therefore be considered painful, normal parturition is painful—that is the way things are. Endorsement of this motif can be said to come from none other than the Lord Himself, who, in fact, made it that way by edict: "I will greatly multiply your pain in childbearing; in pain you shall bring forth children" (Genesis 3:16). It may be noted as an aside that, being cast in the image of chauvinistic man, He ordained on the contrary that Adam be free from such discomfort while Eve was delivered from his rib: "And the Lord God caused a deep sleep to fall upon Adam, and he slept" (Genesis 2:21).

Pain is unpleasant and therefore undesirable to the recipient. Amid all discussions, past or present, of the pain of labor, one participant has seldom dissented from pleas for relief—namely, the mother. We are dealing, however, with a condition which in most instances will resolve spontaneously with good results. We must weigh seriously, therefore, *any* risk involved through our anesthetic or analgesic ventures against the excellent result likely to occur without our efforts. The balance may, of course, shift when a problem occurs. There are obstetric complications in which an anesthetic may facilitate or make possible an operative delivery, at times diminishing trauma to the mother or baby, at times contributing to the salvage rate of mother or baby or both. We must keep in mind the needs of the mother as well as her wishes. We must be familiar with the risks of anesthesia and balance the anesthetic needs against the hazards. We must know when to give anesthesia and which technique will answer our needs with the least risk. However, we must also know when *not* to give anesthesia; this may be our chief contribution to some patients.

Risks of Anesthesia

"Female, married; six times pregnant; had taken [anesthesia] at each confinement. Her pains commenced at 2:00 A.M. No one but a nurse was in attendance. About 20 minutes to 8 A.M., expulsive pains came on, when she called for [anesthesia]. After breathing it a few times, she threw herself violently back, gave a gasp or two, a slight gurgle was heard in her throat, and respiration and pulse instantly ceased. Her physician arrived on the spot ten minutes later, and found her dead. . . . No autopsy was performed."[16]

This death occurred on September 20, 1858—over 100 years ago. Has there been progress since then? Of course; but the sad fact remains that such mishaps are still occurring in hospitals in this country. Several things strike us about the case cited: (1) this multigravida would quite likely have been alive with a good baby had she not received anesthesia; (2) this patient would probably have been alive if an intelligent attendant had evaluated the situation and decided upon the choice of anesthetic; and (3) this patient would probably have been alive *if an intelligent physician had been present during labor and delivery.*

Childbirth is painful, and we are in an era when most American women consider some chemical means of pain relief an accepted part of the delivery process. Whether it is safe for themselves or for their babies they seldom question—nor are they likely to if their attendant physician doesn't. There is a wide range—sometimes minimal, sometimes great—of anesthetic needs. There are times when, after withholding anesthesia, only a recollection of short-lived personal discomfort remains. In other situations delivery is a brutal experience without anesthesia; again, there are times when delivery is impossible without anesthesia, death of the mother or baby or both being the probable outcome without its use. There is risk associated with every treatment, every drug, every anesthetic. We must be aware of the risks involved and take them into account with every delivery, balancing them against the needs of the particular patient. As suggested above, there are times when unquestioning acquiescence with the patient's wishes regarding anesthesia would not be in her best interests.

Death of the mother, of course, is the most serious complication that can result from our anesthetic ventures. Most data on obstetric mortality in this country derive from community maternal study committees; such projects are now active in 44 states and the District of Columbia.[17] The revised edition of the Guide for Maternal Death Studies was published in 1964 by the Committee on Maternal and Child Care of the American Medical Association,[2] and the outline in this guide is used by most of the study committees. It lists five direct causes of obstetric deaths: anesthesia, hemorrhage, infection, toxemia, and other (this included vascular accidents).

A review of 455,553 live births in the city of Baltimore[23] revealed that anesthesia was the contributing factor in 78 of the 427 deaths, or 18 per cent of the total; practically every anesthetic agent and technique was implicated. The most frequent problems cited were respiratory complications and circulatory failure following major conduction block, such as in spinal anesthesia. Respiratory problems were a factor in 60 of the 78 anesthesia-related deaths, and 24 of these resulted from aspiration of vomitus.

The major role of aspiration of vomitus in obstetric anesthesia mortality is confirmed by data from other sources. Basing their estimates upon a review of

2.5 million live births, Merrill and Hingson[19] calculated that there are about 100 maternal deaths in the United States each year from this cause alone. A review of 1000 deaths associated with anesthesia in Great Britain showed that over 50 per cent of all obstetric anesthesia mishaps were due to aspiration of vomitus,[5] and recent reports indicate that the incidence of aspiration of vomitus in maternal deaths is increasing.[27]

La Salvia and Steffen reported that 40 per cent of one group of obstetric patients vomited during or immediately following inhalation anesthesia.[15] Pregnancy alone had little effect on the emptying time of the stomach; sedation, however, decreased motility, and sedation during labor caused a 20 to 43 per cent reduction in gastric emptying time at the end of three hours. In 50 per cent of patients sedated during labor, a fluid level was found in the stomach 5 to 11 hours after ingestion of a test meal.

Crawford has recently discussed measures to prevent such fatalities.[3] Although the hazard of aspiration of vomitus in obstetric anesthesia is well documented, the sole emphasis in the British literature is placed upon safeguards to be carried out with general anesthesia; curiously, there is little reference to methods of avoiding the problem with the use of regional anesthesia. Conduction anesthesia in obstetrics would seem to be a more reasonable approach to pain relief in the parturient with gastric contents than would the continuous challenge of general anesthesia.

In the United States it is generally accepted as a rule of thumb that, if there is to be a reasonable chance that the stomach is empty, a 6 hour interval is imperative between ingestion of food or milk-containing products and the onset of labor. Regardless of the time after a meal, gastric juices collect when labor and fasting are prolonged; these can be vomited or regurgitated during anesthesia, causing a chemical pneumonitis. No patient in active labor, therefore, can really be trusted to have an empty stomach, and the indications for general anesthesia should be clear before an obstetric patient is exposed to the risk of this technique.

Death from spinal or epidural anesthesia usually results from hypotension associated with sympathetic blockade. Hypotension is a physiological response to spinal anesthesia. Although it is more marked with spinal anesthesia for cesarean section than for vaginal delivery, because of a more extensive block, the phenomenon should be recognized and treated without mishap.

A prerequisite to the intelligent treatment of hypotension is a clear concept of the factors normally involved in maintaining blood pressure. The most important of these are: cardiac output, blood volume, and peripheral resistance. We best maintain homeostasis by correcting or adding support to the factor or factors we find to be inadequate. Thus, if there is low cardiac output, we augment the cardiac output. If the patient is hypovolemic, we need to increase the blood volume. If dilatation of the peripheral vascular tree is the prime factor, we need to constrict these vessels. This simple outline serves as the basis for managing hypotension in the obstetric patient.

Howard and associates[13] demonstrated in 1953 that pressure of the uterus on the inferior vena cava can impair blood return to the heart in term parturients in the supine position. This is followed by inadequate cardiac output and a falling arterial blood pressure. Kennedy and his colleagues[14] noted that, although 17.7 per cent of obstetric patients became hypotensive following spinal anesthesia, the problem was resolved in 93.4 per cent of the cases by displacement of the uterus to the left, relieving pressure on the vena cava. This physiological entity is not related to the cardiovascular response to spinal anesthesia per se, but the hypotensive effects of the two are additive and should be considered together in their effect on the patient.

Wollman and Marx[29] have proposed preloading the patient with 1000 cc. of an electrolyte solution prior to spinal block for cesarean section. In this manner, we augment the blood volume, thereby compensating for an expanded vascular bed and lessening the discrepancy between the two. It is certainly a valuable adjunct in the prophylactic management of the problem; in addition, it tempers the hypotensive response to spinal anesthesia when it does occur and also makes it easier to correct.

Since the principal cause of spinal hypotension is sympathetic blockade with the resultant peripheral vasodilatation, the best therapeutic approach (physiological) is to correct this transgression. With a limited spinal or epidural block used for vaginal delivery, hypotension is rarely a problem, and it usually results from vena caval compression rather than the block itself. It can be disturbing, however, with spinal anesthesia for cesarean section. The drop in pressure can be minimized, nonetheless, with a prophylactic dose of 10 mg. of methoxamine (Vasoxyl) intramuscularly—in the deltoid, since this muscle is easier to find than the muscles in the buttocks of most pregnant women. The injection should be given as preparations are being made to administer the spinal anesthesia. Needless to say, a large-bore catheter should be well placed in a vein, in addition to following Wollman and Marx's preloading technique, whenever possible. If hypotension does occur after the block, the uterus is displaced to the left. If there is no response, 2 mg. of methoxamine is given intravenously, and repeated after two minutes if necessary. If there is still no response, it must be presumed that the hypotension stems from some other factor than loss of peripheral resistance, and another cause is sought.

Moya and Smith in 1962 reported that in a series of 1593 patients who received spinal anesthesia for cesarean section, only one failed to respond to vasopressors.[20] The problem in this case was corrected immediately after delivery of the baby, suggesting that it was caused by vena caval compression. These authors called attention to possible adverse affects of methoxamine on the fetus owing to uterine artery constriction and impaired uterine artery blood flow. Greiss[9,10] and also Shnider,[25] both working with pregnant ewes, have demonstrated a reduction in uterine artery blood flow with peripheral vasoconstrictors. Greiss reported a more favorable response to infusion of dextrose and water than to Neosynephrine, with improvement in systemic blood pressure without compromising uterine artery blood flow.

Most clinicians, including Moya and Smith, agree that arterial blood pressure is better controlled with methoxamine than with other vasopressors or with fluids alone. Finster reported maternal hypotension in 7 of 16 human patients who received 10 mg. of methoxamine prophylactically, 11 of 16 who received 100 mg. of ephedrine, and 15 of 16 who received electrolyte solution alone (Table 6–1). In addition, Apgar Scores and blood gas studies on the umbilical artery indicated no adverse effect of methoxamine on the fetus. This work refutes the several studies on sheep that suggest that methoxamine might be an indirect hazard owing to uterine artery constriction. The summary observations suggest

TABLE 6–1.   *Spinal Anesthesia for Cesarean Section Management of Hypotension*

PROPHYLACTIC TREATMENT	MATERNAL HYPOTENSION	1 MIN. APGAR	UMBILICAL ARTERY pH
1000 cc Lactated Ringers	15 of 16	8.2	7.248
100 mg Ephedrine	11 of 16	8.0	7.241
10 mg Methoxamine	7 of 16	7.7	7.271

that this drug corrects the basic problem, namely, peripheral vasodilation, that it is a valuable clinical adjunct in the control of blood pressure, and that it is without undue deleterious effects on either the mother or the fetus.

Anesthetic and analgesic regimes cause problems other than death of the mother; these can occur during the first stage of labor in addition to the delivery period itself. The obstetrician must monitor the progress of labor if he is to get maximum benefit from the drugs while minimizing the side-effects. Friedman[8] has plotted graphically the pattern of labor in primigravida (Figure 6–1) and multigravida. Some labor suites have a graphic record available for each patient, whereby cervical dilatation is plotted against time. Certainly, most obstetricians take into account the progress of labor before administering analgesic drugs; often, however, this aspect of management is heavily weighted by pleas from the patient or family.

The latent phase is associated with very little discomfort. It is a period, also, during which premature intervention with either systemic or regional drugs can delay the onset of the acceleration phase. It is therefore wise to withhold all but the most minimal amount of sedation until the second leg of the acceleration phase—until labor is progressing into the phase of maximal slope. After this point, properly managed analgesia (systemic, paracervical, epidural) is less likely to disrupt the normal progress of labor.

A summary of the highlights of one case will help point out the problems encountered when the attendant disregards these basic tenets relating to the pattern of labor. The patient was a 22 year old primigravida, wife of one of the residents. She entered the hospital at 9:00 A.M., cervix 2 cm. dilated, after 5 to 6 hours of desultory labor at home. Eight compassionate relatives were on hand, and, along with the patient, they were greeted in turn by the obstetrician. This

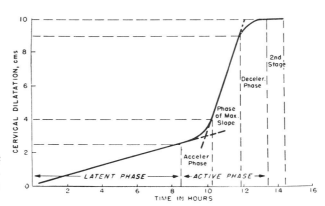

Figure 6-1.   Patterns of labor in primigravida and multigravida. (From Friedman, E. A.: Obstet. Gynec. 6:567, 1955).

sympathetic physician had once volunteered that he felt toward all of his patients as he did toward his own children—he could not bear to see them have any discomfort. The patient was promptly sedated, after which she became more vocal with each contraction. This led to more concern by the family, more calls to the obstetrician, more sedation. At 4:00 P.M., contractions were somewhat harder, but the rhythm was irregular, and little progress had been made. Pelvimetry confirmed the clinical impression that the pelvis was adequate. Oxytocic stimulation was instituted to "coordinate" uterine activities. At 6:00 P.M. a cesarean section was performed for fetal distress. This patient might have been spared an abdominal delivery if her labor had been allowed to progress without premature intervention by an overly solicitous attendant, influenced by a solicitous family.

Charting the course of labor is one of many forms of monitoring that are invaluable, indeed imperative, during the course of labor and delivery. Pulse, blood pressure, and respirations of the mother, cervical dilatation and station of the head, and fetal heart rate—the more frequently these are observed and recorded, the greater the likelihood that problems will be detected promptly. It is of course important that these recordings be made for a period immediately after the administration of any drug. We are all well aware of the possibility of hypotension after epidural block, fetal bradycardia after paracervical block (also associated with maternal hypotension from any cause), or diminution in intensity of uterine contractions following epidural block We must be cognizant of the complications that can occur and of the presenting signs and symptoms. Proper management is possible only if the patient is adequately observed and if the attendant obstetrician is present to interpret data that are recorded.

There are risks associated with all analgesic and anesthetic agents and techniques. The need for pain relief varies from patient to patient, and patients' wishes vary even more. Attendants must be aware of the possible risks and observant of the needs; with them, then, rests the task of balancing the two.

Personnel Required

In the hospital, the removal of a brain tumor in an elderly patient calls for a surgeon with two assistants, scrub nurse, and two circulating nurses, and an anesthetist. The patient's prognosis is about 18 months and the hospital investment is tremendous.

In contrast, the birth of a new baby at 4:00 A.M. is more often attended by one physician, no scrub nurse, one circulating nurse, and inadequate or haphazard anesthesia coverage. As a profession we seem to be committed to the fallacy that to be interesting one has to be an adult, fully developed, and preferably degenerating.[1]

This view of Dr. Allan Barnes in 1963 would suggest little progress since the comments of Dr. Branforth Brown in 1895, 68 years before.[4] Dr. Brown wrote that anesthesia in his era was "often administered by ignorant nurses, husbands, bystanders, even patients themselves, and not infrequently, recklessly and injudiciously by the attending physicians." He continued that "it is wonderful that evil results are so rare"; we marvel with him in 1973.

There is documentation too of the current sad state of anesthetic care for the obstetric patient. In 1961 the Maternal Welfare Committee of the American Society of Anesthesiologists reported the results of a survey.[24] In general, the extent of anesthetic coverage was related to the size of the hospital. There were, however, striking improvements when the service reached 2000 or more births per year. For instance, there was an anesthesiologist in the hospital at all times in 13.3 per cent of the hospitals with 1500 to 1999 deliveries, and in these the anesthesiologist administered anesthesia for vaginal deliveries. There was an anesthesiologist in the hospital at all times in 31 per cent of the hospitals with over 2000 deliveries, and in 35.7 per cent of these he administered anesthesia for vaginal deliveries. It is startling to note that in 27.4 per cent of the hospitals at that time, persons with no training administered anesthesia for vaginal deliveries. It is even more alarming to note that in 20.3 per cent of the hospitals, nontrained persons administered anesthesia for cesarean sections. Nurse anesthetists were responsible for anesthesia in 30.9 per cent of the hospitals and the obstetrician in 22.3 per cent.

Ten years later (1971) the American College of Obstetricians and Gynecologists sponsored a national study of maternity care; this survey included anesthesia techniques and coverage.[21] Few changes had occurred during the ensuing decade. Again, standards were notably superior in hospitals with over 2000 deliveries per year. In one-third of these hospitals an anesthesiologist was on the premises at all times. It's an interesting commentary that in only half this number (one-sixth of the hospitals) was there an obstetrician in the hospital at all times. In hospitals with fewer than 2000 deliveries, coverage by both specialties tapered off notably. In addition, in three of the 2000 plus hospitals there was no anesthesiologist on call, and in 16 of these there was no obstetrician. This review suggests that there is room for improvement in *both* anesthetic *and* obstetric coverage.

Interesting data are presented by Flowers in a survey in North Carolina in 1963.[6] Over 40 per cent of the hospitals seldom or never had any formal anesthesia coverage. In 16.8 per cent there was no anesthesia coverage by nurses, and in 66.3 per cent there was no medical anesthesia coverage. Twenty per cent of the hospitals relied only on nurses on general hospital duty and 9 per cent entrusted this service to licensed practical nurses and aides. It is remarkable, even alarming, that *two-thirds of the obstetricians responding to the survey felt that there were no problems of anesthesia coverage.*

Several factors contribute to the relatively small number of personnel trained in obstetric anesthesia. There is a disproportionately high investment in seemingly more "glamorous" fields, such as heart surgery, lung surgery, brain surgery, kidney transplants, and so forth. Also, the great bulk of surgical anesthesia is performed during the daytime hours, whereas the obstetric anesthetic needs are distributed around the clock. This latter factor alone would certainly make obstetric anesthesia among the least attractive of the anesthetic subspecialties. Furthermore, there seem to be divided opinions among obstetricians regarding the need for improved obstetric anesthesia coverage—indeed, maybe even the need for improved obstetric care.

Dr. William Mengert has recently pointed out that no analgesic or anesthetic drug can satisfy all the requirements of an ideal agent.[18] However, he continued, whereas the intelligent use of available drug combinations can satisfy many of the requirements, it must not be overlooked that the continued presence of an obstetrician throughout labor remains mandatory. Even with the growing movement toward conservation of physicians' time by utilizing allied medical personnel, Dr. Mengert seems to believe that the obstetrician can still make a most important contribution during labor.

The anesthesiologist agrees. It adds little to the zeal or morale of the obstetric anesthesiologist to stay in the hospital for the entire course of labor of a patient, only to await the obstetrician who arrives just before, during, or after the delivery. The foregoing, of course, applies only to some of the private services; fortunately, there are still many for which the obstetrician is in the hospital upon arrival of the patient. Another factor deserving consideration is the fact that many of the house services do little to encourage participation by anesthesiologists. It is certainly not a stimulating experience for an anesthesiologist (or anyone else involved) to administer anesthesia to a ward patient while a medical student accomplishes the delivery, assisted by an intern, instructed by a resident who is not scrubbed—with the attending obstetrician on the service remaining at the office or in bed, awaiting a call only if there is a problem.

Practicing obstetricians maintain that they are far too busy with their private patients to spare time to supervise deliveries of non-private patients, or to teach residents. This means, of course, a need for more practitioners if we are to close the broad chasm that exists between care of private and non-private patients. Willson[28] maintains that there is declining interest in obstetrics and that there are too few students entering the field. He also suggests that many training programs exist principally to meet a need rather than to provide excellence in training, and that possibly there has been a disproportionate concern over the number of practitioners as opposed to their "quality." He points out, however, that some medical schools recruit 10 to 12 per cent of their graduating classes into the specialty of obstetrics, while others recruit almost none. This does suggest that the caliber of the teaching programs may have a long-term influence on the quantity of practitioners choosing a specialty.

Pearse[22] questions the need for more obstetricians and suggests that we should not use previous methods and figures to predict the needs for the future. He points out that there have been unpredictable changes during the past five years, largely related to concern with population growth, a case which he admits may have been oversold. Along with stabilization of the birth rate, there have been changes in mores, so that "A pregnant woman is apologetic rather than proud. . . . Abortion is a *right*. . . . Men boastfully wear vasectomy pins." Although these reactions do not represent a universal attitude toward pregnancy and the family, there are zealots among our obstetrical colleagues who seem to give more attention and publicity to eliminating rather than nurturing the products of conception, referring to to the fetus as a "glob of amorphous protoplasm." Fosterage by obstetricians of the above concepts as the modish approach to obstetric practice would seem to do little to raise their image in the public eye; in turn, it might detract from efforts to entice into the field physicians from allied specialties.

There is a definite need for personnel skilled in obstetric anesthesia; this need encompasses physicians who can offer not only skills but also knowledge and judgment so as to provide pain relief safely. Anesthesiologists should consider obstetrics a legitimate field in which to offer their services, but enthusiasm will wane, or never be born, without encouragement from their obstetrical colleagues. The latter can help most by setting an example—that is, by being present during labor and delivery for private and non-private patients alike. In addition, and most important, the obstetrician must present an image of a skilled specialist, whose role during labor is so important that it cannot be entrusted to trainees and nurses.

Summary

Labor is a natural phenomenon, and pain is a normal part of this process. Since pain is an unpleasant sensation, usually caused by a pathological state, the patient predictably welcomes relief from both the problem and the symptom. However, the pain of labor is unique and contrasts with that of *other* disease states (DeLee has called pregnancy a disease of women). It serves as a valuable guide to the onset and progress of labor; in addition, it accompanies a condition that is usually self-resolving without medical intervention.

Do no harm! Most parturients welcome relief from the pain of labor; their wishes are understandable and should be given consideration. There are problems associated with every form of anesthesia and analgesia, however; injudicious choice or management of any technique can act to the detriment of mother or baby or both. Labor is a dynamic process and an intelligent analgesic regime is possible only if the attending physician is present throughout to interpret observations both on the progress of labor and on other vital signs. He should also be familiar with possible adverse effects of analgesic drugs on the parturient and fetus. Agents and techniques should then be selected in the context of the particular case. It is difficult to justify any regimen that will pose a risk for a normal delivery. On the other hand, an anesthetic may be admittedly hazardous, yet imperative for a life-saving operative delivery.

Properly handled, obstetric anesthesia requires not only technical facility, but also medical judgment, and the latter can be offered only by physicians. Labor is a continuing process; the course often changes suddenly and problems occur unexpectedly. Only if the attendant is constantly present can these be recognized and treated promptly and adequately. Obstetric patients certainly deserve better total care, and are entitled to be managed by more qualified persons than is presently the case.

Since the obstetrician is the primary physician for the parturient, he has a major responsibility in making adequate anesthesia coverage available. He can help by his example. An obstetric service on which an obstetrician is present, not just for delivery but during the entire labor, will greatly raise the morale of anesthesiologists. Their participation should be offered without regard to the financial status of the patient. Anesthesiologists have a deep responsibility to patients in all services of the hospital; their commitment should be firm and independent of the performance of the various other departments.

The obstetric patient is a very important citizen. Despite the hue and cry of population control enthusiasts, the growing fetus is a fact of life, without which the race would not continue. Once gestation is established, once the mother comes for medical guidance, the fetus should be given the best environment possible. This should include expert care, both obstetric and anesthetic, for all patients. We might heed the advice given to physicians by Lord C. P. Snow: "I believe we have to act as if each individual life were significant."[26]

REFERENCES

1. Barnes, A. C.: Quoted in Medical Tribune 4:24, November 11, 1963.
2. Committee on Maternal and Child Care of the Council on Medical Services: A guide for maternal death studies. Chicago, American Medical Association, 1964.

3. Crawford, J. S.: The anaesthetist's contribution to maternal mortality. Brit. J. Anaesth. 42:70–73, 1970.
4. Duffy, J.: Anglo-American reaction to obstetrical anesthesia. Bull. Hist. Med. 38:32–44, 1964.
5. Edwards, G., Morton, H. J. V., Pask, E. A., and Wylie, W. D.: Deaths associated with anaesthesia: A report on 1000 cases. Anaesthesia 11:194–220, 1956.
6. Flowers, C. E., Jr.: Anesthesia and analgesia: Result of a survey in District IV of the American College of Obstetricians and Gynecologists. Obstet. Gynec. 22:729–738, 1963.
7. Freedman, L. Z., and Ferguson, V. M.: The question of "painless childbirth" in primitive cultures. Amer. J. Orthopsychiatry 20:363–372, 1950.
8. Friedman, E. A.: Primigravid labor: A graphicostatistical analysis. Obstet. Gynec. 6:567–589, 1955.
9. Greiss, F. C., and Crandell, L. L.: Therapy for hypotension induced by spinal anesthesia during pregnancy: Observations on gravid ewes. J.A.M.A. 191:793–796, 1965.
10. Greiss, F. C., and Van Wilkes, D.: Effects of sympathomimetic drugs and angiotensin on the uterine vascular bed. Obstet. Gynec. 23:925–930, 1964.
11. Hardy, J. D., Wolff, H. D., and Godell, H.: The pain threshold in man. In Pain. Baltimore, Williams & Wilkins, 1943.
12. Heaton, C. E.: The history of anesthesia and analgesia in obstetrics. J. Hist. Med. 1:567–572, 1946.
13. Howard, B. K., Goodson, J. H., and Mengert, W. F.: Supine hypotensive syndrome in late pregnancy. Obstet. Gynec. 1:371–377, 1953.
14. Kennedy, R. L., Friedman, D. L., Katchka, D. M., Selmantz, S., and Smith, R. N.: Hypotension during obstetrical anesthesia. Anesthesiology 20:153–155, 1959.
15. La Salvia, L. A., and Steffen, E. A.: Delayed gastric emptying time in labor. Amer. J. Obstet. Gynec. 59:1075–1081, 1950.
16. Lyman, H. M.: Artificial Anaesthesia and Anaesthetics. New York: William Wood & Company, 1881.
17. Marmol, J. G., Scriggins, A. L., and Vollman, R. F.: History of the Maternal Mortality Study Committee in the United States. Obstet. Gynec. 34:123–138, 1969.
18. Mengert, W. F.: Practical Ob.-Gyn.—the open line. Ob. Gyn. News 7:26, November 1, 1972.
19. Merrill, R. B., and Hingson, R. A.: Study of incidence of maternal mortality from aspiration of vomitus during anesthesia occurring in major obstetric hospitals in United States. Anesth. Analg. 30:121–135, 1951.
20. Moya, F., and Smith, B.: Spinal anesthesia for cesarean section: clinical and biochemical studies of effects on maternal physiology. J.A.M.A. 179:609–614, 1962.
21. National Study of Maternity Care: Survey of obstetric practice and associated services in hospitals in the United States. Chicago, American College of Obstetricians and Gynecologists, 1971.
22. Pearse, W. H.: Recruitment for obstetrics-gynecology? Obstet. Gynec. 40:429–432, 1972.
23. Phillips, O. C., Davis, G. H., Frazier, T. M., and Nelson, A. T.: The role of anesthesia in obstetric mortality: A review of 455,553 live births from 1936 to 1958 in the city of Baltimore. Anesth. Analg. 40:557–566, 1961.
24. Phillips, O. C., and Frazier, T. M.: Obstetric anesthetic care in the United States. Obstet. Gynec. 19:796–802, 1962.
25. Shnider, S. M., DeLorimier, A. A., Asling, J. H., and Morishima, H. O.: Vasopressors in obstetrics. II. Fetal hazards of methoxamine administrations during obstetric spinal anesthesia. Amer. J. Obstet. Gynec. 106:680–686, 1970.
26. Snow, C. P.: The hospital as a humane institution, Address at the dedication ceremonies at St. Barnabas Hospital for Chronic Diseases. Cited in Hospital Tribune 6:1, December 11, 1972.
27. Unnecessary Deaths. Brit. Med. J. 1:437–438, 1970.
28. Willson, J. R.: Recruitment into obstetrics-gynecology. Obstet. Gynec. 40:432–437, 1972.
29. Wollman, S. B., and Marx, G. F.: Acute hydration for prevention of hypotension of spinal anesthesia in parturients. Anesthesiology 29:374–380, 1968.

Preferable Methods of Pain Relief in Labor, Delivery, and Late Pregnancy Complications

BRADLEY E. SMITH

Vanderbilt University

Introduction

"Controversy" at times seems to sum up the normal state surrounding decisions concerning pain relief in labor and the choice of anesthesia both in normal and in complicated pregnancies. This, however, is an encouraging and optimistic indication of the explosion of new knowledge pertinent to these decisions which has become available in the past decade. Important new research discoveries are at times difficult to identify, and even when recognized, may be difficult to translate into the practical clinical setting of our workaday knowledge. As usual in such situations, holders of various beliefs extol their viewpoints and attempt to convert their colleagues.

Because of the sheer number of existing controversies, it is not appropriate to attempt to enumerate or explore all of them here. Therefore, this discussion will intentionally ignore such important discussions as the proper role of psychoprophylaxis ("prepared childbirth") in obstetric analgesia; the advantages and not inconsiderable disadvantages and dangers of continuous extradural block during labor and delivery; the proper choice of analgesia for breech presentations, multiple pregnancies, or pregnancies complicated by cardiac conditions; and numerous others. These important subjects are omitted only to make room for more extensive discussion of current controversies that have urgent clinical implications applicable to "real life" medical practice.

NARCOTIC-ANTINARCOTIC MIXTURES

The first important controversy we will discuss centers on the now universally accepted observation that narcotics administered to the mother for pain relief during labor display a regular, predictable, and dose related adverse effect on the fetus.[24,68] All narcotics, with only slight and negligible variation in degree, are transferred across the placenta to the fetus, who may retain a very significant proportion of the drug.[37,67] In the immediate postnatal period, this transplacentally received and retained narcotic causes potent sedation, respiratory depression, and often acidosis in far greater degree than was attained in the mother from whom the drug was received.[22,45,68] This enhanced effect on the neonatal brain is the result of a biologic immaturity in the cellular structure of the newborn's brain leading to increased susceptibility.

Owing to deficiencies of various fetal enzyme systems, which in the adult act to detoxify, degrade, and excrete the narcotic, this undesirable effect continues for a prolonged period.[24,68]

In an attempt to circumvent the detrimental effects of drugs on the newborn, literally dozens of reports have advocated the simultaneous use of one or another combination of narcotic antagonists to be administered to the mother along with the narcotic. This practice has been repeatedly deplored by experts in pharmacology, obstetrics, and anesthesiology. Telford and Keats have reviewed these studies and emphasize that they do not satisfactorily demonstrate a decrease in the incidence of neonatal respiratory depression.[102]

More recently, Clark and his associates,[22] by careful laboratory studies of 30 women and their babies in an actual clinical setting, showed that there was insufficient protection against the respiratory depressant effect of the narcotic when nalorphine was administered to the mother. Even more alarming was the failure to prevent acidosis and the prolonged recovery from acidosis. In many cases, infants born after the use of this combination continued to have a downhill course into more severe acidosis rather than advance towards recovery.

These findings in humans agree with the careful animal investigation by Moore and Davis.[61] They demonstrated that nalorphine weakly antagonizes the respiratory depressant effect of morphine but is not effective against meperidine. In these experiments levallorphan did not prevent the respiratory depressant effect of either morphine or meperidine.

Similar findings were observed over 15 years ago after careful respiratory volume measurements in a study of 419 human infants by Roberts and colleagues.[77] In actual clinical human use there was no protection against the depression of the minute volume of respiration caused by meperidine when levallorphan was added to the meperidine. Recently, after a sophisticated computerized and automated evaluation of respiratory responsiveness was performed in human adult volunteers, Rouge has concluded that levallorphan in fact is ineffective and displays no antagonism to respiratory depression caused by simultaneously administered meperidine, thus explaining the consistency of this finding in the newborn in careful laboratory studies over nearly two decades.[82] Smith has recently explained these mechanisms clearly.[94] However, he has added that a recently available drug, naloxone, is exceedingly promising.

Owing to insufficient experience in testing, the Food and Drug Administration as yet does not approve of the use of this drug in clinical practice for reversing narcotic induced respiratory depression in the newborn. However, in an approved investigational setting, Clark has indicated very encouraging and optimistic results in reversing this type of respiratory depression in the newborn.[21] Nevertheless, its usefulness in the old manner of levallorphan-meperidine mixtures is doubtful, owing to frequent reversal of the maternal analgesia as well!

Mortality and morbidity after administration of narcotics during labor

The previous discussion on narcotic-antinarcotic mixtures leads directly to a confusing controversy. Despite general agreement that even small doses of narcotics administered during labor can result in some degree of acid-base derangement and respiratory depression in the newborn period, there is embarrassing disagreement as to the ultimate implications of these drug effects!

This controversy can be introduced by examining the report of the recent extensive Canadian Government Perinatal Mortality Study. As predicted, this report demonstrated a greater incidence of low Apgar scores after general anesthesia than after conduction anesthesia. In addition, the perinatal mortality rate was correspondingly far higher after general anesthesia than after conduction anesthesia in all categories except breech delivery.[71] As have other reports, the study also demonstrated the expected direct correlation of the use of narcotics and sedatives with depressed Apgar scores.[73]

Unexpectedly, however, *there was no correlation of perinatal mortality rate with the use of predelivery narcotics.* In fact, there was a statistical implication that the use of narcotics actually may have been associated with a *decreased* incidence of perinatal mortality.[71] These findings are, indeed, contrary to current thought and require explanation and discussion. Can low Apgar scores, in truth, be unrelated to perinatal mortality rates?

Several careful studies have documented the statistical correlation of low Apgar scores with neonatal mortality and abnormal early neurologic development.[24,31] Even so, the common inference from these studies that low Apgar score, regardless of etiology, always has the same prognostic implication, has never been statistically justifiable. The failure of low Apgar score stemming from the pharmacologic action of narcotics, in the absence of intrauterine asphyxia, to correlate with perinatal mortality may, indeed, have escaped detection in many large studies because the general premise of these studies itself failed.

The majority of low Apgar scores are related to intrauterine asphyxia, as evidenced by the characteristic hypoxemic acidosis in cord blood obtained at birth.[68] Therefore, the repeatedly observed direct statistical correlation of low Apgar scores in general with perinatal mortality and neurologic morbidity tends to be heavily weighted and influenced by the serious nature of asphyxia. However, the Apgar score can also be lowered in a far less threatening (although not necessarily benign) manner by direct pharmocologic actions.

Narcotics and anesthetics lower the Apgar score by central nervous system sedation. Decreased crying, muscle flaccidity, and sluggish reflexes are all recorded as "depression" in the Apgar scoring system. These readings can subtract as much as five points from a normal score. However, in the more frequent situation statistically, these points would have been subtracted by the effects of severe hypoxia and acidosis, a far more threatening and less easily reversible etiology.

Thus, in a general statistical sense low Apgar scores do correlate very well with neonatal morbidity and mortality owing to the statistical preponderance of asphyxia in producing the low score. But, in specific cases, low Apgar scores caused by the relatively innocuous pharmacologic action of the narcotic or anesthetic, but without coexisting severe asphyxia, could very well have a much improved prognostic implication. Statistically speaking, even an opposite or "protective" effect could, indeed, have been masked in previous studies by failure to consider that low scores may have very different etiologies.

Recently various authors have contended that this is a logical finding. They further allege that pharmacologic depression of the oxygen requirement by the use of these agents during asphyxia may actually protect the brain from asphyxial damage.[23,83] Secher and Wilhjelm have reported that both halothane and cyclopropane demonstrate this protective effect in fetuses of laboratory animals. In studies of 217 infants whose mothers used inhalation anesthesia, they also conjecture that, even though the Apgar scores were lower than normal, there was an increased survival rate. However, the series is small and controls were not used.

Cockburn and his colleagues have recently proposed that the use of pentobarbital during labor has a protective effect when asphyxia is experienced.[23] However, it should be pointed out that in Cockburn's animal study there was, indeed, only biochemical evidence of favorability in the "protected" animals. In fact, a greater proportion of the pentobarbital treated fetuses died in the neonatal period than did "unprotected" asphyxiated fetuses, usually as a result of respiratory complications.

In relation to this controversy, Sundell has recently reported a correlation between the use of sedatives and anesthetics during labor and a distinct "respiratory distress syndrome, type II."[100] Although there was considerable morbidity, the mortality rate in this syndrome was not high, as is the expected course in classic hyaline membrane disease.

These reports suggest that perhaps anesthetics and sedatives may, indeed, modify the pathologic character of brain damage owing to asphyxia in utero. However, the residual pharmacologic effects of these drugs postnatally may impede the overall ability of the newborn to adapt to life and to recover from the widespread derangements caused by asphyxia and acidosis.

Finally, protection against the neurologic effects of asphyxia and concern over the immediate postnatal reactivity and adaptability of the infant, however important, should not be the sole foci of our attention to the effects of drugs used in labor and delivery. A wealth of recent information indicates that careful testing can reveal impressive psychologic and neuromuscular pathology in babies whose mothers have received narcotics, sedatives, and general anesthetics. Inhibition of growth, depressed alertness, decreased ability to learn, and depression of reflex and spontaneous neuromuscular activity, in some cases persisting as long as one month, have been revealed by many authors.[18]

PARACERVICAL BLOCK ANESTHESIA

The proper role of paracervical block anesthesia in obstetrics is another unresolved raging controversy. Often considered a recent development, analgesia via paracervical block was actually reintroduced into modern obstetrics in 1945 by Rosenfeld.[80] The use of this block became widespread in the United States in the early 1960's for several reasons. It is simple to perform and is relatively safe for the mother. It can be performed by the obstetrician when specialized anesthesiology personnel are not available. It is effective in relieving the discomfort of late first stage and early second stage labor. The controversy concerns, of course, its safety for the fetus.

Soon after its popularity spread, reports began to appear indicating that fetal bradycardia, sometimes quite severe, occurred in from two to 40 or even 70 per cent of the fetuses.[37,85,101] Although this bradycardia at first caused little apprehension, allegations that it may be associated with fetal and newborn acidosis, or even, on rare occasions, intrauterine or neonatal mortality, led to an outcry in many quarters against its continued use.[36,81,103]

Reports by several authors have demonstrated higher than expected concentrations of the local anesthetic in the fetal blood when bradycardia followed paracervical block (dosage, 6 to 15 mg./ml. mepivacaine).[3,4,36] It should be noted in passing that none of the reports have proved a "cause and effect" relationship from this correlation, however.

Contradictory reports continue to confuse the picture. Several groups have reported admirable safety, as judged by perinatal mortality and morbidity rates, despite a small incidence of transient intrauterine bradycardia.[101] On the other hand, others correlate this bradycardia with fetal depression.

Shnider recently studied the course of 845 paracervical blocks and found a high incidence of bradycardia, particularly in primiparity, prematurity, and when fetal distress was preexistent.[85] They noted an increased incidence of depressed Apgar scores at 1 and 5 minutes in infants who had displayed bradycardia, but not in infants who had not reacted with bradycardia. In a subsequent study, the same group confirmed the presence of fetal acidosis in all the studied infants who had developed bradycardia, and in most cases were able to demonstrate unexpectedly high blood levels of the local anesthetics. However, in no case did the concentration of mepivacaine exceed 6.5 mg./ml. in the fetus.[4]

More recently, another group of investigators has reported a similar incidence (24 per cent) of fetal bradycardia.[35] However, they found no correlation between fetal bradycardia and gestational age, parity, fetal weight, or various maternal complications. They also noted fetal acidosis only in those fetuses in which intrauterine bradycardia persisted longer than 10 minutes. Furthermore, they noted complete recovery from this metabolic acidosis in all cases. They also could not identify any relationship between depressed Apgar scores and fetal bradycardia. In addition, fetal bradycardia could not be induced after injection of high doses of mepivacaine directly into three anencephalic fetuses.

Subsequently, members of the group reported on 86 additional patients who had experienced bradycardia following paracervical block and again found no correlation of bradycardia with low Apgar scores at 1 or 5 minutes.[70]

In passing, it is important to point out that some of the reaction against the fetal danger of paracervical block has been aroused by various reports in the European literature. Several of the most unfavorable of these have utilized the drug bupivacaine, which, until recently, had not been available in the United States. In a combined report comprising a total experience of 32,652 paracervical blocks performed in Europe, nearly 20,000 utilized bupivacaine, and approximately 4000 used prilocaine, another drug not commonly administered for paracervical block in the United States.[11]

In this exceedingly large combined experience, infant mortality following the use of bupivacaine and prilocaine averaged 0.16 per cent overall, in contrast to the overall mortality rate of only 0.03 per cent in 4000 cases using the drug more common in the United States, mepivacaine.[11] Here the heavy weighting of the statistics for the extremely unfavorable response to two drugs infrequently used in the United States might be suspected of leading to conclusions not necessarily applicable to clinical practices utilizing mepivacaine.

In summation, we are faced by diametrically opposed conclusions concerning the pathologic significance of fetal bradycardia. The etiology of the fetal bradycardia is not even clearly identified. Yet paracervical block offers many practical advantages in clinical practice. Therefore, considering that there are at least as many favorable reports as cautionary ones, it seems completely justifiable to continue their use in a cautious and knowledgeable manner.

When paracervical block is used, the dose and concentration of the local anesthetic should be limited to that which is sufficient for the desired pain relief. The use of bupivacaine (now available here) is questionable. If possible, the fetal heart rate should be continuously monitored by an electronic recording device. The occurrence of fetal bradycardia should not be disregarded but should alert the physician to possible fetal acidosis and depression of the newborn. However, moderate, nonprogressive fetal bradycardia is frequently quickly reversible and should, therefore, be treated by alert, conservative observation. The watchful obstetrician should be prepared to support the potentially depressed newborn infant with resuscitation and correction of acidosis, and apparently in very rare cases, support the ventilation and circulation.

ENDOTRACHEAL INTUBATION

A growing controversy in obstetric anesthesia is the use of the endotracheal tube in obstetric patients who are to receive general anesthesia for delivery. Aspiration of gastric contents is responsible for between 30 and 60 per cent of the maternal mortality caused by anesthesia in obstetrics.[17,107] The reasons for the existence of this danger are complex and require some statistical insight.[74]

In 81 per cent of all hospitals in the United States and in 97 per cent of large hospitals, almost all obstetric patients receive some form of anesthesia during childbirth. About 1 in 10 obstetric patients has been estimated to vomit under general anesthesia and in nearly one-third of these episodes the incident goes unnoticed.[59] Unfortunately, the availability of qualified anesthesia personnel to administer this huge load is deficient, frequently leading to the use of poorly qualified anesthetists.

Only about 12 per cent of vaginal obstetric anesthetics are administered by physician anesthesiologists, and only approximately 25 per cent by Certified Registered Nurse Anesthetists.[27] Indeed, only 8 per cent of hospitals reported that a physician anesthesiologist was on 24 hour call, and only 16 per cent of hospitals reported that a Certified Registered Nurse Anesthetist was in the hospital on a 24 hour basis for obstetric anesthesia. In fact, in non-teaching hospitals in the United States, only 32 per cent of the hospitals reported that anesthesia for vaginal delivery was most often administered by an individual trained in the specialty, whether nurse anesthetist or physician anesthesiologist.[26]

Furthermore, although this factor is impossible to quantitate, in the past the most inexperienced—or perhaps the least skilled—anesthetist has often been relegated to the obstetric delivery suite. A recent mandate of the Joint Commission on Accreditation of Hospitals, however, which will take effect within the near future, rules that the skill, training, and experience of anesthetists available for obstetrical patients must be equal to those of personnel available for surgical anesthesia in order for that hospital to continue its certification.

In an attempt to reduce this high incidence of death owing to aspiration during anesthesia, many authorities are beginning to advocate routine endotracheal intubation whenever general anesthesia is used in obstetrics.[88] Therein lies another controversy.

Endotracheal intubation is a potentially hazardous and lethal manipulation. Its safety depends directly upon the skill of the anesthetist performing the laryngoscopy and endotracheal intubation. Owing to the factors outlined above, by far the majority of those who receive anesthesia may not have access to anesthetists skilled in this procedure.

In addition, there are several other controversial objections to routine intubation. Unrecognized right endobronchial intubation occurs in a surprisingly high proportion of intubations done by poorly skilled anesthetists. The hazard of dislodged or broken teeth or even aspiration of a tooth fragment may include risk of litigation. These hazards are well known among anesthesiologists.

The advocates of routine endotracheal intubation sometimes overlook the fact that aspiration often occurs during those few moments after induction, before the endotracheal tube is in place.[30,89]

This danger is obvious if one elects to induce anesthesia by an inhalation agent and then inject succinylcholine before intubation. If muscle relaxants are not used, deep planes of surgical anesthesia must be induced for intubation. During this period the patient may well aspirate vomitus. In addition, these deep anesthetics are unnecessarily hazardous for the baby and cause many more cases of fetal respiratory depression than are necessary.

On the other hand, so-called "crash" intubation by the use of thiopental followed by succinylcholine requires the exposure of all babies to thiopental.[68,95] In term infants, this practice may be acceptable during vaginal delivery. However, when prematurity or suspected erythroblastosis fetalis is present, or when narcotics or tranquilizers have been taken, the thiopental passed to the baby can be both an immediate and a long-term hazard to the baby.[18,24,33,34,46]

In actual practice, transient anoxia and asphyxia resulting from inexpert attempts at intubation are quite frequent in unskilled hands. Furthermore, regurgitation and aspiration can actually be caused by inept attempts at intubation.[90]

Methods other than endotracheal intubation that are advocated to prevent aspiration are equally controversial and generally ineffective. Attempts to use gastric tubes to drain the stomach are uniformly fruitless, and the presence of the tube in the pharynx stimulates vomiting and aspiration during induction. Similarly, use of emetics is only partially successful in emptying the stomach, frequently leading to further emesis during induction.[90]

Antiemetics may depress the baby and are only partially effective.[24] Some are liable to cause hypotension.[24] Instillation of an antacid into the stomach before induction of general anesthesia is partially effective in decreasing morbidity following aspiration. However, a false sense of security may be developed, since the improvement enjoyed is only relative.

In view of these problems, the best alternative seems to be to avoid general anesthesia whenever possible. The wisdom of this course can be gauged by the combined Ontario study of 1967. Seventeen cases of severe aspiration of vomitus during general anesthesia occurred in 14,000 patients undergoing this procedure in one year. In the same year there were no aspirations in 7000 patients undergoing spinal and epidural anesthesia![72]

As a dividend, in most situations almost any method substituted for general anesthesia yields better Apgar scores and a lower perinatal mortality rate than does general anesthesia.[16,73]

If general anesthesia cannot be avoided, rather than following a dogmatic course, first evaluate the skill, training, and experience of the specific anesthetist available, along with the needs of the obstetrician and the relative dangers to mother and fetus. Only then can a reliable decision be made to intubate the trachea!

ASPIRATION OF VOMITUS

The discussion of endotracheal intubation logically requires some mention of aspiration pneumonitis and its treatment. Controversies are present even here.

The very high incidence of this problem is, of course, further related to the unpredictable onset of labor in relation to recent ingestion of food. Gastric emptying usually stops with the onset of pain. This tendency is further encouraged by the inhibiting action of pain-relieving narcotics on gastric emptying. In addition, the competence of the "pinchcock" mechanism, which at best inefficiently guards against regurgitation into the trachea, is largely destroyed by the displacement of the stomach upwards and to the left by the encroaching mass of the gravid uterus.[90]

During the induction of general anesthesia by all routes, the protective laryngeal reflexes are depressed by anesthesia, while at the same time the anesthetic frequently stimulates vomiting, particularly in the "second stage" of induction. Simultaneously, anesthetic induction excitement, "bearing down" efforts, or —later—external pressure to the abdomen applied by an attendant in order to speed the birth, all combine to increase intra-abdominal pressure and, thereby, encourage regurgitation.

Several pathophysiologic events occur following the aspiration of gastric contents.[40,57] Severe hypoxemia develops almost immediately with aspiration of even moderate magnitude. This hypoxemia results not only from the obvious obstruction of the airway, blocking the inflow of oxygen, but perhaps even more importantly from immediate bronchospasm, pulmonary circulatory spasm, and rapidly developing, widespread atelectasis. During this period, rales, rhonchi, inspiratory and expiratory wheezes, cyanosis, hypoxemia, hypercapnea, and increased right heart and central venous pressures are characteristic findings, and cor pulmonale may develop.[57,58]

Within the next several minutes to hours following aspiration of gastric contents, a severe "chemical burn reaction" becomes widespread. This reaction is marked by a prominent outpouring of proteinaceous exudate (which may amount to liters of fluid being produced from the trachea within the next 12 hour period). This characteristically pink, frothy proteinaceous exudate often secondarily obstructs the air passageways with froth and "bubbles." Finally, if the patient survives this initial period, the widespread necrosis, atelectasis, and exudation highly favor the development of secondary pulmonary infections, which frequently lead to widespread pneumonia and death. The mortality rate after massive aspiration of gastric contents is probably greater than 50 per cent.[40,57,58]

Emergency phase treatment of "Mendelson's syndrome"[40,90] consists of clearing out food and gastric liquid from the tracheobronchial tree as quickly as possible, followed by prompt and effective ventilation of the lungs with oxygen. Placement of a large diameter tracheal tube provides easy access to the trachea for suctioning as well as positive pressure breathing. These tubes can be maintained for hours or a few days with less risk and disfigurement than is caused by tracheostomy.

Controversy over the desirability of lavage of the upper airway with either saline or alkaline solutions is unresolved. However, several laboratory investigations indicate that the highly acid gastric content may be spread by this procedure and have recommended that lavage be avoided.[8,40]

Institution of prolonged positive ventilation for moderate and severe aspiration is mandatory for several reasons. It is the only effective therapy for the widespread atelectasis and it decreases pulmonary vascular resistance as well, thereby relieving right heart pressure. Maintenance of airway pressure also aids in suppressing further proteinaceous transudation.[40]

Bronchodilator substances such as isoproterenol cannot be delivered to the bronchioles for treatment of bronchospasm in any other effective manner except through nebulization into the inspired airstream. Frequently the persistence of frothy tracheal exudate will be so severe that 30 per cent alcohol must be delivered by nebulization into the positive pressure breathing device in order to disperse the bubbles.[90] This is accomplished by lowering the surface tension of the exudate.

Bronchoscopy may be necessary if large food particles are obstructing the airway. However, bronchoscopy performed during the period of hypoxia and hypercapnea can in itself lead to dangerous cardiac arrythmias, hypoxemia, hypotension, or even cardiac arrest. Therefore, it should be utilized in this early phase only when it is impossible to retrieve solid particles which are occluding major air passages by suctioning.

Tracheostomy may be necessary in those rare cases when very large particles of food cannot be retrieved either by suctioning or by bronchoscopy, and it facilitates suctioning and positive pressure breathing in treatment of the most severe and protracted cases.[69] Hazards of pneumothorax, mediastinitis, tracheal stenosis, and sudden massive hemorrhage from erosion into nearby major vessels are all complications of tracheostomy which should not be overlooked in making this decision.

Although some disagreement exists concerning lack of evidence that corticoids actually do suppress the proteinaceous exudate resulting from the chemical burn reaction, a consensus of authorities has favored intravenous injection of an anti-inflammatory corticoid, such as 200 mg. of hydrocortisone, immediately following suspected aspiration, and repetition of this treatment every four hours several times following aspiration.[38,40,69,90]

The majority of authors writing on aspiration pneumonitis have favored the use of a broad-spectrum antibiotic as prophylaxis against the severe bacterial pneumonias which frequently supervene from one to two days following aspiration. The actual drug and dosage are left to individual choice.

The continued treatment of patients with severe aspiration pneumonitis should be managed in consultation with a specialist specifically experienced in maintenance of artificial ventilation and acute respiratory emergencies, even if this requires referral and transportation of the patient to a more specialized facility. Movement of the patient should, of course, be carefully planned and coordinated in advance.

METHOXYFLURANE NEPHROTOXICITY

Use of methoxyflurane during labor for analgesia, or at delivery for anesthesia, has recently come into controversy because of the realization that methoxyflurane can in some circumstances be nephrotoxic. Because of the simplicity of its administration, the low incidence of nausea and vomiting that occurs, and its nonflammability, methoxyflurane is now administered to well over one million obstetric patients per year in the United States.[14,42] It is particularly efficacious in subanesthetic concentrations, as an inhaled analgesic agent during labor and delivery.[9,43,78,92]

In 1966 Crandell reported a characteristic toxic nephropathy occurring after long exposure to methoxyflurane in some surgical patients, characterized by polyuria; negative fluid balance; increased serum sodium, serum osmolality, and blood urea nitrogen; and lack of response to a fluid deprivation test.[29]

Recent prospective studies by Mazze have demonstrated his ability to induce this same syndrome by the administration of high concentrations of methoxyflurane for a long period of time. These studies have shown, however, that the renal toxicity actually results from free fluoride ions released from the methoxyflurane molecule by biodegradation and metabolism within the body.[55,56]

Although the incidence of renal nephrotoxicity with methoxyflurane is not great, many anesthesiologists are restricting its use in surgical procedures in patients with preexisting renal disease, in the aged, or when a long surgical operation is expected.

However, because of several physiologic and practical factors, there appears to be very little risk of nephrotoxicity after use for obstetric delivery.

Recent prospective investigations have shown that the serum level of free fluoride resulting after the use of methoxyflurane in anesthetic concentrations for one hour or less is far below the toxic level. Clearly, use of methoxyflurane for obstetric delivery usually extends for less than one hour, and in addition very low concentrations are required. Furthermore, even in anesthesia for surgical procedures, the incidence of this type of toxic nephropathy in young patients with good kidney function is the least for all age groups of patients.[55,56]

Resolution of this controversy should be aided by the recent demonstration of the safety of methoxyflurane analgesia in obstetric patients in Great Britain[79] and by the fact that as of February 1972, with the exception of one unproved case, no cases of kidney damage following the use of methoxyflurane in obstetrics have been reported in the literature or filed with the Food and Drug Administration or with the manufacturer.[14]

ANESTHESIA FOR TOXEMIA OF PREGNANCY

A controversy of over 20 years' duration still rages concerning the choice of anesthesia in toxemia of pregnancy. One group feels that the use of general anesthesia aids in the prevention of eclamptic convulsions and that spinal anesthesia in toxemic patients frequently leads to a severe fall in blood pressure, which may compromise chronically ischemic organ systems and, specifically, may precipitate the onset of eclamptic convulsions.

Opposing this view, another group points out that several of the physiologic alterations of general anesthesia, including very common brain swelling secondary to the pharmacologic effects of the anesthesia (particularly inhalation anesthetic), and the frequency of induction excitement,[32] transient hypoxia owing to respiratory obstruction or laryngospasm, and postanesthetic hypotension[1] (which is very frequent, particularly with cyclopropane anesthesia)[19] are perhaps even more likely to cause eclamptic convulsions.[20,91] These exponents would deny that the incidence of hypotension is greater in toxemic than in normal patients. They also cite the major argument that respiratory depression in the newborn is far less after spinal block than with general anesthesia when the mother is toxemic.

Historically, it appears that suspicion of the danger of spinal anesthesia in toxemia of pregnancy may have begun with a few studies involving very high levels of spinal anesthesia, with complete sympathetic nerve block, which were followed by hypotension and transiently decreased glomerular filtration. Because it is a major physiologic trespass, total spinal anesthesia is never used in clinical practice.[5,6,7]

Nonetheless, in contrast, subsequent authors have reported good therapeutic effect on toxemic patients of prolonged regional block in disagreement with the older work.[51,104] In addition, it should be emphasized that general anesthesia itself also causes a similar decrease in renal blood flow and glomerular filtration rate.[60,108] Furthermore, all these earlier reports indicated that the undesirable effects to which they objected were of a transient nature and were in no way a permanent threat to the patient.[5,6,7] Saddle block anesthesia, of course, causes only a limited rather than complete block of the sympathetic nervous system, as was the case in these experimental patients. In the clinical setting, the lithotomy position for vaginal delivery is another important protection against decreased venous return and hypotension.

However, the obstetrician and anesthetist should be aware of the characteristic decrease in serum protein plasma volume and total blood volume.[1,15] Correction of this deficit in total blood volume is an important feature before initiating spinal anesthesia in the toxemic patient, especially prior to cesarean section anesthesia.

Several reports have confirmed the probable safety of spinal anesthesia in mild and moderately severe toxemia.[51,91,104] However, few have attempted to contrast the results of the use of general or spinal anesthesia in comparable groups of patients in a clinical setting. In one of these few studies, the investigators examined 421 patients who received cyclopropane general anesthesia, 163 who received saddle block anesthesia, and 177 who were delivered under pudendal block or local anesthesia alone. There was a higher percentage of toxemic convulsions following general anesthesia than following saddle block anesthesia in these patients, though the difference was not of statistically provable significance.[91]

In this study, when blood pressure was expressed in terms of mean pressure, the incidence and magnitude of hypotension was the same in the groups that received cyclopropane anesthesia, saddle block anesthesia, or pudendal block anesthesia. However, the incidence of hypertension, which is in itself a warning sign and frequently precedes the onset of eclamptic convulsions, was statistically far greater in groups who received cyclopropane and local anesthesia rather than in those who saddle block anesthesia.[91]

By far the most important argument for the use of saddle block anesthesia instead of general anesthesia in toxemic patients is the marked advantage to the newborn infant. In the study already mentioned, endotracheal resuscitation was required in 8 per cent of newborn infants after their mothers received cyclopropane anesthesia, and in 14 per cent of the infants of mothers with more severe toxemia, in whom both cyclopropane anesthesia and constant intravenous infusion with antihypertensive drugs were necessary. However, there was a tremendously lower incidence for the necessity of performing endotracheal resuscitation after saddle block anesthesia in toxemic mothers: only 2 per cent![91]

Neither general nor major regional anesthesia is without danger in toxemia of pregnancy. These discussions have pointed out several advantages to the mother of regional anesthesia and have indicated that great disagreement exists over traditional fears of its use in toxemia of pregnancy. In this regard, the tremendous proven advantages to the infant of the toxemic mother would call for more liberal use of major regional anesthesia in toxemia. Experience with spinal or epidural anesthesia for cesarean section in severe preeclamptic toxemia (particularly with diastolic blood pressure over 112) is not very extensive, however. Spinal anesthesia and epidural anesthesia in these patients may be considered, but should be approached carefully because of the lack of "published experience."[51,91]

VASOPRESSORS IN OBSTETRICS

An extremely important and disruptive controversy arose during the middle 1960's, concerning the use of vasopressors in obstetric patients. It can be hoped that recent reports have laid to rest at last this needless confusion.

As early as 1962, Moya and Smith pointed out that although in their clinical experience with the obstetric patient, methoxamine was more effective in correcting maternal hypotension, ephedrine, rather than methoxamine, was recommended for use in obstetrics.[66] This observation was based on laboratory evidence by Mishrahy that vasoconstriction of the uterine arteries is caused by potent vasoconstrictor ("alpha constrictor") agents such as methoxamine and levoarterenol. The hazard of methoxamine was later confirmed in the pregnant laboratory ewe by Shnider and associates.[86]

Soon thereafter, Greiss and Crandell attempted to simulate spinal hypotension in pregnant laboratory ewes by the use of infused trimethaphan camphorsulfonate given by constant infusion. When hypotension was induced in this manner the use of phenylephrine and levoarterenol (both potent "alpha constrictor" vasopressors) restored the maternal blood pressure but did not restore the uterine blood flow to normal.[39] Unfortunately, they did not study vasopressors with a mixed alpha and beta action, such as metaraminol, ephedrine, or mephentermine. Subsequently, their work was interpreted to indicate that prophylactic or therapeutic use of all vasopressor agents in conjunction with spinal or other regional anesthesia during pregnancy is contraindicated.[96,98] At about the same time, Stenger and his colleagues also failed to point out the distinction between alpha and beta active vasopressors, implying that all vasoconstrictor agents indeed reduce uterine blood flow.[96,98] Subsequently, however, Lucas and colleagues[47] showed that by infusing metaraminol (a mixed alpha and beta stimulating vasopressor agent) during actual spinal hypotension in the pregnant ewe, maternal hypotension was corrected, and uteroplacental circulation and oxygen consumption of the fetus returned to normal control values.

Shnider and associates[87] demonstrated conclusively in 1968 that when ephedrine was used to correct spinal hypotension in the pregnant ewe, the fetal deterioration, which had already occurred during spinal hypotension, was arrested and there was usually an improvement in fetal oxygenation, carbon dioxide elimination, and fixed acid excretion.

Moya and Smith studied the response to hypotension and the use of vasopressor in clinical practice.[65] They studied 590 cesarean section births in which no fetal or maternal complications were known to be present. All patients received similar mild preanesthetic medication and identical management of spinal anesthesia for the cesarean section. In 279 of these patients, systolic blood pressure fell below 90 mm. Hg. In addition to deflection of the uterus to the left, off the vena cava, vasopressor was used in restoration of the blood pressure in all cases (approximately 90 per cent received ephedrine and 10 per cent received several other drugs). In the infants born to these patients, the incidence of depressed Apgar scores (1 to 7) was 18 per cent.

In 202 patients in whom the systolic blood pressure did not fall below 100, the incidence of depressed Apgar scores was 17 per cent. This was not a significant difference statistically from the patients in whom hypotension had existed and been treated with vasopressor. On the other hand, in 109 patients, the lowest systolic pressure was between 90 and 99. In these patients no vasopressor therapy was used. The incidence of depressed Apgar scores in this group was 28 per cent, a highly significant statistical difference from that group in whom the systolic pressure had fallen much lower, but who had been treated with vasopressor.[65]

This study demonstrates two points: that the prompt restoration of low blood pressure resulting from spinal anesthesia by usual clinical methods, including judicious doses of ephedrine, results in an incidence of subsequent fetal depression which does not differ significantly from patients who did not experience hypotension at all. It also demonstrates that in clinical practice the use of ephedrine despite preexisting hypotension did not result in an increased incidence of fetal depression, as has been implied by many.

Maternal hyperventilation

Moya and associates[64] noted severe respiratory and metabolic acidosis and oxygen desaturation in cord blood of two infants born of mothers who had been artificially hyperventilated. The resulting alkalosis averaged pH 7.67 and Pco_2 less than 17 mm. Hg during thiopental nitrous oxide anesthesia for cesarean section. Twelve other infants in whom the maternal arterial blood averaged less than pH 7.60 and in whom the Pco_2 was 19 mm. Hg did not develop pathologic acidosis. In addition, they displayed even less than normal biochemical evidence of the mild asphyxial acidosis usually present in infants at birth. These workers postulated that a reduction in uterine blood flow could occur when maternal Pco_2 falls below a critical level, which they believed to be 17 mm. Hg.[64] Soon afterwards, Motoyama and colleagues presented evidence in pregnant ewes that forced hyperventilation of the mother reduced the oxygen supply to the fetus.[62] The ewes were maintained in severe respiratory alkalosis for an average of 28 minutes each before sampling of the fetal blood. The average fetal oxygen saturation in these severely hyperventilated lamb fetuses was reduced only from 75 to 67 per cent in the fetal artery (8 per cent difference) and from 88 to 82 per cent saturation in the fetal umbilical vein (6 per cent difference). Prolongation of this extremely alkalotic state for 1 and 2 hours in two lambs caused severe hypoxia and acidosis.[62]

In all instances in these laboratory studies, severe alkalosis was maintained nearly twice as long as the average woman is under anesthesia for cesarean section. Despite this, the differences in results, although statistically significant, were clinically of little importance except in the two lamb fetuses in whom alkalosis was maintained for 1 and 2 hours, an extremely abnormal stress.[62]

In contrast to the reports of Moya and of Motoyama, Behrman concluded that in the primate, maternal hyperventilation resulting in an arterial pH of 7.7 and a P_{CO_2} of 12 mm. Hg did not result in untoward effects to the fetus. Although oxygen saturation in the umbilical and uterine venous blood decreased slightly, the amount of oxygen delivered to each fetus remained constant, owing to mild increase in umbilical blood flow and to shifts in the oxygen dissociation curve as a result of alkalosis. Uterine blood flow was also insignificant at this extreme hyperventilation.[12]

This conclusion was further supported when Coleman reported on a series of 14 human mothers intentionally hyperventilated during general anesthesia for cesarean section in whom P_{CO_2} averaged 14 mm. Hg, the highest arterial P_{CO_2} being 17 mm. Hg. Although a few demonstrated mildly decreased umbilical artery pH, umbilical artery P_{CO_2} was similar to control values, although umbilical arterial P_{O_2} appeared to be suggestively decreased.[25]

More significant, however, was the finding that except for one score of 5 and one of 6, all Apgar scores were 7 or greater, indicating no significant clinical effect of maternal hyperventilation on the neonate. In a study of 86 spontaneously hyperventilating mothers, Lumley and her colleagues also failed to demonstrate significant correlation with fetal acidosis or oxygen desaturation in conscious, voluntarily hyperventilating women.[48]

In summary, these studies provide a reasonable basis for assuming that an anesthetist with average skill maintaining positive pressure ventilation during general anesthesia for a cesarean section operation of average duration may rarely, if ever, be responsible for contributing significantly to fetal oxygen desaturation or acidosis in clinical practice. In addition, all studies seem to indicate that judicious, moderate hyperventilation resulting in a maternal arterial P_{CO_2} of 19 mm. Hg or greater may result in some mild biochemical protection to the fetus against the asphyxial stresses of cesarean section delivery.

THE EFFECTS OF OXYGEN ADMINISTRATION TO THE MOTHER ON FETAL HOMEOSTASIS

Several authors, basing their assumptions largely on experiments in sheep, have claimed adverse effects on the fetus when the pregnant mother breathes elevated concentrations of oxygen. These alleged untoward effects of oxygen inhalation have included decreases in umbilical blood flow, fetal oxygen consumption, total surface area of placental capillaries, and oxygen pressure in the fetal arteries.[10,63,76] However, Battaglia and his colleagues,[10] also studying the pregnant ewe, recently reported opposite findings for each of these allegations. These authors pointed out that the net beneficial effect of maternal oxygen inhalation was equivalent to an increase in uterine blood flow. Even previous reports proposing theoretic dangers from the maternal inhalation of high oxygen concentrations agree that in the hypoxemic animal or human (Po_2 less than 60 mm. Hg), oxygen inhalation by the mother results in a striking increase in fetal arterial oxygen pressure.[10]

Support for the benefit of oxygen inhalation in humans has recently been added by Althabe and associates. They have demonstrated a significant increase in fetal muscular oxygen in normal infants when oxygen was inhaled by the mother. They noted that in conditions of fetal distress, inhalation of oxygen corrected fetal tachycardia and fetal electrocardiographic evidence of uteroplacental insufficiency.[2]

Most recently, Marx and Mateo have also demonstrated beneficial effects from increased maternal oxygenation during elective cesarean section under general anesthesia. Fetal oxygenation was lowest, and respiratory function affected most, as measured by delayed onset of breathing if maternal arterial oxygen was below Po_2 100 mm. Hg. Fetal oxygenation was most favorable and onset of neonatal respiration was quickest when maternal arterial oxygen was 300 mm. Hg or greater.[54]

The current status of these findings seems to be easily summarized: a fetus in a good state of oxygenation and acid-base balance derives no benefit but also suffers insignificant harm from maternal inhalation of high concentrations of oxygen. On the other hand, the hypoxemic and acidotic fetus can be consistently demonstrated to receive exceedingly important beneficial effects from maternal oxygen inhalation.

THE CHOICE OF ANESTHESIA IN CESAREAN SECTION

One of the most controversial topics in obstetrical anesthesia has intentionally been reserved for our final topic: Is conduction anesthesia or general anesthesia preferable in cesarean section? Awareness of recent disagreements concerning vasopressors, endotracheal intubation, maternal hyperventilation, the immediate and long-term implications of medications for the fetus, maternal mortality from anesthesia, and a knowledge of the limitations, both in numbers and in skill, of anesthesia personnel available for obstetric anesthesia are all essential background information.

It is also helpful to know that at the present time in the United States, nearly twice as many cesarean sections are performed under spinal anesthesia as are performed under general anesthesia.[26] Seventy-four per cent of all cesarean section anesthetics are presently being administered by physician anesthesiologists and 19 per cent by nurse anesthetists.[27]

The most notable reason for this popularity is probably that in almost every report of clinical experience, conduction anesthesia almost invariably displays a far lower incidence of depression of the newborn than does general anesthesia. Both a decreased subsequent morbidity rate in the infants and a far lower maternal mortality rate have also been reported after conduction anesthesia.[41,97]

The Ontario National Study reported 21.6 per cent fetal depression in 573 cesarean sections performed under general anesthesia and 8.1 per cent fetal depression in 467 anesthetics performed under conduction anesthesia. In the same report, the perinatal infant mortality rate was 63.4 per thousand live births for cesarean sections performed under general anesthesia, compared to only 17.2 per thousand live births under spinal anesthesia.[73]

Data from the National Collaborative Study of Cerebral Palsy have shown an incidence of 38 per cent fetal depression (Apgar score, 0 to 6) at 1 minute after general anesthesia during cesarean section, but only 12 per cent fetal depression after regional anesthesia. With general anesthesia, 15 per cent were still depressed at 5 minutes, but only 4 per cent were still depressed after regional anesthesia.[13]

They noted, in particular, that a fivefold difference in Apgar score depression at 1 minute and a threefold difference at 5 minutes existed between cesarean section and vaginally delivered babies when general anesthesia was used. However, the incidence of such depression was almost the same as that in the vaginal delivery group when regional anesthesia was employed![13]

Neurologic examination at four months after birth revealed that 16 per cent of infants whose mothers had received general anesthesia for cesarean section had findings deviant from normal, as did 11 per cent of the regional group. Neurologic examination of infants in the general anesthesia group at 1 year showed 12 per cent still deviant from the normal, versus only 6 per cent in the regional anesthesia group.[13]

Both better Apgar scores and better neurologic examination results were seen in the regional anesthesia group as a whole, despite the fact that the premature infants received regional anesthesia approximately three times as frequently as general anesthesia, thus heavily weighting the results *against* spinal anesthesia.[13]

In consideration of specific general anesthetic or regional anesthetic methods, obviously only side by side comparison studies should be considered. Currently, only one example of each is in preponderant clinical use, so only these will be discussed. Only a few published reports attempt to compare, in a prospective manner, in a simultaneous study, and in the same institution, the effects on the fetus of spinal anesthesia with the effects of a pentothal–succinylcholine–nitrous oxide sequence general anesthesia.

Marx and colleagues, in a prospective study, compared the effects of spinal anesthesia in 60 cesarean sections with those of thiopental–succinylcholine–nitrous oxide sequence in 28 cesarean sections.[52] They observed frequent instances of hypotension in the spinal anesthesia series but were able to correct it easily, as has been noted by other authors.[66,84,105] Despite this incidence of hypotension, there was a highly significant increase in depression and respiratory embarrassment in newborn infants following thiopental–succinylcholine–nitrous oxide anesthesia over that following spinal anesthesia.[52]

Shnider compared the condition of the newborn infants after 96 consecutive elective cesarean sections performed under thiopental–succinylcholine–nitrous oxide anesthesia with the condition of the newborns in 120 consecutive elective cesarean sections performed under spinal anesthesia.[84] He found that 93 per cent of the babies born under spinal anesthesia, in contrast to only 56 per cent of the babies born under general anesthesia, were vigorous at birth. After spinal anesthesia nearly 100 per cent of the babies breathed normally within 90 seconds after birth. However, only 70 per cent of the babies born after thiopental anesthesia breathed normally at 90 seconds.[84]

Crawford reported that the thiopental–succinylcholine–nitrous oxide sequence results in a lesser degree of fetal acidosis and a more normal composition of blood gases than does spinal anesthesia.[30] Cosmi and Mark[28] and Shnider,[84] on the other hand, both carrying out prospective, controlled studies, found no difference in the acid-base and blood gas status in the umbilical cord blood at birth.

Stenger and associates performed an extensive analysis of cord blood derived from 26 infants born via cesarean section under the thiopental–succinyl-choline–nitrous oxide sequence.[98,99] There was no simultaneous comparison with blood obtained in a similar fashion during spinal anesthesia, however. They concluded that acid-base values were at least as close to the accepted normal ranges as those found in women undergoing cesarean section under spinal anesthesia.[98] This group had previously published a careful study of umbilical blood values in five infants born under spinal anesthesia during cesarean section.[96] In these five infants, umbilical vein pH varied from 7.29 to 7.40 and umbilical vein Pco_2 varied from 34.7 to 47.7 mm. Hg. In two of their five patients who experienced prolonged hypotension (possibly owing to untreated vena cava compression syndrome), the oxygen content of the umbilical vein blood, however, was markedly reduced.[96]

Thiopental–succinylcholine–nitrous oxide sequence can offer some definite advantages over spinal anesthesia in specific obstetric situations. Ueland and associates[105,106] have shown that cardiac output is more frequently depressed in spinal anesthesia than under thiopental sequence. Therefore, Bonica has suggested that in some types of cardiac disease thiopental sequence may be more favorable for the mother.[16] Emergency fetal distress situations, abruptio placentae, and other specific situations may indicate thiopental sequence anesthesia.

When thiopental sequence anesthesia is indeed indicated, some precautions are wise. The total dose of thiopental should be kept under 250 mg. to minimize the drug effect on the baby.[34,46] In addition, more and more evidence has appeared emphasizing the previously unsuspected role of nitrous oxide in fetal depression.[99] Many authors have demonstrated the advantages of minimizing the duration of anesthesia before delivery.[44,49,50,53,75]

Furthermore, because physicians often attempt to minimize the fetal depression from drugs, maternal awareness resulting from insufficient anesthesia is becoming increasingly frequent.[30,89] This is an unsavory condition which must be avoided.

In summary, then, objections to the use of regional anesthesia in the past decade have largely been concerned with the detrimental effects of hypotension and vasopressor drugs on uteroplacental exchange and acid-base status of the fetus. These objections have largely been raised by the results of animal studies of isolated pharmacologic phenomena or by unfortunate experience in limited clinical experience with spinal anesthesia.

Subsequent studies have shown that while certain vasopressors, such as levoarterenol and methoxamine, may indeed have some detrimental effect in the laboratory fetus, ephedrine has very beneficial effects in correcting hypotension both in the laboratory animal and in actual clinical practice. Many studies have shown that hypotension is easily corrected in these circumstances. When studied in a prospective, comparative fashion, oxygenation level and acid-base status of the umbilical blood of the newborn infant are almost identical in both the thiopental–succinylcholine–nitrous oxide sequence and the spinal anesthesia groups.

Finally, it must be stated that the type of anesthesia chosen for cesarean section must be specifically designed to fit the needs of the moment, and no routine should be unswervingly followed. However, with the amassing of a great deal of laboratory evidence calming earlier alarms concerning the acid-base status of the newborn infant after spinal anesthesia, with the consistent demonstration of very unfavorable depression of infants following thiopental–succinylcholine–nitrous oxide sequence in comparison to spinal anesthesia, as well as the vast clinical experience demonstrating the relative safety of spinal anesthesia, it seems difficult to support the routine use of thiopental–succinylcholine–nitrous oxide anesthesia for cesarean section over use of spinal anesthesia.

REFERENCES

1. Alexander, J. A., Rogers, S. F., Jacobs, W. M., and Wells, S. H.: Rapid stabilization by hypotensive drugs followed by early delivery in antepartum eclampsia treatment. Amer. J. Obstet. Gynec. 89:77, 1964.
2. Althabe, O., Schwarcz, R. L., Pose, S. V., Escarcena, L., and Caldeyro-Barcia, R.: Effects on fetal heart rate and fetal Po_2 of oxygen administration to the mother. Amer. J. Obstet. Gynec. 98:858, 1967.
3. Asling, J. H.: Paracervical block anesthesia. In Shnider, S. M. (ed.); Obstetrical Anesthesia. Baltimore, Williams & Wilkins, 1970.
4. Asling, J. H., Shnider, S. M., Margolis, A. J., Wilkinson, G. L., and Way, E. L.: Paracervical block anesthesia in obstetrics. II. Etiology of fetal bradycardia following paracervical block anesthesia. Amer. J. Obstet. Gynec. 107:626, 1970.
5. Assali, N. S., Kaplan, S. A., Fomon, S. J., Souglass, R. A., and Tada, Y.: The effects of high spinal anesthesia on the renal hemodynamics and the excretion of electrolytes during osmotic diuresis in the hydropenic normal pregnant woman. J. Clin. Invest. 30:916, 1951.
6. Assali, N. S., and Prystowsky, H.: Studies on autonomic blockade. III. Effect of high spinal anesthesia on the vasodepressor action of veratrum in human subjects. J. Pharmacol. Exp. Ther. 100:251, 1950.
7. Assali, N. S., and Rosenkrantz, J. G.: Studies on autonomic blockade. V. The inhibition of water diuresis by high spinal anesthesia in the pregnant woman. Surg. Gynec. Obstet. 93:468, 1951.
8. Bannister, W. K., and Satillaro, A. J.: Vomiting and aspiration during anesthesia. Anesthesiology. 23:251, 1962.
9. Barber, I. J., Jr., Barnett, H. A., and Williams, C. H.: Comparison of methoxyflurane and parenteral agents for obstetric analgesia. Anes. Anal. 48:209, 1969.
10. Battaglia, F. C., Meschia, G., Makowski, E. L., and Bowes, W.: The effect of maternal oxygen inhalation upon fetal oxygenation. J. Clin. Invest. 47:548,1968.
11. Beck, L., and Martin, K.: Hazards associated with paracervical block in obstetrics. Germ. Med. Mon. 15:81, 1970.
12. Behrman, R. E., Parer, J. T., and Novy, M. J.: Acute maternal respiratory alkalosis (hyperventilation) in the pregnant rhesus monkey. Pediat. Res. 1:354, 1967.
13. Benson, R. C., Berendes, H., and Weiss, W.: Fetal compromise during elective cesarean section. Am. J. Obstet. Gynec. 105:579, 1969.
14. Biava, C.: Abbott Laboratories, Chicago, Illinois (unpublished communication, 1972).
15. Bletka, M., Hlavaty, V., Trnkova, M., Bendl, J., Bendova, L., and Chytil, M.: Volume of whole blood and absolute amount of serum proteins in the early state of late toxemia of pregnancy. Amer. J. Obstet. Gynec. 106:10, 1970.
16. Bonica, J. J.: Anesthesia in the pregnant cardiac patient. Clin. Obstet. Gynec. 11:940, 1969.

17. Bonica, J. J.: Principles and Practice of Obstetric Analgesia and Anesthesia. Philadelphia, F. A. Davis, 1967.
18. Brackbill, Y. (ed.): The effects of obstetrical medication on fetus and infant, Monographs, Society for Research in Child Development 35: No. 4, Serial No. 137, 1970.
19. Buckley, J. J., Van Bergen, F. H., Dobkin, A. B., Brown, F. B., Jr., Miller, F. A., and Varco, R. L.: Postanesthetic hypotension following cyclopropane: Its relationship to hypercapnia. Anesthesiology 14:226 1953.
20. Chesley, L. C.: The movement of radioactive sodium in normal pregnant, nonpregnant, and pre-eclamptic women. Amer. J. Obstet. Gynec. 106:530, 1970.
21. Clark, R. B.: Transplacental reversal of meperidine depression in the fetus by naloxone. J. Ark. Med. Soc. 68:18, 1971.
22. Clark, R. B., Cooper, J. O., Stephens, S. R., and Brown, W. E.: Neonatal acid base studies. II. Effects of a heavy medication-narcotic antagonist regimen for labor and delivery. Obstet. Gynec. 33:30, 1969.
23. Cockburn, F., Daniel, S. S., Dawes, G. S., James, L. S., Myers, R. E., Niemann, W., Rodriguez de Curet H. and Ross B. B.: The effect of pentobarbital anesthesia on resuscitation and brain damage in fetal rhesus monkeys asphyxiated on delivery. J. Pediat. 175:281, 1969.
24. Cohen, S. N., and Olson, W. A.: Drugs that depress the newborn infant. Ped. Clin. N. Amer. 17:835, 1970.
25. Coleman, A. J.: Absence of harmful effects of maternal hypocapnia in babies delivered at caesarean section. Lancet 1:813, 1967.
26. National Study of Maternity Care: Survey of obstetric practice and associated services in hospitals in the United States. Chicago. American College of Obstetricians and Gynecologists, 1971, Table VII-5. National Study of Maternity Care: Survey of obstetric practice and associated services in hospitals in the United States. Chicago, American College of Obstetricians and Gynecologists, 1971, Table VII-4.
28. Cosmi, E. V., and Marx, G. F.: Acid-base status of the fetus and clinical condition of the newborn following cesarean section. Amer. J. Obstet. Gynec. 102:378, 1968.
29. Crandell, W. B., and MacDonald, A.: Nephropathy associated with methoxyflurane anesthesia. J.A.M.A. 205:798, 1966.
30. Crawford, J. S.: Awareness during operative obstetrics under general anesthesia. Brit. J. Anaesth. 43:179, 1971.
31. Drage, J. S., Kennedy, C., and Schwarz, B. K.: The Apgar score as an index of neonatal mortality. A report from the Collaborative Study of Cerebral Palsy. Obstet. Gynec. 24:222, 1964.
32. Eckenhoff, J. F., Kneale, D. H., and Dripps, R. D.: The incidence and etiology of postanesthetic excitement: A clinical survey. Anesthesiology 22:667, 1961.
33. Finster, M., Mark, L. C., Morishima, H. O., Moya, F., Perel, J. M., James, L. S., and Dayton P. G.: Plasma thiopental concentrations in the newborn following delivery under thiopental-nitrous oxide anesthesia. Am. J. Obstet. Gynec. 95:621, 1966.
34. Finster, M., Morishima, H. O., Mark, L. C., Perel, J. M., Dayton, P. G., and James, L. S.: Tissue thiopental concentrations in the fetus and newborn. Anesthesiology 36:155, 1972.
35. Freeman, R. K., Gutierrez, N. A., Ray, M. L., Stovall, D., Paul, R. H., and Hon, E. H.: Fetal cardiac response to paracervical block anesthesia. Part I. Amer. J. Obstet. Gynec. 110:583, 1972.
36. Gordon, H. R.: Fetal bradycardia after paracervical block: Correlation with maternal blood levels of local anesthetics. New Eng. J. Med. 279:911, 1968.
37. Gottschalk, W.: Principles of obstetric anesthesia. Obstet. Gynec. Ann. 193, 1972.
38. Graham, E. C., and Choy, D.: Corticosteroids in aspiration pneumonia. J.A.M.A. 184:977, 1963.
39. Greiss, F. C., and Crandell, D. L.: Therapy for hypotension induced by spinal anesthesia during pregnancy. J.A.M.A. 191:793, 1965.
40. Hamelburg, W., and Bosomworth, P. P.: Aspiration pneumonitis. Anes. Anal. 43:669, 1964.
41. Hollmen, A., and Jagerhorn, M.: The effects of epidural anesthesia and caesarean section on foetal and maternal acid-base balance at birth. Acta Anaesth. Scandinav. 12:115, 1968.
42. Ivankovic, A. D., Elam, J. O., and Huffman, J.: Methoxyflurane anesthesia for cesarean section. J. Reprod. Med. 6:24, 1971.
43. Jones, P. L., Rosen, M., Mushin, W. W., Jones, E. V.: Methoxyflurane and nitrous oxide as obstetric analgesics. I. A comparison by continuous administration. Brit. Med. J. 3:255, 1969.
44. Kivalo, I., Timonen, S., and Castren, O.: The influence of anaesthesia and the induction-

delivery interval on the newborn delivered by caesarean section. Ann. Chir. Gynaecol. Fenn. 60:71, 1971.

45. Koch, G., and Wendel, H.: The effect of pethidine on the post-natal adjustment of respiration and acid-base balance. Acta Obstet. Gynec. Scand. 47:27, 1968.

46. Kosaka, Y., Takahashi, T., and Mark, L. C.: Intravenous thiobarbiturate anesthesia for cesarean section. Anesthesiology 31:489, 1969.

47. Lucas, W. E., Kirschbaum, T., and Assali, N. S.: Effects of autonomic blockade with spinal anesthesia on uterine and fetal hemodynamics and oxygen consumption in the sheep. Biol. Neonat. 10:166, 1966.

48. Lumley, J., Renou, T., Newman, W., and Wood, C.: Hyperventilation in obstetrics. Amer. J. Obstet. Gynec. 103:847, 1969.

49. Lumley, J., Walker, A., Marum, J.: Time: An important variable at cesarean section. J. Obstet. Gynec. Brit. Comm. 77:10, 1970.

50. Marx, G. F.: Newer aspects of general anesthesia for cesarean section. N. Y. J. Med. 71:1084, 1971.

51. Marx, G. F.: Toxemia and its anesthetic management. Inter. Anes. Clin. 6:829, 1968.

52. Marx, G. F., Cosmi, E. Z., and Wollman, S. B.: Biochemical status and clinical condition of mother and infant at cesarean section. Anes. Anal. 48:986, 1969.

53. Marx, G. F., Joshi, C. W., and Orkin, L. R.: Placental transmission of nitrous oxide. Anesthesiology 32:429, 1970.

54. Marx, G. F., and Mateo, C. V.: Effects of different oxygen concentrations during general anaesthesia for elective caesarean section. Can. Anaesth. Soc. J. 18:587, 1971.

55. Mazze, R. I., Shue, G. L., and Jackson, S. H.: Renal dysfunction associated with methoxyflurane anesthesia: A randomized, prospective clinical evaluation. J.A.M.A. 216:278, 1971.

56. Mazze, R. I., Trudell, J. R., and Cousins, M. J.: Methoxyflurane metabolism and renal dysfunction. Anesthesiology 35:247, 1971.

57. Mendelson, C. L.: Aspiration of stomach contents into the lungs during obstetric anesthesia. Amer. J. Obstet. Gynec. 52:191, 1946.

58. Mendelson, C. L.: Acute cor pulmonale and pregnancy. Clin. Obstet. 11:992, 1968.

59. Merrill, R. B., and Hingson, R. A.: Study of incidence of maternal mortality from aspiration of vomitus. Anes. Anal. 30:124, 1951.

60. Miles, B. E., and DeWardener, H. W.: Renal vasoconstriction produced by ether and cyclopropane anesthesia. J. Physiol. 118:140, 1952.

61. Moore, W. M. O., and Davis, J. A.: Simultaneous administration of narcotic and narcotic antagonist drugs in the newborn rabbit. J. Ped. 71:420, 1967.

62. Motoyama, E. K., Rivard, G., Acheson, F., and Cook, C. D.: Adverse effects of maternal hyperventilation on the fetus. Lancet 1:286, 1966.

63. Motoyama, E. K., Rivard, G., Acheson, F., and Cook, C. D.: The effect of changes in maternal pH and P_{CO_2} on the P_{O_2} of fetal lambs. Anesthesiology 28:891, 1967.

64. Moya, F., Morishima, H. O., Shnider, S. M., and James, L. S.: Influence of maternal hyperventilation on the newborn infant. Amer. J. Obstet. Gynec. 91:76, 1965.

65. Moya, F., and Smith, B. E.: Maternal hypotension and the newborn infant. Proceedings of the Third World Congress of Anesthesiology, Sao Paulo, 1:94, 1964.

66. Moya, F., and Smith, B. E.: Spinal anesthesia for cesarean section: Clinical and biochemical studies of effects on maternal physiology. J.A.M.A. 179:609, 1962.

67. Moya, F., and Smith, B. E.: Uptake, distribution, and placental transport of drugs and anesthetics. Anesthesiology 26:465, 1965.

68. Moya, F., and Thorndike, V.: The effects of drugs used in labor on the fetus and newborn. Clin. Pharmacol. Ther. 4:628, 1963.

69. Nicholl, R. M., Holland, E. L., and Brown, S. F.: Mendelson's syndrome: its treatment by tracheostomy and hydrocortisone. Brit. Med. J. 2:745, 1967.

70. Paul, R. H., and Freeman, R. K.: Fetal cardiac response to paracervical block anesthesia. Part II. Amer. J. Obstet. Gynec. 113:593, 1972.

71. Ontario Perinatal Mortality Study Committee: Second Report of the Perinatal Mortality Study. Toronto, Ontario Department of Health, 1967, Table 99.

72. Ontario Perinatal Mortality Study Committee: Second Report of the Perinatal Mortality Study. Toronto, Ontario Department of Health, 1967, Table 122.

73. Ontario Perinatal Mortality Study Committee: Second Report of the Perinatal Mortality Study. Toronto, Ontario Department of Health, 1967, Table 113.

74. Phillips, O. C.: The role of anesthesia in obstetric mortality in obstetric complications. In International Anesthesiology Clinics, Vol. VI. Boston, Little, Brown & Co., 1968.

75. Reis, R. A., Gerbie, A. B., and Gerbie, M. V.: Reducing hazards to the newborn during cesarean section. Surg. Gynec. Obstet. 130:124, 1970.

76. Rivard, G., Motoyama, E. K., Acheson, R. M., Cook, C. D., and Reynolds, E. O. R.: The

relation between maternal and fetal oxygen tensions in the sheep. Amer. J. Obstet. Gynec. 97:925, 1967.

77. Roberts, H., Kane, K. M., Percival, N., Snow, P., and Please, N. W.: Effects of some analgesic drugs used in childbirth. Lancet 1:128, January 19, 1957.

78. Rosen, M.: Recent advances in pain relief in childbirth. I: Inhalation and systemic analgesia. Brit. J. Anaesth. 43:837, 1971.

79. Rosen, M., Latto, P., and Asscher, H. W.: Kidney function after methoxyflurane analgesia during labour. Brit. Med. J. 1:81, 1972.

80. Rosenfeld, S. S.: Paracervical anesthesia for the relief of labor pains. Amer. J. Obstet. Gynec. 50:527, 1945.

81. Rosefsky, J. B., and Petersiel, M. E.: Perinatal deaths associated with mepivacaine paracervical block anesthesia in labor. New Eng. J. Med. 278:530, 1968.

82. Rouge, J. C.: Levallorphan and meperidine mixtures. Acta Anaesth. Scand. 13:87, 1969.

83. Secher, O., and Wilhjelm, B.: The protective action of anaesthetics against hypoxia. Can. Anaes. Soc. J. 15:423, 1968.

84. Shnider, S. M. (ed.): Anesthesia for elective cesarean section. In Obstetrical Anesthesia. Baltimore, Williams & Wilkins, 1970.

85. Shnider, S. M., Asling, J. H., Holl, J. W., and Margolis, A. J.: Paracervical block anesthesia in obstetrics. I: Fetal complications and neonatal morbidity. Amer. J. Obstet. Gynec. 107:619, 1970.

86. Schnider, S. M., DeLorimier, A. A., Asling, J. H., and Morishima, H. O.: Vasopressors in obstetrics. II: Fetal hazards of methoxamine administration during obstetric spinal anesthesia. Amer. J. Obstet. Gynec. 106:680, 1970.

87. Schnider, S. M., DeLorimier, A. A., Holl, J. W., Chapler, F. K. and Morishima, H. O.: Vasopressors in obstetrics. I: Correction of fetal acidosis with ephedrine during spinal hypotension. Amer. J. Obstet. Gynec. 102:911, 1968.

88. Smiler, B. G., Goldberger, R., Sivak, B. J., and Brown, E. M.: Routine endotracheal intubation in obstetrics. Amer. J. Obstet. Gynec. 103:947, 1969.

89. Smith, A. M., and McNeil, W. T.: Awareness during anaesthesia. Brit. Med. J. 1:572, 1969.

90. Smith, B. E.: Anesthetic complications in the delivery room. Ill. Med. J. 133:33, 1968.

91. Smith, B. E., Cavanagh, D., and Moya, F.: Choice of anesthesia for vaginal delivery in the patient with toxemia of pregnancy. Anes. Anal. 45:853, 1966.

92. Smith, B. E., and Moya, F.: Inhalational analgesia with methoxyflurane for vaginal delivery. South. Med. J. 61:386, 1968.

93. Smith, R. W.: Cardiovascular alterations in toxemia. Amer. J. Obstet. Gynec. 107:979, 1970.

94. Smith, T. C.: Pharmacology of respiratory depression. Int. Anes. Clin. 9:125, 1971.

95. Stead, A. L.: The response of the newborn infant to muscle relaxants. Int. Anes. Clin. 6:707, 1968.

96. Stenger, V. G., Andersen, T., De Padua, C., Eitzman, D., Gessner, I., and Prystowsky, H.: Spinal anesthesia for cesarean section—physiological and biochemical observations. Amer. J. Obstet. Gynec. 90:51, 1964.

97. Stenger, V. G., Andersen, T., Eitzman, D., Blechner, J., and Prystowsky, H.: Cyclopropane anesthesia. Physiologic and biochemical effects in human pregnancy. Amer. J. Obstet. Gynec. 96:201, 1966.

98. Stenger, V. G., Blechner, J. N., Andersen, T. W., Eitzman, D. V., Cestaric, E., and Prystowsky, H.: Observations on pentothal, nitrous oxide and succinylcholine anesthesia at cesarean section. Amer. J. Obstet. Gynec. 99:690, 1967.

99. Stenger, V. G., Blechner, J. N., and Prystowsky, H.: A study of prolongation of obstetric anesthesia. Amer. J. Obstet. Gynec. 103:901, 1969.

100. Sundell, H., Garrott, J., Blankenship, W. J., Shephard, F. M., and Stahlman, M. T.: Studies on infants with type II respiratory distress syndrome. J. Pediat. 78:754, 1971.

101. Tafeen, C. H., Freedmann, H. L., and Harris, H.: Combined continuous paracervical and continued pudendal nerve block anesthesia in labor. Amer. J. Obstet. Gynec. 100:55, 1968.

102. Telford, J., and Keats, A. S.: Narcotic-antagonist mixtures. Anesthesiology 22:465, 1961.

103. Teramo, K., and Widholm, O.: Studies of the effects of anesthetics on foetus. I: The effect of paracervical block with mepivacaine upon foetal acid-base values. Acta Obstet. Scand. (Suppl. 2) 46:1, 1967.

104. Turner, H. B., and Houck, C. R.: Renal hemodynamics in the toxemias of pregnancy; alterations of kidney function by regional nerve block. Amer. J. Obstet. Gynec. 60:126, 1960.

105. Ueland, K., Gills, R. E., and Hansen, J. M.: Maternal cardiovascular dynamics. I. Cesarean

section under subarachnoid block anesthesia. Amer. J. Obstet. Gynec. *100*:42, 1968.
106. Ueland, K., Hansen, J., Eng, M., Kalappa, R., and Parer, J. T.: Maternal cardiovascular dynamics. V. Cesarean section under thiopental nitrous oxide and succinylcholine anesthesia. Amer. J. Obstet. Gynec. *108*:615, 1970.
107. Walker, A. L.: Report on Confidential Inquiries into Maternal Deaths in England and Wales, 1955–1957. London, Her Majesty's Stationery Office, 1960.
108. Zunker, H. O., Phillips, L. L., and McKay, D. G.: Sodium transport in the kidney and placenta in normal pregnancy and in experimental toxemia. Amer. J. Obstet. Gynec. *92*:325, 1965.

Preferable Methods of Pain Relief in Labor, Delivery, and Late Pregnancy Complications

JESS B. WEISS

Boston Hospital for Women

Introduction

The vast majority of pregnant women giving birth in our hospitals, especially those who have any of the complications of late pregnancy, will request and require some degree of pain relief during labor and delivery, which varies with circumstances. This is not only true today but will continue to be true in the predictable future (Table 6–2).

TABLE 6–2. *Anesthesia Statistics, Boston Hospital for Women—Lying In Division*

YEAR	TOTAL	EPIDURAL	SPINAL	INHALA-TION	PUDENDAL	LOCAL	NO ANESTHESIA
1960–61	5589	120	3428	1674	120	153	168
1961–62	Complete records unavailable						
1962–63	5415	246	3789	1034	60	164	172
1963–64	5526	224	4146	893	67	230	179
1964–65	5356	281	4200	563	62	211	201
1965–66	5418	395	4097	462	71	332	177
1966–67	6006	755	4337	399	109	393	207
1967–68	6377	977	4559	412	71	306	218
1968–69	6662	1198	4563	256	56	356	233
1969–70	7256	2007	4128	322	35	395	369
1970–71	6654	2299	3145	293	29	339	549

This treatise is based on 15 years' experience in directing an anesthesia service that has provided pain relief for about 80,000 women in labor. During this period, our hospital's neonatal mortality rate has fallen steadily and in recent years has been roughly one-half national average. It is worth mentioning that the rate was slightly lower in the non-private than in the private sector of the hospital population.[1]

Although this view is subject to controversy, it is doubtful that the application of such techniques as hypnosis, psychoprophylaxis in its various forms, natural childbirth, Lamaze, and similar techniques, and even acupuncture can

203

provide adequate pain relief for a successful outcome in more than 15 to 20 per cent of patients. In our society it is usually the white middle or upper class patient who because of economic status has the privilege of having her obstetrician in constant attendance. It is this group in the main who desires to be candidates for the above-mentioned methods.

I am unaware of the existence of any data showing that the elimination of analgesia and anesthesia—as these techniques are practiced today in our institution—would in any way reduce the present maternal and neonatal morbidity and mortality rates. On the contrary, there are data to show that in both premature and term deliveries, perinatal death rates were higher when delivery occurred without anesthesia than when conduction anesthesia was used. These data come from a Canadian study involving 10 university teaching hospitals, and the results are striking.[2,3]

Indeed, it is possible that clinical obstetrics could revert to the plight of the first half of the nineteenth century, when a large part of the frightful morbidity and mortality rates for both mother and infant occurred because methods of pain relief were not available that would permit timely intervention in the complications of pregnancy and labor. Moreover, it is pointless today to have all of the monitoring equipment now available if the hospital environment will not permit a cesarean section or any other operative procedures that may be indicated within minutes of the onset of what might become disturbing and perhaps irreversible damage to the fetus as a result of hypoxia. Obviously patients in such circumstances should have available at all times a method of pain relief that will afford the obstetrician the opportunity to terminate the labor by a procedure that will provide maximum safety to the mother and her infant.

Having thus outlined the importance of modern anesthesia in obstetrics, it now becomes germane to lay a foundation for the specific situations of clinical practice in which various types of analgesia and anesthesia are required, which at the same time will serve to reduce further the perinatal morbidity and mortality. In my clinical practice of the past 15 years, at least two related changes in obstetric anesthesia practice have helped to accomplish these objectives.

First and most important was the establishment of a full-time anesthesia service with a Board certified anesthesiologist available around the clock, whose offices were adjacent to the labor and delivery suites. These individuals have been assigned a primary responsibility to the obstetrical patient and are not subordinated to or shared with other anesthetic needs of the hospital. The pregnant female can no longer remain a second class hospital patient for whom skilled anesthesia is available only after the needs of the surgical suite are fulfilled. In terms of practice, no hospital should be permitted licensure if it cannot meet this basic qualification and need. As has been stated on earlier occasions, this means regional planning, with the emergence of fewer but larger centers that will support and merit the establishment of such anesthetic services.

Certainly the time has long since arrived when the most experienced anesthesiologist should be responsible for obstetric anesthesia administration— rather than the least experienced. In fact, two lives are involved simultaneously, and to jeopardize one may well jeopardize the other. Recognizing that the majority of cases of cerebral palsy and mental retardation result from complications that compromise the intrauterine environment, expediting the infant's escape from this unfriendly milieu without further risk is largely the responsibility of a skilled anesthetist. The question is not whether an individual may travail in labor without pain relief, but rather whether quality analgesia and anesthesia are available at all times for the parturient.

Second in our list of necessary obstetric anesthesia changes was the widespread acceptance of the safety and superiority of all forms of regional or conduction anesthesia over inhalation or general anesthesia. Table 6–2 illustrates the results after instituting these changes under our direction at the Boston Hospital for Women. Indeed, there must have been a direct contraindication to a regional technique before a patient was allowed to undergo general anesthesia. A primary indication for general anesthesia is the anticipated need for uterine relaxation when intrauterine manipulation is required to accomplish delivery.

We contend that every pregnant patient in labor must be treated as if she had a "full stomach." Many years ago we discarded the concept that the gravid patient is ever safe for general anesthesia simply because 6 or more hours had elapsed from her last food ingestion prior to the onset of labor and she therefore had an "empty stomach." Consequently, regional anesthesia in some form is our anesthesia of choice for delivery.

Certainly, in the past, aspiration of regurgitated or vomited gastric contents, which are often highly acid, has been a primary cause of maternal mortality.[5] These events usually have occurred in association with the administration of general anesthesia via face mask and in the absence of endotracheal intubation.

If a contraindication to regional anesthesia exists, if the patient refuses to consent to it, or if general anesthesia is indicated to produce uterine relaxation for an anticipated intrauterine maneuver, then obligatory rapid ("crash") endotracheal intubation is performed in all cases. We utilize head-up position, rapid intravenous thiopental induction in a single dose of 4 mg./kg., cricoid cartilage pressure, rapid intravenous succinylcholine administration to facilitate tracheal intubation, and skillful placement of an endotracheal tube followed quickly by cuff inflation to occlude the trachea.

Essential to successful adoption of this philosophy is a high degree of skill, training, and competence of all personnel administering anesthesia. Eternal vigilance and a thorough understanding of the possible problems and complications that might occur, so that they may be quickly and successfully recognized and treated, are fundamental.

To repeat an earlier statement, the most experienced anesthetist must be responsible for obstetric anesthesia administration, not the least experienced.

Pain Relief During Labor

Pain relief during early labor can be adequately provided for with judicious, individualized use of various pharmacologic agents, including small amounts of barbiturates and tranquilizers. It is well appreciated, however, that these agents quickly traverse the placenta and can cause fetal depression. If the fetus is premature, if it is already in jeopardy because of maternal diabetes, toxemia, other placental pathology, or mechanical problems of cord obstruction, these agents may add to the hypoxia and acidosis already present and hence are contraindicated.

As labor progresses, with dilation of the cervix, pain increases in intensity.

Patients trained for natural childbirth usually do well with no medication during this early phase of labor, but may require some pharmacologic assistance, such as other patients may have received earlier in their labors, often with the addition of moderate amounts of narcotic analgesics.

At this point, regional blocks with local anesthetic agents may be needed. These have become popular and widespread in their application. They can provide more adequate analgesia, do not affect labor, will not depress mother or baby if overdosage, toxicity, or other technical misadventures are not allowed to occur, and allow the mother more actual participation in the events of labor and delivery. Paracervical block, pudendal block, spinal, lumbar epidural, and caudal anesthesia are the useful regional techniques in either single-dose or continuous catheterization methods.

In our clinic, continuous lumbar epidural has become a preferred, widely used technique for providing analgesia during labor, administered to 34.6 per cent of our patients (2299 of 6654) in the 1971 hospital year.

We do not use paracervical block for analgesia during labor. Our experience with the technique produced 43 instances of fetal bradycardia in 100 paracervical blocks. In a total of 300 patients, we had one stillbirth and one neonatal death associated with the use of paracervical block.[6] In an excellent review of the literature on the subject, Thiery and Vroman surveyed the world literature, comprising over 70,000 cases, and found that "even this amount of data has proved insufficient to answer the question concerning the possible fetal hazards." They found bias and inadequate data, as well as lack of controlled studies, to be responsible for this.

Pain Relief for Pelvic Delivery

Pain relief for delivery may be provided in a variety of ways, using many different agents and techniques. A choice for a particular patient is made with due regard to both the patient's and her obstetrician's previous experiences and wishes. Proper consideration must first be given to the presence of any contraindication for a particular drug or technique. Management of a previous labor of the patient may also be a determining factor in the choice of anesthesia. Certainly the presence of any medical complication of pregnancy, such as diabetes mellitus, cardiac disease, and so forth, will merit a role in choosing pain relief techniques for delivery, as will complications of labor or delivery, such as maternal bleeding, persistent occiput posterior position, breech presentation, twin pregnancy and brow or shoulder presentations.

Our preference for regional techniques for providing pain relief during delivery has relegated the use of inhalation anesthesia to the occasional patient who has a contraindication to regional techniques or agents, to the rare patients who will not consent to their use, and to the group of patients for whom we believe there is a positive indication for its use. In these patients, the principal indication for inhalation anesthesia is the anticipated need for uterine relaxation to permit intrauterine manipulation. These patients are all treated as if they had full stomachs, and obligatory rapid endotracheal intubation is performed in all cases. Halothane or diethyl ether is the agent used with this technique to produce uterine relaxation when it is indicated for breech delivery, multiple pregnancies, retained placenta, internal podalic version, or any situation that might require intrauterine manipulation. In our last hospital year, 4.4 per cent of our patients (293 of 6654) were given general anesthesia, all with rapid endotracheal intubation.

For the more complicated pelvic deliveries, which may involve intrauterine manipulation by the obstetrician, such as forceps rotation, breech extraction and delivery, version as with the second twin, manual removal of retained placenta, and other procedures (e.g., internal podalic version), we still will utilize regional anesthetic techniques, such as lumbar epidural or spinal anesthesia, until such time as uterine relaxation is required, if at all. At this point, rapid endotracheal intubation is performed. With the patient continuously inspiring 100 per cent oxygen by mask, she is given, in rapid succession, Pentothal Sodium or Surital intravenously in a single dose of 4 mg./kg., usually comprising 150 to 250 mg., followed quickly by 60 to 100 mg. succinylcholine intravenously. With the patient in a head-up position, and with cricoid pressure, endotracheal intubation is accomplished quickly, and the endotracheal cuff is inflated to occlude the trachea. Two to three per cent halothane is then given with nitrous oxide and oxygen, only for the duration of the need for uterine relaxation.

Anesthesia for Cesarean Section

In considering anesthesia for elective cesarean section, we still in great measure prefer spinal anesthesia, although lumbar epidural and balanced, general anesthesia—particularly the latter—are of late more frequently used. In a predominantly healthy and well-prepared patient population, our choice of anesthetic technique usually is based on the patient's medical or obstetrical problems (if any), her past experiences, and her present desires. We find, in our present patient population, that most of our elective cesarean section patients are well motivated to remain awake at least until the baby is delivered, and will prefer spinal anesthesia.

Those patients who have supine hypotension preoperatively, those who refuse regional anesthesia, who insist on being asleep, and those in whom there is a contraindication to spinal anesthesia will be given a "balanced" anesthetic technique, with rapid endotracheal intubation, after intravenous Pentothal Sodium induction, intravenous succinylcholine, nitrous oxide, and oxygen.

For emergency cesarean section, the kind of emergency and the condition of mother and baby are primary considerations that will indicate a preferable method of providing anesthesia. If the section is being done for lack of progress, dysfunctional labor, cephalopelvic disproportion, malposition or malpresentation, or repeat cesarean section in labor, mother and baby are usually not distressed, and spinal anesthesia is usually our anesthetic technique of choice.

When the emergency section is being done for bleeding, whether it results from either placenta previa or abruptio placentae, in which case hemorrhagic shock is a threat, we prefer light, balanced anesthesia, previously described as safest for both mother and baby. When fetal distress occurs because of uterine tetany, cord compromise, or placental inadequacy, and when it is the primary indication for emergency section, we again prefer light, balanced, general anesthesia to accomplish immediate delivery.

Anesthesia for Toxemia of Pregnancy

Although the etiology of toxemia is not known, it has been—along with hemorrhage and infection—a major cause of maternal morbidity and mortality. It has also been recognized as a major factor in much neonatal mortality. Its pathophysiology is largely that of arteriolar spasm, hypertension, salt and water retention, and renal functional deterioration with albuminuria. These may progress to convulsions, anuria, and death. There is impairment of placental function involved with low birth weight for age, and a higher incidence of premature placental separation. Increased peripheral resistance, increased cardiac output, and increased blood viscosity are often present and can increase cardiac work and in the extreme lead to pulmonary edema, not unlike left ventricular failure.

With this background, we have favored a regional anesthetic technique, either spinal or epidural, for the toxemic patient, but we prefer the latter. The use of lumbar epidural anesthesia during the first stage of labor can obviate use of large doses of depressant narcotics, barbiturates, and ataractics. This regional technique may help reduce an elevated blood pressure.

At this point, however, a word of caution is in order regarding the use of regional techniques in toxemic patients. Hypotension after spinal or epidural anesthesia in such patients, particularly those treated with sedatives, magnesium sulfate, or any of the many antihypertensive agents used in toxemias, may be far more profound in these patients than in non-toxemia patients. This may possibly be a result of the altered vascular reactivity that occurs with this disease, which serves to reduce the extent of the usual cardiovascular compensatory mechanisms operant after sympathetic block. Furthermore, there may well be an additive effect in the treated patients given spinal or epidural anesthesia.

We urge evaluation of the various elements of these processes in each toxemic patient, in order to individualize the anesthetic choice for each.

Anesthesia in Prematurity

Incidence of prematurity has been said to range from 3.5 to 12 per cent in various populations around the world, and neonatal morbidity and mortality rates are high.

Premature labor is a common complication of pregnancy, and management of pain relief may be an important element in the prognosis of the prematurely delivered infant. A primary consideration in the choice of anesthesia is the fact that this is a high-risk situation in which the fetus may already be in jeopardy. After birth, such an infant is more liable to cardiorespiratory and central nervous system depression resulting from use of barbiturates, narcotics, other sedatives, inhalation anesthetic agents, and local anesthetic agents by the mother. The hepatic and renal functions for the metabolism and excretion of these agents may not be as mature as in the full term infant, and these infants are more easily rendered asphyctic and acidotic.

In our management of pain relief in these patients we abstain from using narcotics and favor the use of continuous lumbar epidural analgesia as early in labor as necessary. We prefer this technique to caudal anesthesia because it is more reliable and because it requires a much smaller dosage (50 per cent as much) to produce an equivalent extent and duration of pain relief. When properly administered, epidural anesthesia does not produce fetal depression, and obviates the need for the use of any other analgesic. It produces less hypotension than does spinal anesthesia, and will provide analgesia during labor when a spinal anesthesia cannot yet be administered.

REFERENCES

1. Reid, D. E., Ryan, K. J., Benirschke, K.: Principles and Management of Human Reproduction. Philadelphia, W. B. Saunders Co., 1972.
2. Obstetric anesthesia and perinatal morbidity [editorial]. New Eng. J. Med. 279:941, 1968.
3. Russell, E. S.: Neonatal depression and mortality: influence of anesthesia, sedation and method of delivery. *In* International Congress Series No. 168. Proceedings of the Fourth World Congress of Anesthesiologists: London, September 9–13, 1968. Amsterdam, Excerpta Medica, 1968.
4. Ontario Perinatal Mortality Study Committee. Second Report of the Perinatal Mortality Study. Toronto: Ontario Department of Health, 1967.
5. Bonica, J. J. (ed.): Obstetric analgesia and anesthesia. A manual for physicians, nurses, and other health personnel. Berlin, Springer-Verlag, 1972.
6. Rosefsky, J. B., and Petersiel, M. E.: Perinatal deaths associated with mepivacaine paracervical-block anesthesia in labor. New Eng. J. Med. 278:530, 1968.
7. Thiery, M., and Vroman, S.: Paracervical block analgesia during labor. Amer. J. Obstet. Gynec. 113:988, 1972.

Preferable Methods of Pain Relief in Labor, Delivery, and Late Pregnancy Complications

Editorial Comment

Pain relief in labor is a topic that is fraught with controversy; in an effort to resolve the problem, some philosophy has been brought to bear, and various attitudes toward the conduct of labor and delivery are advocated. Since its introduction into clinical obstetric medicine, anesthesia as a valid tool has been under constant surveillance. Indeed, the history of anesthesia is interwoven with the efforts to provide pain relief in labor and allow for operative delivery in the interests of both the mother and the fetus.

About 1870, Sir James Y. Simpson made a statement that has current applicability: "New rules are required to be established for its use. This is necessary, for the application of anesthesia to midwifery involves many more delicate and difficult problems than its mere application to dentistry and surgery. The effects of these agents upon the action of the uterus, upon the state of the child, and upon the parturient, and the puerperal state of the mother are all required to be accurately studied." Aside from the contributors to this chapter and those cited in their respective lists of references, there is rightful concern over whether other colleagues in the field of anesthesia are cognizant of Dr. Simpson's admonitions. There appears to be general agreement that no one routine suffices, and the selection of the anesthesia must be made with the realization that two lives are simultaneously at stake. Also, the fact that safety is preferable to comfort is amply demonstrated by the critical assessments of the contributors.

The progress in surgery over the past two decades has been made possible in large measure by the advances in anesthesia, which have permitted new and intricate operations to be performed. Prolonged cardiovascular procedures in particular have placed or created enormous demands on the anesthesia services of general hospitals; undoubtedly these demands will increase as more operations are devised and extended, although some physicians criticize the priorities, asserting that the results appear simply to maintain life, rather than improve it.

Moreover, although one may have the most sophisticated monitoring system, it is of little avail if a cesarean section cannot be carried out within minutes after the decision is made that immediate delivery is mandatory. Furthermore, this emergency demands the skill of an experienced anesthesiologist. This is the crucial issue in the use of pain relief in labor and delivery—namely, whether quality anesthesia is available immediately, not whether the normal patient who desires little or no medication for pain relief can negotiate labor to her own satisfaction and that of her obstetrician.

It follows that although the prospectus for pain relief for labor and delivery contains many agents and methods, there are few anesthesia services prepared to administer these to the parturient. At best, it appears that in a general hospital, anesthesiologists respond only to emergency calls and certainly do not care to assist in the management of pain relief during labor. Thus, the obstetrician often must compromise and make do with whatever is available. This is readily illustrated in the case of paracervical and perineal block, which are used not necessarily by preference. Undoubtedly the enthusiastic writings on paracervical and perineal block are influenced in large measure by the fact that there is no other method available.

The reluctance of many obstetricians to accept conduction or regional techniques was based on the possibility that a hypotensive episode might occur. Nothing is of greater threat to the fetal welfare than when the systolic blood pressure falls below 90 mm. Hg. In this event, intravillous blood flow is reduced and placental exchange is compromised. Although balanced anesthesia is a distinct advance, unless the patient is prepared by restriction of food and fluids for several hours prior to labor, inhalation anesthesia has limits to its usefulness. Most obstetricians feel more secure if an intratracheal tube is in place before any operative procedure is attempted, since stimulation of the parasympathetic pelvic innervation, as with a forceps procedure, may precipitate reflex vomiting. If this occurs in the course of a forceps delivery, the latter should be abandoned and the situation reassessed. A regional type of anesthesia might be prudently substituted. This illustrates the necessity for team work by the anesthesiologist and obstetrician.

The prognostic value of the Apgar score in relation to neonatal morbidity has been correctly questioned. In a collaborative study in one New England clinic, where pain relief was a policy in the conduct of labor, the Apgar scores were higher than in a neighboring institution, where drugs for pain relief has limited use. The difference might well be accounted for by the unnecessary prolonged perineal arrest of the fetus in the hope that an unassisted delivery might ensue.

Also, a distinction must be made between acute hypoxia, as in the prolapse of the cord, in which case the Apgar score may be extremely low, and chronic or prolonged hypoxia occurring over several days or weeks, in which case the Apgar score may well be normal. In either situation the fetus may be permanently compromised. In general, an Apgar score of under 6 is unacceptable, but on the other hand it must also be recognized that a high Apgar score is no assurance that the neonate is free of the ill effects of chronic hypoxia.

The question is commonly posed as to whether methods of pain relief impede labor. Actually, the elimination of fear and anxiety by appropriate medication may change what is an ineffective labor or a labor without progress to one with progress. Much has been said—and much of it is nonsense—that pain in labor may be one of the effects of an industrialized society, implying that inhabitants of underdeveloped countries and so-called primitive people do not suffer this pain. Careful studies on this subject are meager and results are unconvincing. In caring for the economically less privileged patients, however, one is struck by their desire for pain relief. Indeed, they tend to place themselves under the care of hospitals that are prepared to provide a comfortable labor totally consistent with the welfare of the mother and her unborn child.

One of the contributors decries the unfortunate trend of many obstetrician-gynecologists who seek to relinquish their responsibilities for the total care of the parturient, directing their energies and efforts only toward the care or management of abnormal cases. Needless to say, these all too often cannot be anticipated. Therefore, every patient in labor is entitled to have an obstetrician present in the hospital at all times to meet any emergencies.

The notion that there is need for fewer obstetricians and gynecologists ignores (at least) the latter's role in the overall care of women. That fewer students are entering the field may no longer be true—indeed, there may be an upsurge. The concept of obstetrics-gynecology as a medical surgical specialty within a family practice setting is appealing to many present-day students whose strong social conscience is one of their many attributes.

As one contributor suggests: let the image of obstetrics and gynecology be based on maintaining a healthy balance between relevant research, teaching, and patient care. Granted that this is very necessary, an additional proposal seems to be in order. Anesthesia personnel must be motivated to place medical priorities above personal comfort and satisfactions and give equal weight to needs of obstetric practice that are at least of equal importance to surgical needs. Certainly it is not too much to request that an anesthesiologist totally free of other duties in the hospital be assigned to meet any emergency, obstetric or otherwise, supervise closely nurse anesthetists, and teach residents the fundamentals of pain relief in labor and delivery. The number of anesthesiologists so engaged under this arrangement would be determined by the size of the obstetrical service, with these individuals rotating on a daily or weekly basis. It is only through a cooperative team effort of many disciplines that any appreciable reduction can be made in the incidence of cerebral palsy and mental retardation—and quality anesthesia is basic to this effort.

7

Preferable Management of Gestational Trophoblastic Disease: Benign and Malignant

Alternative Points of View:

By John I. Brewer and Thomas R. Eckman

By Donald P. Goldstein

By Charles B. Hammond

Editorial Comment

Preferable Management of Gestational Trophoblastic Disease: Benign and Malignant

Early Detection and Treatment of Invasive Mole and Choriocarcinoma Associated with Hydatidiform Mole

JOHN I. BREWER and THOMAS R. ECKMAN

Northwestern University–McGraw Medical Center

A prospective study has been conducted to determine our ability to detect the presence of invasive mole and choriocarcinoma associated with termination of hydatidiform mole at the earliest possible time and to evaluate the results of therapy started at this early date. In designing this study 10 years ago, there were two recognized factors that prevented the establishment of a perfect design. Hydatidiform mole is relatively infrequent (1:2000 to 3000 deliveries in United States), which means that only approximately 1200 to 1500 new cases are encountered in the United States per year, and of these, the number of patients we might examine and test would be relatively few each year or every few years. Another factor was the fact that a prospective study such as this had not previously been made and there were no guides to follow. As a result, each patient had to be studied on a prospective rather than retrospective basis, decisions regarding the presence of progressive disease (invasive mole, choriocarcinoma) had to be made without established criteria, and those patients to be treated had to be selected by clinical judgment. Not until the study was completed would it be possible to evaluate our ability to make a correct diagnosis of progressive disease and to evaluate the results of early therapy. Only one criterion was established at the onset of the study—namely, that a decision regarding the presence or absence of invasive mole or choriocarcinoma would be made by 60 days after termination of the hydatid mole, and that patients who were to be treated would be selected and have treatment started between 60 and 70 days after termination of the molar pregnancy.

This study was supported by United States Public Health Service Research Grant CA 12109, and by grants from the Obstetrical and Gynecological Assembly of Southern California and the American Association of Obstetricians and Gynecologists.

A second objective of this study was to observe the natural history of hydatidiform mole on a prospective rather than a retrospective basis. In order to obtain this objective, patients could not be treated prophylactically with chemotherapy, since this could interfere with the natural course of the disease. Presented here are the results of the study.

MATERIAL AND METHODS

Comprising this report are the data of 139 consecutive patients studied over an 8 year period, with a subsequent 2 year minimum follow-up period for all patients, and a maximum of 10 years follow-up for the first patient studied.

Within 24 hours prior to termination of the hydatidiform mole the patient is examined, including x-rays of the lungs, and a quantitative human chorionic gonadotropin (HCG) test is performed as a baseline for future examinations. The HCG levels are determined and physical examinations are conducted at 10, 20, 30, 45, and 60 days after termination of the molar pregnancy. On each of these days, the titer levels and physical examination findings are evaluated, and at 60 days (earlier if necessary) a final decision is made regarding the necessity of instituting therapy. Indications for treatment are a rising titer at 60 days, a persistently high titer at that time, or evidence of metastatic disease. The latter was seldom encountered by the sixtieth day postmole. It is desirable to perform a curettage 10 to 14 days after termination of the mole to determine if there is residual molar tissue in the cavity of the uterus. If none is present, the follow-up with titer determinations is more meaningful, since a rise in titer level under this circumstance would more positively indicate the existence of progressive disease. If a curettage is not done, the rise in titer level might indicate only the presence of residual molar tissue in the cavity of the uterus, not necessarily the presence of invasive mole or choriocarcinoma.

At the beginning and all through the study, the mouse uterine weight bioassay was utilized to determine HCG levels. A sensitive test method is necessary, since in the spontaneous resolution of a hydatidiform mole, the level of the hormone will eventually reach a point below the sensitivity range of the usual commercial tests and in some instances both invasive mole and choriocarcinoma may be associated with HCG titers below the range of commercial titers, contrary to popular belief. We have demonstrated these phenomena in a previous study of 137 patients followed—by serial commercially available HCG titers—from the termination of hydatidiform mole to the time invasive mole or choriocarcinoma was diagnosed (Table 7–1). It is obvious that these tests were inadequate to

TABLE 7–1.   *Study of Commercially Available HCG Tests in the Follow-up of 137 Patients with Hydatidiform Mole*

	INVASIVE MOLE (26 PATIENTS)*	CHORIOCARCINOMA (26 PATIENTS)*
Tests positive all times tested	2 (8%)	4 (15%)
Tests negative all times tested	10 (38%)	6 (23%)
Tests negative at one or more times	14 (54%)	16 (62%)

* This is not a true incidence of invasive mole and choriocarcinoma (26 of 137 patients for both categories) associated with hydatidiform mole, since there was a bias in selection: These patients were sent to us because they had or were thought to have invasive mole or choriocarcinoma.

permit the accurate and reliable diagnosis of choriocarcinoma and invasive mole in patients following the termination of molar gestations. In a similar manner, these tests are not sufficiently specific for use in following the results of therapy in those patients who respond favorably, since the HCG titers will eventually reach low levels not detectable by commercial tests. Commercial tests are adequate as long as they are positive, but when they become negative, either in the follow-up of patients with hydatidiform mole or in following the effectiveness of therapy, it is necessary that more sensitive test methods be employed. We are now using a radioimmunoassay in place of the mouse uterine weight bioassay, since it is sensitive, accurate, cheaper, and less time-consuming.

Chemotherapy has been employed in those patients requiring treatment. Either methotrexate or actinomycin D is used in the following manner: methotrexate, 25 mg. intramuscularly, daily for 5 days; actinomycin D, 10 μg. per kg. body weight per day, intravenously, for 5 days. Toxic manifestations are monitored daily (bone marrow depression, oral and gastrointestinal reactions, dermatologic lesions, and so forth).

RESULTS AND COMMENT

The results of the HCG titer determinations on Day 30 and Day 60 following termination of the hydatidiform moles in 139 patients shown in Table 7–2. Physical and x-ray examinations did not aid materially in establishing the existence of invasive mole or choriocarcinoma, since a rise in the titer level preceded physical or x-ray evidence of disease. Thus, the titer determination is a most valuable procedure in detecting the progression of disease.

A total of 28 (20 per cent) of the 139 patients required treatment. This percentage is consistent with the generally accepted incidence of patients with hydatidiform mole who develop invasive mole and choriocarcinoma—namely, 19.5 per cent. These data are remarkably similar, especially in view of the fact that the data were gathered by a retrospective study in one instance and by a prospective study in the other instance. In the latter, the decision of the need for treatment was made upon serial titer level characteristics for each patient encountered during the 8 years of this study, and was made without past experience to guide us.

TABLE 7–2.   *Human Chorionic Gonadotropin Titer Data in 139 Patients Followed After Termination of Hydatidiform Molar Pregnancies*

	DAYS AFTER TERMINATION OF MOLAR GESTATION	
HCG TITERS	30	60
Normal	42 (30.2%)	90 (64.7%)
Elevated	97 (69.8%)	49* (35.3%)*
Patients treated	0	28†
Patients not treated	0	21‡

* Six of the 49 were not eligible for testing on Day 60, since they had sudden rises in titer levels at Day 45 after termination of hydatidiform mole, and therapy was started prior to Day 60.

† Twenty-two of the 28 patients were selected for treatment as a result of titer levels on Day 60 (in the other six, treatment was started prior to Day 60).

‡ Twenty-one patients with elevated titers at Day 60 had had declining titers each time tested, had low levels on Day 60, and were not treated. The titers became normal 72 to 142 days postmole, without need of treatment, and all have remained free of disease.

Of the 28 patients treated, three had proved choriocarcinoma and 25 had presumed invasive mole. In order that we keep data concerning choriocarcinoma as precise as possible, we place a patient in the choriocarcinoma category only if it can be proved that she has this disease. If this cannot be proved, she is placed in the diagnostic category of invasive mole. Such empirical division is required since chemotherapy is utilized for treatment and, as a result, adequate surgical specimens are seldom available from which a pathologic diagnosis can be made. The incidence of choriocarcinoma following hydatidiform mole in this study was 2.1 per cent, which closely coincides with the generally accepted 2.5 per cent incidence of choriocarcinoma developing after a molar pregnancy. The incidence of invasive mole in our study of 18 per cent is in close agreement with 17 per cent established by retrospective studies.

Of the three patients with choriocarcinoma, two developed demonstrable metastatic disease; of the 25 patients with invasive mole, three developed metastatic disease.

All of the 28 patients treated have attained permanent remissions. The remaining 111 of the 139 patients, who were not treated, are living and well, without evidence of disease.

These results seem to indicate that a regimen such as employed in this study is a most appropriate method for the management of patients subsequent to the termination of a molar gestation. It has an advantage over the prophylactic chemotherapy of patients with hydatidiform mole in that chemotherapeutic agents are administered only to those who need them. Another essential point is that even if prophylactic chemotherapy is used during the time of evacuation of a molar pregnancy, the HCG testing regimen described here must be carried out to determine the presence or absence of progressive disease. It is apparent that prophylactic chemotherapy, as now employed, does not prevent the development of progressive disease—namely, invasive mole and choriocarcinoma—in all instances, and that some patients do require subsequent therapy. Although we strongly advocate chemotherapy in trophoblastic disease, it is not considered desirable to administer these agents unless they are really required. On rare occasions, even an 80 per cent dose regimen has in our experience caused severe toxic manifestations and, in one instance, death.

Preferable Management of Gestational Trophoblastic Disease: Benign and Malignant

Donald P. Goldstein

Harvard Medical School, Boston Hospital for Women, and New England Trophoblastic Disease Center

It is now nearly two decades since the first patient with metastatic choriocarcinoma was treated at the National Cancer Institute. Since that time, the use of chemotherapy for trophoblastic disease has become the accepted means of treatment not only for patients with metastatic disease but also for patients with locally invasive disease who desire to preserve their reproductive function.

Despite the widespread use of chemotherapy, however, some misunderstandings remain regarding indications for treatment, drug regimens, and the role of surgery. The confusion arises in part because of the multiplicity of terminology used and the variations in interpretation, not only of the clinical symptoms but also of the morphologic criteria. Though most obstetrician-gynecologists have seen the disastrous effects of invasive mole or metastatic choriocarcinoma, the myth still persists that some forms of trophoblastic disease are "benign" and require only curettage and observation. This attitude arises from experience with patients with molar pregnancy whose pregnancy tests remain positive for months after evacuation, despite the absence of clinical stigmata of trophoblastic disease, and from observations of the rare patients with an invasive mole whose lung lesions regress spontaneously following hysterectomy.

The purpose of this discourse is to attempt to clarify the terminology applicable to trophoblastic disease and to suggest a revised therapeutic classification designed to permit more accurate selection of optimal forms of treatment in a wide variety of clinical situations.

Definition of Benign and Malignant Trophoblastic Disease

We will deal exclusively with trophoblastic disease which arises from pregnancy, i.e., gestational trophoblastic disease (GTD), and omit from the discus-

This study was supported in part by United States Public Health Service Grant CA 08388 from the National Cancer Institute, and the Choriocarcinoma Research Fund.

219

sion any material pertaining to trophoblastic tumors arising in the testis, ovary, or extragonadal sites, which are referred to collectively as nongestational trophoblastic disease.

Included in the category of "gestational trophoblastic disease" are three distinct morphologic entities that are readily distinguishable histopathologically —namely, hydatidiform mole, chorioadenoma destruens (invasive mole), and choriocarcinoma. The distinguishing feature of these tumors is the degree of retention of recognizable villous structures, or, stated in another way, the degree of differentiation of the neoplastic chorionic tissue. Hence, in those instances in which the entire tumor mass is confined to the uterine cavity and is made up of hydatidiform mole with minimal to moderate trophoblastic overgrowth, the lesion is called *hydatidiform mole*. When the tumor invades the uterine wall or adjacent extrauterine structures but retains the ability to differentiate villi from the residual trophoblastic tissue, it is termed *chorioadenoma destruens (invasive mole)*. When the trophoblastic tissue mass has become sufficiently anaplastic so as to lose its ability to differentiate villous structures and its growth is now associated with invasiveness, hemorrhage, and necrosis, the tumor is termed *choriocarcinoma*. At this stage the disease is highly malignant and the clinical situation quite serious.

Despite these apparently clear-cut morphologic criteria, there still exists a vast amount of confusion in everyday clinical practice with respect to the prognostic significance of these entities. It is well recognized that in over 50 per cent of patients with what ultimately proves to be choriocarcinoma there is a clear history of previous hydatidiform mole. Furthermore, numerous patients with a prior histologic diagnosis of invasive mole subsequently develop choriocarcinoma. This has created the inevitable controversy over whether this "benign" tissue changes morphologically during its growth or whether malignant tissue was already present at the inception of the disease. The situation is further complicated by the fact that the maternal host possesses the inherent capacity to reject the invading fetal tissue, thus leading to rare but well-documented instances of spontaneous regression of the tumor process; this is associated with complete absence of residual disease in some cases, and merely partial regression of an isolated metastasis in others. Accordingly, any prognostic inferences or any therapeutic claims in relation to gestational trophoblastic disease must involve a large number of cases carefully evaluated on clinical, morphological, and hormonal grounds, with full appreciation being given to the highly varied and complex dynamic interrelationships between these and the several forms of the tumor.

Because of this confusion in morphologic interpretation of the various forms of GTD, the concept of using the clinical status of the patient rather than the known histopathology has been adopted. Thus, GTD is considered nonmetastatic if the tumor has not spread beyond the confines of the uterus, and metastatic when there is clinical, laboratory, or radiological evidence of extension or spread beyond the confines of the uterus, either locally to adjacent or contiguous pelvic structures, or distantly, to extrapelvic locations.[1]

Therapeutic Classification

We have utilized the above-mentioned generally accepted taxonomy as the basis for a revised therapeutic classification of gestational trophoblastic disease, which takes into consideration the following factors: histopathology, duration of the disease from the antecedent pregnancy (or, where this is unknown, the onset of symptoms), initial gonadotropin titer prior to institution of therapy, depth of myometrial invasion, and location of metastases. This classification has been used clinically for about four years in the management of over 300 patients at the New England Trophoblastic Disease Center and has proved to be of considerable value in selecting the optimal therapeutic regimen in individual patients.

The proposed therapeutic classification for GTD is as follows: *

Class 1.   Molar pregnancy
    a. Pre-evacuation
    b. Post-evacuation (< 8 weeks)
Class 2.   Noninvasive trophoblastic disease
    a. Hydatidiform mole
    b. Choriocarcinoma
Class 3.   Invasive trophoblastic disease
    a. Hydatidiform mole
    b. Choriocarcinoma
Class 4.   Low-risk metastatic trophoblastic disease
    a. Hydatidiform mole
    b. Choriocarcinoma
Class 5.   High-risk metastatic trophoblastic disease

Preferable Management of Class 1 (Molar Pregnancy)

DIAGNOSIS

Class 1 includes all patients with molar pregnancy diagnosed either prior to evacuation (1a) or within eight weeks after evacuation (1b).

For Class 1a, a positive diagnosis of molar pregnancy is made on the basis of clinical, laboratory, or radiologic evidence. Clinically, unevacuated molar pregnancy is characterized by a number of signs and symptoms, which may include vaginal bleeding, rapid uterine enlargement, hyperemesis gravidarum, toxemia of pregnancy, theca lutein cysts, hyperthyroidism, and trophoblastic embolization.[2] In most instances, the chorionic gonadotropin (HCG) titer will be markedly elevated (Figure 7-1). The most accurate means of diagnosis, however, utilize the relatively new techniques of amniography and ultrasonography. Injection of radiopaque dye transabdominally into uteri larger than that characteristic of 14 weeks' gestation will clearly outline the molar vesicles (Figure 7-2), in contrast to the appearance of a normal single (Figure 7-3) or multiple (Figure 7-4) pregnancy. Similarly, the use of B scan ultrasonography will reveal the characteristic picture of molar pregnancy (Figure 7-5), in contrast to the easily distinguishable fetal sac (Figure 7-6). Amniography has the advantage of being readily available in every radiology department, but the disadvantages of requiring invasion of the uterus and radiation exposure to a normal fetus if present. Ultrasonography is advantageous in being completely safe for the patient and a normal fetus, but has

---

* Categories *a* and *b* in each class are based on available pathologic material.

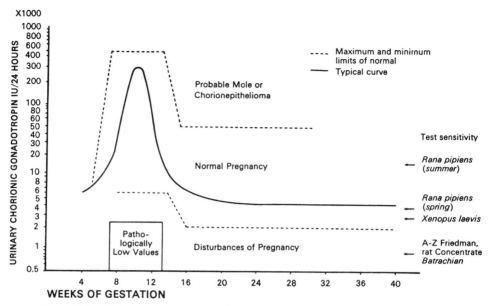

Figure 7-1. Urinary chorionic gonadotropin excretion in patients with molar and normal pregnancy. (After Hon: Pregnancy Testing. New Haven, Yale University Press, 1955.)

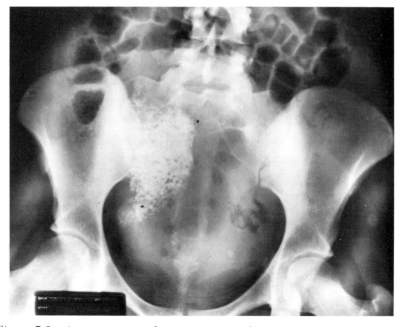

Figure 7-2. Anteroposterior plane amniogram of intrauterine dye study in a patient with molar pregnancy showing the "moth-eaten" or "honeycombed" pattern of the vesicles.

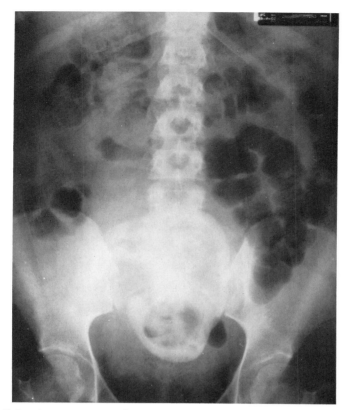

Figure 7-3.   Anteroposterior plane amniogram of intrauterine dye study in a patient with a normal single fetus.

the disadvantage of requiring expensive equipment and highly trained personnel not generally available in most community hospitals.

For Class 1*b*, the diagnosis of molar pregnancy is made at evacuation and confirmed pathologically, but in these cases an insufficient period of time has lapsed to be certain whether or not the patient will develop proliferative trophoblastic sequelae.

TREATMENT

The preferable method of evacuation in cases of Class 1*a* molar pregnancy depends upon the patient's wishes regarding preservation of reproductive function. When future pregnancies are desired, the method of choice for evacuation is the use of suction curettage regardless of the uterine size. If a suction aspirator is unavailable, sharp curettage should be performed when the uterus is of a smaller size than that of a 12 to 14 weeks' gestation, and abdominal hysterotomy utilized in patients in whom the uterus is larger than that of a pregnancy of 12 to 14 weeks. In rare instances, there may be justification for inducing spontaneous passage of the molar pregnancy by the use of intravenous oxytocics in a patient whose uterus is larger than that characteristic of 12 to 14 weeks' gestation and whose condition is too critical for anesthesia. In these uncommon situations, the goal is to reduce the size of the uterus by removing most of its contents and then

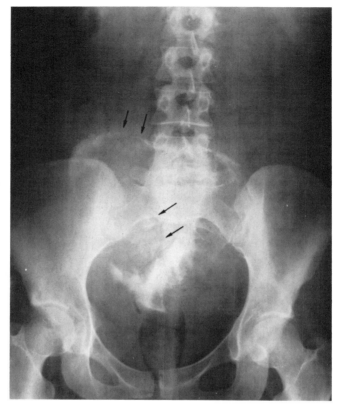

Figure 7-4. Anteroposterior plane amniogram of intrauterine dye study in a patient with twins.

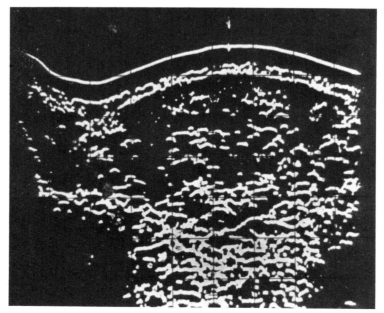

Figure 7-5. Lateral ultrasonogram of a patient with molar pregnancy.

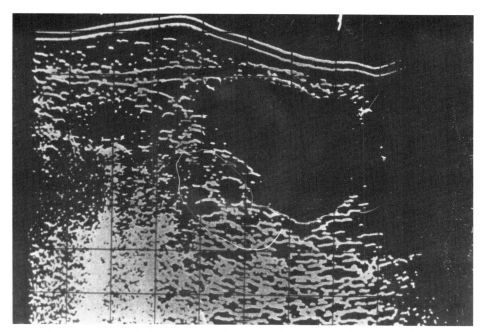

Figure 7-6. Lateral ultrasonogram of a patient showing an early gestational sac.

completing the evacuation by sharp curettage when the patient's clinical status has improved.

When future pregnancies are no longer desired, the preferable method of evacuation is abdominal hysterectomy because removal of the uterus with the mole in situ eliminates the complication of locally invasive disease and substantially reduces the likelihood that the patient will develop metastases.[3]

In patients with unevacuated molar pregnancy (Class 1*a*), in whom early diagnosis is made and evacuation carried out electively, the use of chemotherapy prophylactically virtually eliminates metastatic sequelae and substantially reduces the incidence of nonmetastatic complications without producing serious toxicity.[4] The recommended protocol calls for the use of a five day course of actinomycin D (Cosmegen), 12 μg. per kg. body weight per day, intravenously, with evacuation performed on the third day. The use of prophylactic chemotherapy in Class 1*b* patients has not yet been evaluated.

In all Class 1 patients, careful evaluation of both the molar specimen and endometrial curettings using the criteria of Hertig and Sheldon[5] is important, with particular attention paid to the histologic grade and the degree of invasion. A histologic diagnosis of invasive mole or choriocarcinoma is an indication for chemotherapy. Furthermore, it is important to obtain a chest film for use as baseline and to institute a program of gonadotropin follow-up in order to achieve early detection of proliferative trophoblastic sequelae. The *sine qua non* for adequate follow-up of *all* patients with molar pregnancy is a weekly determination of the gonadotropin level using a sufficiently sensitive assay system to permit measurement of gonadotropin levels down to normal endogenous pituitary levels (Figure 7-7). This is best accomplished by the use of the new radioimmunoassay methods which utilize serum.[6] If the gonadotropin titer drops to normal pituitary

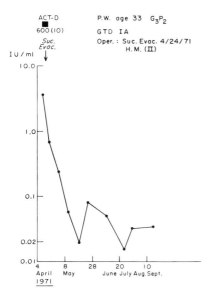

Figure 7-7. Clinical data from a patient with molar pregnancy following evacuation.

levels and remains in the normal range for three consecutive weeks, the patient is considered to be in remission. At this point follow-up gonadotropin titers are obtained at monthly intervals for *six* months, during which time careful contraception should be practiced. Oral contraceptives are desirable because they tend to lower and stabilize endogenous pituitary gonadotropin output. If the gonadotropin titer remains normal for six consecutive months, then a subsequent pregnancy is permitted. On the other hand, if the post-evacuation gonadotropin level plateaus over two or more weeks, becomes reelevated, or metastases appear during follow-up, the patient should be reevaluated and further therapy instituted.

PROGNOSIS

The prognosis for Class 1 patients depends on whether the patient undergoes elective evacuation with prophylactic actinomycin D chemotherapy (Class 1*a*), or whether evacuation is carried out without drug cover (Class 1*b*). As noted above, termination of the molar pregnancy by abdominal hysterectomy, in contrast to curettage or hysterotomy, also influences prognosis.

Table 7–3 summarizes the overall results in 200 patients with molar pregnancy. In Class 1*a* the use of prophylactic actinomycin D in 100 patients was

TABLE 7–3.   *Overall Results in 200 Patients with Class 1 (Molar Pregnancy)*

OUTCOME	TREATED*	UNTREATED†
Normal involution	98	84
Persistent disease‡		
Nonmetastatic	2	12
Metastatic	—	4
Total Patients	100	100

* Actinomycin D administered at the time of evacuation.
† Follow-up was begun no later than two weeks after evacuation.
‡ Gonadotropin level elevated eight weeks or longer after evacuation.

associated with a 2 per cent incidence of nonmetastatic trophoblastic disease. In a comparable group of 100 patients evacuated without prophylactic actinomycin D (Class 1b), 12 per cent developed non-metastatic disease and 4 per cent were found to have metastases. This difference is statistically significant ($P < 0.01$). Trophoblastic sequelae were not encountered in the 13 patients who underwent hysterectomy regardless of whether or not chemotherapy was utilized. (These figures are based on the premise that the gonadotropin level is an accurate means of determining the outcome when a patient with molar pregnancy either completely resolves residual trophoblastic tissue or develops proliferative trophoblastic sequelae. In this study, if an elevated serum gonadotropin level persists beyond eight weeks, rises, or plateaus for two or more weeks before this time, the patient is considered to have trophoblastic disease.)

Preferable Management of Class 2 (Noninvasive Trophoblastic Disease)

DIAGNOSIS

Class 2 of gestational trophoblastic disease includes all patients who exhibit uterine subinvolution, vaginal bleeding, and an elevated gonadotropin level for more than eight weeks after evacuation of a molar pregnancy or termination of an abortal or term pregnancy. Theca lutein cysts may or may not be present. Metastases to the lungs, brain, vagina, liver, and other organs are *not* present, neither is there evidence of deep myometrial invasion on pelvic angiography (Figure 7-8). Curettage should be performed to determine whether the residual trophoblastic tissue is molar (Class 2a) or choriocarcinoma (Class 2b).

THERAPY

The preferable treatment of Class 2 disease depends upon whether the patient desires future pregnancies rather than on the histologic diagnosis. If she does, treatment should consist of one course of chemotherapy, either methotrexate (0.4 mg. per kg. body weight per day, intramuscularly) or actinomycin D (12 μg. per kg. body weight per day, intravenously), administered for five days according to well established guidelines.[7] Diagnostic curettage should be performed during this course of treatment to avoid dissemination of viable trophoblastic tissue.[8]

When preservation of reproductive function is no longer desired, the preferable treatment is total abdominal hysterectomy (with or without oophorectomy). If hysterectomy is elected, one course of chemotherapy should be given to reduce the likelihood that viable trophoblastic tissue will be spread. After completion of therapy (whether alone or in combination with surgery), careful monitoring of the gonadotropin titers should be instituted utilizing the principles outlined previously.

When normal pituitary gonadotropin levels are achieved, assays should be performed monthly for six months and bimonthly for six months, during which time careful contraception should be practiced. After one year of normal gonadotropin titers pregnancy is permissible.

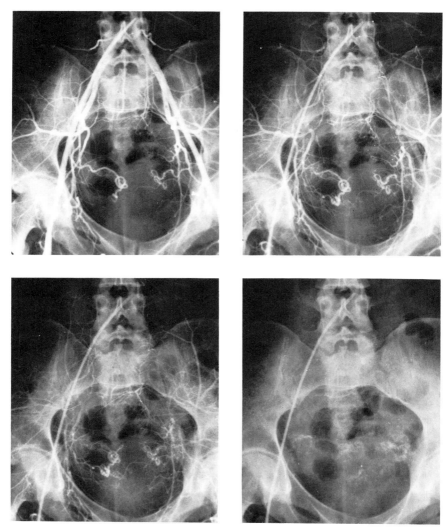

Figure 7-8.   Transfemoral pelvic angiogram in a patient with a normal uterus.

Prognosis

Table 7–4 summarizes the results of treatment in 11 patients with Class 2 disease. All patients are living and well without clinical, hormonal, or radiological evidence of disease, regardless of histologic diagnosis, agent(s) utilized, or whether or not the uterus was removed.

It should be stressed that if the patient has been properly classified, no further therapy should be required. It is inevitable that in the occasional patient, pathologic review of the histologic material will reveal the presence of unsuspected deep myometrial invasion or choriocarcinoma. When this situation arises, careful monitoring of the gonadotropin level will provide an adequate measure of the presence of residual disease. Further therapy may be safely withheld pending the outcome of these studies.

TABLE 7–4. *Results of Treatment in Class 2 (Noninvasive Gestational Trophoblastic Disease)*

THERAPY AND OUTCOME	HYDATIDIFORM MOLE (10 PATIENTS)	CHORIOCARCINOMA (1 PATIENT)
Remission Therapy		
Methotrexate	3	0
Actinomycin D	5	1
Both	0	0
Hysterectomy*	2	0
Outcome		
Remission	10	1
Death	0	0

* Surgery performed with adjunctive chemotherapy.

Preferable Management of Class 3 (Invasive Trophoblastic Disease)

DIAGNOSIS

Class 3 includes patients who have clinical, hormonal, and radiological evidence of persistent trophoblastic disease deeply invading the myometrium, without evidence of distant metastases. Invasion may be reliably determined by pelvic angiography (Figure 7-9) or curettage. This syndrome is characterized by uterine enlargement, vaginal bleeding, and elevated gonadotropin titers after evacuation of a molar pregnancy or termination of an abortal or term pregnancy.

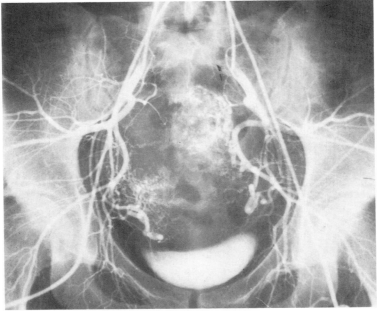

Figure 7-9. Transfemoral pelvic angiogram in a patient with invasive mole.

Persistent theca lutein cysts are seen only in the patients with antecedent molar pregnancy. Class 3a consists of patients with an histologic diagnosis of hydatidiform mole, while Class 3b patients have choriocarcinoma.

TREATMENT

In Class 3 disease as well, the preferable treatment depends upon whether or not preservation of reproductive function is desired by the patient. In this group, it is important to determine as precisely as possible the histologic nature of the invading trophoblastic tissue because of the increased morbidity rates associated with the presence of choriocarcinoma.[9] Despite this increased morbidity, Class 3a or 3b patients are managed according to the same principles.

Patients who desire future pregnancies should be treated with sequential methotrexate and actinomycin D according to the intermittent intensive regimen reported by Ross and co-workers.[10] Diagnostic curettage, when performed, should be carried out during the first course of therapy for the same reason as is outlined above. Methotrexate is administered intramuscularly in five day courses in doses ranging from 0.3 to 0.5 mg. per kg. body weight per day, and actinomycin D is administered intravenously in five day courses in doses ranging from 10 to 12 μg. per kg. body weight per day.

Response to chemotherapy is based solely on the gonadotropin response as determined weekly by serum radioimmunoassay. Therapy is continued until the gonadotropin titer is in the normal pituitary range for three consecutive weeks. At this point, a final course of chemotherapy, consisting of the last effective drug, should be administered to reduce the likelihood of relapse. Further follow-up should consist of measuring monthly gonadotropin titers for six months and bimonthly determinations for six months, during which time careful contraception should be practiced. After one year of normal gonadotropin titers, pregnancy is permitted. Gonadotropin assays should be performed every six months until pregnancy is achieved.

When systemic chemotherapy proves ineffective or excessively toxic so as to preclude adequate therapy, hypogastric artery infusion should be instituted.[11] Combination chemotherapy such as triple therapy is contraindicated in this group of patients because of its increased morbidity and mortality rates. When resistance to sequential therapy is encountered, the treatment of choice is hysterectomy.

In Class 3 patients who no longer desire to preserve fertility, hysterectomy is advisable. Surgery should always be performed in conjunction with chemotherapy to reduce the chance of tumor spread. Gonadotropin follow-up following surgery is the same as when chemotherapy alone is utilized.

PROGNOSIS

Table 7-5 summarizes the results of treatment in 55 patients with Class 3 disease. All patients are living and well, without clinical, hormonal, or radiological evidence of disease, regardless of histologic diagnosis, agent(s) utilized, or whether or not the uterus was removed. Three patients (all with a histologic diagnosis of choriocarcinoma) required hysterectomy because of chemotherapy failure, whereas surgery was performed in four patients because they no longer desired children. Eight patients achieved remission with hypogastric artery infu-

TABLE 7–5.   *Results of Treatment of Class 3 (Invasive Gestational Trophoblastic Disease)*

THERAPY AND OUTCOME	HYDATIDIFORM MOLE (46 PATIENTS)	CHORIOCARCINOMA (9 PATIENTS)	TOTAL PATIENTS (55)
Remission Therapy			
Methotrexate	24	2	26
Actinomycin D	9	2	11
Both	9	2	11
Hysterectomy*	4	3	7
Outcome			
Remission	46	9	55
Death	0	0	0

* Surgery performed with adjunctive chemotherapy.

sion instituted because of excessive toxicity or unsatisfactory response to systemic chemotherapy at the dose level. In five of these eight patients, diagnosis of choriocarcinoma was confirmed. Two patients relapsed during the 12 month follow-up period and required treatment. In both, an histologic diagnosis of choriocarcinoma was made. One of these patients subsequently developed pulmonary lesions, which responded to therapy. When remission therapy is considered, it is apparent that the presence of choriocarcinoma is associated with higher drug requirements, increased need for surgery, and a greater morbidity rate.[12]

Preferable Management of Class 4 (Low-risk Metastatic Trophoblastic Disease)

DIAGNOSIS

Class 4 includes patients with clinical, radiologic, and hormonal evidence of persistent trophoblastic disease beyond the confines of the uterus when the duration of the disease is less than four months from the termination of the antecedent pregnancy or the onset of symptoms, and the initial gonadotropin titer is less than 100,000 I.U./24 hours (or the equivalent). Only patients with metastases to the lungs, vagina, and pelvis are included. Class 4a consists of patients with an histologic diagnosis of hydatidiform mole, while Class 4b patients have choriocarcinoma. Approximately 50 per cent of patients in this group show no evidence of uterine involvement.

TREATMENT

The preferable treatment of Class 4 patients is chemotherapy regardless of the desire to preserve reproductive function. Chemotherapy should consist of sequential administration of methotrexate and actinomycin D as already outlined. Once again response to chemotherapy is based solely on the weekly determinations of gonadotropin response. Therapy is continued until the gonadotropin titer is in the normal pituitary range for three consecutive weeks. A final course of the last effective drug should be administered to reduce the likelihood of relapse. If resistance to sequential therapy is encountered, triple therapy should be utilized, consisting of methotrexate (0.3 mg. per kg. body weight per day), actinomycin D

(10 μg. per kg. body weight per day), and cyclophosphamide (3 mg. per kg. body weight per day), given simultaneously in five day courses.[13] Hysterectomy is reserved for surgical indications such as an enlarged tumor-filled uterus, palpable adnexal spread, sepsis, or heavy bleeding. Bowel metastases should be surgically excised because of the danger of bleeding, obstruction, and poor response to drugs. Open thoracotomy is rarely justified—unless persistent pulmonary bleeding is encountered—because of the multiple nature of most pulmonary spread.[14]

PROGNOSIS

Table 7–6 summarizes the results of treatment in 47 patients with Class 4 disease. All patients are living and well, without clinical, hormonal, or radiological evidence of disease, regardless of histologic diagnosis, agent(s) utilized, or whether or not the uterus was removed. In 10 patients hysterectomy was required because of surgical indications. Two patients relapsed during the 12 month follow-up period and were successfully re-treated. In both, a histologic diagnosis of choriocarcinoma was confirmed. When remission therapy is considered, it is apparent that the presence of choriocarcinoma is associated with higher drug requirements, increased need for surgery, and increased morbidity.[12]

Preferable Management of Class 5 (High-risk Trophoblastic Disease)

DIAGNOSIS

Class 5 includes patients with clinical, radiologic, and hormonal evidence of trophoblastic disease beyond the confines of the uterus, when the duration of disease is longer than four months from the termination of the antecedent pregnancy or the onset of symptoms, and the gonadotropin titer is higher than 100,000 I.U./24 hours (or the equivalent). Patients with brain or liver metastases are limited to this group. All patients in this group have an histopathologic diagnosis of choriocarcinoma. Approximately 50 per cent of patients show no evidence of residual uterine involvement.

TABLE 7–6.   *Results of Treatment of Class 4 (Low-Risk Metastatic Gestational Trophoblastic Disease)*

THERAPY AND OUTCOME	HYDATIDIFORM MOLE (27 PATIENTS)	CHORIOCARCINOMA (20 PATIENTS)	TOTAL PATIENTS (47)
Remission Therapy			
Methotrexate	7	4	11
Actinomycin D	11	4	15
Both	7	8	15
Triple	2	4	6
Outcome			
Remission	27	20	47
Death	0	0	0

Treatment

The preferable treatment of Class 5 patients is chemotherapy regardless of the desire to preserve reproductive function. Since the results of therapy with sequential methotrexate and actinomycin D have been uniformly poor, optimal treatment should consist of triple therapy. It should be emphasized that the mortality rate of this therapy as a result of gram-negative septicemia, secondary to marrow suppression, runs as high as 15 per cent. Hysterectomy should be performed when there is evidence of intrauterine or adnexal tumor, sepsis, or bleeding. When brain metastases are diagnosed by neurologic examination, brain scan, and electroencephalography, whole head irradiation using approximately 2000 to 3000 rads is imperative because of the danger of sudden hemorrhage. Liver metastases should be treated with local irradiation followed by systemic therapy. Local resection of liver lesions is of limited value for the same reason that pulmonary resection fails—namely, because of the presence of multiple foci. In our experience, hepatic infusion using triple therapy has proved to be of value in two patients with solitary liver lesions.

Prognosis

Table 7–7 summarizes the results of treatment in 10 patients with Class 5 disease. Since the use of primary triple therapy is a recent innovation, there is insufficient data to report meaningful survival figures. It is of interest, however, that the two patients with Class 5 disease who did survive were treated with triple therapy after sequential methotrexate and actinomycin D regimen failed.

Conclusions

The dramatic change which has occurred in the management of patients with gestational trophoblastic disease during the past 15 years has stimulated renewed enthusiasm for using chemotherapy with other tumors. The reason why this tumor responds so spectacularly to the agent(s) commonly used less successfully against other tumors eludes us. It is not clear what role immunology—or for that matter, the genetic heterogeneity which is characteristic of trophoblastic cells—plays in this regard. Furthermore, there are still a number of unanswered questions, such as the etiology of molar pregnancy and the reasons for its geographic and socioeconomic variations.

TABLE 7–7. *Results of Treatment in Class 5 (High-Risk Metastatic Gestational Trophoblastic Disease)*

THERAPY AND OUTCOME	NUMBER OF PATIENTS
Remission Therapy	
Methotrexate	0
Actinomycin D.	0
Both	0
Triple*	2
Outcome	
Remissions	2
Death	8

* Always used after sequential therapy with methotrexate and actinomycin D.

Nonetheless, the lessons learned from trophoblastic disease are many. For the first time in oncology it has become possible to apply the same principles that have been developed for the treatment of infections to the treatment of tumors. The unusual ability of trophoblastic tissue to consistently produce a polypeptide hormone with gonadotropin properties similar to that produced by natural placental tissue and the pituitary gland provides us with remarkably sensitive and reliable ways to detect, or to follow, trophoblastic cell growth and regression in relation to both the natural history of the tumor and its response to chemotherapy. Thus the use of the gonadotropin assay permits early detection, a means of monitoring the effectiveness of therapy, and a means of reliable follow-up to detect the rare instances of relapse owing to inadequate therapy. Studies of the natural history of trophoblastic tumor have culminated in the very suggestive evidence, already cited, that this tumor may have an in situ phase which can be prevented by the use of prophylactic therapy. Thus, early diagnosis, adequate therapy, careful follow-up—and now prophylaxis—make the day seem not too distant when death from trophoblastic tumors will have been eliminated.

REFERENCES

1. Holland, J. F., and M. M. Hreshchyshyn, M. M. (Eds.): Choriocarcinoma: Transactions of a Conference of the International Union Against Cancer. Appendix I. New York, Springer-Verlag, 1967.
2. Goldstein, D. P.: Five years' experience with the prevention of trophoblastic tumors by the prophylactic use of chemotherapy in patients with molar pregnancy. Clin. Obstet. Gynec. 13:945, 1971.
3. Chun, D., Lu, T., and Chung, H. K.: Observation of the prophylactic use of chemotherapy after termination of hydatidiform mole. In Holland, J. F., and Hreshchyshyn, M. M. (Eds.): Choriocarcinoma: Transactions of a Conference of the International Union Against Cancer. New York, Springer-Verlag, 1967.
4. Goldstein, D. P.: Prophylactic chemotherapy of patients with molar pregnancy. Obstet. Gynec. 38:817, 1971.
5. Hertig, A. T., and Sheldon, W. H.: Hydatidiform mole—a pathologicoclinical correlation of 200 cases. Amer. J. Obstet. Gynec. 53:1, 1947.
6. Goldstein, D. P., Miyata, J., Taymor, M. L., and Levesque, L.: A rapid solid-phase radioimmunoassay for the measurement of serum luteinizing hormone and human chorionic gonadotropin activity in very early pregnancy. Fertil. Steril. 23:817, 1972.
7. Hertz, R., Lewis, J. J., Jr., and Lipsett, M. B.: Five years' experience with the chemotherapy of metastatic choriocarcinoma and related trophoblastic tumors in women. Amer. J. Obstet. Gynec. 82:631, 1961.
8. Lewis, J., Jr., Gore, H., Hertig, A. T., et al: Treatment of trophoblastic disease with rationale for the use of adjunctive chemotherapy at the time of indicated operation. Amer. J. Obstet. Gynec. 96:710, 1966.
9. Brewer, J. I., Smith, R. T., and Pratt, G. B.: Choriocarcinomas: Absolute five year survival rates of 122 patients treated by hysterectomy. Amer. J. Obstet. Gynec. 85:841, 1963.
10. Ross, G. T., Goldstein, D. P., Hertz, R., et al.: Sequential use of methotrexate and actinomycin D in the treatment of metastatic choriocarcinoma and related trophoblastic disease in women. Amer. J. Obstet. Gynec. 93:223, 1965.
11. Goldstein, D. P., Couch, N. P., and Hall, T. C.: The role of infusion therapy in the treatment of patients with choriocarcinoma and related trophoblastic tumors. Surg. Forum 18:426, 1967.
12. Goldstein, D. P.: The chemotherapy of gestational trophoblastic disease. J.A.M.A. 220:209, 1972.
13. Li, M. C., Whitmore, W. F., Jr., Goldberg, R., et al.: Effects of combined drug therapy on metastatic cancer of the testis. J.A.M.A. 174:1291, 1960.
14. Shirley, R. L., Goldstein, D. P., and Collins, J. J., Jr.: The role of thoracotomy in the treatment of patients with chest mestastases from gestational trophoblastic disease. J. Thor. Cardiovasc. Surg. 63:545, 1972.

Preferable Management of Gestational Trophoblastic Disease: Benign and Malignant

CHARLES B. HAMMOND

*Southeastern Regional Center for Trophoblastic Disease
and Duke University Medical Center*

Introduction

Prior to the introduction of chemotherapy, the survival rate for patients with gestational trophoblastic neoplasms, choriocarcinoma, and related tumors was unusually poor.[1,2] However, in 1956 a patient with metastatic choriocarcinoma was successfully treated chemotherapeutically and a new era in tumor therapy began.[3] Many reports followed in rapid succession, including a 10 year study by Hertz and co-workers in Bethesda, who investigated the effects of various chemotherapeutic agents upon nearly 200 patients with these malignancies.[4,5,6] From all these studies came several conclusions: first, a significant number of these patients can be cured with chemotherapy; second, early disease is more often limited in amount and is associated with higher cure rates and less therapy; third, the toxic side-effects of chemotherapeutic agents are predictable and rarely fatal if the person administering them is experienced with their use and both clinical and laboratory expertise are available; finally, less than adequate therapy often results in the subsequent development of resistant disease.[7]

Equal in importance to aggressive therapy of patients with gestational trophoblastic neoplasms (GTN) is the availability of an accurate laboratory in which the human chorionic gonadotropin (HCG) levels may be measured. This hormone is produced in essentially all patients with these tumors.[8] Through precise measurement of the amount of HCG present, one can accurately follow the progress of therapy, document remission, and maintain follow-up. Precise and sensitive assays, including radioimmunoassay and bioassays on concentrates of 24 hour urine collections, are necessary if tragic consequences are to be avoided.

In the past several years several treatment centers have been developed to treat and investigate patients with these tumors. This chapter will attempt to review our concept of adequate therapy for patients with both benign and malignant trophoblastic disease, and to discuss several newer treatment methodologies.

Benign Trophoblastic Disease

By benign trophoblastic disease we mean primary hydatidiform mole, a gestation which usually lacks an intact fetus and is characterized by cystic swelling of the chorionic villi. The histopathologic criteria of hydatidiform mole are edema of the villous stroma, loss of the vascular pattern, and varying degrees of trophoblastic proliferation. The frequency of mole has marked geographic variation, and the best estimates of incidence in the United States are 1:1000 to 2000 pregnancies. Approximately 50 per cent of patients with metastatic gestational trophoblastic neoplasms, and 75 per cent of GTN patients without metastases, initially had molar pregnancies.

DIAGNOSIS

In the early stages of gestation, hydatidiform mole has no characteristics to distinguish it from normal pregnancy. Uterine bleeding is the single outstanding sign, and may vary from spotting to profuse hemorrhage. Anemia is a common finding. Early abortion may occur, but if not, the uterus may enlarge disproportionately to that expected. Abortion is most likely to occur near the seventeenth week of gestation and rarely after the twenty-eighth week. Massive enlargement of the ovaries may occur owing to theca lutein cyst formation. Toxemia of pregnancy is seen in 10 to 15 per cent of patients with hydatidiform mole and hyperemesis is a common complaint.

The diagnosis of mole may be quite easy, owing to the passage of molar vesicles, but usually it is more difficult to achieve. If the uterus is enlarged to adequate size, useful diagnostic findings include: palpation of fetal parts or movement, detection of a fetal heart by auscultation or electrocardiography, or x-ray visualization of the fetal skeleton. Positive evidence is reliable, but negative findings may be misleading. Amniography, using transabdominal instillation of a radiopaque dye into the uterine cavity, is probably the best diagnostic test, as a classic "honeycomb" pattern is produced by the dye around the dilated vesicles. Ultrasound patterns are also quite useful for diagnosis of hydatidiform mole. Tests for human chorionic gonadotropin (HCG) usually show significant elevations over those seen in normal pregnancy, but we must remember that no single HCG value can be diagnostic. Repeated high HCG titers are quite suggestive of hydatidiform mole. Assays for leucine aminopeptidase, placental lactogen, and estrogens have been of little use.

MANAGEMENT

The mortality rate in primary molar pregnancy should be quite low with aggressive management. Primary therapy should be aimed at correction of anemia, management of superimposed medical complications, and uterine evacuation. Data now suggest that the route or method of uterine evacuation does not influence the ultimate outcome of patients with molar pregnancy in respect to the incidence of postevacuation malignancy, which occurs in 10 to 20 per cent of these patients. The decision to evacuate the uterus by oxytocic infusion, followed by curettage, suction curettage, hysterotomy, or hysterectomy, is dependent upon the status of the patient with regard to labor, bleeding, uterine size, age, parity, and the patient's wishes concerning further reproduction. We have suggested primarily either suction dilatation and curettage or hysterectomy, depending upon whether or not the patient desires future pregnancies.

Several studies have demonstrated that there is a 10 to 20 per cent chance that patients with hydatidiform mole will later develop malignant trophoblastic disease.[9,10] The initial histopathology is of little aid in predicting which particular patients will develop malignancies.[11] Classical findings such as prompt uterine involution, regression of cystic ovarian enlargement, and cessation of bleeding are all favorable clinical signs, but a definitive follow-up of the patient after evacuation of hydatidiform mole is made with HCG assays to detect residual or proliferating trophoblastic malignancy. For such follow-ups the assay must be sufficiently sensitive and specific to measure levels of HCG well into normal pituitary gonadotropin ranges. Bioassays on concentrates of 24 hour urine samples or radioimmunoassays are required for these levels of sensitivity. Pregnancy tests are of use *only when positive*.[12] We suggest that HCG assays be performed at 1 to 2 week intervals after the evacuation of the mole. Delfs has well shown that the persistent secretion of HCG 6 to 8 weeks after molar evacuation is associated with a great likelihood that malignant trophoblastic disease is present or will develop.[9] If the HCG titer fails to decline, rises, or plateaus by 6 to 8 weeks after evacuation, or if metastases are noted, we suggest that systemic therapy be instituted. If the HCG titer falls to nonmeasurable levels, follow-up is instituted with HCG assays at 1 to 2 month intervals for one year. We have not found that repeated curettage was of assistance in follow-up or management of these patients.

PROPHYLACTIC CHEMOTHERAPY

Several authors have reported a reduction in the incidence of post-molar trophoblastic malignancy if patients received systemic chemotherapy at the time of evacuation of the mole.[13,14] To date, however, these studies have been small and conducted by experts in the use of these agents; even these have not totally eradicated the malignant sequelae of hydatidiform mole. We have seen several patients who received such "prophylactic therapy" administered by community physicians not familiar with these potent agents, and the subsequent toxicity was severe. Fortunately, no deaths have occurred. It will be shown later in this chapter that the 10 to 20 per cent of patients who develop malignant disease after molar pregnancy can be readily identified at 6 to 8 weeks after molar evacuation by HCG assay and by the clinical course of their disease, and that such early diagnosis can be equated with a cure rate of essentially 100 per cent with appropriate therapy.[15] For these reasons, we have not recommended prophylactic chemotherapy for all patients with hydatidiform mole, which means treating 80 to 90 per cent of these patients unnecessarily. This is not to condemn a needed experimental approach by qualified investigators; instead, it is an effort to reduce unnecessary morbidity and mortality for most of these patients.

Malignant Trophoblastic Disease

The spectrum of disease in the category of GTN includes malignancies under the pathologic terms of hydatidiform mole (after initial evacuation), invasive mole (chorioadenoma destruens), and choriocarcinoma. All are preceded by some type of pregnancy, although over 50 per cent initially were molar gestations. The follow-up of patients with hydatidiform mole has been described in the previous section, but once therapy is indicated in these patients, or if a diagnosis of either invasive mole or choriocarcinoma is made, then treatment should be promptly initiated.

Once the diagnosis of GTN is made we determine the HCG level and attempt to determine if metastases are present. We have found these studies to be particularly useful: thorough history, physical and pelvic examinations; chest x-ray; electroencephalogram; liver and brain isotopic scans; intravenous pyelogram; and complete hematologic and chemical evaluations.

Nonmetastatic Trophoblastic Disease

Nonmetastatic GTN, or disease confined to the uterus without evidence of distant metastases, will be seen with a greater frequency if the examiner's index of suspicion is high! In approximately 75 per cent of patients the diagnosis will be achieved during follow-up of individuals who have had molar pregnancy, and the remainder will follow other types of pregnancy. In both situations, abnormal gestational tissue may be discovered on curettage and gonadotropins will be elevated. It is important to diagnose histopathologically one of the various categories of trophoblastic disease, and the patient is then best followed by monitoring gonadotropin titers. Metastatic staging studies, as outlined above, should be carried out. The patient and physicians should then come to a decision for or against further reproduction, as the choice will influence her management. If the reproductive potential is to be preserved, the patient is then begun on single agent methotrexate or actinomycin D as outlined in Table 7–8. Therapy is continued with repetitive courses of either agent, utilizing the response of the HCG titer as the primary index of oncolytic effectiveness. Treatment is maintained in this fashion until the HCG titer is reduced to nonmeasurable levels. If the HCG titer fails to decline, if it rises, or if metastases appear, then therapy is switched to the alternative drug.

If the patient with *nonmetastatic GTN* does not desire further pregnancies we suggest the uterus be removed by total abdominal hysterectomy on the third day of the initial five-day course of chemotherapy. Lewis and others have reported no increase in postsurgical morbidity among patients receiving these agents, who were submitted to a variety of surgical procedures.[16] Repetitive courses of chemotherapy must be continued in the postoperative period in similar fashion to that which would have been carried out had surgery not been performed. If treatment is not continued in the postsurgical period, a tumor which has either been disseminated during the procedure or which was present but unidentified at the time of surgery may be given the opportunity to expand.

A small percentage of patients with nonmetastatic GTN will fail to achieve remission with systemic chemotherapy. Pelvic arteriography may demonstrate a focus of trophoblastic disease deep in the myometrium, and resistant disease is manifested by persistent elevation of the HCG titer despite repetitive systemic chemotherapy. In these patients one can consider either arterial infusional chemotherapy in a last attempt to preserve the uterus or hysterectomy during chemotherapy.

TABLE 7–8.   *Method of Single Agent Chemotherapy*

1. Repetitive 5 days courses: Methotrexate, 15 to 25 mg. intramuscularly q.d., or actinomycin D, 10 to 13 μg./kg. body weight intravenously q.d.
   a. Consider hysterectomy during first course of chemotherapy if further reproduction is not desired.
   b. *Minimum* interval between courses: 7 days.
   c. Maximum interval between courses: 14 days (unless laboratory values are too low).
   d. Consider oral contraception for pituitary suppression.
2. Continue repetitive 5 day courses of the *same drug* until:
   a. If HCG titer drops to normal pituitary range, then cease therapy.
   b. If HCG titer "plateaus" and is elevated ⎫
   c. If HCG titer rises by tenfold   ⎬change to alternate drug.
   d. If new metastases appear   ⎭
3. Monitor oncolytic effect by *weekly* HCG titers, chest x-rays, and pelvic examinations.
4. Treatment is terminated when HCG titer is within *normal pituitary ranges*. Three consecutive normal weekly HCG titers are necessary to diagnosis remission.
5. Treatment safety factors (done daily during therapy regimen, less frequently between courses). Do not start, continue, or resume a dose of medication if:
   a. White blood count is less than 3000/mm.³
   b. Polymorphonuclear leukocytes number less than 1500/mm.³
   c. Platelets number less than 100,000/mm.³
   d. Significant elevations of BUN, SGOT, or SGPT occur.
6. Follow-up:
   a. HCG titers monthly for six months, bimonthly for six months, then every 6 months thereafter.
   b. Physical, pelvic exams, chest x-rays, blood survey every three months for 1 year, every 6 months thereafter.
   c. No pregnancy for 1 year.

It is now anticipated that esssentially all patients with nonmetastatic GTN can be cured. In 1966, the Bethesda group reported that 98 per cent of a series of 58 patients achieved cure with the methods outlined previously.[6] In 1972, Hammond and associates reported cures in all of a group of 100 patients[15] (Table 7–9). In both of these series, over 90 per cent of patients who desired to preserve reproductive capacity were able to do so. In neither series were there any toxic deaths

TABLE 7–9.   *Patients Treated for Nonmetastatic Trophoblastic Disease (9/1/66 to 8/31/71)*

TYPE OF THERAPY	PRIMARY THERAPY	REMISSIONS AFTER PRIMARY THERAPY	SECONDARY THERAPY	REMISSIONS AFTER SECONDARY THERAPY	DEATHS
Single Agent Chemotherapy Alone*	73	61	—	—	0
Single Agent Chemotherapy with Initial Hysterectomy†	26	26	—	—	0
Pelvic Arterial Infusional Chemotherapy	1	0	6	6	0
Single Agent Chemotherapy with Secondary Hysterectomy‡	—	—	7	7	0
TOTALS	100	87	13	13	0

Remissions: 100/100 patients (100%).

  * Chemotherapy: Methotrexate or actinomycin D (see text).

  † Initial hysterectomy: Total abdominal hysterectomy done during the first course of chemotherapy.

  ‡ Secondary hysterectomy: Total abdominal hysterectomy done only after developing resistance to single agent chemotherapy.

owing to therapy, nor have there been any recurrences up to the time of this report. Ross and others have reported normally successful reproduction rates in this group.

Metastatic Trophoblastic Disease

Patients with GTN in whom metastases are present beyond the uterus are classified as having "good" or "poor" prognosis. This categorization is based on data from the Bethesda study which demonstrated that a successful outcome to chemotherapy was greatly influenced by the duration of disease, the height of the initial pretreatment HCG titer, and the presence or absence of either cerebral or hepatic metastases. Patients who were diagnosed promptly, even those with metastases beyond the uterus (other than cerebral and hepatic) and who had none of the other signs and findings giving a poor prognosis could expect a 90 per cent cure rate with chemotherapy. For the patients who had these "poor prognosis" signs and findings, the survival rate was less than 30 per cent.[4,5] Thus, if a patient has metastatic GTN and a pretreatment HCG titer in excess of 100,000 I.U. per 24 hour urine sample, or cerebral or hepatic metastases, or a duration of symptoms attributable to the disease for longer than four months, it is felt she has "poor prognosis metastatic disease."

GOOD PROGNOSIS METASTATIC DISEASE

Patients with good prognosis metastatic GTN are treated in similar fashion to those with nonmetastatic disease (Table 7–8). We continue to utilize methotrexate as our initial drug in patients if they have received recent blood transfusions and if renal and hepatic function is normal. Despite the fact that actinomycin has seemed to be somewhat less toxic than methotrexate, one must recall that approximately half of these patients will ultimately require treatment with both agents, owing to development of resistance to one of the drugs. We have chosen to utilize methotrexate initially, but change to actinomycin D in case serum hepatitis develops.

After institution treatment one continues repetitive five day courses of chemotherapy, and the patient's progress is monitored by weekly HCG assays. Treatment is switched to the alternate drug if a patient fails to show a significant decline through two courses of chemotherapy. It appears that peripheral metastases in patients with good prognosis GTN are usually even more sensitive to these drugs than is deep-seated myometrial disease. Experimental data are accumulating that hysterectomy done during the first course of therapy may influence the outcome for patients who do not desire further pregnancies and in whom there is either curettage evidence or arteriographic signs of uterine disease. It must be stressed that this technique remains in experimental stages. If a patient desires to preserve her reproductive potential, or if local uterine disease cannot be identified, then systemic chemotherapy also is continued. If resistance to both agents develops, delayed hysterectomy with chemotherapy or arterial infusional chemotherapy with the uterus in situ may be indicated. In any of these situations in which surgery is performed, repetitive courses of the drugs are

TABLE 7–10.   *Patients Treated for "Good Prognosis" Metastatic Trophoblastic Disease (9/1/66 to 8/31/71)*

TYPE OF THERAPY	PRIMARY THERAPY	REMISSIONS WITH PRIMARY THERAPY	SECONDARY THERAPY	REMISSION WITH SECONDARY THERAPY	DEATHS
Single Agent Chemotherapy Alone*	53	47	—	—	1
Single Agent Chemotherapy with Initial Hysterectomy†	18	18	—	—	0
Pelvic Arterial Infusional Chemotherapy	—	—	3	3	0
Single Agent Chemotherapy with Secondary Hysterectomy‡	—	—	2	2	0
TOTALS	71	65	5	5	1

Remissions: 70/71 patients (98%). One patient treated elsewhere with single agent chemotherapy died at the medical center of hematopoietic toxicity.

  * Chemotherapy: Methotrexate or actinomycin D (see text).

  † Initial hysterectomy: Total abdominal hysterectomy done during the first course of chemotherapy.

  ‡ Secondary hysterectomy: Total abdominal hysterectomy done only after developing resistance to single agent chemotherapy.

continued postoperatively until the HCG titer falls into the normal pituitary gonadotropin range. Hysterectomy must be approached with extreme caution if there is evidence of extrauterine pelvic extension of tumor. Hemorrhage may be severe during such a procedure. Table 7–10 shows our results with these forms of therapy for patients with "good prognosis GTN."[15]

POOR PROGNOSIS METASTATIC DISEASE

Earlier in this section the findings in patients with metastatic GTN that mark poor prognosis were listed. Since the prognosis for such patients has remained so poor with conventional single-agent chemotherapy, we have recently completed a study in which more vigorous initial therapy was carried out. We now suggest that these patients be initially treated with high-dose combination chemotherapy consisting of methotrexate (15 mg. intramuscularly), actinomycin D (10 μg. per kg. body weight intravenously), and Chlorambucil (8 mg. orally), all given daily for five days per course. The same safety criteria listed in Table 7–8 are used, except the between-course interval is increased to a minimum of 12 days. After two or three courses of this combination therapy the treatment is diverted to single-agent actinomycin D in standard fashion. If cerebral or hepatic metastases are present, the patient is begun on 2000 rads whole liver or brain irradiation, simultaneous with the start of chemotherapy. Weekly monitoring with HCG assay is utilized. Toxic results from this approach are a major hazard, and this more radical form of therapy should be undertaken only by an experienced physician with considerable laboratory and therapeutic support available. Extreme caution must be used when the patient has impaired renal or hepatic function. Results from our studies comparing conventional therapy with more vigorous initial therapy are shown in Table 7–11.[15]

TABLE 7–11. *Patients Treated for "Poor Prognosis" Metastatic Trophoblastic Disease (9/1/66 to 8/31/71)*

	PATIENTS TREATED PRIMARILY WITH COMBINATION CHEMOTHERAPY (10 PATIENTS)	PATIENTS TREATED SECONDARILY WITH COMBINATION CHEMOTHERAPY (7 PATIENTS)
Cured	7	1
Died	3	6
	(1 toxicity, 2 disease)	(3 toxicity, 3 disease)
Total Cured	7 (70%)	1 (17%)
Total Patients Cured	8/17 (47%)	

* Combination chemotherapy: Methotrexate, actinomycin D, and chlorambucil given simultaneously. Also whole liver or brain irradiation if metastases are present (see text).

Comment

Regardless of the type of therapy utilized, the treatment of malignant trophoblastic disease is continued until the HCG titer has returned to normal by an assay sensitive enough to measure well into normal pituitary gonadotropin ranges. Pregnancy tests are of use only when positive, then full range assays must be utilized. Early and accurate diagnosis can be achieved with frequent and repeated use of such sensitive and precise HCG assays. High remission rates and successful therapy are dependent upon the use of such assays. We also have utilized pituitary gonadotropin suppression via oral contraceptives in all patients who do not have contraindications to these agents. This allows a more accurate determination of remission by HCG assays, which also react with pituitary LH.[15]

Systemic, single-agent chemotherapy with methotrexate or actinomycin D remains the primary treatment modality for patients with gestational tropho-blastic disease. The clinical identification of these patients as to the presence or absence of metastases and the subdividing of the group with metastases into "good" and "poor" prognosis patients are of major aid in determining the initial method of therapy most likely to achieve remission with the least toxic hazard. The use of arterial infusion chemotherapy and of hysterectomy in conjunction with chemotherapy are now being studied, and both certainly seem to warrant further use. The initial therapy of the poor prognosis patient with combination chemotherapy (with and without cerebral or hepatic irradiation) seems to improve the salvage rate markedly, while such therapy administered after resist-ant disease has developed offers little in the way of improving mortality rates. The recurring point these data seem to raise is that the type of initial therapy must be tailored to each individual patient.

Hysterectomy performed during the first course of chemotherapy in patients who have clinical evidence of uterine disease and who do not desire further reproduction has been associated with high cure rates and less need for chemotherapy. Arterial infusion of chemotherapeutic drugs may provide an alter-native to hysterectomy for selected patients. The role of prophylactic chemo-therapy for pre- and post-evacuation of a hydatidiform mole seems promising, but we feel that the toxic hazard outweighs the possible reduction in malignant per-sistence. Both of these treatment methodologies require further investigation before widespread clinical use is acceptable.

One can only anticipate that in the future there will be more effective agents and regimens to further increase remission rates for patients with malignant trophoblastic disease. It is also anticipated that such agents and techniques will also be associated with reduced toxicity, which remains a most desirable goal. The demand for more rapid, more easily available, and less expensive HCG assays remains. Despite the possibility that all these improvements will be made in the future, however, it now appears that malignant trophoblastic disease is amenable to nearly complete control with the therapeutic modalities currently available.

REFERENCES

1. Brewer, J. I., Rinehart, J. J., and Dunbar, R.: Choriocarcinoma. Amer. J. Obstet. Gynec. 81:574, 1961.
2. Greene, R. R.: Chorioadenoma destruens. Ann. N.Y. Acad. Sci. 80:143, 1959.
3. Li, M. C., Hertz, R., and Spencer, D. B.: Effects of methotrexate therapy upon choriocarcinoma and chorioadenoma destruens. Proc. Soc. Exp. Biol. Med. 93:361, 1956.
4. Hertz, R., Lewis, J. L., Jr., and Lipsett, M. B.: Five years' experience with the chemotherapy of metastatic choriocarcinoma and related trophoblastic tumors in women. Amer. J. Obstet. Gynec. 82:631, 1961.
5. Ross, G. T., Goldstein, D. P., Hertz, R., Lipsett, M. B., and Odell, W. D.: Sequential use of methotrexate and actinomycin D in the treatment of metastatic choriocarcinoma and related trophoblastic diseases in women. Am. J. Obstet. Gynec. 93:223, 1965.
6. Hammond, C. B., Hertz, R., Ross, G. T., Lipsett, M. B., and Odell, W. D.: Primary chemotherapy for nonmetastatic gestational trophoblastic neoplasms. Am. J. Obstet. Gynec. 98:71, 1967.
7. Lewis, J. L., Jr.: Chemotherapy for metastatic gestational trophoblastic neoplasms. Clin. Obstet. Gynec. 10:330, 1967.
8. Odell, W. D., Hertz, R., Lipsett, M. B., Ross, G. T., and Hammond, C. B.: Endocrine aspects of trophoblastic neoplasms. Clin. Obstet Gynec. 10:290, 1967.
9. Delfs, E.: Quantitative chorionic gonadotropin; prognostic value in hydatidiform mole and chorionepithelioma. Obstet. Gynec. 9:1, 1957.
10. Brewer, J. I., Smith, R. T., and Pratt, G. B.: Choriocarcinoma. Amer. J. Obstet. Gynec. 85:841, 1962.
11. Hammond, C. B., and Parker, R. T.: Diagnosis and treatment of trophoblastic disease. Obstet. Gynec. 35:132, 1970.
12. Hammond, C. B., Hertz, R., Ross, G. T., Lipsett, M. B., and Odell, W. B.: Diagnostic problems of choriocarcinoma and related trophoblastic neoplasms. Obstet. Gynec. 29:224, 1967.
13. Holland, J. F., Hreshchyshyn, M. M., and Glidewell, O.: Controlled clinical trials of methotrexate in the treatment and prophylaxis of trophoblastic neoplasia. Abstracts, 10th International Cancer Congress, Houston, May 1970. Detroit, Medical Arts Publishing, 1970.
14. Goldstein, D. P., and Reid, D. E.: Recent developments in the management of molar pregnancy. Clin. Obstet. Gynec. 10:313, 1967.
15. Hammond, C. B., Borchert, L. G., Tyrey, L., Creasman, W. T., and Parker, R. T.: Treatment of metastatic trophoblastic disease: good and poor prognosis. Am. J. Obstet. Gynec. 115:451, 1973.
16. Lewis, J. L., Jr., Gore, H., Hertig, A. T., and Goss, D. A.: Treatment of trophoblastic neoplasms. With rationale for the use of adjunctive chemotherapy at the time of indicated operation. Amer. J. Obstet. Gynec. 96:710, 1966.

Preferable Management of Gestational Trophoblastic Disease: Benign and Malignant

Editorial Comment

Despite the remarkable advances in the management of patients with gestational trophoblastic disease there are several unresolved questions that have bearing on clinical management. Although there are differences in nomenclature that add somewhat to the reader's woes, there now appears to be a thread of universality running through these contributions from three of the major trophoblastic disease centers in this country. Certain procedures now recommended follow those previously advocated by overseas authorities, particularly those in the Far East, where for reasons still to be clarified molar pregnancy occurs some seven or eight times more frequently than it is encountered in countries of the Western world. More specifically, these treatment procedures include the more liberal use of hysterectomy and repeat curettage, which perhaps contribute to a higher cure rate.

To insure as far as is possible that all of the tissue in the uterine cavity had been removed, recurettage on the seventh to tenth day is advocated. The uterus is now involuted sufficiently to permit a more vigorous curettage not possible when molar evacuation is done, at which time the uterus is notoriously fragile and more easily perforated. The value of a second curettage may be even more desirable when suction curettage has been employed, for which there is a greater likelihood that trophoblastic tissue might still remain in the uterus. Also, if molar tissue was obtained, it might offer some histologic criteria for subsequent patient management. For, as Hertig and Sheldon emphasize in their studies, directed toward establishing criteria for determining the benignity or malignancy potential of the mole, the tissue adjacent to the myometrium is the most valuable in attempting to answer the question.

Regardless of the fact that the classification of the patient's disease may differ from clinic to clinic, those cases with a guarded prognosis have now been defined. Whether patients are placed in the category termed "poor prognosis metastatic disease" (Hammond) or in the so-called "high risk metastatic trophoblastic disease" group (Goldstein), it is within this same group that the mortality resides. In these patients the disease has been present for longer than four months, the pretreatment gonadotrophin titer is over 100,000 I.U./24 hours, and there may be cerebral or hepatic metastasis. Whatever else, the time is at hand when a universal classification of the disease should be forthcoming.

Several assumptions were made that would be challenged by both pathologists and clinicians. One might question how it can be proved whether or not molar tissue can become metastatic and in so doing change its behavior and histopathology to assume characteristics not unlike those of choriocarcinoma. Many statements are made and ideas conveyed that can only be proved by histologic examination of the source of the tumor—i.e., the uterus. Since the introduction of chemotherapy this organ has rarely been available for such examination. It is indeed an assumption that the myometrium is free of disease when curettage fails to divulge evidence of trophoblastic disease.

Disagreement continues over the value of preevacuation prophylactic chemotherapy. Drs. Brewer and Eckman, on the basis of a prospective study, are of the opinion that the natural history of molar pregnancy supports their conclusion that such therapy is unnecessary and hence unwarranted. Dr. Hammond agrees, but regards this as an open-ended question, subject to further study in a trophoblastic disease center. This makes one wonder whether preevacuation chemotherapy would have averted persistent disease within the group listed as patients with local invasion. Presumably these are referral cases, but whatever else, they illustrate how difficult it is to assess the value of prophylactic chemotherapy.

Certainly, when advocating a type of treatment one must ensure that the therapy can be managed in all hospitals and by nonspecialists. There should be acceptance of the fact that when complications arise from trophoblastic disease the patient should be referred to a trophoblastic disease center. However, it seems a bit unrealistic to believe that patients with molar pregnancies, once diagnosed, will always be sent to a trophoblastic disease center in the undelivered state—indeed, the patient's condition may demand emergency measures even at the time she is initially seen. The degree of bleeding and previous blood loss may demand prompt therapy without chemotherapy coverage. As suggested, the risks of such therapy administered outside of trophoblastic disease centers may well negate any possible value.

8

Preferable Management of Complications of the Venous System in Pregnancy and the Puerperium

Alternative Points of View:

By Leonard A. Aaro and John L. Juergens

By Stephen J. Healey

By Jack W. Pearson

Editorial Comment

Preferable Management of Complications of the Venous System in Pregnancy and the Puerperium

LEONARD A. AARO and JOHN L. JUERGENS
Mayo Clinic and Mayo Foundation

For more than 300 years, obstetricians have been concerned about thrombosis of the veins of the lower extremities. Mauriceau,[1] in 1668, first described the swollen leg of the puerpera and believed that the swelling represented an abnormal reflux of the lochia. Almost a century later, Puzos[2] first used the term "milk leg" for the condition we now know as thrombosis of the iliofemoral vein. He believed that the swelling was caused by an abnormal accumulation of milk in the leg because lactation often became suppressed when the leg swelling began. Even now, about 200 years later, the term "milk leg" is still employed by some laymen. Davis,[3] in 1823, first described the pathologic basis of the condition after he found extensive thrombosis and inflammation of the iliac veins in postmortem studies.

Today, for many reasons—including better prenatal care, less traumatic delivery, earlier ambulation, and better means of combating infection—thrombophlebitis probably is less commonly associated with pregnancy than in former years. Although less prevalent than in the past, venous thrombosis is a complication of approximately 1 in every 70 pregnancies.[4] This relatively common disorder may present the obstetrician with difficult therapeutic, if not diagnostic, problems.

For both prognostic and therapeutic reasons, we believe that it is important to distinguish between superficial and deep venous thrombosis. However, we do not attempt to distinguish between thrombophlebitis and the so-called phlebothrombosis. We have not found the latter term diagnostically or prognostically useful, and we prefer the term "thrombophlebitis" when there are sufficient local clinical signs to permit the diagnosis of venous thrombosis. A full description of the symptoms and signs of acute superficial and deep thrombophlebitis is available in a standard text.[5]

The most common type of venous thrombosis associated with pregnancy is superficial thrombophlebitis, and this usually occurs in the varices that so frequently accompany pregnancy. If recognized and treated promptly, the process rarely becomes serious or disabling. However, if the condition is allowed to progress, it may become painful and even dangerous.

Although less common, deep venous thrombosis may occur in either the antepartum or the postpartum state. It occurs most frequently in the veins of the lower extremities and pelvis. Below the knee these include the muscular veins of the calf (sural veins) and the tibial veins. The thrombophlebitis may extend proximally and involve the popliteal, femoral, or iliofemoral veins. Thrombophlebitis of the pelvic veins is seen most frequently with postpartum infection and sepsis. Thrombophlebitis in the deep veins is always serious and calls for prompt and careful treatment.

Prevalence

A review of more than 32,000 pregnancies at the Mayo Clinic[4] revealed that superficial thrombophlebitis occurred during the antepartum period in 1 of every 622 pregnancies, and during the postpartum period in 1 of every 95 patients. Deep venous thrombosis was diagnosed during pregnancy in 1 of every 1902 pregnancies and during the postpartum period in 1 of every 668 patients. The overall prevalence for all types of thrombophlebitis associated with pregnancy was 1 in 70 (1.4 per cent). Fortunately, pulmonary embolism occurred in only 1 of every 2488 pregnancies.

Superficial Thrombophlebitis

Although common during the postpartum period, superficial thrombophlebitis is rare during pregnancy. It may occur at any time during pregnancy but is most frequently found during the third trimester. The time of onset after delivery is usually rapid, with approximately 40 per cent of the instances occurring within 24 hours and more than 85 per cent developing within three days of delivery.[6]

Patients with a history of thrombophlebitis are likely to develop the disorder again. Approximately 40 per cent of patients who develop superficial thrombophlebitis associated with pregnancy have had previous superficial or deep thrombophlebitis.[4]

Almost all patients who develop superficial thrombophlebitis associated with pregnancy have readily visible varicose veins, but we have been impressed with the many patients with minimal varicosities who develop this disorder. Most frequently, superficial thrombosis involves one leg or one leg and thigh. Bilateral involvement occurs in only approximately 10 per cent of cases.

Patients with obvious varicose veins should ensure adequate elastic support for their lower extremities during pregnancy and the postpartum period by wearing either heavy elastic stockings or elastic bandages of the Ace type. Many of the sheer and thin so-called support hose do not give enough support for incompetent veins of the lower extremities.

More than 90 per cent of women who develop postpartum superficial thrombophlebitis have had normal labor and delivery.[6] It is difficult to determine what effect delivery-table stirrups might have in traumatizing superficial veins and thus contributing to the development of venous thrombosis. We have thought that metal stirrups with multiple constricting leg straps and metal contact points might be an etiologic factor in thrombophlebitis, and we have, therefore, tried various stirrup modifications employing foam rubber padding. At present, stirrups with a single foot strap and a single foam-padded contact point adjacent to the lower medial part of the calf seem the most successful in preventing postpartum superficial thrombophlebitis.

We believe that local heat, rest in bed, and elevation of the involved extremity should constitute the primary therapy plan for acute superficial thrombophlebitis. On rare occasions when there is a severe associated periphlebitic reaction, we employ short-term therapy with an anti-inflammatory drug such as phenylbutazone. Since there is no reliable evidence that bacterial infection contributes to this type of thrombophlebitis, we do not recommend antibiotic therapy. Likewise, we do not recommend anticoagulant therapy for superficial thrombophlebitis during pregnancy unless the process becomes severe, fails to respond to local therapy, or threatens to extend to the deep veins, or unless pulmonary embolism occurs.

However, during the postpartum state, we have commonly employed anticoagulant therapy, especially for those with severe or rapidly progressing superficial thrombophlebitis. Anticoagulants also have been administered prophylactically after delivery to patients who have a history of previous severe superficial or deep venous thrombosis, as well as to those who have a history of previous pulmonary embolism. In our experience, because of the shortness of the interval between delivery and the onset of thrombophlebitis, prophylactic anticoagulant therapy with an orally administered coumarin compound should be started immediately after delivery. If anticoagulants are to be used to treat severe and rapidly extending superficial thrombophlebitis, we usually begin therapy with both intravenous heparin and oral coumarin compounds; the latter are employed alone once the patient's prothrombin time has been recorded as reaching therapeutic levels. It is our present practice to give 5000 units of heparin intravenously every 4 hours, until the coumarin drug has brought the prothrombin time between two and two and a half times normal. This can usually be accomplished within 48 hours. For patients with severe superficial thrombophlebitis after delivery, anticoagulant therapy may be continued on an outpatient basis for 4 to 6 weeks after hospital dismissal. Effective and safe anticoagulant therapy with the coumarin drugs, even for a short time, requires frequent and reliable prothrombin time tests. The possibility that coumarin will interact with other drugs and the small calculated risk of major bleeding must be considered.

Deep Thrombophlebitis

Deep thrombophlebitis is rare during pregnancy and uncommon during the postpartum state. As with superficial thrombophlebitis, it may occur at any time during pregnancy, but it is more frequent during the third trimester. Deep thrombophlebitis usually starts shortly after delivery. About 50 per cent of all cases are detectable within 48 hours of parturition.[7]

Approximately 35 per cent of those who develop deep thrombophlebitis after delivery have had previous significant superficial or deep thrombophlebitis. In about 50 per cent of patients, the deep veins of the calf are the primary site of the thrombus, and in approximately 25 per cent, the iliofemoral veins are the chief site of clinical involvement.[7] The popliteal, femoral, and pelvic veins are less commonly involved. There seems to be little relationship between the presence of varicosities and the development of deep venous thrombosis.

In our experience, more than 25 per cent of the patients who develop deep thrombophlebitis after delivery have had some type of obstetric complication during labor and delivery.[4] These complications include such difficulties as prolonged labor, cesarean section, toxemia, difficult forceps delivery, and hemorrhage.

Local heat, rest in bed, and elevation of the involved extremity are recommended in the treatment of deep thrombophlebitis associated with pregnancy. We also believe that anticoagulant therapy is indicated for both pregnant and postpartum patients who have deep venous thrombosis. Our present management of these patients includes the immediate administration of both intravenous heparin and oral coumarin compounds. Intermittent intravenous heparin is given via an indwelling plastic needle until the coumarin compounds have brought the prothrombin time to therapeutic levels. The anticoagulant therapy is continued until the tenderness disappears and the patient has been ambulatory for at least three or four days. Often we continue the use of anticoagulants longer than this, on an outpatient basis, if we feel a recurrence is likely. In patients with severe or repeated antepartum venous thrombosis or pulmonary embolism, anticoagulant therapy is continued until just before labor begins or is induced. In most instances, vitamin K_1 should then be given to correct the prothrombin deficiency before delivery; this minimizes the danger of hemorrhage for both the mother and the fetus.

Heparin, with a high molecular weight, apparently is incapable of crossing the placental barrier.[8] Several investigators[9-12] have recommended heparin as the anticoagulant of choice for antepartum thrombophlebitis. Objections to the use of heparin alone rest mostly with the inconvenience of long-term administration, as this medication must be given parenterally. Orally administered coumarin compounds, with lower molecular weights, may pass through the placenta and enter the fetal circulation.[8,10] Indeed, a few cases of fetal hemorrhage and even fetal death after coumarin administration to the mother during pregnancy have been reported.[10,13,14] It has also been suggested that coumarin therapy might be an etiologic factor in the production of fetal anomalies.[12] We believe that the danger to the fetus is minimal when coumarin compounds are carefully administered and prothrombin times are well controlled within the therapeutic range. However, we always discontinue anticoagulant therapy during labor and delivery to minimize the danger of hemorrhage for the mother and the fetus.

Pulmonary Embolism

Pulmonary embolism is only very rarely associated with pregnancy,[8,15] but obstetricians must constantly be aware that it may occur at any time during pregnancy or after delivery. It must be considered in the differential diagnosis of chest pain associated with pregnancy. Only with prompt diagnosis can proper therapy be instituted. In our experience, definite pulmonary embolism is associated with approximately 1 in every 2500 pregnancies.[4]

We have found that almost all instances of pulmonary embolism occurred in association with clinical evidence of deep thrombophlebitis. In only one instance can we recall a pulmonary embolism occurring after delivery in a patient who had only superficial thrombophlebitis. More than 75 per cent of cases of pulmonary emboli associated with pregnancy occur during the postpartum period,[4] and these commonly occur after difficult or traumatic delivery, especially if there is an associated hemorrhage.

All patients with pulmonary embolism are treated in the hospital with rest in bed, anticoagulant therapy, and local application of heat to the area affected with thrombophlebitis. Analgesics and oxygen therapy are administered as indicated; hypotension, if present, should be treated with pressor agents. Heparin and coumarin are used at the beginning of therapy, but once the patient's prothrombin time reaches therapeutic levels, only the coumarin compounds are administered. If antepartum pulmonary embolism occurs at or near term pregnancy, the patient may be given heparin therapy alone until after delivery. However, if the antepartum pulmonary embolism occurs early in pregnancy, we prefer to continue with coumarin therapy until term. Then the patient can be given vitamin K_1 to correct the prothrombin deficiency, and labor may be induced. After delivery, anticoagulants should be given during the postpartum period. If recurrent pulmonary embolization occurs despite anticoagulant therapy, or if there is major hemorrhage which contraindicates continued anticoagulants, a transvenous placement of a Mobin-Uddin type of caval umbrella may be indicated.[5]

Comment

We prefer to treat both pregnant and postpartum patients who develop superficial thrombophlebitis with local heat, rest in bed, and elevation of the involved extremity. Anticoagulant therapy often is not necessary during pregnancy for the treatment of superficial thrombophlebitis, and we generally avoid its use because of the danger (even though rather remote) of fetal or maternal hemorrhage. However, during the postpartum period, we are more likely to employ anticoagulant therapy, especially for severe or rapidly progressing superficial thrombophlebitis.

In our opinion, anticoagulant therapy is indicated for both pregnant and postpartum patients who develop deep venous thrombosis. Surgical thrombectomy has not been shown to have advantages over medical therapy and, in our opinion, caval ligations or plications are rarely necessary. The anticoagulant therapy includes the immediate administration of both heparin and coumarin compounds; the coumarin compounds alone generally are sufficient once the patient's prothrombin time has reached therapeutic levels.

We believe that postpartum prophylactic anticoagulant therapy is indicated not only for those who have had deep thrombophlebitis or pulmonary embolism but also for those who have had severe or repeated episodes of superficial thrombophlebitis in order to prevent serious venous thrombosis. Because of the rapid onset of either superficial or deep thrombophlebitis after the termination of pregnancy, prophylactic anticoagulant therapy, to be of maximal value, should begin immediately after delivery.

Pulmonary embolism, as we have stated, is very rarely associated with pregnancy, but when it occurs, it usually appears after obstetric complications, including trauma and hemorrhage. Thus, one should be especially alert for this complication after a difficult labor or delivery. For patients who develop pulmonary embolism, we favor prompt therapy with anticoagulants, analgesics, oxygen, and other supportive measures.

REFERENCES

1. Mauriceau: Cited by Davis.[3]
2. Puzos: Cited by Davis.[3]
3. Davis, D. D.: An essay on the proximate cause of the disease called phlegmasia dolens. Trans. R. Med.-Chir. Soc. (Lond.) 12:419, 1823.
4. Aaro, L. A., and Juergens, J. L.: Thrombophlebitis associated with pregnancy. Am. J. Obstet. Gynec. 109:1128, 1971.
5. Fairbairn, J. F., Juergens, J. L., and Spittell, J. A.: Peripheral Vascular Diseases. 4th Ed. Philadelphia, W. B. Saunders Co. 1972.
6. Aaro, L. A., Johnson, T. R., and Juergens, J. L.: Acute superficial venous thrombophlebitis associated with pregnancy. Am. J. Obstet. Gynec. 97:514, 1967.
7. Aaro, L. A., Johnson, T. R., and Juergens, J. L.: Acute deep venous thrombosis associated with pregnancy. Obstet. Gynec. 28:553, 1966.
8. Finnerty, J. J., and MacKay, B. R.: Antepartum thrombophlebitis and pulmonary embolism: report of a case and review of the literature. Obstet. Gynec. 19:405, 1962.
9. Blum, M.: Anticoagulant treatment of phlebothrombosis during pregnancy. Am. J. Obstet. Gynec. 73:440, 1957.
10. Cegelski, F. C., DeWeese, J. A., and Lund, C. J.: Deep iliofemoral venous thrombosis during pregnancy: treatment with anticoagulants and thrombectomy. Am. J. Obstet. Gynec. 89:510, 1964.
11. Quenneville, G., Barton, B., McDevitt, E., et al.: The use of anticoagulants for thrombophlebitis during pregnancy. Am. J. Obstet. Gynec. 77:1135, 1959.
12. VillaSanta, U.: Thromboembolic disease in pregnancy. Am. J. Obstet. Gynec. 93:142, 1965.
13. Gordon, R. R., and Dean, T.: Foetal deaths from antenatal anticoagulant therapy. Brit. Med. J. 2:719, 1955.
14. Mahairas, G. H., and Weingold, A. B.: Fetal hazard with anticoagulant therapy. Am. J. Obstet. Gynec. 85:234, 1963.
15. Moore, J. G., O'Leary, J. A., and Johnson, P. M.: The changing impact of pulmonary thromboembolism in obstetrics: value of the isotopic perfusion scan. Am. J. Obstet. Gynec. 97:507, 1967.

Preferable Management of Complications of the Venous System in Pregnancy and the Puerperium

Thromboembolism in Pregnancy and the Puerperium

STEPHEN J. HEALEY

Boston Hospital for Women, Peter Bent Brigham Hospital, and Harvard Medical School

Although thromboembolism is a common occurrence in medical and surgical patients, it is a rare complication in pregnancy. The apparent rarity of this condition in the antepartum period, its high mortality, and the special hazards of anticoagulant treatment at this time have led to confusion and controversy in its management. This paper presents the current method of management of thromboembolism in pregnancy and the puerperium employed at the Boston Hospital for Women.

INCIDENCE

It is commonly thought that the incidence of thromboembolism is increased during pregnancy. This is not strictly correct, as the incidence is increased only after delivery. The incidence of deep vein thrombosis in nonpregnant females is 31 cases per 100,000 women per year. This rate is based on patient visits to the physician and includes women with and without predisposing causes.[1] In a retrospective review of over 200,000 pregnant patients, the incidence of deep phlebitis when extrapolated from a 9 to 12 month period was found to be the same as in the nonpregnant female.[2] After delivery, however, the incidence increased thirteenfold to 3.9 cases per 1000 (390 per 100,000) deliveries.[2] Most important is the fact that pulmonary embolism occurred in 20 per cent of this group with overt thrombophlebitis.[3,4]

PREDISPOSING CAUSES

The special inquiries by the Ministry of Health into maternal deaths in England and Wales have identified a group of patients who are at increased risk during pregnancy and the puerperium.[5] Included are elderly primigravidas, women over 34 years of age, obese women, those who suffered trauma at delivery, or those undergoing cesarean section, all of who have been shown to have a significantly increased risk of thromboembolism.

A possible cause of increased puerperal thrombosis may be the administration of oral diethylstilbestrol. A recent study notes a tenfold increase of deep phlebitis in nonlactating mothers whose lactation was suppressed by diethylstilbestrol, compared to lactating mothers.[6] In 60 per cent of the maternal deaths reported from England and Wales, estrogens had been administered post partum.

The incidence of thromboembolism is increased fourfold by the addition of postpartum tubal ligations.[7] A final group of patients at considerable risk are those with a previous history of thrombosis or embolism or those who have suffered either of these during a current pregnancy.[8] Immediate postpartum sterilization or the use of estrogens would be contraindicated in these patients.

DIAGNOSIS

Despite the rarity of pulmonary embolism in pregnancy, it remains one of the major causes of maternal death. It is the second most common cause of maternal deaths in England and Wales, and it is responsible for 10 per cent of all maternal deaths in Massachusetts. Since studies have shown that multiple nonlethal embolic events may precede the lethal embolism, diagnosis of these early embolic showers is essential to reduce maternal mortality.[9]

The diagnosis of overt, deep thrombophlebitis is usually not difficult. The patient complains of an ache or heaviness in the leg associated with worsening of the symptoms on dependency. She may note a limp and a swelling. Examination will show a measurable increase in the affected calf's circumference. There may be induration of the calf and local tenderness over the deep veins. Homan's sign may be present.

Most necessary for the diagnosis of embolism is that it be considered when any patient is thought to have pneumonia or atelectasis. Clinical phlebitis is present in fewer than 50 per cent of these patients with clinical embolism. Unexplained dyspnea or collapse should especially alert the physician to the possibility of embolism. Once embolism arises as a diagnostic possibility, the patient should be started on intravenous heparin infusion and continued on it while appropriate diagnostic tests are being done.

In the pregnant patient or puerpera, who is usually a healthy young person, pulmonary embolism will cause dyspnea and pleuritic chest pain in 90 per cent and cough and hemoptysis in 50 per cent.[10] Overt phlebitis will be present in 50 per cent of the patients and a pleural rub or splinting in 25 per cent. Arterial blood gases may be of aid in screening patients with symptoms suggestive of pulmonary embolism. Recent studies have determined that an arterial Po_2 of greater than 90 mm. Hg will rule out pulmonary embolism in a symptomatic patient.[11,12] A chest x-ray may be normal in 30 per cent of patients with pulmonary emboli. When the clinical setting is highly suggestive of embolism, radioactive lung scanning should be performed to establish a diagnosis. Pulmonary angiogram is indicated in those patients in whom the scan is not diagnostic.

Management

The mortality of antepartum thromboembolism has been reported to be about 15 per cent in untreated patients, compared to less than 1 per cent in patients treated with anticoagulants.[3,4] All available evidence suggests that anticoagulant therapy significantly reduces mortality in antepartum thromboembolism. The management of antepartum thromboembolism, however, presents the special problem of the effect of these anticoagulants on the fetus.

Heparin is a potent anticoagulant. It is a large molecule which does not cross the placenta and presents no special risks to the fetus. Use of heparin is impractical when prolonged administration is necessary, however, because it requires hospitalization and parenteral administration. On the other hand, coumarin derivatives are anticoagulants that may be taken orally on an outpatient basis, but they are small molecules that cross the placenta and can anticoagulate the fetus. A high incidence of intrauterine fetal deaths has been reported with the use of these drugs.[3] In addition, these oral anticoagulants may produce teratogenic effects, especially if given in the first trimester.[12,13]

In our experience—and that of others as well—the preferred method of treatment for antepartum deep phlebitis is the use of intermittent intravenous heparin.[14,16] From 1960 to 1970, 25 patients were treated for antenatal thromboembolism at the Boston Hospital for Women.[17] Twenty-one of these patients were treated with heparin anticoagulation for 10 to 14 days. In 18 of these 21 patients there was remission of the phlebitis for the duration of their prenatal course, and they delivered healthy babies. Recurrences of phlebitis occurred in two patients; one responded to a second course of heparin and the other to femoral vein ligation. Only one patient, of 12 weeks' gestation, who had a left iliofemoral phlebitis, developed pulmonary emboli when the anticoagulant was discontinued. Interruption of this patient's inferior vena cava was performed using a Teflon clip. Her prenatal course was then uneventful and she delivered a normal baby. There were no deaths or major bleeding complication in these 21 patients treated with heparin anticoagulation. All the mothers were discharged with normal babies and all were given prophylactic anticoagulants immediately post partum.

If the patient presents with embolism or develops it after a course of anticoagulants in pregnancy, inferior vena cava interruption is performed. This is accomplished by placing a serrated Teflon clip on the inferior vena cava just below the right renal vein. The use of the Teflon clip helps avert any distal venous hypertension or fluid sequestration which might pose a risk to the mother or fetus. This procedure can be performed with minimal risk and provide prolonged protection against further embolism.[18] The hazard of anticoagulation with coumarin derivatives is avoided. Femoral vein ligation provides less sure protection, as emboli may originate from veins proximal to the inguinal ligament.

The therapy of the patent with postpartum phlebitis and embolism generally presents no special problems. These patients are treated with intermittent doses of intravenous heparin during the acute stage and, after discharge, with a coumarin derivative for continued protection for two to three months. Venous interruption is restricted to the postpartum patient in whom anticoagulation is contraindicated, recurrent embolism occurred despite adequate anticoagulation, or in whom the initial embolism was massive and life-threatening.

From 1960 to 1970, 45 patients were treated for thromboembolism in the postpartum period.[17] Forty-three of these patients were treated with anticoagulants. Three patients had a venous interruption performed. There was no mortality in this group. Marked vaginal bleeding occurred in two patients seven and ten days after initiation of anticoagulant treatment, which required their discontinuance.

Summary

Antenatal thrombophlebitis can be effectually and safely treated with a limited course of heparin anticoagulation. The use of coumarin derivatives, with their potential risks to the fetus, does not appear justified. Vena caval interruption with a Teflon clip is recommended for proven cases of embolism in pregnancy. Postpartum thromboembolism is best treated by a combination of heparin and coumarin derivatives.

REFERENCES

1. Records Unit and Research of the Royal College of General Practitioners: Oral contraception and thromboembolic disease. J. Coll. Gen. Practit. 13:267, 1967.
2. Drill, A.: Oral contraceptives and thromboembolic disease. J.A.M.A. 219:583, 1972.
3. Villasanto, V.: Thromboembolic disease in pregnancy. Amer. J. Obstet. Gynec. 93:142, 1965.
4. DeVito, V. T., Wiener, L., and Massumi, R.: Antepartum thrombophlebitis and pulmonary embolization. Med. Ann., D. C. 34:177, 1965.
5. Confidential Enquiries into Maternal Deaths in England and Wales: Ministry of Health Reports on Public Health and Medical Subjects. London, Her Majesty's Stationery Office, 119:1964–1966, 1969.
6. Daniel, D. G., Campbell, H., and Turnbull, A. C.: Puerperal thromboembolism and suppression of lactation. Lancet 2:287, 1967.
7. Turner, G., and Hooper, N.: Sterilization and thromboembolism. J. Obstet. Gynec. Brit. Comm. 78:737, 1972.
8. Kakkar, V. V., Howe, C. T., Nicholaides, A. N., Renney, J. T. G., and Clarke, M. B.: Deep vein thrombosis of the leg. Am. J. Surg. 120:527, 1970.
9. Smith, G. T., Damin, G. J., and Dexter, L.: Postmortem arteriographic studies of the human being in pulmonary embolization. J.A.M.A. 188:143, 1964.
10. Sasahara, A. A., Cannilla, J. E., Morse, R. L., Sidd, J. J., and Tremblay, G. N.: Clinical and Physiological studies in pulmonary thromboembolism. Amer. J. Cardiol. 20:10, 1967.
11. Szucs, M. M., Brooks, H. L., Grossman, W., Banas, J. S., Meister, S. G., Dexter, L., and Dales, J. E.: Diagnostic sensitivity of laboratory findings in acute pulmonary embolism. Ann. Int. Med. 74:161 1971.
12. Kerber, I. J., Warr, O. S., and Richardson, C.: Pregnancy in a patient with a prosthetic mitral valve. J.A.M.A. 203:157, 1968.
13. Laros, R. K., Hage, M. L., and Hayashi, R. N.: Pregnancy and heart valve prostheses. Obstet. Gynec. 35:241, 1970.
14. Wingfield, J. G.: Anticoagulation for antenatal thromboembolic disease. J. Obstet. Gynec. Brit. Comm. 76:518, 1969.
15. Dale, A. W., and Lewis, M. R.: Heparin control of venous thromboembolism. Arch. Surg. 101:744, 1970.
16. Quenneville, G., Barton, B., McDevitt, E., and Wright, I.: The use of anticoagulants for thrombophlebitis during pregnancy. Am. J. Obstet. Gynec. 77:1135, 1959.
17. Healey, S. J.: Unpublished data.
18. Crane, C.: Femoral vs. caval interruption for venous thromboembolism. New Eng. J. Med. 270:819, 1964.

Preferable Management of Complications of the Venous System in Pregnancy and the Puerperium

JACK W. PEARSON
William Beaumont General Hospital

Complications or compromise of the venous system associated with pregnancy are frequently seen in the obstetrician's office. The problems that present range from a patient's complaint of pain, swelling, and cosmetic disfiguration to the more serious and even life threatening problems associated with thrombophlebitis and thromboembolic phenomena. Close attention must be paid, at the time of the patient's initial visit, to any past history of thrombophlebitis or embolization that may have occurred either in prior pregnancies or while on oral contraceptives, and these patients are followed in our high-risk clinic. Although individual clinicians' anxiety levels vary, as do criteria for seriousness of the observed disease process, the impression gained is that the incidence of venous complications in pregnant women ranges from five per cent to 33 per cent. Parity, age, degree of symptoms considered significant, and the amount of time one spends with the patient on a routine prenatal visit contribute to the number of problems recognized. The purpose of this section will be to point out and to attempt to place in proper perspective the significance of these complications and to present a method of management in each situation. Our primary purpose will be to discuss the efficacy of medical management in the vast majority of these patients. There will be no attempt to discuss in any depth the pathogenesis of venous disease or predisposing factors in pregnancy, as this has been well done in many other texts and articles considering this subject.

Varicose Veins in Pregnancy

Among the most frequent and aggravating problems for the pregnant patient are those related to varicose veins which develop in pregnancy. The patient's complaints are primarily those of cosmetic disfiguration, leg pain, and swelling which occur as the pregnancy progresses. The problem is obviously self-

259

limited and we consider conservative management to be optimal in these circumstances. We recommend daily rest periods with the legs elevated, emphasizing that the patient lie on her side rather than supine to further facilitate venous return from the lower extremities. Angiographic studies have shown the detrimental effect of the supine position on venous return in the pregnant patient. In the more severe cases we will also prescribe full leg support, usually with panty support hose.* According to Nabatoff and Pincus, 20 per cent of patients with varicose veins in the lower extremities in pregnancy will demonstrate associated vulvar varicosities. In most cases we have found that support of the perineal area can be obtained by use of these same panty support hose.

Several articles have been published, particularly from European countries, advocating a surgical attack on the varices in pregnancy, using the same indications as for nonpregnant patients. The majority of American physicians and surgeons, however, feel that any consideration of surgical correction of the varices appearing in or aggravated by pregnancy should be postponed from six weeks to three months subsequent to parturition. The preponderance of literature indicates that both injection techniques and surgical techniques, even including the so-called radical surgical approach have less optimal results in pregnant than in nonpregnant patients. In view of the fact that conservative measures are so effective and the transient nature of pregnancy so certain, there should be little question that the conservative approach is by far the best. However, it goes without saying that these patients are at significant risk in terms of developing more serious complications and, therefore, close attention must be paid to persisting or recurrent symptoms that might indicate a change in clinical status.

Over the past four years we have prophylactically administered 500 cc. of low molecular weight Dextran during labor and for each of the next three post partum days to these patients at greater risk. This is done to prevent the occurrence of puerperal thrombophlebitis. During this period of time, 7220 patients have been delivered at our hospital (William Beaumont General Hospital). The incidence of postpartum thrombophlebitis has been negligible, and there have been no instances of pulmonary embolus. Similar methods have been applied at our affiliated hospital (R. E. Thomason General Hospital) by our resident staff, and over the same time an additional 6569 patients have been delivered, again with no instances of postpartum thromboembolism. We feel that the administration of low molecular weight Dextran has no risk, and there have been no side effects of consequence noted in conjunction with its administration. The obvious precautions must be taken in those cases of severe cardiovascular disease in which the blood volume expansion inherent in the Dextran administration would present a threat of decompensation.

Superficial Thrombophlebitis

If the patient develops symptoms and findings of superficial phlebitis either ante partum or post partum, our approach and management remains the same. In all cases we try to rule out deep thrombophlebitis using techniques that we will describe below. After this is done, bed rest is prescribed and the patient is advised to lie on either side but not on her back. The foot of the bed is elevated and local heat, elastic bandages, and bed exercises are prescribed. The patient is

---

* Available through Jobst Institute, Inc., P.O. Box 653, Toledo, Ohio 43601.

ambulated as soon as she no longer experiences leg pain. In addition to this, she is given 500 ml. of Dextran daily for three days. We have been impressed by the fact that in the vast majority of cases the patient's symptoms disappear within 12 to 24 hours after therapy is instituted. The patient is discharged to the high-risk clinic in three to five days from the time of initiation of therapy. We do not use anticoagulation therapy in these cases and feel that surgery is certainly contra-indicated.

Deep Thrombophlebitis

Perhaps the most significant aspect in considering deep thrombophlebitis of pregnancy is the importance of an accurate diagnosis. The patient who has significant varices during the present gestation or who has a significant past history of complications of the venous system in a previous pregnancy (or while on oral contraceptives) should be made aware of what the significant symptoms of venous complications in pregnancy are when she is seen for her initial obstetric clinic visit, in order that she may seek medical care at the earliest possible moment if these symptoms develop. The symptoms and findings to be emphasized in education of the patient are: extremity swelling, whether unilateral or bilateral; acute leg pain; chest pain; chronic cough or hemoptysis. The incidence of these has been variously reported to be between 0.018 per cent and 0.29 per cent. As noted in Table 8–1, our recent combined experience would indicate an approximately 0.073 per cent incidence. Methods we routinely use in establishing the diagnosis of deep thrombophlebitis are as follows:

1. Physical examination, with particular emphasis on observation and documentation of any areas of redness or cord formation in the peripheral venous system and also auscultation of the lungs.

2. Careful documentation of comparable leg measurements are taken 6 cm. above and below the patella on each leg and carefully recorded in the patient's chart.

3. The Lowenberg blood pressure cuff test is utilized bilaterally and any difference noted in terms of the pressure necessary to produce leg pain in each leg.

4. We use the technique of Doppler assessment of the venous system, placing the transducer cephalad to the apparent area of involvement and noting presence or absence of increased venous flow when pressure is applied over the muscle mass of the calf.

TABLE 8–1. *Incidence of Deep Thrombophlebitis*

NUMBER OF DELIVERIES	NUMBER OF CASES OF DEEP THROMBO-PHLEBITIS	INCIDENCE OF ANTEPARTUM DEEP THROMBO-PHLEBITIS	MATERNAL MORTALITY	EMBOLIZA-TION	FETAL DEATH
13,789	10	0.73/1000	0	0	1
13,500	7	0.52/1000	0	1*	0

* Episode occurred when heparin treatment was discontinued and phlebitis recurred.

We have not used phlebography techniques or scanning with radioactive fibrinogen to further document the disease process, as the Doppler technique has been shown to correlate well with these studies and is far more accessible to the clinician. Upon establishing the diagnosis of deep thrombophlebitis our policy is to treat the patient with anticoagulation throughout the remainder of her pregnancy. Our technique is as follows:

The patient is admitted to the hospital and an intravenous catheter of the pediatric disposable type* is utilized. Over the first 24 hours sodium heparin is administered intravenously every four hours to establish a coagulation time between two and three times control levels when measured one half hour before the administration of the next injection. Over the next 24 to 48 hours, the patient is educated in the technique of self-administration of intravenous heparin, and from that point on she administers the heparin to herself through the indwelling catheter, with doses of between 10,000 and 12,000 units every six hours. This is continued throughout the remainder of her pregnancy (Figure 8-1). The patient is ambulated as soon as she is relatively asymptomatic, and when she is fully ambulatory she is discharged from the hospital. She maintains her therapy while being followed with weekly visits to the outpatient clinic until delivery. We have found that the indwelling catheter technique is satisfactory and that the catheters need to be replaced at intervals of two weeks to three monhs. There have been no instances of infection occurring at the catheter site or manifestations of systemic infection. The catheters have been cultured routinely when they have had to be replaced and we have had no instances of positive catheter cultures. We have personal experience with 10 cases and know of at least 12 others in which the technique has been utilized at other institutions, with one fetal death in asso-

---

* Available through Endo Laboratories, Inc., 1000 Stewart Ave., Garden City, New York 11530.

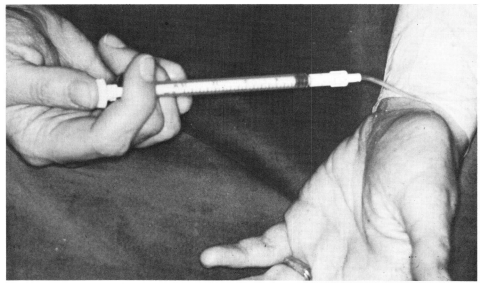

Figure 8-1. Demonstration of technique in which patient administers heparin with intracath in place.

ciation with our only serious maternal complication. Seven of these were reported by Gurll and associates[16] and the other five were disclosed in personal correspondence with the physicians concerned.

We are aware of no instances of recurrence of the disease process during the pregnancy when therapy has been continuous and there have been no reports of embolization while this regimen is followed. The anticoagulation is continued throughout pregnancy, labor, and the first 24 to 48 hours of the puerperium, with a coumarin derivative subsequently being utilized for the first six weeks postpartum. We feel strongly that this type of long-term therapy is indicated, as it has been reported that 24 per cent of the patients with deep antenatal thrombophlebitis will develop pulmonary emboli if their condition is not treated, with an associated death rate of 15 to 18 per cent. The incidence of embolization is decreased to 4.5 per cent in those patients who are receiving anticoagulants, and the death rate drops to 0.7 per cent. We feel that the self-administration of heparin is quite safe and is analogous to the case of diabetic patients, who traditionally have administered insulin to themselves and treated their own disease with medical supervision and guidance. We have had no maternal mortality in association with this regimen, and there has been only one instance in which there has been significant maternal morbidity. In this case, a massive retroperitoneal hematoma, secondary to trauma, developed in a 300 pound patient in the early third trimester of pregnancy. In this instance, the mother did well but the attendant maternal hypovolemia caused fetal hypoxia and death. There have been no significant bleeding complications in labor or the puerperium. In two instances in which lochia was somewhat increased, anticoagulation therapy was continued and bleeding was controlled with the administration of methergine. The cases we have discovered in the literature in which intravenous heparin therapy was used throughout pregnancy are summarized in Table 8–1.

We recognize that anticoagulation with coumarin derivatives has been advocated in several publications, but we have also noted that there has been significant fetal loss in association with this regimen from both fetal and neonatal bleeding as well as from associated maternal complications, such as in our single fetal loss. A high incidence of abortion and some suggestion that fetal deformity may also be associated with coumarin treatment have strengthened our belief that heparin therapy is the preferred approach to management. Fogarty and co-workers have recommended thrombectomy as an optimal means of management, particularly in cases of deep iliofemoral thrombophlebitis. In view of the fact that recurrence of thrombosis is not uncommon, the only circumstances in which we feel surgery might be indicated are those cases in which recurrent embolism complicates the disease process in spite of therapy. Up to the present this has not been a complication of our anticoagulant approach.

Pelvic Thrombophlebitis

Puerperal pelvic or ovarian thrombophlebitis is a serious complication and is an extremely difficult diagnosis to establish. We feel that any puerpera in whom fever and pelvic tenderness indicate presence of endometritis and parametritis which do not resolve within 48 to 72 hours after the initiation of systemic antibiotic therapy should be considered to have pelvic phlebitis, whether or not the diagnosis is apparent on pelvic or abdominal examination. In these circumstances, the patient is treated with intravenous heparin therapy, which is continued from five to 10 days, with conversion to coumarin therapy. This in turn is continued on an empiric basis for six weeks. If resolution of the fever and pelvic complaints are not apparent 48 to 72 hours after initiation of the heparin therapy, one must consider the possibility of adnexal abscess or other surgical complications of the puerperium, and laparotomy is indicated.

Thromboembolic Disease

The diagnosis of embolic phenomena, particularly pulmonary, requires firm documentation before or during the institution of a therapeutic approach. The patient's symptoms are significant and close attention should be paid to any complaint of chest pain, chronic cough, or hemoptysis, even in the absence of apparent thrombophlebitis in the extremities or pelvis. It has been reported that up to 50 per cent of postpartum patients with pulmonary embolization have few signs of distal thrombophlebitis. The usual diagnostic measures of enzyme studies, EKG, auscultation, and x-ray assessment of the chest should be performed. Pulmonary angiographic studies should be obtained to confirm the diagnosis in order to effectively document and treat these patients. Scanning techniques utilizing radioactive substances have been shown to be particularly inaccurate in the postpartum patient. We feel that the first line of defense and management is anticoagulation, and until the patient's course in the hospital is well established, we rely entirely upon intravenous heparinization to attempt to control the disease process and prevent further embolic phenomena. Coumarin is not to be utilized in this phase of treatment. If repeat embolization occurs despite adequate anticoagulation, a surgical approach may be necessary. In this case, the anticoagulation achieved by heparin is readily reversed, whereas that obtained with coumarin derivatives presents definite hazards to the patient in the operating room. We further feel that the coumarins are a poor second choice to heparin as an immediate and early agent of anticoagulation in these patients because of their delayed action and questionable value in preventing repeat embolization. In view of the fact that no embolizations have occurred in our patients who have had deep thrombophlebitis treated as just described, our experience to date is that there is no need for surgical intervention in our pregnant population.

The following selected bibliography of pertinent articles has been of value in preparing this section and is recommended to the interested reader.

REFERENCES

1. Aaro, L. A., and Juergens, J. L.: Thrombophlebitis associated with pregnancy. Amer. J. Obstet. Gynec. 109:1128, 1971.
2. Barner, H. B., William, V. L., Kaiser, G. C., and Hanlon, C. R.: Thrombectomy for iliofemoral venous thrombosis. J.A.M.A. 208:2442, 1969.
3. Bates, M. M.: Venous thromboembolic disease and ABO blood type. Lancet 1:239, 1971.
4. Beller, F. K.: Thromboembolic disease in Pregnancy. Clin. Obstet. Gynec. 11:290, 1968.
5. Bonnar, J., and Walsh, J.: Prevention of thrombosis after pelvic surgery by British Dextran 70. Lancet 1:615, 1972.
6. Brown, T. K., and Munsick, R. A.: Puerperal ovarian vein thrombophlebitis: a syndrome. Amer. J. Obstet. Gynec. 109:263, 1971.

7. Burnstein, R., Alkjaersig, N., and Fletcher, A.: Thromboembolism during pregnancy and the postpartum state. J. Lab. Clin. Med. 78:838, 1971.
8. Byrne, J. J.: Thrombophlebitis in pregnancy. Clin. Obstet. Gynec. 13:305, 1970.
9. Crane, C., Hartsuck, J., Birtch, A., Couch, N. P., Zollinger, R., Matloff, J., Dalen, J., and Dexter, L.: The Management of major pulmonary embolism. Surg. Gynec. Obstet. 128:27, 1969.
10. Dale, W. A., and Lewis, M. R.: Heparin control of venous thromboembolism. Arch. Surg. 101:744, 1970.
11. Dodson, M. G., Mobin-Uddin, K., and O'Leary, J. A.: Intracaval umbrella-filter for prevention of recurrent pulmonary embolism. South. Med. J. 64:1017, 1971.
12. Duncan, I. D., Coyle, M. G., and Walker, J.: Management and treatment of 34 cases of antepartum thromboembolism. J. Obstet. Gynaec. Brit. Comm. 78:904, 1971.
13. Evans, D. S., and Cockett, F. B.: Diagnosis of deep-vein thrombosis with an ultrasonic Doppler technique. Brit. Med. J. 2:802, 1969.
14. Fogarty, T. J., Wood, J. A., Krippaehne, W. W., and Dennis, D. L.: Management of iliofemoral venous thrombosis in the antepartum state. Surg. Gynec. Obstet. 128:546, 1969.
15. Fogarty, T. J., and Hallin, R. W.: Temporary caval occlusion during venous thrombectomy. Surg. Gynec. Obstet. 122:1269, 1966.
16. Gurll, N., Helfand, Z., Salzman, E. F., and Silen, W.: Peripheral venous thrombophlebitis during pregnancy. Amer. J. Surg. 121:449, 1971.
17. Haeger, K.: The treatment of varicose veins in pregnancy by radical operation or conservatively. Acta Obstet. Gynec. Scand. 47:233, 1968.
18. Henderson, S. R., Lund, C. J., and Creasman, W. T.: Antepartum pulmonary embolism. Amer. J. Obstet. Gynec. 112:476, 1972.
19. Hill, W. C., and Pearson, J. W.: Outpatient intravenous heparin therapy for antepartum iliofemoral thrombophlebitis. Obstet. Gynec. 37:785, 1971.
20. Hirsh, J., Cade, J. F., and O'Sullivan, E. F.: Clinical experience with anticoagulant therapy during pregnancy. Brit. Med. J. 1:270, 1970.
21. Hirsh, J., Cade, J. F., and Gallus, A. S.: Anticoagulants in pregnancy: a review of indications and complications. Amer. Heart. J. 83:301, 1971.
22. Hushni, E. A., Leopoldo, I. P., and Lenhert, A. E.: Thrombophlebitis in pregnancy. Amer. J. Obstet. Gynec. 97:901, 1967.
23. Ikard, R. W., Ueland, K., and Folse, R.: Lower limb venous dynamics in pregnant women. Surg. Gynec. Obstet. 132:483, 1971.
24. Jick, H., Westerholm, B., Vessey, M. P., Lewis, G. P., Slone, D., Inman, W. H., Shapiro, S., and Worcester, J.: Venous thromboembolic disease and ABO blood type. Lancet 1:539, 1969.
25. Juergens, J. L.: Venous thromboembolism. Cardiovasc. Clin. 3:233, 1971.
26. Mavor, G. E., and Galloway, J. M. D.: Iliofemoral venous thrombosis. Brit. J. Surg. 56:45, 1969.
27. Moncrief, J. A., Darin, J. C., Canizdro, P. C., et al.: Use of dextran to prevent arterial and venous thrombosis. Ann. Surg. 158:553, 1963.
28. Mueller, M. J., and Lebherz, T. B.: Antepartum thrombophlebitis. Obstet. Gynec. 34:874, 1969.
29. Nabatoff, R. A., and Pincus, J. A.: Management of varicose veins during pregnancy. Obstet. Gynec. 36:928, 1970.
30. Olwin, J. H., and Koppel, J. L.: Anticoagulant therapy during pregnancy. Obstet. Gynec. 34:847, 1969.
31. Ross, M., Nowicki, K., and Rangarajan, N. S.: Asymptomatic pulmonary embolism during pregnancy. Obstet. Gynec. 37:131, 1971.
32. Sher, M. H.: Management of antepartum thrombophlebitis. Amer. Surg. 37:587, 1971.
33. Talbot, S., Ryrie, D., Wakley, E. J., and Langman, M. J. S.: ABO blood groups and venous thromboembolic disease. Lancet 1:1257, 1970.
34. Turnbull, A. C., Daniel, D. G., and McGarry, J. M.: Antenatal and postnatal thromboembolism. Practitioner 206:727, 1971.
35. Villasanta, U.: Thromboembolic disease in pregnancy. Amer. J. Obstet. Gynec. 93:142, 1965.
36. Wallach, R. C.: Dextran therapy for pregnancy-associated deep thrombophlebitis. Amer. J. Obstet. Gynec. 112:613, 1971.
37. Weekes, L. R., and Deukmedjian, A. G.: Thromboembolic disease in pregnancy. Amer. J. Obstet. Gynec. 107:649, 1970.
38. Thrombo-embolic disease in obstetrics and gynaecology. Med. J. Australia 2:1283, 1969.
39. Antenatal thromboembolism. Brit. Med. J. 1:249, 1970.

Preferable Management of Complications of the Venous System in Pregnancy and the Puerperium

Editorial Comment

Venous problems in women often begin with a pregnancy. Although the antepartum incidence of thromboembolic disease is reputedly not increased over that of nonpregnant women, the frequency increases seven- to eightfold in the postpartum period. Some 8 to 10 per cent of maternal deaths result from thromboembolism,[1] but this represents only a portion of the story, for varicosities that begin in pregnancy, with their attendant threats of complications, continue throughout the lifetime of the individual. Thus, when considering deaths from embolism in women, cognizance should be taken of the possibility that varicosities and subsequent superficial thrombophlebitis may have originated during a pregnancy. Certainly, there seems to be general agreement that pregnant patients or those recently pregnant are at greater risk of developing a deep thrombophlebitis or thromboembolism if they have previously been plagued by varicosities and superficial thrombophlebitis. It would follow logically that the prevention of varicosities could remove this risk.

Discussions of preventive measures for varicosities in pregnancy have in large measure fallen on deaf ears, for, as in the nonpregnant individual, sclerosing solutions placed at the proper venous location will prevent the spread or extension of beginning varicosities, remove the need for further treatment, and prevent the complications alluded to above. Why then is the pregnant patient treated differently from the nonpregnant? In any maternity clinic concerned principally with the care of the nonprivate patient, the ultimate condition is seen all too often in women who have had many pregnancies and are afflicted with enormous and disabling varicosities owing in large measure to neglect in previous pregnancies. Not only are these patients incapacitated but they are also at high risk. Also at risk is the fetus, for the amount of the blood volume sequestered in the legs may be a factor in reducing intravillous blood flow, which may thereby compromise the fetal environment. Undoubtedly, the number of these neglected patients will decrease somewhat with limitations of family size.

With few exceptions, surgeons and even vascular surgeons show little interest in preventing diseases of the veins in pregnancy, probably because the prophylactic care is tedious, unspectacular, and requires frequent patient visits— and hence many man-hours of work. According to patients referred to vascular surgeons, they are commonly told to "come back after you have finished having your family. I will do a vein stripping if necessary and that will fix you."

So the obstetrician and most surgeons continue to use the ancient approach of binding the legs—modified, to be sure, by utilizing more sophisticated materials. Whether this so-called time honored method decreases the spread of varicosities or reduces superficial phlebitis is open to question, but apparently this is what the majority of physicians believe. However, sclerosing substances also can accomplish this objective. One of the editors of this volume can testify, having observed this approach to patient care, that this method of therapy will prevent varicosities and their spread and hence decrease the risk of developing superficial thrombophlebitis. Of course, this treatment has no value when the varicosities are already extensive because of previous neglect. Again, vein stripping should not be done until after delivery, but the procedure can be carried out on the fourth or fifth day post partum, thus avoiding a later hospital admission, which is never propitious for these patients, many of whom have large families. Hence, any sizeable maternity service deserves to have a vascular or vein clinic whose major objective is to prevent varicosities and thus block the chain reaction leading from superficial or deep thrombophlebitis in some patients to thrombo-embolism.

The controversy in the management of thromboembolism and thrombophlebitis appears to center on the diagnosis and the approach to the use of anticoagulants. Lung scanning, if extended, may reveal that the incidence of pulmonary embolization ante partum is greater than that reported. This seems to hold true in the differential diagnosis of cardiovascular problems and in other fields as well. Also, lung scanning may reveal startling findings when other types of emboli occur in pregnancy, notably wandering trophoblastic tissue from molar pregnancy and amniotic fluid embolism. The Doppler test likewise has a place in diagnosis. The use of tagged fibrinogen is being evaluated, but it appears not to be as helpful or reliable as originally thought. Pulmonary arteriography and phlebography have their indications.

Unfortunately, deep pelvic thrombophlebitis can be silent, and a fatal embolism literally can occur "like a bolt from the blue." A review of the patient's chart after the event may reveal that tachycardia had been present for several hours without evidence of any changes in the patient's other vital signs. Hence, an unexplained sharp increase in pulse rate (tachycardia) occurring in the puerperium should at least raise the question of a possible pelvic thrombophlebitis or of small thromboemboli coming to lodge in the pulmonary system.

The demonstration that ambulatory heparinization is feasible has provided a ready method of continuing therapy throughout pregnancy. When pregnancy itself represents a hypercoagulable state once anticoagulant therapy is instituted, it should not be discontinued until sometime in the postpartum period. Heparin administration should be carefully monitored by determining the partial thromboplastin time and performing other appropriate tests. Undoubtedly, the heparin dosage should be decreased somewhat during labor and delivery but promptly increased to a therapeutic level through the tenth postpartum day at least. Excessive bleeding from the placental site in this period has been observed as the decidua and spiral arterioles slough away. In fact, alarming uterine bleeding can occur if the patient is near total heparinization, as for example in renal dialysis. This undesirable effect of heparin is readily negated by protamine and the bleeding will cease promptly after its administration. When substituting warfarin for heparin, the former should be started in advance of the discontinuation of the heparin.

REFERENCES

1. Henderson, S. R., Lund, C. J., and Creasman, W. T.: Antepartum pulmonary embolism. Am. J. Obstet. Gynec. *112*:476, 1972.

9

The Clinical Spectrum and Management of Acquired Coagulopathy in Pregnancy

Alternative Points of View:

By Fritz K. Beller

By James J. Corrigan

By Donald G. McKay

Editorial Comment

The Clinical Spectrum and Management of Acquired Coagulopathy in Pregnancy

FRITZ K. BELLER
New York University School of Medicine

Acquired coagulation defects in pregnancy are a manifestation of the intravascular coagulation syndrome. The trigger for the activation of this system may vary in different clinical situations, but the pathophysiological end result is identical. Various constituents of the system, such as platelets, fibrinogen, factor V, and factor VIII, are consumed during this process, and the term *consumption coagulopathy* is being used with increasing frequency. However, additional pathogenic factors are required to deposit fibrin in the microcirculatory bed, for which condition we use the term *disseminated intravascular coagulation* (DIC). These factors are not too well known and require further research. Evidence is accumulating for the existence of organ specificity.

Consumption coagulopathy is associated not only with a decrease in coagulation factors but also with an increase in fibrin derivatives. During the early stage of activation of the coagulation system, fibrinogen monomers aggregate to form high molecular weight derivatives (weight up to 1,000,000). These derivatives do not yet have the characteristics of a fibrin clot and are removed from the circulation by a variety of defense mechanisms, including the reticuloendothelial system (RES). High molecular weight derivatives of fibrinogen or fibrin resulting from fibrinolysis are now differentiated by a variety of frequently used immune techniques. The presence of fibrin derivatives, therefore, is diagnostic of the fibrinolytic digestion of fibrin deposits only when determined by specified techniques. This explains the difficulty in differentiating between primary enzyme activation of the coagulation system and primary hyperfibrinolysis. Primary hyperfibrinolytic states, however, are rare under obstetrical conditions. This applies especially to the clinical entity of premature separation of the normally implanted placenta and septic shock.

The differentiation between the presence of consumption coagulopathy without glomerular fibrin deposition on the one hand, and DIC with fibrin deposition, especially in the glomerular capillaries, appears to be of greater clinical significance for the obstetrician. We have shown that the concentration of plasma hemoglobin is most closely correlated with glomerular fibrin deposition. An increase in plasma hemoglobin by more than 100 per cent indicates fibrin deposition in the microcirculation.

Administration of the following agents has been proposed for treatment: (1) blood, (2) fibrinogen, (3) heparin, and (4) fibrinolytic inhibitors (epsilon amino caproic acid, or EACA). Each of these modalities is, to a degree, controversial.

It should be remembered that patients hemorrhage as a result of a consumption coagulopathy only after delivery and not during labor. Even a reduced concentration of plasma fibrinogen does not indicate hemorrhage from the placental implantation site. It is estimated that only about 25 per cent of patients with a consumption coagulopathy will eventually bleed, depending, of course, on the degree of the coagulation defect. This applies to such clinical conditions as abruptio placentae, dead fetus syndrome, postpartum hemorrhage after normal deliveries, and the recently recognized consumption coagulopathy during termination of second trimester pregnancy by the instillation of hypertonic saline.

BLOOD

Whole fresh blood contains approximately 0.5 g. of fibrinogen per unit of blood. A plasma fibrinogen level of not more than 100 mg. per 100 ml. is required for hemostasis. Four grams of fibrinogen are needed to raise the plasma fibrinogen concentration from 0 to 100 mg. per 100 ml., or 2 g. to increase the level from 50 to 100 mg. per 100 ml. From this quantitative evaluation, it can be calculated that the decreased plasma fibrinogen concentration can be raised by two to three units of blood, provided that the fibrinogen level is between 50 and 90 mg. per 100 ml., and that there is no further blood loss. These considerations apply especially to patients with premature separation of the placenta, who may have had considerable bleeding into the uterine cavity. This may be estimated by measuring central venous pressure, urinary output, and hematocrit level. The timely infusion of whole blood before delivery corrects not only the hypovolemia (hemorrhagic shock) but also the consumption coagulopathy. Catastrophic hemorrhagic events result from the failure of the obstetrician to recognize the amount of blood lost. The continuous blood loss is frequently of a larger volume than that which is substituted, and this applies especially to fibrinogen.

Although the platelet count may be quite low in a patient with consumption coagulopathy or DIC, we have rarely seen the need for platelet substitution. This may be a result of the fact that patients with idiopathic thrombocytopenia rarely hemorrhage from the placental implantation site, indicating the significance of fibrinogen for producing hemostasis in the area of uterine contractility.

Platelet substitution may be required, however, if large quantities of "old" blood from the blood bank are used. Platelets in bank blood older than 6 hours are reduced in numbers and become qualitatively insufficient. Infusion of such blood may, therefore, result in a degree of dilution superimposed on a low platelet count. We prefer, therefore, to use one unit of fresh blood for every five units of old blood to correct for platelet deficiencies. One unit of fresh blood (not older than 6 hours) raises the platelet count by 10,000 to 15,000/mm.[3] if the mechanism for the consumption coagulopathy has ceased and blood loss has been controlled.

Fibrinogen

Commercially available fibrinogen is not a purified substance. It is in fact an undefractionated Cohn fraction I. Many preparations contain salt for stabilization purposes. The potential danger of producing serum hepatitis will be reduced in the future by scanning of donors using the Australian antigen technique. The quantitative aspects of the fibrinogen method have already been evaluated, and they indicate that very little fibrinogen is needed for substitution. We prefer to substitute fibrinogen in small quantities (1 to 2 g. in severe abruptio placentae), in addition to blood substitution, to achieve an uneventful delivery.

Recently an additional objection to fibrinogen substitution was raised. Provided that the trigger system for the coagulation activation is still present, fibrinogen would "pour fuel on the flames," since it provides additional substrate. This controversial consideration is closely related to similar objections to the use of heparin and will be discussed in this context.

Heparin

Heparin acts as an antithrombin agent, inhibiting thrombin formation. From a theoretical point of view, it should interfere in some way with the sequence of the coagulation activation. For reasons not fully understood, this concept has not been proved valid at the present time. There is ample clinical evidence for the assumption that the trigger system is exhausted in the acute phenomenon of consumption coagulopathy, as for instance in abruptio placentae. The heparin-induced antithrombin effect seems then to be superimposed on the already present consumption coagulopathy, explaining severe hemorrhagic episodes, which were observed by various investigators, including this group. We have, therefore, failed to see the beneficial effect of primary heparin application or of "shielding" fibrinogen substitution with additional heparin when obstetrical hemorrhage occurs.

Heparin has been shown, however, to be of therapeutic value for the chronic activation of the coagulation system in the dead fetus syndrome. In this instance consumption coagulopathy progresses slowly over weeks. An infusion with low dosages of heparin interrupts the gradual activation and raises the plasma fibrinogen level in 24 hours by stimulating endogenous synthesis of fibrinogen.

There is also clinical evidence to indicate beneficial effects of heparin if given prophylactically in patients with febrile and septic abortions. In most instances, septic shock results from gram-negative infection and endotoxemia. There is, of course, no diagnostic test available at present to identify patients who will progress from low-grade endotoxemia into septic shock. It was therefore proposed to use a low dosage of heparin infusion in patients who had chills and fever above 101° F., associated with a subnormal platelet number. Curettage as well as hysterectomy can be performed without fear of hemorrhagic episodes provided that the clotting time is not longer than 20 minutes.

Recent evidence has indicated that DIC is part of the pathophysiologic derangement in toxemia. Previous attempts with short-term heparin treatment were disappointing. Long-term treatment has not yet been tried, and the indication, dose relationship, length of treatment, and timing must be studied further.

Fibrinolytic inhibition

The discovery that breakdown products of fibrin are biologically active as inhibitors of the coagulation system stirred up the controversy regarding fibrinolytic inhibitors. Epsilon amino caproic acid (EACA; Amicar) is available commercially, although a variety of more potent inhibitors are under investigation. However, for a variety of reasons, enthusiasm for EACA treatment has diminished. Breakdown products must circulate in large quantities to inhibit the coagulation system. Such large quantities can result from hyperfibrinolysis, but this is an exception under obstetrical conditions. Fibrinolysis, on the other hand, is the most effective defensive system for digesting fibrin deposition and freeing the microcirculation. Significantly, the quantity and duration of deposited fibrin is directly related to organ necrosis, as for instance renal cortical necrosis. Tissue activator is released from ischemic cells, activating fibrinolysis locally and digesting fibrin. The EACA, however, is metabolized in the kidney and is basically an inhibitor of tissue activator. Under experimental conditions, and especially in pregnancy, it has been shown that consumption coagulopathy may progress into DIC with glomerular fibrin deposition if EACA is administered. Not surprisingly, then, reports have suggested that partial renal cortical necrosis was related to the administration of this inhibitor. It is, therefore, generally accepted that EACA is contraindicated in any condition related to consumption coagulopathy or DIC.

Only occasionally have we seen a need for administration of EACA in patients who gave evidence that there were large amounts of circulating activator. Clinical experience shows that the best candidates for EACA treatment are patients who deliver uneventfully and begin to hemorrhage 30 to 60 minutes later from a contracted uterus. We consider using EACA if 4 g. of fibrinogen fails to provide a plasma fibrinogen concentration of 100 mg. per 100 ml., as indicated by unclotted venous blood or clots which dissolve by shaking the tube.

The recognition of the role of DIC in the development of irreversible organ necrosis and the significance of organ fibrinolysis as a significant defense system have initiated a new controversy where treatment is concerned. A few groups have begun to treat patients in irreversible shock with fibrinolytic activators, such as streptokinase or urokinase. It will, however, take several years before indications, dosage, and side-effects are sufficiently evaluated to know whether this method will be beneficial.

The controversy in treatment stems from the fact that the obstetrical patient may have acquired a consumption coagulopathy requiring only the substitution of fibrinogen. Further elucidation must be made of the conditions under which consumption coagulopathy progresses into fibrin deposition, especially glomerular fibrin deposition. Clearly it is not simply a quantitative problem.

REFERENCES

1. Bang, N., Beller, F. K., Deutsch, E., and Mammen, E. (eds.): Thrombosis and Bleeding Disorders. New York, Academic Press, 1971.
2. Beller, F. K.: Treatment of coagulation disorders in pregnancy. Clin. Obstet. Gynec. 7:372, 1964.
3. Beller, F. K.: Physiologic aspects of circulating endotoxin in septic abortion. Internat. J. Gynec. Obstet. 812:617, 1970.

4. Hardaway, R. M.: Syndromes of disseminated intravascular coagulation. Springfield, Ill., Charles C Thomas, 1966.
5. Jiminez, J. M., and Pritchard, J. A.: Pathogenesis and treatment of coagulation defects resulting from fetal death. Obstet. Gynec. 32:449, 1968.
6. Kuhn, W., and Graeff, H.: Gerinnungsstoerungen in der Geburtshilfe. Stuttgart, G. Thieme, 1971.
7. McKay, D. G.: Disseminated intravascular coagulation. New York, Hoeber, 1964.
8. Selye, H.: Thrombohemorrhagic phenomena. Springfield, Ill., Charles C Thomas, 1965.

The Clinical Spectrum and Management of Acquired Coagulopathy in Pregnancy

James J. Corrigan, Jr.
University of Arizona Medical Center

Introduction

Acquired coagulopathy connotes a change in the coagulation or fibrinolytic systems that is secondary to an underlying disease and produces in the patient either an increased or decreased ability to form thrombi. These coagulopathies can result from activation of the coagulation/fibrinolytic systems or from inadequate synthesis of the blood platelets and plasma procoagulants. Activation of the blood coagulation mechanism may lead to the increased tendency to form thrombi, the so-called "hypercoagulable state." This risk appears to be substantial when other defense mechanisms are impaired, e.g., when there is an inadequate fibrinolytic system, the presence of vascular stasis, a poorly functioning reticuloendothelial system, and so forth. In addition, activation of the coagulation system may be such that the utilization of the platelets and coagulation factors is so great that synthesis cannot keep abreast with it; thus, these factors fall below hemostatic levels and the patient may paradoxically manifest a bleeding diathesis.

Although liver disease, aplastic anemia, idiopathic thrombocytopenic purpura, systemic lupus erythematosus, and so forth, are seen in the obstetrical patient the purpose of this article is to focus on those acquired coagulopathies which are complications of and, many times, peculiar to pregnancy. Furthermore, those situations in which the patient manifests a bleeding state secondary to an active coagulation or fibrinolytic system (coagulation failure of pregnancy) are emphasized, since these are the most common.[1-7]

Changes in the Hemostatic Mechanism in Normal Pregnancy

The physiological and biochemical events that lead to normal hemostasis will not be outlined in detail here since they have been the subject of excellent recent reviews. It is sufficient to say that following blood vessel injury two events occur: the production of a platelet plug (primary hemostasis) and the formation of a fibrin thrombus (secondary hemostasis). The first event utilizes vascular constriction, platelet adhesion, platelet aggregation, and finally the production of a platelet plug which insures adequate early hemostasis. The second event proceeds by two pathways. On tissue injury, tissue factor is released, which in the presence of calcium activates the extrinsic or tissue coagulation pathway. Tissue factor activates plasma coagulation factor VII, which in turn activates factor X. Activated factor X, in the presence of factor V, calcium, and phospholipid, converts factor II (prothrombin) to active factor II (thrombin). Thrombin then acts on factor I (fibrinogen) to remove two small peptides, leaving a molecule called fibrin monomer, which then polymerizes to fibrin. Thrombin also activates factor XIII (fibrin stabilizing factor). This enzyme is necessary to insure stability of the fibrin thrombus. The second mechanism is called the intrinsic or plasma coagulation pathway. Factor XII (Hageman) is somehow activated, perhaps by the exposed subendothelial collagen fibers, and it activates factor XI, which in turn activates factor IX. Activated factor IX, with factor VIII (antihemophilic factor, or AHF), phospholipid, and calcium, then activates factor X, and the sequence leading to fibrin formation follows the same route as in the extrinsic system. The presence of natural inhibitors helps keep the production of fibrin in check. The fibrinolytic system is composed of activators, inhibitors, and the inactive enzyme plasminogen. The conversion of plasminogen to plasmin is usually accomplished by an increase in activator activity, either locally or systemically. Plasmin degrades and dissolves fibrin, but if it becomes systemically overactive may also attack factor VIII, factor V, fibrinogen, and other plasma proteins.

In normal pregnancy a number of changes occur.[7-12] The mechanisms responsible for these alterations are unknown. They may result from hormonal influences and stress, but whether they are due to altered synthesis, utilization, in vivo activation or a combination of these is unexplained. Many studies done during pregnancy, labor, and the puerperium have been reported and are summarized by Kleiner and associates.[7] Compared to normal nonpregnant adults, the obstetrical patient tends to demonstrate elevated levels of fibrinogen and of factors VII, VIII, IX, and X. The platelet count and the levels of factors II and V are usually no different in pregnant and nonpregnant persons, but factor XI has been reported to be reduced in pregnancy.[11] Platelet adhesiveness (to glass beads) has been noted to range from normal to elevated. As far as the fibrinolytic mechanism is concerned, the pregnant woman has elevated levels of plasminogen, long euglobulin clot lysis time, but mild elevation of the serum fibrin split products.

TABLE 9–1. *Comparison of Platelet Counts, Factor II, Factor V, Factor VIII, and Fibrinogen Levels Between Normal Pregnant Women and Normal Nonpregnant Adults*

	NORMAL PREGNANCY	NORMAL ADULTS
Platelet Count (per cubic millimeter)	220,000–237,000*	275,000*
Factor II (per cent)	107	100
Factor V (per cent)	106–108	100
Factor VIII (per cent)	196–288	100
Fibrinogen (mg. per 100 ml.)	400–530	325

* Results are expressed as mean values from published data.[7, 9, 10, 11]

These changes appear to be fully developed by the third trimester; however, the data are incomplete with regard to the early gestational periods.

These data are relevant for at least two reasons. First, because of the elevated activity of many coagulation factors and the possible reduction in systemic fibrinolytic activity, the obstetrical patient is in a "hypercoagulable state." Second, from a diagnostic and therapeutic point of view, the coagulation data obtained from sick obstetrical patients must be compared with values from normal pregnant patients and not normal nonpregnant adults, if one is to adequately delineate a normal from an abnormal change.

Acquired Coagulopathy in Pregnancy

DIAGNOSIS

Acquired systemic coagulopathy may result from disseminated intravascular coagulation, massive bleeding, or, rarely, systemic hyperfibrinolysis. Furthermore, all three may be operative in the same patient at the same time.

Disseminated intravascular coagulation (DIC) is an abnormality in which the production of fibrin is accelerated.[1,6,13] Since fibrin is formed from the soluble plasma protein fibrinogen, it follows that fibrinogen consumption or utilization occurs in DIC. In addition, other plasma coagulation factors and the blood platelets are utilized during this process. If the consumption exceeds the patient's ability to produce these procoagulants, then the resultant level of platelets or of any one of the coagulation factors will be lower than normal. If they are reduced below hemostatic levels, they may produce a hemorrhagic state—thus the terms "consumption coagulopathy" and "defibrination syndrome." The two main consequences of DIC are bleeding and impairment of the microcirculation from fibrin deposition. The bleeding manifestations range from a few petechiae or bruises to troublesome bleeding from venipuncture or cutdown sites, to massive hemorrhage, particularly from the uterus in the pregnant patient. In the latter instance, significant anemia is the rule rather than the exception. Fibrin deposition may or may not lead to local or diffuse tissue damage. Although most patients with DIC have some form of bleeding, in many of the cases the data are not clear as to how significant a problem fibrin deposition can be. A few patients with DIC will manifest neither bleeding nor a thrombotic state. The onset of DIC may be acute (as in abruptio placentae), subacute (as in retained dead fetus), or chronic (as in malignancy).

Coagulation failure, with massive hemorrhage in the obstetrical patient, may occur by either of two mechanisms. First, in the process of formation of a massive retroplacental hematoma, the circulating plasma becomes depleted of clotting factors. Second, patients with hemorrhagic shock from any cause may have an acquired coagulopathy, which is probably the result of DIC, as has been emphasized by Hardaway.[14]

In systemic hyperfibrinolysis, hypocoagulability exists because of the inability to lay down adequate amounts of fibrin. This occurs because the fibrin is lysed rapidly, and other coagulation factors are subjected to enzymatic degradation by plasmin.

TABLE 9–2.   *Similarities and Dissimilarities of Coagulation Data in Obstetrical Patients with Prolonged Coagulation Screening Tests, Compared to Normal Pregnant Patients*

	DISSEMINATED INTRAVASCULAR COAGULATION	MASSIVE BLEEDING	MASSIVE VOLUME REPLACEMENT	HEPARIN	SYSTEMIC HYPERFI-BRINOLYSIS
Platelets	R	R	N–R	N	N
Factor II	R	R	N–R	N	N
Factor V	R	R	R	N	R
Factor VIII	R	R	R	N	R
Fibrinogen	R	R	N–R	N	R
Fibrin Split Products	E	E	N	N	E
Plasminogen	R	R	R	N	R
Euglobulin Lysis Time	N	N	N	N	S
Partial Thromboplastin Time	P	P	P	P	P
Prothrombin Time	P	P	P	P	P

R = Reduced; E = Elevated; N = Normal; P = Prolonged; S = Short.

When acquired coagulopathy is suspected clinically, the diagnosis is ultimately based on laboratory reports. Strict criteria must be followed, for bleeding may occur for many different reasons. Although "screening tests" help identify that a hemostatic problem exists, specific studies with proper controls are necessary. As shown in Table 9-2, the partial thromboplastin time and prothrombin time indicate that something is wrong, but not what it is.

Diagnosis of classical DIC is not difficult, since these patients have the characteristic findings of hypofibrinogenemia, low plasma levels of coagulation factors II, V, and VIII, fibrinolytic split products in the serum, and thrombocytopenia. It must be remembered, however, that the level of the platelets or any of the coagulation factors measured at one point in time may be misleading, as it depends on previous levels, rate of production, and rapidity of consumption. In acute DIC, the fall in levels of platelets, fibrinogen, and factors II, V, and VIII is precipitous. Production cannot keep up with the destruction, so that the levels are usually lower than in normal nonpregnant adults. In subacute and chronic DIC, the levels can be normal or below normal for pregnancy, and on occasion below normal adult ranges. Nevertheless, bleeding can occur if there is severe reduction in platelets or one or all of the factors. If changes occur that are characteristic of DIC but the levels are only mildly reduced, the patient may not bleed at all. Other supporting laboratory findings in DIC include the presence of fragmented red blood cells in the blood smear and positive ethanol gelation test.

If these laboratory tests are not readily available or if only one or two of the coagulation abnormalities exists, then one should exert caution in diagnosing DIC. In such instances the clinical setting should be carefully evaluated and other laboratory aids used. For example, in the absence of severe hepatocellular disease, the finding of thrombocytopenia, hypofibrinogenemia, and fibrin split products is strong evidence for DIC. In addition, by using sequential factor studies or by determining the turnover rates of isotopically tagged platelets and fibrinogen, one can identify excessive utilization. The giving of a "trial of heparin" is another method sometimes used to test if DIC is present or not. This is potentially hazardous and is not generally recommended. The utmost caution is to be exercised in patients who have defects in hemostatic mechanism that are not due to DIC, but who still have abnormal screening tests. In Table 9–2 the similarities and dissimilarities between these entities and DIC are shown. These must be ruled out before anticoagulant therapy is attempted, which can be done only by the use of specific laboratory studies. Perhaps the most common situation is the one of massive volume replacement in the obstetrical patient with bleeding or septic infection. If, in such situations, volume replacement consists solely of packed red blood cells, whole blood that is not fresh, stored plasma, albumin, dextran, or purified protein fractions (PPF), it is possible that dilutional thrombocytopenia or reduction in the coagulation factors shown in Table 9–2 may occur. Platelets are inadequate in all of these. Coagulation factors are not present in albumin, dextran, and PPF, and factors V and VIII are significantly reduced in stored plasma and nonfresh whole blood. Thus, simple replacement therapy is all that is necessary for treatment of this condition. The most perplexing situation is the obstetrical patient with serious uterine blood loss and the findings shown in Table 9–2 prior to any therapy. As already mentioned, patients with hemorrhagic shock may develop DIC. In abruptio placentae, three mechanisms could account for the observed coagulation changes: (1) development of DIC from the postulated release of thromboplastic material into the maternal circulation from the placenta; (2) DIC resulting from hemorrhagic shock; or (3) massive deposition of fibrin in the retroplacental space, with resultant depletion of plasma platelets and procoagulants. The obstetrical patient who has been given heparin for thrombophlebitis will have an abnormal partial thromboplastin time and prothrombin time. Similarly, it is common practice to put heparin in intravenous catheters to "keep the line open." Blood samples obtained through this catheter, if not washed thoroughly, will contain enough heparin to give abnormal screening test results and thus may provide an erroneous diagnosis.

Finally, knowing the clinical states in which DIC is associated is of fundamental importance for reaching a correct diagnosis in this pathophysiological response.

TREATMENT

The obstetrical conditions in which acquired coagulopathy exists are shown on Table 9–3. The predominant mechanism responsible for the coagulopathy in these disorders is presumed to be intravascular coagulation. The evidence will not be reviewed here, but it is sufficient to say that there are many studies which support the concept of DIC as the mechanism for abruptio placentae,

TABLE 9–3.   *Obstetrical Conditions Associated with Acquired Coagulopathy*

Abruptio placentae
Septic abortion
Intrauterine fetal death
Amniotic fluid embolism
Uterine rupture
Intra-amniotic injection of hypertonic saline
Hydatidiform mole
Placenta accreta
Transfusion reaction (hemolytic)
Toxemia

retained dead fetus syndrome, septic abortion (especially with shock), transfusion reactions, and intra-amniotic injection of hypertonic saline. Fragmentary and incomplete data exist for the remainder of the patients, especially those with toxemia.

The therapy in these obstetrical settings is fairly clear. This consists of eliminating the precipitating cause, replacing the depleted procoagulants, and in selected cases medically interrupting the DIC.

ABRUPTIO PLACENTAE. This condition, the premature separation of the normally implanted placenta, has been extensively studied.[4,7,15,16] It appears that this abnormality occurs in 1:85 to 1:250 pregnancies, and of these about 1 in 5 or 10 patients progresses to a hemorrhagic diathesis. Furthermore, the incidence of renal cortical necrosis is high in this group. However, it is not clear if the responsible mechanism for the renal disease is the fibrin generated from DIC or a preexisting kidney disease plus vascular spasm owing to hypovolemia. As is true for all conditions with DIC in pregnancy, the removal of the products of conception is of fundamental therapeutic importance to abolish DIC. Whether this is accomplished by cesarean section or by amniotomy, with eventual pelvic delivery, is an obstetrical judgment. In the meantime, the control of bleeding can be accomplished by replacement therapy. Depending on the need, this may consist of platelet concentrates, fresh frozen plasma, fresh whole blood, or fibrinogen. Since the coagulopathy is thought to result from DIC, heparin has been advocated by some. In addition, some investigators question the prudence of giving coagulation factors to a patient with DIC without first anticoagulating with heparin. Although this may be a very real precaution, our experience, as well as that of a number of other investigators, does not support this view. Controlled studies with and without heparin have not been published, and no general recommendation can be made. However, the onset of abruptio placentae is so swift it is doubtful if heparin could be beneficial; indeed, it could complicate definitive obstetrical management. It would appear that rapid diagnosis, replacement therapy, and prompt obstetrical care is the management of choice.

INTRAUTERINE FETAL DEATH (RETAINED DEAD FETUS SYNDROME).[4,17-19] Between three and four weeks after death of the fetus the fibrinogen concentration begins to decline, and hypofibrinogenemia occurs if the period of retention approaches five weeks or longer. It has been estimated that 2 to 10 per cent of all cases of fetal death have associated maternal hypofibrinogenemia, and 33 per cent are affected if the retention is greater than five weeks. The available evidence suggests that the reduced fibrinogen levels result from DIC and not underproduction. Frequently other coagulation changes may also be found (e.g., thrombocytopenia) in this subacute DIC state. Heparin has been shown to be beneficial in this syndrome and in selected cases has definite advantages. In women with serious hypofibrinogenemia (< 150 mg. per 100 ml.) heparin may be infused, intravenously, until the fibrinogen concentration reaches an adequate hemostatic level (200 mg. per 100 ml. or greater). The heparin then can be stopped or neutralized with protamine sulfate and the appropriate obstetrical procedure carried out to remove the dead fetus. Replacement therapy alone has also been used successfully.

AMNIOTIC FLUID EMBOLISM WITH AND WITHOUT UTERINE RUPTURE.[4] Defibrination with evidence of an active fibrinolytic system is seen in amniotic fluid embolism. Unfortunately, the mortality rate is very high and therapy unsatisfactory. Although heparin has been recommended, its value has not been established. In addition to supportive care (oxygen, and so forth), the coagulopathy has been treated with fresh whole blood, plasma, and fibrinogen. In addition, the severe thrombocytopenia that develops should be corrected with platelet concentrates. Although an active fibrinolytic response is seen in amniotic fluid embolism, the etiology of its activation is not known. It could be a response to DIC or to the shock. In any event, the efficacy of antifibrinolytic agents in combating the coagulopathy has not been established.

SEPTIC ABORTION.[4,20,21]   The coagulopathy that occurs with septic abortion is due to DIC. Therapy consists of antibiotics, adequate antishock measures, and removal of the infected contents. There are claims and counterclaims regarding the use of heparin in this setting. However, it is clear that DIC stops when the infected products of conception or the uterus (or both) is removed. In nonpregnant patients with septic shock and DIC, heparin has not been found to be beneficial.[22] The available data suggest that the defibrination syndrome seen in septicemia occurs predominantly in those with shock.[22,23] Since patients with sepsis without shock have evidence of an activated coagulation mechanism (manifested as thrombocytopenia, elevated factors V and VIII, and elevated fibrinogen),[23,24] it has been postulated that this progresses to DIC. In this case the DIC may be responsible for the shock. Thus, heparinization prior to shock has been viewed as perhaps beneficial.[25] Stronger evidence suggests that it is not until blood stasis develops, in the form of shock, that the preexisting activated state progresses to DIC.[22,26] In this case, heparin may not affect the mortality rate from shock but might help correct the hemostatic defects. It has been reported that in patients with septic shock and DIC, the DIC ceases without the use of heparin when the shock has been effectively treated.[26] Thus, the data regarding the beneficial effect of heparin in septic abortion are not clear and more investigations using controlled studies are badly needed before general recommendations can be made.

ABORTION BY INTRA-AMNIOTIC INJECTION OF HYPERTONIC SALINE.   Many reports have shown that mild to moderate changes occur in the platelets, factors V and VIII, and fibrinogen with the use of hypertonic saline.[27-31] The changes are consistent with DIC but seem to be short-lived and without serious consequence. Since they subside spontaneously, without the use of anticoagulants, specific therapy is probably not needed. More experience is necessary before the total spectrum is appreciated.

OTHER COAGULOPATHIES.   The coagulopathies that occur in this group are probably the result of DIC. Incompatible hemolytic transfusion reactions, either fetomaternal or from simple blood transfusion, and hydatidiform mole have been studied in detail and have demonstrated the classic changes in the coagulation mechanism. Therapy has consisted of type-specific blood or plasma replacement and measures to avoid renal shutdown in hemolytic transfusion reactions, and emptying the uterus for therapy of the hydatidiform mole.[32] Heparin has not been used. Hypofibrinogenemia has been noted rarely in cases of placenta accreta and has been treated without heparin.[33,34] No controlled studies using heparin have been reported for toxemia.[4,35,36]

As mentioned above, in selected patients, the treatment of the underlying disease may be inadequate or the replacement therapy ineffective, so that medically interrupting the DIC with anticoagulation must be considered. Heparin has been the drug of choice in view of its rapid action, potent anticoagulating activity, ease of regulation and neutralization, and failure to cross the placenta.[37,38] It can be given on an intermittent or continuous schedule. We use 100 units per kg. body weight intravenously every four hours (e.g., 5000 to 7000 units/4 hours). Blood should be drawn every 4 to 8 hours for coagulation studies to evaluate the effectiveness of therapy. Although the Lee-White clotting time can be used to assess the anticoagulant dose, it is more desirable to have specific coagulation assays to judge the effectiveness and duration of therapy. Individual patients vary in their responses, and the response in the same patient may vary during the course of treatment.

Complications of therapy include serum hepatitis, especially with fibrinogen, volume overload, and bleeding from anticoagulation.

SUMMARY

Acquired coagulopathies peculiar to the obstetrical patient are discussed. The presumed basis of the coagulation failure is disseminated intravascular coagulation. Management consists of effectively removing the underlying cause, coagulation factor replacement therapy, and, in the rare and highly selected patient, medically interrupting the DIC with anticoagulants. The importance of establishing a correct laboratory diagnosis is also discussed.

REFERENCES

1. Hjort, P. F., and Rapaport, S. I.: The Shwartzman reaction: pathogenetic mechanisms and clinical manifestations. Ann. Rev. Med. *16*:135, 1965.
2. Reid, D.: Acquired coagulation defects in pregnancy. Obstet. Gynec. Surv. *20*:431, 1965.
3. Verstaete, M., and Vermylen, J.: Acute and chronic "defibrination" in obstetrical practice. Thromb. Diath. Haemorrh. *20*:444, 1968.
4. Pritchard, J. A.: Treatment of defibrination syndromes of pregnancy. *In* Ratnoff, O. D. (ed): Treatment of Hemorrhagic Disorders. New York, Harper & Row, 1968.
5. Fort, A. T.: Hemorrhagic complications of labor and delivery. Obstet. Gynec. *34*:717, 1969.
6. Schneider, C. L.: Disseminated intravascular coagulation. Thrombosis versus fibrination, in clinical disease states. *In* Disseminated intravascular coagulation. Thromb. Diath. Haemorrh. (Suppl.) *36*:1, 1969.
7. Kleiner, G. J., Merskey, C., Johnson, A. J., and Markus, W. B.: Defibrination in normal and abnormal parturition. Brit. J. Haemat. *19*:159, 1970.
8. Pechet, L., and Alexander, B.: Increased clotting factors in pregnancy. New Eng. J. Med. *265*:1093, 1961.
9. Strauss, H. S., and Diamond, L. K.: Elevation of factor VIII (antihemophilic factor) during pregnancy in normal persons and in a patient with von Willebrand's disease. New Eng. J. Med. *269*:1251, 1963.
10. Preston, A. E.: The plasma concentration of factor VIII in the normal population. I. Mothers and babies at birth. Brit. J. Haemat. *10*:110, 1964.
11. Nossel, H. L., Lanzkowsky, P., Levy, S., Mibashan, R. S., and Hansen, J. D. L.: A study of coagulation factor levels in women during labour and in their newborn infants. Thromb. Diath. Haemorrh. *16*:185, 1966.
12. Steihm, E. R., Kennan, A. L., and Schelble, D. T.: Split products of fibrin in maternal serum in the perinatal period. Am. J. Obstet. Gynec. *108*:941, 1970.
13. Merskey, C., Johnson, A. J., Kleiner, G. J., and Wohl, H.: The defibrination syndrome: clinical features and laboratory diagnosis. Brit. J. Haemat. *13*:528, 1967.
14. Hardaway, R. M.: Disseminated intravascular coagulation in experimental and clinical shock. Am. J. Cardiol. *20*:161, 1967.
15. Sutton, D. M. C., Hauser, R., Kulapongs, P., and Bachmann, F.: Intravascular coagulation in abruptio placentae. Am. J. Obstet. Gync. *109*:604, 1971.

16. Pritchard, J. A., and Brekken, A. L.: Clinical and laboratory studies on severe abruptio placentae. Am. J. Obstet. Gynec. 97:681, 1967.
17. Jimenez, J. M., and Pritchard, J. A.: Pathogenesis and treatment of coagulation defects resulting from fetal death. Obstet. Gynec. 32:449, 1968.
18. Phillips, L., Skrodelis, V., and King, T. A.: Hypofibrinogenemia and intrauterine fetal death. Am. J. Obstet. Gynec. 89:903, 1964.
19. Waxman, B., and Gambrill, R.: Use of heparin in disseminated intravascular coagulation. Am. J. Obstet. Gynec. 112:434, 1972.
20. Pritchard, J. A., and Whalley, P. J.: Abortion complicated by *Clostridium perfringens* infection. Am. J. Obstet. Gynec. 111:484, 1971.
21. Smith, L. P., McLean, A. P., and Maughan, G. B.: *Clostridium welchii* septicotoxemia. A review and report of 3 cases. Am. J. Obstet. Gynec. 110:135, 1971.
22. Corrigan, J. J., Jr., and Jordan, C. M.: Heparin therapy in septicemia with disseminated intravascular coagulation. Effect on mortality and on correction of hemostatic defects. New Eng. J. Med. 283:778, 1970.
23. Corrigan, J. J., Jr., Ray, W. L., and May, N.: Changes in the blood coagulation system associated with septicemia. New Eng. J. Med. 279:851, 1968.
24. Goldenfarb, P. B., Zucker, S., Corrigan, J. J., Jr., and Cathey, M. H.: The coagulation mechanism in acute bacterial infection. Brit. J. Haem. 18:643, 1970.
25. Margulis, R. R., Dustin, R. W., Lovell, J. R., Robb, H., and Jabs, C.: Heparin for septic abortion and the prevention of endotoxic shock. Obstet. Gynec. 37:474, 1971.
26. Corrigan, J. J., Jr.: Cessation of intravascular coagulation in septicemia without the use of heparin. Blood 36:836, 1970.
27. Stander, R. W., Flessa, H. C., Glueck, H. I., and Kisker, C. T.: Changes in maternal coagulation factors after intra-amniotic injection of hypertonic saline. Obstet. Gynec. 37:660, 1971.
28. Brown, F. D., Davidson, E. C., and Phillips, L. L.: Coagulation changes after hypertonic saline infusion for late abortions. Obstet. Gynec. 39:538, 1972.
29. Halbert, D. R., Buffington, J. S., Crenshaw, C., Jr., Brame, R. G., and Silver, D.: Consumptive coagulopathy with generalized hemorrhage after hypertonic saline-induced abortion. A case report. Obstet. Gynec. 39:41, 1972.
30. Goodlin, R. C.: Intravascular coagulation after intra-amniotic saline. Obstet. Gynec. 39:163, 1972.
31. Beller, F. K., Rosenberg, M., Kolker, M., and Douglas, G. W.: Consumptive coagulopathy associated with intra-amniotic infusion of hypertonic salt. Am. J. Obstet. Gynec. 112:534, 1972.
32. Talbert, L. M., Easterling, W. E., Flowers, C. E., Jr., and Graham, J. B.: Acquired coagulation defects of pregnancy—including a case of a patient with hydatidiform mole. Obstet. Gynec. 18:69, 1961.
33. Koren, Z., Zuckerman, H., and Brzezinski, A.: Placenta previa accreta with afibrinogenemia. Obstet. Gynec. 18:138, 1961.
34. Ochshorn, A., David, M. P., and Soferman, M. Placenta previa accreta. A report of 9 cases. Obstet. Gynec. 33:677, 1969.
35. Preston, F. E., Malia, R. G., Tipton, R. H., and Smith, A. J.: Intravascular coagulation and pre-eclamptic toxaemia. Lancet 1:34, 1972.
36. Wardle, E. N.: Intravascular coagulation and pre-eclamptic toxaemia. Lancet 1:262, 1972.
37. Hirsh, J., Cade, J. F., and Gallus, A. S.: Anticoagulants in pregnancy: A review of indications. Am. Heart J. 83:301, 1972.
38. Pitney, W. R., Pettit, J. E., and Armstrong, L.: Control of heparin therapy. Brit. Med. J. 4:139, 1970.

The Clinical Spectrum and Management of Acquired Coagulopathy in Pregnancy

Physiological Intravascular Coagulation in Normal Pregnancy

Donald G. McKay

University of California School of Medicine and San Francisco General Hospital

For those who regard normal pregnancy as a disease, the terms "physiological" and "normal pregnancy" will probably appear as contradictory or even mutually exclusive. It is not surprising to them that chronic intravascular coagulation occurs in normal pregnancy. Those who regard pregnancy as a normal event, however, will find the idea distasteful that a disease process such as intravascular coagulation can be considered a physiological component of gestation. Both these attitudes have merit, but whether or not one regards pregnancy as physiological or pathological, the evidence shows that it is accompanied by chronic local intravascular coagulation. It is the purpose of this communication to document this evidence.

Physiologic Alterations in the Coagulation System in Normal Pregnancy

It has long been known that concentrations of certain components of the blood coagulation system are elevated in normal pregnancy.

FACTOR I (FIBRINOGEN). At least since 1922 (Gram[1]), it has been known that circulating fibrinogen levels are higher in pregnant than in nonpregnant females. Numerous subsequent studies,[2-4] using a variety of techniques, have confirmed this fact and have also shown that fibrinogen levels increase progressively from the first to the third trimester of pregnancy. Todd and associates[5] found levels of 315 mg., 357 mg. and 391 mg. per 100 ml. in the first, second, and third trimesters, respectively.

FACTOR VII (PROCONVERTIN). In 1952, Loeliger and Koller[6] were the first to demonstrate an elevation of factor VII in the blood of pregnant women, and in

---

This study was aided by United States Public Health Service Grant HL-12033-05, National Institutes of Health.

1956 Alexander and colleagues[3] confirmed this observation. The test used at that time actually measured both factor VII and factor X (Stuart-Prower factor) which had been discovered in the intervening years. In a subsequent study, separating these two factors, Pechet and Alexander[7] observed a mean value of 160 per cent over normal levels of factor VII in pregnant compared to normal nonpregnant women.

FACTOR X (STUART-PROWER FACTOR).   In the same study, Pechet and Alexander observed that factor X was also elevated, on an average to 130 per cent of that of normal nonpregnant women. Todd and co-workers[5] observed increases to 152 per cent, 235 per cent, and 251 per cent in the first, second, and third trimesters, respectively.

FACTOR II (PROTHROMBIN).   Alexander and associates[3] and Todd and co-workers[5] found a very slight increase in prothrombin to 111 per cent of values for normal nonpregnant women. Ratnoff and Holland[8] found a moderate increase to 121 per cent of normal.

FACTOR IX (PLASMA THROMBOPLASTIN COMPONENT).   In 1959, Ratnoff and Holland[8] demonstrated a marked increase in factor IX activity in pregnant women. Todd and associates[5] found the increase to average 118 per cent in the third trimester.

FACTOR VIII (ANTIHEMOPHILIC FACTOR).   In 1963, Strauss and Diamond[9] observed an increase in levels of factor VIII in pregnant women. This was confirmed in 1964 by Kasper and co-workers,[10] who found an increase to a mean of 192 per cent of normal values in the third trimester. These authors also demonstrated that mean levels rose to 109 per cent, 147 per cent, and 192 per cent in the first, second, and third trimesters, respectively.

FACTOR V (PROACCELERIN).   Conflicting data exist on the effect of normal pregnancy on the blood concentration of factor V. Talbert and associates[11] found no significant change. Todd and co-workers[5] observed lower concentrations in pregnant than in nonpregnant women. On the other hand, Kasper and his group[10] found levels of 108 per cent and 109 per cent over normal in the second and third trimesters. Whatever the true value may be, the change is minimal.

The results of these studies are presented in Table 9–4.

PROTHROMBIN TIME.   Talbert and colleagues[11] observed a progressive shortening of the Quick prothrombin time during normal pregnancy from 13.5 seconds to 11 seconds at term.

PARTIAL THROMBOPLASTIN TIME.   Talbert and colleagues[11] also observed a progressive shortening of the partial thromboplastin time. Shortening of both the prothrombin time and the partial thromboplastin time were confirmed by Reid and associates[12] and probably reflect the effect of elevated levels of components of the coagulation system.

The increased levels of these coagulation factors indicates that the blood of normal pregnant women is hypercoagulable. This interpretation was made in 1956 by Alexander and co-workers,[3] who suggested that the hypercoagulability played an important role in the increased tendency to thrombosis in otherwise normal pregnant women. However, until now, no satisfactory explanation of the mechanism of the elevation had been adduced.

It is of equal interest to note that the coagulation factors show a *progressive increase* throughout pregnancy, which is documented in Table 9–5. This progressive increase is of importance since it is directly related to the progressive increase

TABLE 9-4. *Concentrations of Certain Components of the Coagulation System in Pregnancy Compared with Nonpregnant Levels**

	FACTOR I (FIBRINOGEN) (MG. PER 100 ML.)		FACTOR II (PROTHROMBIN) (PER CENT)		FACTOR V (PROACCELERIN) (PER CENT)		FACTOR VII (PROCONVERTIN) (PER CENT)		FACTOR VIII (ANTIHEMOPHILIC FACTOR) (PER CENT)		FACTOR IX (PLASMA THROMBOPLASTIN COMPONENT) (PER CENT)		FACTOR X (PER CENT)	
	NP	P	NP	P	NP	P	NP	P	NP	P	NP	P	NP	P
Kasper et al.[10]		432 (367–505)		117 (104–132)		109 (71–176)		206 (170–208)		192 (123–240)		244 (180–344)		165 (90–240)
Todd et al.[5]	322 ± 32	391	100 ± 8.5	111	100 ± 25	82	100 ± 17	380	100 ± 23	147	100 ± 19	118	100 ± 27	251
Pechet and Alexander[7]								162 (70–260)						130 (72–200)
Alexander et al.[3]			98 (58–128)	111 (58–219)										
Ratnoff and Holland[8]	300	440		121									100	300

* Most of the data are from the third trimester of pregnancy.
P = Pregnant.
NP = Nonpregnant.

TABLE 9–5.   *Examples of the Progressive Increase in Certain Coagulation Factors During Normal Pregnancy*

	NONPREGNANT	PREGNANT		
		First Trimester	Second Trimester	Third Trimester
Fibrinogen (mg. per 100 ml.)	322*	315	357 (336)†	391 (432)
Prothrombin (per cent)	100	113	102 (111)	111 (117)
Factor V (per cent)	100	98	93 (108)	82 (109)
Factor VII (per cent	100	110	310 (174)	380 (206)
Factor VIII (per cent)	100 (108)	114 (109)	116 (147)	147 (192)
Factor IX (per cent)	100	92	121	118 (244)
Factor X (per cent)	100	152	235 (134)	251 (165)

* Open figures are from Todd *et al.*[5]
† Figures in parentheses are from Kasper *et al.*[10]

in the size of the placenta, which is the locus for the alterations in the coagulation factors.

PLATELETS. Todd and colleagues[5] found a slightly elevated number of platelets in the first two trimesters of pregnancy (284,000 per cubic millimeter), followed by a slight decrease in the third trimester (253,000 per cubic milimeter). Talbert and associates[11] observed a progressive decrease in average platelet count during normal pregnancy.

In addition to the slight decrease in numbers, there is further evidence that mild damage occurs to circulating platelets. In 1964 we presented evidence that platelets are damaged to a slight extent in normal pregnancy.[13] This was shown by an increase in the platelet adhesiveness index compared to that of nonpregnant women (Table 9–6).

When this study was done we were mainly interested in the fact that preeclamptic patients showed an even greater increase in platelet adhesiveness

TABLE 9–6.   *Platelet Adhesiveness Indices in Normal Pregnancy**

	NUMBER	MEAN INDEX	STANDARD ERROR
Nonpregnant women	10	0.98	±0.029
Pregnant women			
First Trimester	5	1.03	±0.043
Second Trimester	5	1.09	±0.056
Third Trimester	5	1.12	±0.058

* From McKay, D. G., *et al.*: Platelet adhesiveness in toxemia of pregnancy. Am. J. Obstet. Gynec. 90:1315, 1964.

and suggested at that time that the cause was a chronic low-grade process of intravascular coagulation caused by damaged trophoblast.

This is essentially the same interpretation we are now making for normal pregnancy, at a quantitatively lower level. The progressive increase in the platelet adhesiveness index is noteworthy and to be compared with the progressive increase in the coagulation factors. Although our own platelet adhesiveness data for normal pregnancy lacked statistical significance, this thesis has been confirmed recently for normal pregnancy (third trimester) by Reid and Associates,[12] who used a different technique.

THE FIBRINOLYTIC ENZYME SYSTEM

Although they are separable in the test tube, the plasminogen and coagulation systems are inextricably related to each other in vivo. It has been known for some time that normal pregnancy is associated with an "inhibition of fibrinolysis." That is, the plasminogen system is more difficult to activate in normal pregnancy. The precise mechanism by which this effect occurs has been the subject of debate. Brakman[4] has observed normal levels of plasminogen throughout normal pregnancy. However, he found a slight decrease in the fibrinolytic activity of the plasma euglobulins, which represent activator activity. Thus, one explanation for the decrease in fibrinolysis might be a diminution in activator substance. In a search for a possible inhibitor of fibrinolysis in the plasma, he found a progressive increase in the ability of plasma from pregnant women to inhibit urokinase activity (Brakman and Astrup[14]). The problem of interpreting this finding remains, since no such inhibitory influence was exerted on streptokinase or on tissue activator. Whatever the precise mechanism may be, whether it is based on presence of an inhibitor or on diminished amounts of an activator, there is general agreement that an impairment of activation of the fibrinolytic enzyme systems does occur during pregnancy.

SOLUBLE FIBRIN

Appearance in the circulating blood of pregnant women of a cold-insoluble protein similar to fibrinogen was first observed by Morrison.[15] The material was obtained from the plasma of pregnant or acutely ill patients by precipitation with 16.6 per cent ammonium sulfate and was referred to as "contractinogen." Contractinogen was reversibly cold-insoluble and showed an unusual propensity to clot spontaneously, and then to retract markedly. Morrison suggested that contractinogen represented a qualitative alteration of fibrinogen—perhaps partial polymerization—occurring as a result of disease.

The next observations to be made in relation to this topic were those of Thomas and colleagues,[16] who found that a protein material similar to fibrinogen was precipitated when the plasma of rabbits, exposed to bacterial endotoxin intravenously, was allowed to stand in the cold. This material was precipitated in the presence of heparin as the anticoagulant and was therefore referred to as heparin precipitable fraction (HPF). Small amounts were found in the blood of normal rabbits.

It was found that, after the precipitate is washed and redissolved at 37° C., this protein migrates in a manner similar to fibrinogen during paper electrophoresis. Smith and von Korff[17] examined the cryoprecipitate and found that its solubility was favored by increased ionic strength, elevated temperature, alkaline pH, and the absence of calcium or magnesium ions. This substance is absent from serum, is clottable with thrombin, and moves in a manner similar to fibrinogen.

Smith[18] subsequently devised a quantitative technique for the determination of HPF (heparin precipitable fraction) and noted that this material appeared in normal human plasma in mean amounts ranging from 0.101 to 0.144 g. per 100 ml., depending on the individual's age and sex. Higher levels were observed in females than in males, and in adults than in children. Smith observed gradually rising values during gestation and even higher levels in patients with preeclampsia, although actual amounts were not reported. In our own study of cryofibrinogen in pregnancy we confirmed Smith's findings with respect to toxemia, but we failed to demonstrate the rise during normal gestation, probably because the number of cases studied was too small.

In studies of the effect of incompatible blood transfusion on the blood clotting mechanism, we had observed the appearance of this precipitate at 4° C. when oxalate rather than heparin was used as the anticoagulant.[19] Therefore, cold rather than heparin was the major precipitating factor, although a greater amount of precipitation occurs with heparin than with oxalate. Cryofibrinogen is now referred to as "soluble fibrin," which generally is a better term. Soluble fibrin can also be demonstrated by precipitation or gelation with protamine sulfate and ethanol, although these latter appear to be considerably less sensitive techniques for detecting small amounts of intravascular coagulation than the cold precipitation method. The exact chemical nature of soluble fibrin is not clear. For many years it has been thought to represent a molecule of fibrin monomer closely associated with a molecule of fibrinogen. It is possible that it actually is partially polymerized fibrin, as originally suggested by Morrison. Whatever its precise chemical architecture, an increased amount in the circulating blood is evidence of intravascular coagulation and is most likely the effect of small amounts of thrombin activity in vivo.

SERUM FIBRIN DEGRADATION PRODUCTS

Serum fibrin degradation products (or fibrin split products) are elevated in normal pregnancy. Woodfield and associates,[20] using the tanned red cell technique, observed a progressive increase in fibrin degradation products from the first to the third trimester (Table 9–7).

TABLE 9–7.   *Estimation of Serum Fibrin Degradation Products in 169 Pregnant and 43 Nonpregnant Patients**

	NONPREGNANT	PREGNANT		
		First Trimester	Second Trimester	Third Trimester
Mean fibrin degradation products (μg./ml.)	6.5±2.1	6.6±2.6	8.2±4.1	14.0±6.9

* From Woodfield, D. G., et al.: Serum fibrin degradation products throughout normal pregnancy. Brit. Med. J. 4:665, 1968.

Using the staphylococcal clumping test, Henderson and colleagues[21] obtained comparable results, although the absolute figures differed somewhat. They found a rise from 1.9 ± 0.37 μm./ml. in the first trimester to 4.8 ± 0.70 μm./ml. in the third trimester.

Fibrin degradation products are derived from the enzymatic splitting of fibrin and fibrinogen by plasmin. However, in spontaneous disease in the human they are indicative of intravascular coagulation. This is simply because in spontaneous disease (or in this instance normal pregnancy) fibrinolysis occurs secondary to intravascular coagulation. In other words, the appearance of increased fibrin degradation products does not occur (except in artificial or experimental conditions) as a result of "primary" fibrinolysis, even though these fractions are enzymatic degradation products of fibrinolysis.

SUMMARY

The alterations in normal pregnancy in the coagulation system and in the so-called "para-coagulation" factors can be summarized as follows:
1. There are above normal values of fibrinogen and other components of the coagulation system, including factors II, V, VII, VIII, IX, and X.
2. There are decreased numbers of circulating platelets and increased platelet adhesiveness.
3. There are increased amounts of soluble fibrin (partially polymerized fibrin).
4. There are increased amounts of serum fibrin degradation products.
5. There is inhibition of fibrinolysin activation (diminished amounts of fibrinolysin activator and increased amounts of urokinase inhibitor.)

The Anatomy of the Placenta

The explanation for these changes in the coagulation system comes from the histologic examination of the normal placenta, which shows intravascular coagulation in the maternal circulation (the intervillous spaces) from early in pregnancy until term.

Large amounts of fibrin are laid down in the "floor" of the placenta, and this has been called "Nitabuch's fibrin layer." This fibrin deposit lines the intervillous space at the base of the placenta, and lies upon and within the mixture of decidual and cytotrophoblastic cells of this region. In relation to the intervillous space, it represents a mural deposit of fibrin or "mural thrombosis" (Figure 9–1).

Similar mural deposits, which are also composed of decidual and cytotrophoblastic cells and represent extensions upward of the floor or base of the placenta (Figure 9–2), are found lining the intervillous space along the placental septae.

Another site of fibrin deposition in the placenta is on the surface of the villi (Figure 9–3). These focal fibrin deposits bind many villi together in the late stages of gestation and make the anatomic dissection of intact villi extremely difficult. These deposits lie upon and beneath the syncytial trophoblast and in the past have been referred to as "subsyncytial fibrinoid." By use of the fluorescein labeled antibody technique, McCormick and his colleagues[22] have clearly shown that these deposits are immunologically identical to fibrinogen.

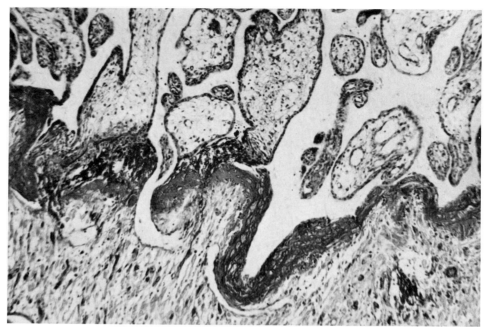

Figure 9-1. Normal placenta at 17 weeks of gestation. The dense wavy line at the junction of the villi and decidua consists of fibrin, which lines the maternal vascular space of the "floor" of the placenta and is referred to as "Nitabuch's fibrin layer." (×50. Periodic acid–Schiff stain.)

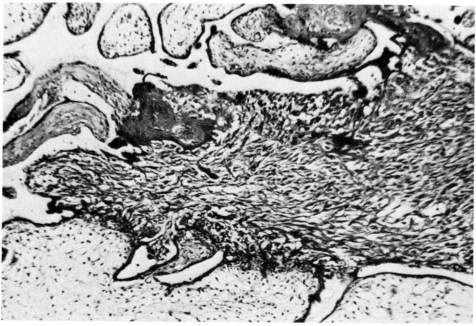

Figure 9-2. Normal placental septum at 15 weeks of gestation. The villi are in part anchored to the septum by dense deposits of fibrin. Some are adherent to each other because of fibrin in the intervillous space. (×50. Periodic acid–Schiff stain.)

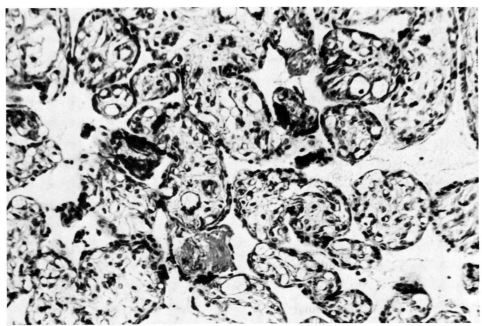

Figure 9-3. Normal placental villi at 35 weeks of gestation. Fibrin deposits can be seen binding villi together. (×50. Periodic acid–Schiff stain.)

Two other changes (i.e., types of fibrin deposits) are found in some, but not all, normal placentas of normal pregnancies: (1) placental infarcts, and (2) intervillous thrombi. Placental infarcts are associated with—in fact caused by—large deposits of fibrin which intertwine between the villi, cutting off the maternal circulation and leading to necrosis of villi. These are referred to as "white infarcts" from the standpoint of naked-eye examination. Intervillous thrombi are large deposits of laminated fibrin and red cells, platelets, and leukocytes, which push aside villi and which generally do not cause infarction. Both infarcts and inter-villous thrombi represent large, rapidly accumulated deposits of fibrin in the intervillous space (i.e., the maternal circulation of the placenta).

Another site of intravascular clotting is in the veins of the decidua and the uterine muscle at the endomyometrial junction. These deposits are usually mural, but some actually amount to thrombi which occlude the lumen of the vessels and which become organized and recanalized.

Thus, the placenta is the site of chronic local intravascular coagulation in the maternal circulation in normal pregnancy. An important corollary is the fact that the amount of intraplacental clotting progressively increases from the first trimester to term. Nitabuch's layer in the floor of the placenta not only covers a larger and larger area as the placenta increases in size but it also becomes thicker. The number of focal deposits on the syncytial trophoblast of the villi increases throughout gestation. The increase in surface area of the placental villi during gestation is even greater than the increase in placental weight. This anatomic demonstration of a progressive increase in fibrin deposits is directly related to the progressive changes in the coagulation mechanism.

Anatomic–Physiologic Correlation

The histologic demonstration of fibrin deposits in the maternal blood channels of the normal placenta constitutes proof that intravascular coagulation is a physiological process in normal pregnancy. An understanding of the anatomy of the placenta is also essential in order to comprehend that the clotting is local. In some 400 autopsies on pregnant women I have not seen any evidence by light microscopy of intravascular clotting in any other organ in patients who could be considered to have had a normal pregnancy and whose death was not related to the blood coagulation system. Not only is the clotting local, but it is also of several months' duration, and therefore chronic. It starts in the first trimester and progressively increases as the placenta increases in size. These anatomic observations are essential to understanding this process. Test tube studies of the circulating blood indicate that intravascular coagulation is occurring and can estimate its extent, but they cannot indicate the location of the clotting.

Confirmation of the anatomic observations comes from finding increased levels of soluble fibrin and fibrin degradation products in the maternal circulation. The degree of elevation is small and increases progressively during pregnancy, serving as a rough measure of the rate of clotting at the different stages of pregnancy.

The platelet alterations are also indicative of a low-grade intravascular coagulation. There is a slight but perceptible decrease in the number of circulating platelets and an increase in the platelet adhesiveness index. Platelets are essential for clotting and a small percentage are damaged as they circulate through the maternal channels of the placenta.

The elevation in levels of the clotting factors I, II, V, VII, VIII, IX, and X is somewhat more difficult to understand when viewed as evidence of chronic intravascular coagulation. This is largely a result of the fact that in the past most of our studies have been concentrated on *acute disseminated intravascular coagulation*, in which the levels of these factors are decreased. The elevations are not difficult to understand when the homeostatic mechanism is taken into account. The primary consideration is the rebound to above normal levels of these coagulation factors following a *single massive* clotting episode. This rebound phenomenon is illustrated in Figure 9–4, which also shows that the recovery rate for the various clotting factors is not the same. The rebound represents an overproduction of coagulation factors following a period of decreased utilization.

We have recently described the effect of chronic intravascular coagulation on these clotting factors.[23] In this condition, the stimulus to clotting is mild and occurs repeatedly or continuously (Figure 9–5). Initially, there is a slight decrease in fibrinogen and in most of the other coagulation factors. This is followed by a rebound to above normal levels when a second mild clotting episode occurs. When this happens, a second slight decrease occurs, but because the stimulus to clotting is quantitatively small, the blood concentration of the coagulation factor fails to drop below the normal level. This process is repeated or continues and keeps these factors fluctuating at above normal values. The degree to which any one is elevated is dependent on its "half-life" or on its rate of synthesis, so that some factors are present in relatively greater amounts than others. Platelets are the exception to this process and their numbers tend to remain below normal levels during chronic intravascular coagulation. This may be a result of the fact that

ALTERATIONS IN THE CLOTTING FACTORS

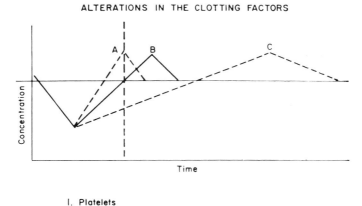

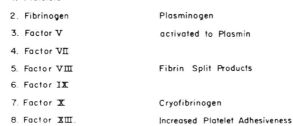

I. Platelets

2. Fibrinogen   Plasminogen

3. Factor V   activated to Plasmin

4. Factor VII

5. Factor VIII   Fibrin Split Products

6. Factor IX

7. Factor X   Cryofibrinogen

8. Factor XIII.   Increased Platelet Adhesiveness

Figure 9-4. Effect of a single episode of acute massive disseminated intravascular coagulation on the coagulation system. The top horizontal line represents 100 per cent concentration of blood levels of all factors. Initially, all factors fall proportionately. After the decrease, they recover and rise to above normal values. The rate of return and overshoot is dependent on the rate of regeneration of each individual factor. Line A represents Factor VIII; line B, fibrinogen; line C, platelets. The arbitrarily drawn vertical dashed line shows that a single determination of these factors at this time may yield a high level of Factor VIII, a normal level of fibrinogen, and a low platelet count.

only small quantities of thrombin are needed to aggregate large numbers of platelets, as well as the fact that platelets are more slowly replaced in the circulating blood than are the other clotting factors.

Thus, the coagulation factors are maintained at above normal values by the process of a continuous increase in rate of production, which in turn results from a continuous overutilization in the chronic clotting process. This basic principle is of general significance and can be observed in a variety of diseases totally unrelated to pregnancy.

The alteration in the fibrinolytic system has also been observed in chronic intravascular coagulation in diseases not associated with pregnancy. In some of these diseases, the "inhibition of fibrinolysis" or impaired activation of the fibrinolytic system can be related to a diminution in amounts of fibrinolysin activator. When intravascular coagulation occurs, activator is consumed. The location, extent, and duration of clotting in any single disease state or condition determines the effect on activator. Activator is found predominantly in vein endothelium[24] and this is true for the uterus as well as for other organs. A wide variety of agents or activities cause release or loss of activator from vein endothelium,[25] and mural thrombosis is one of these. As noted above, some of the normal clotting in pregnancy occurs in the decidual and myometrial veins of the uterus. It is possible that this local trauma is sufficient to reduce the amount of activator in the vein

ALTERATIONS   IN   COAGULATION   MECHANISM
IN   CHRONIC   INTRAVASCULAR   COAGULATION

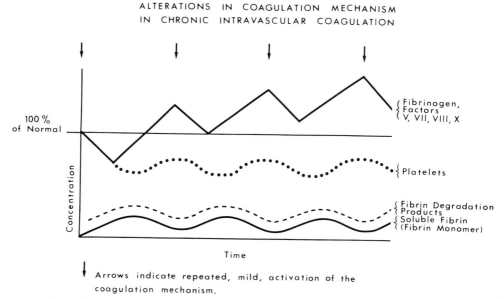

Figure 9-5. Chronic intravascular coagulation: the characteristic pattern of the coagulation system in this condition is: above normal levels of fibrinogen, Factors V, VII, VIII, IX, X; paradoxically low platelet counts; and increased levels of soluble fibrin and serum fibrin degradation products.

endothelium and thus reduce its availability to the circulating blood. It could equally well be that activator in the blood is simply used up during clotting in the placenta, thus reducing its concentration in the circulating blood. What role the increased amounts of urokinase inhibitor (Brakman and Astrup[14]) may play in the intravascular plasmin system in pregnancy remains to be determined.

The Mechanism of Intraplacental Coagulation

Perhaps the most interesting biological question relating to this process is the nature of the proximate cause which activates coagulation. The most obvious answer would be that the clotting occurs as a result of exposure of the blood to the tissue thromboplastin of the trophoblast and decidua. The placenta, as well as the uterus, increases progressively in size and undergoes a constant remodeling of its architecture during pregnancy. In this process there is proliferation of the cells of the cytotrophoblast in the floor, the septae, the chorion of the roof of the placenta, and the chorion laeve.[26] There is also a concomitant death or necrosis of some of these cells, as well as of the decidual cells at the base of the placenta. Cell death in the decidual layer is a prominent feature of a normal pregnancy, and large patches of necrotic decidua are associated with an accumulation of large numbers of polymorphonuclear leukocytes. With the constant remodeling of the placenta, these decidual and trophoblastic cells, which in many places line the maternal vascular channels, are exposed to the circulating blood and the release of tissue thromboplastin from the dying cells induces local clotting. Years ago, Schneider[27] demonstrated that trophoblast and decidua contain the highest relative concentrations of "tissue thromboplastin" of any cells in the body. Thus, small amounts of these tissues are potent triggers of the clotting system. Tissue thromboplastin is an essential component of the cell cytoplasm and is a very heavy, sedimenting material which does not diffuse across living cell membranes. In order for it to reach the circulating blood there must be disruption of cells or blood vessels or both.

This process in normal pregnancy should not be misconstrued as a propulsion of tissue thromboplastin into the general circulation of the mother. Such an event seems to occur in some patients with premature separation of the placenta, but not in normal pregnancy. Intraplacental clotting in normal pregnancy is largely a "mural coating" phenomenon. The exposure of dead or dying individual cells or groups of cells to the circulating blood induces immediate deposition of fibrin at the site, walling off and isolating the locally released tissue thromboplastin from the maternal circulation.

The activation of clotting by tissue thromboplastin has been referred to as the "extrinsic prothrombin activator" system. It activates in sequence factors VII, X, V, II, and I. If the extrinsic system alone were involved in this local clotting, one would expect that, since the "intrinsic" or "contact" system had been bypassed, there would be no alteration in the concentration of the factors that compose the "intrinsic" system. However, actual measurements have shown that there is a change in factors VIII and IX. This suggests that the contact system (intrinsic prothrombin activator) is also being triggered.

Several considerations make this more plausible than it might appear at first sight. In the first place, Matsuoka and associates[28] have presented evidence that tissue thromboplastin activates the contact system in vivo. Second, electron microscope studies by Hufnagel and Riddle[29] of samples of tissue thromboplastin revealed a variety of membrane-like structures. These included collapsed spherules (200 to 360 nm. in diameter), small membranous fragments, and large pleated sheets, as well as particulate matter. Bjorklid and Otnaess[30] observed "spherulites" of concentrically arranged vesicles which underwent a variety of changes when treated with phospholipase C and concomitantly lost coagulant activity. Since the contact system is activated by "surface contact," it may be that these membranous structures are capable of activating Hageman factor as well as the extrinsic prothrombin activator system.

In essence, there is evidence that both the extrinsic and the intrinsic prothrombin activator systems are triggered, presumably by the exposure of the blood to tissue thromboplastin of the trophoblast and decidua of the placenta.

Intravascular Coagulation in Other Species

Intravascular coagulation in the maternal circulation of the placenta occurs in mammalian species other than man. Mural deposits of fibrin are found in the normal placenta of the rhesus monkey, the rabbit, and the rat.[31] Although my personal observations are limited to these species and man, it is quite likely that most mammalian species share this property. A complete study of all mammals from the standpoints of fibrin deposits in the placenta and alterations in the coagulation system in normal pregnancy has not yet been done, but it seems quite safe to generalize from the observations thus far made that chronic local intravascular coagulation is a physiologic component of pregnancy in most species of mammals.

Exogenous Progestational Agents

Because of the increased incidence of thromboembolic disease in women taking exogenous progestational agents, a great deal of attention has been paid to the effect of these synthetic steroids on the blood coagulation system. It has been known for some time that certain of these steroids cause an elevation in the circulating levels of some of the components of the coagulation system. Because of the great variability in chemical structure of these agents, there is wide variation in the effects they exert. Nevertheless, some steroids in common use produce an effect on the coagulation system which is similar to that of pregnancy, but to a lesser degree. The study of Todd and co-workers[5] is illustrative. In 12 patients who had taken oral contraceptives for periods ranging from 9 months to 5½ years they found a slight shortening of the prothrombin time, an elevation of the concentrations of prothrombin, factor VII, and factor VIII, no change in factor IX, and a decrease in factor X. These alterations are far from identical to those observed in normal pregnancy, and the study did not include observations on platelet adhesiveness, soluble fibrin, and fibrin degradation products. Most recently it has been proposed that the estrogenic component of these medications is the responsible factor.

The general interpretation of these studies has been that the steroids cause the changes in the coagulation system through some direct stimulatory action on the rates of synthesis of the clotting factors. Although this remains a possibility, it is also clear that some of the patients are victims of chronic local intravascular coagulation in the uterus and that this may be a significant stimulus to elevation of clotting factors.

The first evidence of this came from the studies of Ryan and associates,[32] who demonstrated thrombi in the small vessels of the uterus or ovary in three patients who had been taking exogenous steroids. We have confirmed this observation many times on examination of endometrial currettings from similarly treated patients (Figure 9-6). The basic reason for thrombosis of the small vessels of the endometrium is stasis. When ovulation is inhibited, menstruation does not occur, and the vessels (particularly venules) of the endometrium become dilated and thrombosed. Thus, at least in part, the effect of these steroids on the coagulation system is indirect, through their effect on the vessels of the endometrium. This same phenomenon can be observed in so-called "cystic hyperplasia of the endometrium," in which necrosis produced by the thrombosis is the basic cause of bleeding in these anovulatory patients.

This mechanism of local intravascular coagulation in patients on synthetic steroids could easily account for the alterations in the coagulation factors in these patients. On the other hand, the possibility that some of these steroids may have a direct effect, stimulating an increased rate of synthesis, has not been ruled out. It is possible that both mechanisms are in operation, but confirmation of this will probably have to await the development of more sensitive methods of measuring these quantitative changes.

In comparing these patients with normal pregnant women, it is obvious that the amount of intravascular clotting in the pregnant uterus far exceeds any that occurs in the small nonpregnant uterus or endometrium. This correlates roughly with the fact that the changes in the coagulation mechanism in pregnancy greatly exceed those induced by exogenous steroids.

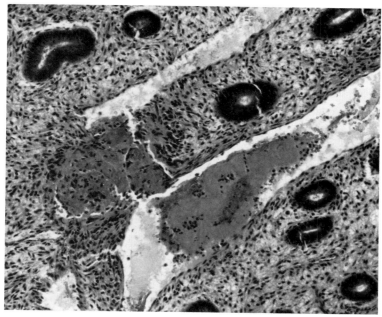

Figure 9-6. Endometrium from patient treated with exogenous progestational agent. The vessels are dilated and each contains a small thrombus composed of platelets and fibrin. (×100. Hematoxylin and eosin stain.)

Historical Perspective

Those interested in the way in which new knowledge is evolved will find the development of the concept that normal pregnancy is accompanied by physiological intravascular coagulation to be of interest. This contribution to the physiology of pregnancy was a direct result of the study of disease. In 1953, we demonstrated that one of the basic pathogenetic mechanisms of eclampsia is *acute massive disseminated intravascular coagulation.*[33] This conclusion was based on the anatomic demonstration of thrombi in the microcirculation of many organs, and has subsequently been confirmed by observations on the coagulation mechanism.[34]

Since eclampsia is usually preceded by preeclampsia, the next question was whether or not intravascular coagulation occurs in this premonitory syndrome as well. In 1964 we presented evidence that intravascular coagulation does occur in preeclampsia but that it is of a different order of magnitude and duration—i.e., it is essentially a low-grade *chronic disseminated intravascular coagulation.*[35] The evidence was both anatomical and physiological, and was based on the observation of increased amounts of clotting in the placenta, granular fibrin deposits in the renal glomeruli, alterations in the coagulation mechanism, increased amounts of circulating soluble fibrin, and an increased platelet adhesiveness index. Preeclampsia was the first disease in which chronic disseminated intravascular coagulation was recognized as a pathogenetic mechanism of disease.

Recognition that intravascular coagulation is part and parcel of normal pregnancy has also been dependent on correlating both anatomic and physiologic findings. Observation of the deposits of fibrin on the mural surface of maternal vascular channels of the normal placenta is all that is necessary to prove that chronic intravascular coagulation accompanies normal pregnancy. These deposits have been observed by pathologists and anatomists for decades, but the correct interpretation was delayed for many years. This delay was occasioned in part by the fact that previous observers traditionally referred to these deposits as "fibrinoid" rather than fibrin. The difference in terminology might sound trivial—however, the word "fibrinoid" carried with it the implication that although it was "fibrin-like," it was not actually fibrin but some other unidentified or mysterious substance. Under these circumstances it would be difficult to interpret the deposits as derivatives of fibrinogen of the maternal blood.

The hematologic data which confirm the anatomic findings in normal pregnancy were all derived from the "control" samples from studies of toxemia. Perhaps the most cogent evidence is the progressive elevation of soluble fibrin and of serum fibrin degradation products. These changes can only be interpreted as the result of a progressive increase in intravascular coagulation.

The proper interpretation of the elevation of the coagulation Factors I, II, V, VII, VIII, IX, and X has been dependent on the knowledge that this elevation is the result of chronic intravascular coagulation in disease processes in general, whether or not they are associated with pregnancy.[23]

While recognizing the significant contributions of basic science studies to clinical medicine in the past century, it is equally important to recognize the contributions of pathology and the study of disease processes to fundamental biological knowledge. As Castle[36] has stated, "The pathway between physiology and clinical medicine, today a broad highway, has long been at least a two-way lane."

SIGNIFICANCE

The major significance of physiological intravascular coagulation in the normal placenta is that it is responsible for the hypercoagulable state of normal pregnancy. It is the explanation for the long-standing knowledge that certain blood coagulation factors are elevated in normal pregnancy. The hypercoagulability is surely a contributing factor to the relatively high incidence of thromboembolic disease in pregnant women.

The physiological significance of the hypercoagulability may lie in the fact that separation of the placenta involves severance of large vascular channels at the uteroplacental junction, and an increased tendency to clotting aids in sealing off these vessels, thus protecting the maternal organism against excessive blood loss.

Intravascular coagulation also has bearing on diseases of pregnancy. Such conditions as eclampsia, amniotic fluid embolism, premature separation of the placenta, septic abortion, and premature rupture of the membranes with chorioamnionitis are all associated with acute disseminated intravascular coagulation. It is now clear that these conditions are superimposed upon a preexisting chronic local intravascular coagulation in the placenta, which renders the blood hypercoagulable and leaves pregnant women more susceptible to any exposure to procoagulant substances or activities in the bloodstream. This is well illustrated by studies in experimental pathology.

The basic principle involved may be found in our definition of "hypercoagulable." This principle, which can be illustrated by thrombosis of the micro-circulation in the Shwartzman reaction, holds that a secondary activator which fails to produce a thrombus in the presence of a normal coagulation system will do so in the presence of hypercoagulable blood.

In the local Shwartzman reaction, the injection of a small dose of bacterial endotoxin into the skin produces an acute inflammation with a very small amount of fibrin deposition in the local microcirculation, which is detectable only by electron microscopy. The injection of a second dose of endotoxin intravenously activates the coagulation mechanism systemically, and occlusive thrombi localize at the skin site of the first injection, resulting in hemorrhagic necrosis of the area. Without the production of hypercoagulable blood by the intravenous injection, the local inflammatory site heals completely, with no formation of thrombi.

In the generalized Shwartzman reaction, the first intravenous injection of endotoxin causes a minor clotting episode with capillary thrombi appearing in the liver, lungs, and spleen, but not in the kidney. The decrease in circulating fibrino-gen levels is so small as to be barely detectable. The animals usually survive but are left with hypercoagulable blood. A second, properly timed injection of endo-toxin results in a much more extensive clotting, with deposition of fibrin in every renal glomerular capillary.[37] This extensive clotting is associated with a 40 per cent decrease in circulating fibrinogen. In essence, the second activation of the coagulation mechanism by an identical amount of bacterial endotoxin in the same animal results in a clotting episode of much greater magnitude when the blood is hypercoagulable as a result of the first injection. In this reaction, the period of hypercoagulability is known and lasts from 6 to 72 hours after the first intra-venous injection of endotoxin.

Pregnant rabbits develop the extensive clotting with glomerular capillary thrombosis of the generalized Shwartzman reaction with only one injection of bacterial endotoxin.[38] These animals are already "prepared" for the generalized Shwartzman reaction by the chronic hypercoagulable state induced by the "physi-ological" clotting in the placenta. Of equal interest is the fact that nonpregnant rats will not develop the Shwartzman reaction with two injections of endotoxin, but will do so with only one injection when they are pregnant.[39] Thus, pregnancy induces a chronic hypercoagulable state at least in several species.

For the future, the knowledge that chronic local intravascular coagulation is part of the normal physiology of pregnancy will serve as a basis for studies of the physiological significance of a variety of substances intimately related to the clotting mechanism, such as serotonin, histamine, fibrin degradation products, kallikrein, and complement.

REFERENCES

1. Gram, H. C.: The results of a new method of determining the fibrin-percentage in blood and plasma. Acta Med. Scand. 56:107, 1922.
2. Phillips, L. L.: Fibrinolysis and thrombosis during pregnancy and hormone treatment. In Astrup, T., and Wright, I. S., eds.: Symposium on Blood Coagulation, Thrombosis and Female Hormones. Washington, D.C., James F. Mitchell Foundation, 1968, p. 33.
3. Alexander, B., Meyers, L., Kenny, J., Goldstein, R., Gurewich, V., and Grinspoon, L.: Blood coagulation in pregnancy: proconvertin and prothrombin, and the hypercoagulable state. New Eng. J. Med. 254:258, 1956.
4. Brakman, P.: Fibrinolysis in blood during pregnancy and hormone treatment. In Astrup,

T., and Wright, I. S., eds.: Symposium. Washington, D.C., James F. Mitchell Foundation, 1968, p. 27.

5. Todd, M. E., Thompson, J. H., Jr., Bowie, E. J. W., and Owen, C. A., Jr.: Changes in blood coagulation during pregnancy. Mayo Clin. Proc. 40:370, 1965.

6. Loeliger, A., and Koller, F.: Behavior of factor VII and prothrombin in late pregnancy and in newborn. Acta Haemat. 7:157, 1962.

7. Pechet, L., and Alexander, B.: Increased clotting factors in pregnancy. New Eng. J. Med. 265:1093, 1961.

8. Ratnoff, O. D., and Holland, T. R.: Coagulation components in normal and abnormal pregnancies. Ann. N. Y. Acad. Sci. 75:626, 1959.

9. Strauss, H. S., and Diamond, L. K.: Elevation of factor VIII (antihemophilic factor) during pregnancy in normal persons and in a patient with von Willebrand's disease. New Eng. J. Med. 269:1251, 1963.

10. Kasper, C. K., Hoag, M. S., Aggeler, P. M., and Stone, S.: Blood clotting factors in pregnancy: Factor VIII concentrations in normal and AHF-deficient women. Obstet. Gynec. 24:242, 1964.

11. Talbert, L. M., and Langdell, R. D.: Normal values of certain factors in the blood clotting mechanism in pregnancy. Am. J. Obstet. Gynec. 90:44, 1964.

12. Reid, D. E., Frigoletto, F. D., Tullis, J. L., and Hinman, J.: Hypercoagulable states in pregnancy. Am. J. Obstet. Gynec. 111:493, 1971.

13. McKay, D. G., de Bacalao, E. B., and Sedlis, A.: Platelet adhesiveness in toxemia of pregnancy. Am. J. Obstet. Gynec. 90:1315, 1964.

14. Brakman, P., and Astrup, T.: Selective inhibition in human pregnancy blood of urokinase induced fibrinolysis. Scand. J. Clin. Lab. Invest. 15:603, 1963.

15. Morrison, I. R.: Qualitative changes in fibrinogen which influence the erythrocyte sedimentation rate and the clot retraction time. Am. J. Med. Sci. 211:325, 1946.

16. Thomas, L., Smith, R. T., and von Korff, R. W.: Cold precipitation by heparin of a protein in rabbit and human plasma. Proc. Soc. Exper. Biol. Med. 86:813, 1954.

17. Smith, R. T., and von Korff, R. W.: A heparin precipitable fraction of human plasma. I. Isolation and characterization of the fraction. J. Clin. Invest. 36:596, 1957.

18. Smith, R. T.: A heparin precipitable fraction of human plasma. II. Occurrence and significance of the fraction in normal individuals and in various disease states. J. Clin. Invest. 36:605, 1957.

19. McKay, D. G., Hardaway, R. M., Wahle, G. H., Edelstein, R., and Tartock, D. E.: Alterations in the blood coagulation mechanism after incompatible blood transfusion. Am. J. Surg. 89:583, 1955.

20. Woodfield, D. G., Cole, S. K., Allan, A. G. E., and Cash, J. D.: Serum fibrin degradation products throughout normal pregnancy. Brit. Med. J. 4:665, 1968.

21. Henderson, A. H., Pugsley, D. J., and Thomas, D. P.: Fibrin degradation products in pre-eclamptic toxaemia and eclampsia. Brit. Med. J. 3:545, 1970.

22. McCormick, J. N., Faulk, W. P., Fox, H., and Fudenberg, H. H.: Immunohistological and elution studies of the human placenta. J. Exp. Med. 133:1, 1971.

23. McKay, D. G.: "Intravascular Coagulation—Acute and Chronic; Disseminated and Local." Presented as the Fifth Jessie Horton Koessler Memorial Lecture. Joint meeting of the Chicago Institute of Medicine and Chicago Pathological Society, The Drake Hotel, April 17, 1972.

24. Todd, A. S.: The histological localization of fibrinolysin activator. J. Path. Bact. 78:281, 1959.

25. Silver, D.: Vascular injury: its effect on thrombolysis. J. Trauma 9:668, 1969.

26. McKay, D. G., Hertig, A. T., Adams, E. C., and Richardson, M. V.: Histochemical observations on the human placenta. Obstet. Gynec. 12:1, 1958.

27. Schneider, C. L.: Thromboplastin complications of late pregnancy. In Toxemias of Pregnancy, Human and Veterinary. A Ciba Foundation Symposium. Philadelphia, Blakiston, 1950.

28. Matsuoka, M., Zinbo, C., Tachikawa, M., and Watanabe, T.: Triggers in the initiation of intravascular coagulation syndrome. In Abstracts, XIII International Congress of Hematology, Munich, August 1970, p. 202.

29. Hufnagel, L. A., and Riddle, J. M.: Electron microscopy of bovine brain thromboplastin. In Abstracts, III Congress, International Society on Thrombosis and Haemostasis, Washington, D.C., August 1972, p. 102.

30. Bjorklid, E., and Otnaess, A-B.: The effect of phospholipase C on tissue thromboplastin—an electron microscopical study. In Abstracts, III Congress, International Society on Thrombosis and Haemostasis, Washington, D.C., August 1972, p. 68.

31. McKay, D. G.: The placenta in experimental toxemia of pregnancy. Obstet. Gynec. 20:1, 1962.

32. Ryan, G. M., Jr., Craig, J., and Reid, D. E.: Histology of the uterus and ovaries after long term cyclic norethynodrel therapy. Am. J. Obstet. Gynec. 90:715, 1964.

33. McKay, D. G., Merrill, S. J., Weiner, A. E., Hertig, A. T., and Reid, D. E.: The pathologic anatomy of eclampsia, bilateral renal cortical necrosis, pituitary necrosis, and other acute fatal complications of pregnancy, and its possible relationship to the generalized Shwartzman reaction. Am. J. Obstet. Gynec. 66:507, 1953.

34. McKay, D. G.: Hematologic evidence of disseminated intravascular coagulation in eclampsia. Obstet. Gynec. Surv. 27:399, 1972.

35. McKay, D. G.: Clinical significance of the pathology of toxemia of pregnancy. Circulation 30 (Suppl. 2): 30:66, 1964.

36. Castle, W. B.: Advances in physiology derived from the study of anemia in man. In H. K. Beecher, ed.: Disease and the Advancement of Basic Science. Cambridge, Harvard University Press, 1960.

37. McKay, D. G., and Shapiro, S. S.: Alterations in the blood coagulation system induced by bacterial endotoxin. I. In vivo (generalized Shwartzman reaction). J. Exp. Med. 107:353, 1958.

38. McKay, D. G., Wong, T. C., and Galton, M.: Effect of pregnancy on the disseminated thrombosis caused by bacterial endotoxin. Fed. Proc. 19:246, 1960.

39. McKay, D. G. and Wong, T. C. The effect of bacterial endotoxin on the placenta of the rat. Am. J. Path. 42:357, 1963.

The Clinical Spectrum and Management of Acquired Coagulopathy in Pregnancy

Editorial Comment

Alterations in the clotting mechanism may be divided into two categories: (1) those producing a hypercoagulable state and (2) those producing a hypocoagulable state. The hypercoagulable state may be regarded as preliminary to the latter but in many, if not most, instances—as in severe or total placental separation and amniotic fluid embolism—the changes in the clotting mechanism may occur so rapidly that the patient may appear to bypass the hypercoagulable state. However, hypercoagulability can be identified in the dead baby syndrome, in impending endotoxic shock, and possibly in an insidious or a chronic phase of placental separation. The acceleration of the clotting mechanism in these situations must be interpreted in the light of the normal changes of pregnancy, in which a relative hypercoagulable state exists compared to the situation in the nonpregnant individual. However, changes beyond the normal values for pregnancy can be ascertained before a consumption coagulopathy reaches a hypocoagulable state. As summarized by one of the contributors, "the patient has either an increased or a decreased ability to form thrombi."

To illustrate this approach, the clinical management of two patients will be presented briefly. The first patient is an example of the rare but well documented cases in which the placenta tends to separate in each and every pregnancy. One infant born to this patient had been salvaged by cesarean section at the onset of placental separation and three fetuses were stillborn, owing to complete placental separation. The so-called "game plan" for this pregnancy was to hospitalize the patient at 37 weeks' gestation and, assuming she remained free of symptoms, to deliver the infant by elective cesarean section one week later. Amniocentesis was performed 48 hours prior to the scheduled operation and the lecithin/sphingomyelin ratio was found to be 1.7. The cesarean section was unfortunately postponed and rescheduled for a later date. A complete placental abruption occurred 72 hours after the amniocentesis, and despite a hysterotomy 1 hour after the initial symptom was noted, a stillborn infant of 6 lb. 5 oz. was delivered. There was a mild, transient clotting defect that was self-correcting with blood replacement. During the preoperative period of hospitalization observation, the blood platelets numbered well below 200,000 on several occasions. One may question whether or not the patient had some degree of chronic placental separation without outward symptoms. In this instance, procrastination led to the mistake of waiting for "the laboratory findings to catch up to one's clinical judgment." In retrospect, the decrease in platelets should have served as a warning.

304

The second patient, with a threatened abortion associated with an in situ intrauterine shield, showed a diminished platelet count (125,000) and a rise in the partial thromboplastin time (PTT). The patient's vital signs were normal except for mild fever. The intrauterine device was removed, and a curettage with minimal blood loss was performed. The patient responded with a slight fall in blood pressure, diminished urine output, and tachycardia. These were only transient, and recovery was rapid. The blood values described were a factor in the decision to terminate the pregnancy before endotoxin shock developed, with possible consumption coagulopathy.

One of the more controversial aspects of this subject is the role of heparin in the management of patients with disseminated intravascular clotting. To the internist-hematologist, heparin heads the list of therapeutic agents in the treatment of a consumption coagulopathy. Accordingly, to administer fibrinogen is to add fuel to the fire. However, the clotting factors may have already been utilized or consumed totally when the patient is observed initially. Blood replacement is urgent—perhaps fibrinogen also, together with heparin coverage.

The investigations of one of the contributors (Dr. Corrigan) have revealed that heparin, when used in treating disseminated intravascular clotting associated with sepsis, fails to alter the prognosis or to influence favorably the coagulation mechanism unless the infection can first be brought under control.

A recent maternal death which supports this conclusion was called to our attention. In brief, the patient became pregnant with an intrauterine shield and developed vaginal bleeding at 16 weeks, associated with intrauterine infection. She was treated vigorously with heparin and antibiotics. However, the product of conception—the nidus of the infection—was not removed until late in her clinical course. The patient failed to respond and died soon thereafter from sepsis with endotoxin shock and a profound consumption coagulopathy, despite heparinization and blood replacement. The blood contained enormous amounts of fibrin split products. Heparin is not the complete answer to correcting a disseminated intravascular clotting in the presence of severe intrauterine infection. Certainly, in the management of the obstetrical patient who already has or is threatened by a consumption coagulopathy, the obstetrician must not relinquish his responsibility of decision making.

Much is to be learned with respect to overall patient management in monitoring these clotting changes, particularly in the chronic states of intravascular clotting wherein bleeding need not occur, such as pregnancy toxemia, the dead baby syndrome, and the early phase of placental separation and septic shock. A hematologic profile, which should include glass silicone clotting time, the partial thromboplastin time (PTT), and platelet count, may assist in the hour-to-hour management of these potentially seriously ill patients. Consistent with good practice, it is far better to anticipate these complications rather than to have to treat them after the fact. This is best illustrated in the case just cited, in which hysterectomy would have been life saving, provided that it was done not as a last resort measure, but prior to the development of full-blown consumption coagulopathy.

10

Preferable Medical and Surgical Methods of Conception Control

Alternative Points of View:

> By William E. Crisp and William S. Bazley

> By Daniel R. Mishell, Jr.

> By Mamdouh Moukhtar and Seymour L. Romney

Editorial Comment

Preferable Medical and Surgical Methods of Conception Control

WILLIAM E. CRISP

University of Arizona College of Medicine and Maricopa County Hospital

WILLIAM S. BAZLEY

University of Florida College of Medicine

Despite the variety, the availability, and the reliability of contraceptive methods, more women today are undergoing surgical sterilization than ever before. Contraceptive failures, dissatisfaction with contraceptive methods because of inconvenience or associated symptoms, fear of possible complications, decreased libido, associated guilt with repeated use of contraception, and a social conscience regarding overpopulation are some of the reasons for patients requesting surgical sterilization.

It is estimated that 180,000 women each year in this country have a surgical procedure which renders them sterile, and over 50 per cent of these procedures are performed specifically for sterilization.

Interestingly, some women view conventional contraceptive practices as interfering with their "nature" or physiology, but do not necessarily have the same feeling toward surgery. Contrariwise, some women regard menstruation as a badge of femininity and will not consider hysterectomy for conception control per se.

The mortality rates of tubal ligation and hysterectomy are virtually the same (0.1 per cent to 0.2 per cent). The morbidity of the two procedures, however, varies considerably. Vaginal hysterectomy is associated with morbidity rates that vary from 28 to 31 per cent, while tubal ligation or laparoscopic tubal fulguration carries a morbidity rate of 2 per cent. Hospitalization for simple vaginal hysterectomy alone averages 4.8 days, versus 6 hours for tubal sterilization.

Operative procedures, however, should not be selected primarily on the basis of morbidity statistics, length of hospitalization, or cost, but also on individual considerations of a particular patient's overall needs.

The procedure of choice for woman should be based primarily on medical indications, both immediate and long-term, psychosexual acceptance in the light of her particular social environment, and lastly, convenience and economics.

Tubal sterilization is a convenient and immediate solution to someone seeking permanent sterilization, and it has been considered an almost benign procedure. However, granted that the associated morbidity is low and the contraceptive failure rate varies from 1 to 3 per cent, what other surgical procedure would be considered benign that produces—within 5 years—associated symptoms that require additional major surgery in a significant number of individuals? These sequelae are, in order of frequency, abnormal uterine bleeding, pelvic pain, and symptoms of descensus, and they occur in 15 per cent of post-tubal ligation patients within three years. Of these women, 24 per cent underwent a hysterectomy within five years, and 34 percent within 10 years.

In evaluating these figures, it must be emphasized that the statistics quoted have been taken from series that were compiled when tubal ligation was a more restricted procedure, confined by medical mores to multiparas—the very group of women who predictably would have a higher incidence of gynecologic problems that would lead to additional surgery. Under the most liberal indications for hysterectomy the expected incidence in this same group of women would be in the range of 8 per cent in five years, and 18 per cent at 10 years. Perhaps the post-tubal sterilization statistics will change when new data gathered on younger women with fewer children, utilizing different techniques, are analyzed.

Although surgical sterilization in most hospital services may now be obtained after the personal decision and request of the patient, in consultation with the physician, and not by a committee review—which is as it should be—the method of surgical sterilization is still not as individualized as it might be. As physicians, we should not be pressured by society or patients to do a procedure without also evaluating the operation in relation to the individual patient. It is recommended that hysterectomy, as well as tubal ligation, be considered as a primary method of sterilization.

Hysterectomy: Which Method? When?

Hysterectomy for sterilization may be done at the time of cesarean section, in the immediate postpartum period, or as an interval procedure following uterine involution.

As with any elective operative procedure, to avoid unnecessary morbidity and mortality, certain criteria must be met before subjecting the patient to surgery. We insist that the woman ask for surgical sterilization and that she fully understand the procedure. In addition, there must be physical or socioeconomic indications for hysterectomy. The patient must be suitable and properly prepared emotionally and physically for surgery, with no limiting systemic disease.

The psychological implications have been one of the primary objections to this operation as a contraceptive method. Although there is no solid evidence that the uterus has any endocrine or metabolic function, as previously implied it is an organ with high ego-image value and the site of many women's sense of identity and femininity.

For the past 10 years, we have asked patients who have had hysterectomies to fill out a psychologically designed questionnaire and return it with or without identification, as they desire; 500 returned questionnaires have been evaluated. The most important factors found in the analysis of these data are directly related to psychological acceptance of hysterectomy, which means, we suspect, retention of female identity. Thus, there must be a preoperative discussion with both the patient and her husband of what a hysterectomy involves, including basic anatomy, physiology, sexuality, menopause, and so forth. Many times the husband's misconceptions are a cause of psychological nonacceptance. In addition to this preoperative discussion, the nurse in charge of the gynecology service should reiterate many of the basic points made by the physician, which the patient may not have understood. If there are any major problems, the nurse alerts the resident or the patient's physician. Certainly preoperative counseling is most important and usually cannot be replaced by postoperative reassurance. When the patients and their husbands are properly counseled prior to their decision, there is minimal risk of untoward psychological effects.

Two interesting exceptions to the above discussions were noted in our study. One small group of patients (3 per cent) have been identified by this survey who do not achieve sexual satisfaction unless there is a "risk of getting pregnant." These are the same women who are not reliable in their contraceptive practices and probably make up the bulk of those patients who feel they have lost their femininity and eventually seek psychiatric help. Perhaps these women would have been better served with tubal ligation, which would have allowed them to act out their sexual fantasies.

Another 1 per cent of the patients had misgivings after surgery because of a change in their domestic relationship (loss of a child, divorce, and so forth) which they psychologically at least relate to the hysterectomy. We feel that this, too, could be obviated by better emotional preparation of the patient.

Although serious morbidity varies from 2 to 4 per cent, a certain percentage of morbidity is unavoidable. Both serious and unavoidable complications can be reduced by careful selection of patients and the timing of hysterectomy.

An important factor that must be balanced against the morbidity of hysterectomy is the percentage of patients with uterine pathology which would not have been eliminated by tubal sterilization. Data on 330 patients, both private and nonprivate, showed that 19 per cent (62 patients) had significant uterine pathology at the time of sterilization hysterectomy. This ran the gamut, from submucous leiomyomata, cancer in situ, and adenomyosis to ovarian pathology that may or may not have been noted at the time of tubal sterilization, depending on the technique used.

Just as cesarean section is indicated for sound obstetrical indications, cesarean hysterectomy also has its generally acceptable indications. Most of the large series of cesarean hysterectomies reported have been composed of both emergency and elective cases. In the emergency cases, hysterectomy was not anticipated at the time of cesarean section but became necessary because of unexpected operative findings (uterine scar, postpartum hemorrhage, placenta accreta, adnexal disease, or an unanticipated technical problem). These are readily acceptable indications. Elective cesarean hysterectomy, however, has been questioned because of the related morbidity, associated primarily with blood loss, which accounts for 80 per cent of the 20 to 30 per cent morbidity rate.

A review of the literature and of our own data has demonstrated that elective cesarean hysterectomy has an associated morbidity rate similar to that for elective hysterectomy for benign uterine disease. For our 80 elective cesarean hysterectomies, the morbidity rate was 28.2 per cent. The major complications were urinary tract infections, vaginal cuff cellulitis, atelectasis, and wound abscess. Twenty-eight per cent of these patients received transfusion, with twice the amount of blood than needed for an interval hysterectomy.

A major contributing factor to morbidity is the number of hours that patient has been in labor before cesarean section was done. Those patients who had been in labor for over eight hours had a 55 per cent morbidity rate. There have been no maternal deaths.

In our experience, elective cesarean hysterectomy is justified in those women who require a cesarean section for sound obstetrical reasons and who desire sterilization for socioeconomic or other reasons, provided that their labors have not exceeded eight hours.

As indicated, cesarean hysterectomy is associated with increased blood loss. In attempting to identify the cause of this loss, it was found that most of it occurs if routine hysterectomy techniques are used.

Following hemostasis of the cesarean uterine incision, no attempt is made to dissect the bladder further until it is necessary to uncover the cervix. This avoids considerable early blood loss from possible varicosities beneath the bladder.

In addition, the operator must recognize that the uterus immediately post partum not only has the usual hypertrophied external blood supply, but also has an active internal myometrial blood supply.

It is very apparent in the operative procedure that uterine areas above the ligated ovarian and uterine vessels will continue to bleed until the cervix is secured. We have arrested this blood loss by placing several loops of No. 1 chromic ligatures around the cervix after the uterine vessels have been ligated. This controls the internal circulation of the uterus and also helps to define the anatomy of the cervix so that a dissection can be readily accomplished at the site of the vaginal cuff.

Postpartum abdominal hysterectomy may also be indicated in selected individuals in the immediate postpartum period, usually the third day following vaginal delivery. These are the same multiparous women who desire surgical sterilization, who have associated gynecologic problems, personal beliefs that rule out tubal ligation or other forms of contraception, and a long history of not returning for medical care until the third trimester of the next pregnancy. Study of 102 women with these characteristics has established that the third postpartum day was the optimum time for elective hysterectomy. The average postpartum uterus weighs approximately 1100 g. immediately after delivery. Uterine involution during the first three days is dramatic, with an average decrease in uterine weight of 300 g. This is associated with a relative decrease in vasculization and restitution of normal anatomy. After the third day, uterine weight loss drops to approximately 25 g. a day until involution is nearly complete.

Hospitalization time averaged 6.9 days for cesarean hysterectomies and 4.8 days for the postpartum hysterectomies.

In reviewing the data of women who had vaginal hysterectomies (112 cases) either immediately post-abortal or later, but within 12 weeks postpartum, no particular technical difficulties were encountered, but pelvic hematomas and vaginal cuff abscesses were increased. These are now being avoided with greater emphasis given to hemostasis. Despite the fact that the uterus was well involuted, the tissues were more friable and the vascularity greater than expected with routine hysterectomy. In this group of patients, the morbidity was 35 per cent with hysterectomy alone, increasing to 46 per cent with anterior plastic repair of urethrocystocoele. This was comparable to the morbidity rate of the routine non-pregnant hysterectomy, which approximated 30 per cent with hysterectomy alone, and 34 per cent when vaginal repair was also performed. The only exception has been a small group of patients with IUD in situ, in whom the morbidity rate has been 42 per cent. All IUD's are now removed for at least one menstrual cycle prior to surgery.

Conclusion

The method of female surgical sterilization should be a decision based on all aspects of the woman's life, both medical and socioeconomic, and it should go beyond her immediate problem and consider her long-term health.

Any attempt to adopt a single approach or method as a solution to all the medical, emotional, and gynecological problems will certainly not be in the best interests of either the woman or her husband.

With proved criteria and careful patient selection, hysterectomy for elective sterilization is justifiable. Once the uterus has served its reproductive function, it becomes a potential liability and unnecessary inconvenience in many women. Only with hysterectomy can a woman enjoy the emotional, physical and sexual freedom that has been the exclusive privilege of the male.

REFERENCES

1. Atkinson, S. M., and Chappell, S. M.: Vaginal hysterectomy for sterilization. Obstet. Gynec. 39:759, 1972.
2. Brenner, P., et al.: Evaluation of cesarean section hysterectomy as a sterilization procedure. Amer. J. Obstet. Gynec. 108:335, 1970.
3. Bazley, W. S., and Crisp, W. E.: Postpartum hysterectomy (in press).
4. Hofmeister, F. J.: Tubal ligation versus cesarean hysterectomy. Clin. Obstet. Gynec. 3:676, 1969.
5. Muldoon, M. J.: Gynecological illness after sterilization. Brit. Med. J. 1:84, 1972.
6. Nichols, E. E.: Current practices in female sterilization in the United States. Am. J. Obstet. Gynec. 101:345, 1968.
7. Wright, R. C.: Hysterectomy: past, present, and future. Obstet. Gynec. 33:560, 1969.

Preferable Medical and Surgical Methods of Conception Control

Daniel R. Mishell, Jr.

University of Southern California School of Medicine

There are many different types of contraceptives available, but the two most effective methods of contraception are the oral steroid drugs and the intra-uterine devices. The diaphragm, condom, and vaginal foam are also good contraceptives and should be used by some couples who are not able or willing to use contraceptive steroids or the IUD. It must be realized, however, that the failure rate of these traditional methods is approximately five times that of oral contraceptives or IUD. New, improved vaginal foams have a pregnancy rate of about 3 per cent if used consistently prior to each coital act.[1] If the rhythm method is utilized, the woman should take her daily basal temperature each morning. The couple should abstain from intercourse until 48 hours after the basal body temperature shift. Even with this technique, the failure rate of the rhythm method is estimated to be about 7 per cent.[2]

HORMONAL CONTRACEPTIVES

There are two basic types of oral steroid contraceptives: combination and sequential. The former is made up of estrogen and a progestogen combined in a single tablet, given continuously for 3 weeks, whereas the latter utilizes a regimen of estrogen alone, for about 2 weeks, followed by a course of combination tablets for 1 week as in combination therapy. Progestogens are used in oral contraception instead of progesterone, which is inactive orally. The progestogens utilized are modified mainly at the C-17 and C-3 positions so that they are not inactivated as rapidly as progesterone and thus are effective when taken orally.

There are two major chemical prototypes of progestogens; one is chemically related to progesterone, the other has 19-nortestosterone as its basic component. Various modifications of this latter type of progestogen are used in the only oral steroidal contraceptives now available in the United States. These progestogens vary in potency depending on their chemical structure. One cannot

314

predict their pharmacological activity solely upon the weight of the compound present in the particular contraceptive steroid; the biological activity of the various progestogens has also to be considered. Biological assays have been performed in animals as well as humans to determine the potency of these compounds. One human bioassay is the Swyer-Greenblatt test of delay of menses.[3] In this test women are given 0.1 mg. of ethinylestradiol together with the progestogen. The least amount of progestogen that delays the onset of menses for 2 weeks is used as the basis for comparing potency of these progestogens.

Greenblatt[4] has reported that norethindrone and norethynodrel are approximately equal in activity, while norethindrone acetate is twice as active as these two. Ethinyldiol diacetate is 15 times as potent and norgestrel is about 30 times as potent as norethindrone. The activities of these compounds differ because of modifications in their chemical structures that prevent norgestrel and ethinyldiol diacetate from being hydroxylated and conjugated as easily as norethindrone.

The estrogenic component of the oral contraceptive pills likewise consists of orally active synthetic estrogens, instead of natural estrogens such as 17β-estradiol. The two types of estrogenic compounds present in oral contraceptives are ethinylestradiol and ethinylestradiol-3-methylether, or mestranol. Similar to the various progestogens, these two estrogens have different biological activity in the human. Delforge and Ferin[5] have shown that ethinylestradiol is about 1.7 to 2 times as potent as mestranol. Heinen[6] has recently compared the activity of the oral contraceptive steroids currently being marketed, using as criteria both weight and biologic activity. He has indicated that certain compounds with a lower total weight of steroid are actually more potent than other compounds containing a greater amount of less active steroids. When prescribing contraceptive steroids for patients, it is important to evaluate both these factors, quantity and activity, especially if the patient develops breakthrough bleeding or amenorrhea when taking one type of pill. It is best to increase the estrogen in amount or type in treating women who develop breakthrough bleeding and decrease the progestogenic component in treating amenorrhea.

Although some individuals suggest prescribing preparations with greater amounts of progestogens for "estrogen dominant" women and greater amounts of estrogens for "progestogen dominant" women, there is little evidence that the incidence of side-effects is significantly reduced by such therapy. It would appear best to utilize basic principles of pharmacology and initially prescribe the preparations with the lowest steroid activity, since all available hormonal contraceptives are nearly completely effective in preventing pregnancy. After initial therapy with these preparations, if side-effects such as breakthrough bleeding occur, then the dosage of steroid can be increased or a more potent steroid can be used. Government regulatory agencies have reported that preparations containing 50 μg. of estrogen are associated with a significantly reduced incidence of thromboembolism. It would appear prudent to prescribe initially compounds containing this dosage of estrogen.

The combined type of oral contraceptive is the most effective method of contraception currently available. Provided the patient remembers to take every tablet, the pregnancy rate is less than 0.2 per cent per 100 woman-years. This effectiveness stems partially from the fact that these compounds act in many different ways to prevent conception.[7] Their primary mechanism of action is inhibition of ovulation. In addition, the cervical mucus is altered so that it remains thick and viscid and interferes with sperm penetration. The endometrium is altered so that the glands do not produce sufficient glycogen to optimally support the blastocyst during the time it remains in the endometrial cavity prior to implantation. The ovary is changed so that it is less responsive to the same amount of gonadotropins. In addition, there are effects on the oviduct and the uterine muscles which probably interfere with both sperm and ovum transport.

The sequential type of contraceptive therapy is not as effective as the combination type[8] and should only be utilized in rare instances. Although the mid-cycle gonadotropin surge and ovulation are prevented by the combination type of pill, both these events occur with some frequency during treatment with the sequential method. Since the alterations of the cervical mucus and of the endometrium are not as great with sequential therapy, the pregnancy rate associated with this type of oral contraception is twice as high as that with the combined form. In addition, the sequential type of contraception provides a higher dose of estrogen and is associated with a greater incidence of side-effects than the combined type. Thus fewer patients continue on sequential oral contraceptives than continue on the combination pill.[8]

In addition to affecting the female genital tract, both the estrogen and the progestogen components of the oral contraceptives have some effect on nearly every organ system of the body. As a result, patients taking these medications frequently obtain undesirable symptoms, such as nausea and vomiting, breakthrough bleeding, bloating, weight gain, and edema, as well as central nervous system symptoms such as headache, nervousness, fatigue, dizziness, psychological changes, and decreased libido. Other symptoms include hypomenorrhea or amenorrhea, breast tenderness, and facial pigmentation. One of the reasons for the relatively high incidence of side effects is the fact that steroids are administered to most women in excessive doses. This is the result of three main factors:

1. The dose that is administered is large enough to inhibit ovulation instead of only preventing fertility; presumably, a larger dose of steroid is needed to inhibit ovulation than to prevent conception.

2. The pills are packaged in a uniform dosage. Although different types of pills have different potencies, the dosage range is relatively narrow and each woman receives a uniform dosage of most preparations.

3. The medication is given once a day. The steroid blood level rises rapidly after oral administration and then slowly declines throughout the next 24-hour period. Yet the steroid blood levels must still be high enough to prevent pregnancy 24 hours after ingestion.

More than 50 metabolic changes associated with the use of oral contraceptives have been reported in the literature.[9] Although unwanted symptoms associated with oral contraceptive therapy are not infrequent, *serious* complications associated with their use is relatively rare. Effects other than contraception can be classified into three categories: (1) effects on the primary target organs of the female reproductive system, (2) effects on other endocrine organs, and (3) effects on nonendocrine organ systems.

    1. Effects on organs of female genital tract:

        A. *Ovary.* In the ovary, stromal fibrosis has been reported. It is usually transitory and disappears after contraceptives are stopped.

        B. *Myometrium.* Fibromyomata enlarge with oral contraceptive use. They can enlarge to a great extent and become symptomatic.

Their presence constitutes one of the contraindications to the use of contraceptive steroids.

C. *Endometrium.* Alterations occur in the endometrium so that amenorrhea, or lack of withdrawal bleeding, may occur, in addition to intermenstrual bleeding.

D. *Cervix.* An increased amount of cervical mucus has been reported with contraceptive steroids, especially of the sequential type. A polypoid hyperplasia of the endocervical glands has also been noted. This change is not malignant or premalignant. There is no evidence that oral contraceptives cause an increased incidence of epidermoid carcinoma of the cervix or carcinoma in situ. Stern and associates[10] have shown that patients who choose oral contraceptives have a higher incidence of abnormal cervical cytology than women who choose other types of contraception.

E. *Vagina.* There have been numerous reports of bacterial changes in the vagina, with an increase in vaginitis (especially moniliasis) in women receiving contraceptive steroids. However, a prospective study by Spellacy and colleagues[11] indicates that contraceptive steroids do not cause an increased incidence of monilial vaginitis.

F. *Breasts.* There is an increased incidence of breast tenderness, mainly related to the estrogenic component of the pill. In addition, there is a change in lactation, as both the amount of milk produced is diminished and the quality of the milk is altered by contraceptive steroids. Hormonal contraceptives both reduce the concentration of protein in human milk and are themselves found in measurable amounts in the milk. Oral contraceptives are therefore not advised for patients who wish to nurse their babies. Development of galactorrhea is also an uncommon side-effect associated with hormonal contraceptives.

2. Effects of oral contraceptives on other endocrine organs:

A. *Adrenal and Thyroid.* Both the estrogen and progestogen components alter the concentration of various serum proteins. There is an increase in corticosteroid binding globulin, with a resultant decrease in excretion of 17-ketosteroids, 17-hydroxysteroids, and aldosterone, although there is no evidence that the oral contraceptives change the function of the adrenal cortex. Likewise, there is an increase in thyroid binding globulin similar to that which occurs in pregnancy. As a result, there is an alteration in the thyroid function tests similar to the changes that are found in pregnancy. However, there is no evidence that oral contraceptives alter the function of the thyroid gland.

B. *Pancreas.* There is evidence that alterations in glucose metabolism occur with oral contraceptives. It has not been definitely established whether these changes are related to the estrogen or progestogen component of the pill, or to both. There is some indication that different progestogens may have a varying effect upon glucose tolerance.[12] Women who have taken oral contraceptive steroids for long periods of time have an increased incidence of abnormal glucose tolerance tests. For this reason, oral contraceptives are not advised after pregnancy for patients who develop gestational diabetes, because there is an increased likelihood that oral contraceptives will induce the same alterations in glucose metabolism which developed in these individuals during pregnancy. Because of the increased risk of developing altered glucose metabolism, it is suggested that a glucose tolerance test be performed annually in all women receiving this type of contraceptive.

C. *Hypothalamus.* Since oral contraceptive steroids inhibit the release of LRF and thus prevention of ovulation may be said to occur at the hypothalamic-pituitary level, this inhibition persists in some individuals after stopping the pill, and "post-pill" amenorrhea develops. The incidence of this type of amenorrhea is quite low in patients who discontinue taking oral contraceptives, but it is probably higher in patients who have oligomenorrhea or amenorrhea prior to starting oral contraceptive therapy than in those with regular menses. Therefore, the use of combined oral steroid contraception is contraindicated for patients who have oligomenorrhea or amenorrhea. If steroid therapy was proposed because these individuals desire regular menses, treatment with a progestogen alone for 5 days each month is usually sufficient to induce menses without suppressing hypothalamic function. For contraception, a method other than hormonal steroids is preferred, but if steroid contraceptives are used, it is best to utilize the sequential type of pill, which causes less hypothalamic inhibition than the combined steroids.

3. Effect on other organ systems:

A. *Lipids.* Treatment with oral contraceptives can cause an increase in serum lipids, particularly serum triglycerides, and a change in the atherogenic index to a male type of pattern.[13] These changes, combined with changes in glucose metabolism, might lead to an increase in atherosclerosis in women receiving these contraceptive steroids for prolonged periods of time. At the present time no evidence exists for an increased incidence of atherosclerosis, but it may be too early to determine the incidence of this long-term effect.

B. *Liver.* There is an increased incidence of abnormalities in some liver function tests in oral contraceptive users, mainly those tests dealing with bile excretion, such as bromsulphalein (BSP) retention. The steroids adversely affect the function of the enzymes aiding excretion of bile, similar to the changes which occur in pregnancy. Those individuals who develop idiopathic recurrent jaundice of pregnancy frequently develop jaundice when treated with oral contraceptive steroids, and their use is thus contraindicated in these individuals. Active liver disease is also a contraindication to hormonal contraceptive therapy, but these agents are not contraindicated in individuals who have a past history of hepatitis and normal liver function at present.

C. *Thromboembolism*. Studies by Vessey and Doll[14] in England and Sartwell and associates[15] in the United States revealed a significant but low increase in thromboembolic disease in oral contraceptive users, estimated to be about 4.4 times greater than in non-users. Mortality from thrombolic disease associated with the use of hormonal contraceptives is estimated to be about 3 per 100,000 women per year. A causal relation has thus been established and appears to involve changes in blood clotting factors induced by the estrogenic component of the pill. There is evidence that this increased incidence of thromboembolism is related to the amount of estrogen and that pills containing 50 μg. or less of the estrogen component are associated with a lower incidence of thromboembolic phenomena. Therefore, it is best not to prescribe pills with a greater amount of estrogen than this unless it is necessary to prevent breakthrough bleeding. It is not necessary for patients to have clinical evidence of deep vein thrombophlebitis of the lower extremities to develop pulmonary thromboembolism while receiving oral contraceptives. Individuals who develop chest pain should discontinue oral contraceptive therapy as well as have further diagnostic studies, including a lung scan.

D. *Skin*. Melasma, similar to that which develops in pregnancy, occurs in some patients receiving oral contraceptives. This change is accentuated by exposure to sunlight and takes a long time to disappear after stopping the oral contraceptives.

E. *Central Nervous System*. There is an increased incidence of nausea, as well as headache, depression, and change in libido in women receiving oral contraceptives. There is some indication that women receiving this medication have an increased incidence of cerebrovascular accidents, owing mainly to arterial thrombi, although the incidence is extremely low and a definite causal relation has not been established. Nevertheless, if patients develop an increased incidence of headache while they are taking the pill or develop any peripheral neurological changes, it is prudent to discontinue its use.

F. *Kidney*. Use of oral contraceptives can increase levels of plasma-renin substrate, with resultant alteration in renin-angiotensin balance. In certain individuals these changes can cause a significant but reversible hypertension. The incidence of hypertension associated with oral contraceptive therapy is very low; however, the blood pressure of all individuals receiving this medication should be monitored regularly.

G. *Body Weight*. Because these progestogens are chemically related to testosterone, they are anabolic and in some women there will be an increase in body weight beyond the 3 to 5 pound gain resulting from retention of fluid. Balance studies have shown an increase in nitrogen retention in individuals receiving oral contraceptives. Thus, if a woman gains more than 10 pounds in a year, oral contraceptives should be discontinued or an agent containing a less potent progestogen should be utilized.

H. *Other Organ Systems.* Several studies have been published consisting of a few case reports indicating possible changes in the gastrointestinal tract related to oral contraceptives—mainly, an increased incidence of mesenteric thrombosis and possibly ulcerative colitis. Patients developing these disease entities while receiving oral contraceptive therapy should discontinue medication. Changes in vitamins A and B$_6$ metabolism with oral contraceptive therapy have also been reported, but their clinical significance has not been established.

One must also realize that there are potential harmful effects in *not* taking oral contraceptive therapy, and those of an unwanted pregnancy are relatively great. The risk of morbidity and death associated with therapeutic abortion is greater than that associated with hormonal contraceptive use. When prescribing oral contraceptives, the physician must weigh the benefits against risks for the individual patient. In the opinion of the U.S. Food and Drug Administration, the oral contraceptives are safe inasmuch as their benefits outweigh their risks.[16] Nevertheless, there are certain absolute contraindications to their use. These contraindications include cancer of the breast and uterus, fibromyomata, pregnancy, active liver disease, and a past history of gestational diabetes or thromboembolic phenomena. In addition, all individuals receiving these potent pharmaceutical agents should be seen and examined regularly by a physician, at least 3 months after initiating therapy and annually thereafter. At these intervals, a pelvic examination should be performed, and the patient's blood pressure and weight recorded. In addition to this procedure, a breast examination and a 2-hour postprandial blood sugar test should be performed. By performing these routine examinations in all women—and realizing that these women are receiving potent pharmacologic agents—one can hopefully avoid some of their serious but recurring side-effects. Provided that the physician follows this good medical practice, patients can continue to receive oral contraceptive steroids until age 50 without interruption. There is no necessity for stopping oral contraceptive therapy for any interval (except for any pregnancies the patient may desire) prior to the menopausal age. No benefit is derived from intermittent stopping of therapy before this, and there is a risk of unwanted pregnancy. At age 50 their use should be discontinued for an interval, and if the patient is menopausal, she can be given replacement low doses of an estrogen alone, if desired. If she is still ovulating at this age, oral contraceptive therapy should be continued. During this interval without steroid contraceptives, alternative methods of contraception, such as the condom, diaphragm, or foam, should be used to prevent an unwanted pregnancy.

INTRAUTERINE DEVICE

The intrauterine device (IUD) is the other most effective method of contraception. Although the IUD is not as effective as oral contraceptives, this method of contraception has several advantages. In contrast to oral contraceptives, with their ubiquitous action through the body, the effects of the IUD in the human are limited to the female genital tract. In addition, the IUD need only be inserted once and then continues to act as a contraceptive for years, in contrast to the necessity of daily ingestion of oral steroids. Furthermore, in contrast to the relative paucity of good clinical data concerning hormonal contraceptives in their first decade of use, an abundance of reliable epidemiologic information about the IUD was made available soon after the new plastic devices were first produced and used clinically. These important clinical data were made available by a Cooperative Statistical Program (CSP) established in 1965 by Christopher Tietze at the request and with the support of the Population Council. The Ninth Progress Report of the Cooperative Statistical Program for the Evaluation of Intrauterine Devices, published in 1970, provided information obtained from 29 investigators evaluating various devices inserted into 31,767 women for 546,787 woman-months of use.[17] Life table techniques were used to analyze these data, and the following information was obtained: Pregnancy rates varied slightly among different devices. The Lippes loop D has a 2.7 per cent pregnancy rate at the end of the first year. For any type of device, the pregnancy rate is greater in the first year than in the second, and pregnancy rates are higher for smaller devices than for larger devices of the same design. When pregnancies do occur with an IUD in situ, the device is never located within the amniotic sac, as implantation occurs in the endometrium not immediately adjacent to the IUD.

The incidence of congenital defects in babies born to mothers with an IUD in situ is no greater than that in the general population. The incidence of fetal death also is not increased, but spontaneous abortion is significantly more frequent. A report by Lewit[18] indicated that the abortion rate was significantly higher in women who become pregnant with an IUD in situ than in women of the same population group who become pregnant after expelling an IUD. It is frequently asked whether the device should be removed in an individual who becomes pregnant with an IUD in the uterus. If the appendage is visible, it is best to remove the IUD, as the abortion rate is lower after removal of the device than if it is left in situ. However, if the appendage is not visible, one should not attempt to probe the cavity to remove the IUD.

The IUD reduces the incidence of both intrauterine and ectopic pregnancies, but it is more effective in preventing intrauterine pregnancies. In the Cooperative Statistical Program during a period of 244,000 woman-months, about 229 to 343 ectopic gestations would be expected to occur. However, there were only 34 ectopic pregnancies in this time period. Thus, the IUD would appear to prevent ectopic pregnancies at a rate of about 90 per cent, in contrast to preventing intrauterine pregnancies at a rate of about 97 to 98 per cent. Nevertheless, if a patient becomes pregnant with an intrauterine device in situ, she has about a 1 in 20 chance of having an ectopic pregnancy. Thus the physician should be aware of the fact that in every patient who becomes pregnant with an IUD in situ there is a substantial risk that the pregnancy is ectopic. Patients who have a therapeutic abortion for an IUD failure should have the uterine contents examined histologically to be certain that the gestation was intrauterine.

One of the problems with the IUD is expulsion of the device, especially if the expulsion is not noticed by the wearer. In the Cooperative Statistical Program, about 20 per cent of the expulsions were unnoticed and, therefore, could be followed by an unwanted pregnancy. About one-third of pregnancies in IUD users occur after an unnoticed expulsion, indicating that it is important to have an appendage attached to the IUD so that the user can be sure the device has not been expelled.

Expulsions are highest in the first few months after insertion and higher in the first year than in the second year of use. The expulsion rate is also higher with smaller than with larger devices of the same design, and higher in younger individuals and in women who have not had children. The expulsion rate has been found to vary inversely with the age of the woman and also with the number of pregnancies. If noticed by the patient, expulsion is not a great problem because the patient has a good chance of retaining the device following reinsertion. For the loop D, the expulsion rate for first insertions is about 11.3 per cent. If reinserted, the patient has about a 68 per cent chance of retaining it; after two expulsions, she has a 34 per cent chance of retaining the third device.

The major problem with the IUD is removal for medical reasons, mainly bleeding and pain. The incidence of removal is approximately the same for all devices, about 15 per cent during the first year and 7 per cent during the second year of use. Removal for medical reasons is the most common cause for discontinuing this method of contraception, accounting for more than 50 per cent of all discontinuations. Insertion is best performed at the time of the menstrual period because patients are not as worried by a slight amount of excess bleeding at that time of the cycle. In order to lessen the incidence of complaints of pain, the patient should be informed that a foreign body is going to be inserted and that her body will have to adjust to it, similar to the adjustment that must be made to false teeth or contact lenses.

Discontinuation rates for IUD's are approximately the same for all devices —about 20 to 30 per cent in the first year and about 10 to 15 per cent in the second year. Most experience has been obtained with the loop D, for which reliable data are available for 6 years of use. At the end of the first year, 22.6 per cent of the women will have discontinued use of this device, another 15.3 per cent will stop using it in the second year, 13.6 per cent in the third, 11.9 per cent in the fourth, 8.6 per cent in the fifth, and 6.3 per cent in the sixth. Thus, at the end of 6 years, 42.6 per cent of women originally inserted with a loop D will still be wearing it. Of the discontinuations, 5.4 result from pregnancy. Although the incidence of expulsion is about 10 per cent during the first year, most of these women will have the IUD reinserted. Therefore, at the end of 6 years, only 7 per cent will have discontinued using the loop D because of expulsion. About 50 per cent, or 31.3 per cent of the 57.4 per cent, who discontinue using it do so because of bleeding and pain and other medical reasons. New types of IUD's are being developed in an attempt to reduce this incidence. There is no need to change an IUD unless after a period of time the patient develops increased bleeding. Calcium salts are deposited on the plastic in time, and their roughness can cause ulceration and bleeding of the endometrium. If increased bleeding develops after the IUD has been in the uterus for a year or more, the old IUD should be removed and a new one inserted.

One of the major problems with an IUD is perforation of the uterus. The incidence of perforation for the loop is about 1 per 2500 insertions and for the shield about 1 per 350 insertions.[19] Perforation initially occurs at the time of insertion and can best be prevented by straightening the uterine axis with a tenaculum and then probing the cavity with a uterine sound prior to IUD insertion. Sometimes only the distal portion of the IUD penetrates the uterine muscle at the time of insertion, and then the uterine contractions over the next few months force the IUD into the peritoneal cavity. One should always suspect that perforation has occurred if a patient states she cannot feel the appendage but did not notice if the device was expelled; it should not be assumed that an unnoticed expulsion has occurred. Frequently the device has rotated 180 degrees and the appendage is withdrawn into the cavity. In this situation, after the pelvic examination is performed, and unless pregnancy is suspected, the uterine cavity should be probed. If the device cannot be felt with a uterine sound or biopsy instrument, an X-ray should be obtained. In order to determine the location of the IUD, it is best to take a lateral X-ray with contrast media inside the uterine cavity. The perforated IUD may be located in the cul-de-sac and the diagnosis may be missed with an ordinary anteroposterior film. Intraperitoneal IUD's are probably best removed, although there is no evidence that leaving a loop within the peritoneal cavity is harmful. Intraperitoneal IUD's can usually be removed by laparoscopy.

Another problem associated with the IUD is upper genital tract infection. It was originally believed that the IUD, acting as a foreign body, allowed continual contamination of the uterine cavity with bacteria. Several years ago a study was performed whereby transfundal cultures of the endometrial cavity were obtained from uteri removed from patients who had had an IUD inserted for 3 hours to 7 months prior to hysterectomy.[20] Samples of endometrium were removed, homogenized, placed in eight different culture media, and incubated under aerobic and anaerobic conditions for 5 days. The cultures were reported to be sterile only if no bacteria grew in any of these media. Only 10 of the 61 hysterectomy specimens had positive cultures of the endometrial cavity; however, all five specimens in which the IUD had been in place for 24 hours or less grew bacteria. In each instance, the organism in the endometrium was identical to that cultured from the cervical mucus. In the next 24 hour period, 80 per cent of endometrial cultures were found to be sterile, and 30 days after IUD insertion all cultures of the cavity were sterile. In specimens with sterile cavities, cultures taken from the IUD itself and from the threads within the endometrial cavity were also sterile, indicating that the appendages do not provide access for the bacteria to enter the endometrial cavity. This study indicated that an IUD should not be placed in a patient who has evidence of salpingitis because additional bacteria would be introduced. It also revealed that most infections which occur after an IUD has been in place for 30 days are unrelated to the IUD itself, as the device is not the causative factor for these venereal infections. There is no reason to remove the IUD when treating salpingitis occurring more than 30 days after insertion. The results of this study have been confirmed by the clinical findings of the Cooperative Statistical Program. The incidence of pelvic inflammatory disease was substantially higher in the first month after insertion, and the rate during the first 2 weeks after insertion was significantly greater than at later times during the first 6 years post-insertion.

Histologically, evidence of chronic endometritis persists for long periods of time in endometrial specimens obtained from IUD users.[21] Thus, pathologic evidence of inflammation persists after the bacterial infection disappears .

Neutrophils, mononuclear cells, and plasma cells are greatly increased in numbers in the endometrium during the first 6 months after insertion. Thereafter, mononuclear cells are moderately reduced in quantity, but tissue concentrations remain elevated for at least 5 years. Plasma cells are seen as a transient invader of endometrial tissue, disappearing in most patients 5 months after IUD insertion. Flushings of endometrial cavities with an IUD in place show increased numbers of inflammatory cells, as well as a high content of protein. These cells all represent a sterile, inflammatory reaction to the foreign body.

We have postulated that this sterile tissue reaction in the endometrial cavity is the main causative factor for the contraceptive effect of the IUD in the human female. This reaction is transitory so that when the IUD is removed the foreign body reaction ceases. The monthly incidence of conception in the first years after removal of an IUD is the same as that after stopping usage of condoms or diaphragm. At the end of one year, 90 per cent of those patients who wish to conceive have done so.

Several long-term studies have shown that there is no clinical evidence that the IUD causes an increased incidence of adenocarcinoma of the endometrium. Likewise, there is no evidence that the IUD causes an increased incidence of carcinoma of the cervix. In the Cooperative Statistical Program, the incidence of cervical carcinoma and carcinoma in situ in IUD users remained constant during the first 6 years after insertion of the IUD.

Because the IUD is not a perfect means of contraception, having a 2.5 per cent first year pregnancy rate and a 15 per cent first year removal rate for medical reasons, attempts have been made to improve the design and composition of the IUD's. There have been a few reports from individual clinics that one of the newer devices, the Dalkon shield, has lower failure or complication rates than the loop or double coil. Nevertheless, widespread epidemiological data for this device are unavailable. A recent multiclinic study indicates that the expulsion rate and medical removal rate for the Dalkon shield are lower than the rates for the loop, but the pregnancy incidence is higher, reaching 3.8 per cent in the first year.[19] Comparative studies using this device and the loop are currently under way, but thus far the evidence does not indicate that the Dalkon shield is significantly better than its plastic predecessors.

The most exciting development in IUD design is the T-shaped device originated by Tatum. The plastic T devices had a high pregnancy rate, but Zipper's discovery that the addition of copper wire was more effective in preventing pregnancy led to the development of the copper T. A comparative study of the TCu 200 and the Lippes loop indicated that copper T device has both a lower pregnancy rate and a lower removal rate for bleeding and pain.[22] The TCu 200 is especially suitable for nulliparous women in whom the removal rate is high for pain with other devices. The shape of the T, together with its ease of insertion, has provided the nulliparous woman with an effective alternative to the oral contraceptive steroids. A device of similar design, the copper 7, has pregnancy or complication rates similar to the TCu 200 and can also be used by the nulliparous woman.[23] Studies are being initiated with the plastic T in which progesterone and other agents are impregnated on the vertical arm in an effort to produce an IUD without side-effects. All these devices, including the copper T, will have to be removed at varying intervals, probably after one or more years' duration, as the metal or steroid is steadily released from the device.

Studies are also ongoing to develop new methods of steroidal and nonsteroidal contraceptives, such as subdermal Silastic implants and vaginal rings. Their availability for clinical usage is several years distant. The daily regime of a minidose of progestogen is associated with a relatively high incidence of irregular bleeding episodes and a pregnancy rate of 2 to 8 per cent per year. Thus, at the present time, the combination type of oral contraception and the IUD are the contraceptives of choice for most women. The less effective diaphragm, condom, and vaginal foam are optimal contraceptive methods for a minority of couples. In choosing a contraceptive for a patient the physician should state the advantages and disadvantages of each and allow the patient to choose the method she prefers, unless there is a definite medical contraindication. Women will then participate in the decision and will be better motivated to continue use of the contraceptive of choice. Continued use of any contraceptive technique is a more important factor in preventing unwanted pregnancy than the differences in effectiveness of the various contraceptive methods now available.

REFERENCES

1. Bernstein, G. S.: Clinical effectiveness of an aerosol contraceptive foam. Contraception 3:37, 1971.
2. Marshall, J.: A field of trial of the basal-body-temperature method of regulating births. Lancet 2:8, 1968.
3. Swyer, G. I. M., Sebok, L., and Barns, D. F.: Determination of the relative potency of some progestogens in the human. Proc. Soc. Med. 53:435, 1960.
4. Greenblatt, R. B.: Progestational agents in clinical practice. Med. Sci. 10:37, 1967.
5. Delforge, J. P., and Ferin, J.: A histometric study of two estrogens: ethinylestradiol and its 3-methyl-ether derivative (mestranol); their comparative effect upon the growth of the human endometrium. Contraception 1:57, 1970.
6. Heinen, G.: The discriminating use of combination and sequential preparations in the hormonal inhibition of ovulation. Contraception 4:393, 1971.
7. Diczfalusy, E.: Contraceptive steroids and their mechanism of action. In Diczfalusy, E., and Borell, U., eds:. Control of Human Fertility. Stockholm, Almqvist and Wiksell, 1971.
8. Feldman, J. G., and Lippes, J.: A four-year comparison between the utilization and use-effectiveness of sequential and combinal oral contraceptives. Contraception 3:93, 1971.
9. Metabolic effects of oral contraceptives. Lancet 2:783, 1969.
10. Stern, E., Clark, V. A., and Coffelt, C. F.: Contraceptives and dysplasia; higher rate for pill choosers. Science 169:493, 1970.
11. Spellacy, W. N., Zaias, N., Buhi, W. C., and Birk, S. A.: Vaginal yeast growth and contraceptive practices. Obstet. Gynec. 38:343, 1971.
12. Spellacy, W. N., Buki, M. S., and Birk, S. A.: The effect of estrogens on carbohydrate metabolism: glucose, insulin, and growth hormone studies on 171 women ingesting premarin, mestranol and ethinylestradiol for 6 months. Amer. J. Obstet. Gynec. 114:378, 1972.
13. Wynn, V., Doar, J. W. H., and Mills, G. L.: Some effects of oral contraceptives on serum-lipid and lipoprotein levels. Lancet 2:720, 1966.
14. Vessey, M. P., and Doll, R.: Investigation of relation between use of oral contraceptives and thromboembolic disease: a further report. Brit. Med. J. 2:651, 1969.
15. Sartwell, P. E., Masi, A. T., Arthes, F. G., Greene, G. R., and Smith, H. E.: Thromboembolism and oral contraceptives: an epidemiologic case-control study. Amer. J. Epidemiol. 90:365, 1969.
16. Hellman, L. M.: The oral contraceptives in clinical practice. Family Planning Perspectives 2:13, 1969.
17. Tietze, C., and Lewit, S.: Evaluation of intrauterine devices: ninth progress report of the Cooperative Statistical Program. Studies in Family Planning, No. 55, p. 1, July 1970.
18. Lewit, S.: Outcome of pregnancy with intrauterine devices. Contraception 2:47, 1970.
19. Snowden, R., and Williams, M.: The use-effectiveness of the Dalkon-shield in the United Kingdom. Contraception 7:91, 1973.
20. Mishell, D. R., Jr., Bell, J. H., Good, R. G., and Moyer, D. L.: The intrauterine device: a bacteriologic study of the endometrial cavity. Amer. J. Obstet. Gynec. 96:119, 1966.
21. Moyer, D. L., and Mishell, D. R., Jr.: Reactions of human endometrium to the intrauterine foreign body. II Long term effects on the endometrial histology and cytology. Amer. J. Obstet. Gynec. 111:66, 1971.
22. Tatum, H. J.: The first year of clinical experience with the copper T intrauterine contraceptive system in the United States and Canada. Contraception 6:179, 1972.
23. Bernstein, G. S., Israel, R., Seward, P., and Mishell, D. R., Jr.: Clinical experience with the Cu-7 intrauterine device. Contraception 6:99, 1972.

Preferable Medical and Surgical Methods of Conception Control

Surgical Sterilization in the Female

MAMDOUH MOUKHTAR and SEYMOUR L. ROMNEY

Albert Einstein College of Medicine and the
Bronx Municipal Hospital Center

The changing social, cultural, and economic trends, as well as greater awareness of ecology and the influence of overpopulation, have all resulted in a greater demand for methods of family planning. The trend has included increasing requests for permanent sterilization as a method of birth control. This evolution of thought has been shared equally by the medical community and the general population, as reflected in the changed prerequisites for sterilization recommended by The American College of Obstetricians and Gynecologists. In the Manual of Standards (1968), the criteria for voluntary sterilization were: (1) any woman 25 years of age who has or will have five living children at termination of the present pregnancy; (2) any woman 30 years of age who has or will have four living children with the present pregnancy; (3) any woman 35 years of age who has or will have three living children with the present pregnancy.[1] In August, 1970, The American College of Obstetricians and Gynecologists policy was changed, and the number of children a woman had was abolished as a relevant factor.[2] The procedure is now regarded as a medical decision to be carried out in the best interests of the health of the patient, as with any other surgical procedure. Informed consent of the patient and her husband is requested. Although a husband's consent is not legally required in a number of jurisdictions, physicians may guard against future legal action by securing the husband's consent whenever it can be reasonably obtained. It is further recommended that gynecological consultation, either by a single consultant or by the committee method, be obtained for these procedures. This last point has not been universally accepted by hospital services; the feeling being that the decision to undergo and perform sterilization involves only patient, her husband, and the surgeon. However, although not explicitly stated in the policy, it is implied that whenever vaginal hysterectomy is utilized for the purpose of sterilization, the skill and experience of the surgeon must be considered.

326

The management of sterilization in the female has thus become an important consideration for the obstetrician-gynecologist. The decision becomes a critical one because, at the present time, methods for sterilization in the female must be considered irreversible, notwithstanding the occasional claim to reversibility by some. The general use of hysterectomy solely for voluntary sterilization is to be criticized.

The approaches to definitive sterilization which have been employed involve abdominal or vaginal tubal ligation and abdominal or vaginal hysterectomy. More recently, endoscopic techniques are being utilized. The purpose of this discussion is to provide an overview of the general subject of surgical sterilization, including its controversial aspects, and to present guidelines that would appear to be medically sound and socially responsible.

MEDICAL INDICATION

Sterilization for medical indications has long been accepted. The critical issue in such cases is the selection of a method that will be safest for the patient with her particular disease. For example, a patient whose cardiac status is precarious should have the simplest sterilization procedure.

AGE, PARITY, AND FAMILY SIZE

While it is easier for the physician to reach the decision to perform sterilization in women in the late reproductive years, an evaluation of the unique circumstances of each patient should be the ultimate determining factor. For example, the number of previous pregnancies, family size desired, cultural influences, and personal preferences should be considered and thoroughly discussed in arriving at a decision. There are women who with their husbands have made a decision and want a two child family. In such circumstances, sterilization, regardless of age and parity, can be properly indicated and represents the patient's preference to this operation rather than being chained in long-term commitment to contraceptive techniques. When questions are raised as to the possibility of death of her husband or of existing children and how surgical sterilization might influence remarriage, the opinion frequently expressed by these women is that adoption is an acceptable alternative. Emotional maturity and judgment may be independent of chronologic age, and this is a critical issue for the physician to assess in the decision making process. Sterilization has long been acceptable for grand multiparas because of the increased risk of ruptured uterus, postpartum atony, and hemorrhage. In general, the availability and implementation of effective family planning programs have resulted in fewer grand multiparas. In large measure, this is related to the nature of the educational and counseling component received with the obstetric care both ante partum and post partum, as well as the availability of family planning services. When considering sterilization for grand multiparas, awareness that these patients have a greater incidence of pelvic pathology requires that the method selected be given more thought. This has been emphasized by follow-up studies which show a disproportionate number of grand multiparas having tubal ligations and needing subsequent surgery.[3,4] The obstetrician-gynecologist should not attempt to sit in judgment on the validity of a couple's decision to obtain sterilization on the basis of only an office visit or two. If there is ambivalence on the part of the physician or a genuine inability to accede to the couple's request for personal reasons, the couples should have the opportunity for additional counseling and consultation.

MARITAL STATUS

The changing status of women in society and the increasing awareness of their independence and rights has resulted in larger numbers of single women requesting sterilization. The decision to sterilize a woman, regardless of her marital status, must be based on a careful appraisal of her physical health, her emotional maturity, and her social circumstances. That desire and ability to become pregnant and to assume child rearing responsibilities are independent of marital status must be recognized. A reappraisal of the role of women in our culture is going on, with considerable evidence that the paternalistic, chauvinistic value system has been effectively challenged.

In summary, the functional control of a woman's fertility is independent of her age and marital status as long as she has a clear understanding of basic reproduction, anatomy, and physiology, and provided that she is well motivated and certain of her desire to undergo sterilization.

Demography of Sterilization

Campbell reported on a nationwide survey done in 1960 by the Scripps Foundation that 8 per cent of white American married women between the ages of 18 and 39 have had a procedure that rendered them sterile.[5] Approximately 50 per cent of these were for the express purpose of preventing pregnancy, with the other 50 per cent becoming sterile secondary to being treated for other pathology. It is estimated that approximately 180,000 sterilizing operations are performed each year, involving approximately 1 per cent of the 19 million married women between the ages of 18 and 39. Another indication of the frequency of sterilization was provided by Starr and Kosasky, who reported a nationwide instance of approximately 3.2 per cent for puerperal sterilization.[6] Moore and Russell, comparing the number of sterilization procedures to number of deliveries, found an incidence of 1.6 per cent in four hospitals in Los Angeles.[7] This study was completed 9 years ago, and undoubtedly the number of sterilization procedures performed has increased considerably since then. Lang and Richardson, in the United Kingdom, reported more than a doubling of the rate of sterilization compared to deliveries, from 1.0 per cent in 1962 to 2.4 per cent in 1966.[4] With liberalized abortion laws and adequate counseling in family planning, an increasing segment of women of lower socioeconomic status have learned of the existence and safety of permanent surgical sterilization, and also that such procedures do not interfere with their sexuality. A note of caution is indicated because there is the inclination to combine abortion with sterilization, with an unfortunate increase in morbidity rates in two essentially safe procedures.[8]

Methods and Selection of Procedures

In present gynecological practice, surgical techniques are the generally accepted methods of sterilization. These include (1) tubal sterilization, either abdominal or vaginal, (2) hysterectomy, abdominal or vaginal, and (3) oophorectomy. Oophorectomy is not acceptable as a primary surgical procedure for sterilization. Wood and Leeton recently advocated ovariotexy as a method of temporary sterilization.[9] However, since a sterilization procedure should not be considered anything but permanent, the need for such procedure must be very limited. Review of the literature reveals that obstetrician-gynecologists are still far from forming a consensus about the best method of achieving sterilization. Certain guidelines may help in deciding which methods would be more applicable and have the best results. The considerations to be noted are: (1) the method must be safe and generally require no specialized skills outside the surgical competence of a well-trained gynecologist; (2) it must be effective as a method of sterilization and the incidence of failure and complications must be lower than with any other procedure; (3) the procedure must have no long-term complications, either physical or psychological.

TUBAL STERILIZATION

It is our contention that in the absence of pelvic pathology, the safest and best method of achieving sterilization is by tubal surgery. The failure rate of various procedures involving tubal surgery is remarkably low. With careful safeguards to avoid the known pitfalls of inadvertently mistaking the round ligament for the fallopian tube, and with diligent selection of cases suitable for ligation, these procedures approach the ideal as methods of permanent sterilization. The criticisms which have been directed against tubal sterilization are: (1) there is a small but definite number of failures; (2) large numbers of patients with tubal sterilization develop subsequent gynecologic problems which require surgery; (3) if the uterus is left behind, bereft of its reproductive function, there is needless exposure of the patient to the risk of cervical or endometrial carcinoma or other uterine pathology.

The long-term follow-up of patients with tubal sterilization does not, on the whole, validate these criticisms. However, the criticisms leveled fail to consider the comparative risks of ligation and hysterectomy, nor do they take into account the psychological impact of hysterectomy in some women. We will therefore review these reservations about tubal surgery.

FAILURE OF TUBAL STERILIZATION.   That pregnancy can occur after tubal

TABLE 10–1. *Tubal Ligation Failures**

TECHNIQUE	NUMBER	PER CENT FAILURE
Madlener	7829	1.44
Cornual resection	311	2.89
Pomeroy	5477	0.4
Irving	1056	0.0

* From Garb, A. E.: A review of tubal sterilization failures. Obstet. Gynec. Surv. 12: 291–305, 1957.

sterilization is well known. However, the incidence of such failure is not widely known.

Lee and associates reported 1169 tubal sterilizations, with an overall 1 per cent failure rate. All the failures were in patients in whom the Madlener technique was employed. These authors report a failure rate of 2 per cent for tubal ligation at the time of cesarean section.[11]

The high incidence of failure at the time of cesarean section was also reported by Prystowsky and Eastman, who reported that the Pomeroy technique, performed at the time of hysterotomy and cesarean section, had a failure rate of 1 in 57, compared to 1 in 340 for puerperal sterilization.[12]

Boyson and McRae suggested that the puerperal state per se may be a factor in many of the tubal ligation failures, and that failures are solely the result of the technique employed.[34] Briefly, the causes of failure may be related to:

1. Error in technique.
   a. Error in identification, such as mistaking the round ligament for the fallopian tube.
   b. Incomplete resection of tube.
   c. Use of nonabsorbable suture ligature and ligation under tension, which can facilitate the formation of new canal.
2. Employment of the Madlener technique at the time of cesarean section or hysterotomy.

Lee and associates found no difference in the failure rate between abdominal and vaginal tubal ligation.[11]

It is prudent to submit the excised tube for pathological examination and have definite proof that the tube had been properly identified and resected.

NEED FOR SUBSEQUENT SURGERY AND DEVELOPMENT OF UTERINE PATHOLOGY AFTER TUBAL STERILIZATION. The answer to questions about these sequelae must be discerned from long-term follow-up of a large number of cases. Lu and Chun,[13] in a long-term study of 1055 cases of puerperal tubal sterilization performed in Hong Kong in the 6 year period from 1957 to 1962 inclusive, reported patient follow-up for periods varying from 3 to 8 years. They noted the following:

1. *Pelvic Pathology.* At follow-up examination, hydrosalpinx or peritubal adhesion was suspected in 5.9 per cent of patients because of clinical evidence of thickening and small tender masses with slight fixity. None required operative treatment.

2. *Menstrual Changes.* Some menstrual changes were noted in 51.8 per cent of patients, involving either length of the cycle, duration of the flow, or amount of blood loss. However, most of the changes were of mild degree. Menorrhagia of such severity to require hysterectomy was observed in only four patients.

3. *Patient Satisfaction.* Of the 1055 patients, 98.7 per cent (1041 women) were pleased that they had had the operation; 1.3 per cent (14 patients) were not. Eleven of the 14 dissatisfied patients thought their minor disturbances were a result of the sterilization operation. Two women had an ectopic pregnancy subsequent to the sterilization procedure. One patient, who was 32 years old and had seven children, remarried and regretted having been sterilized.

SUBSEQUENT DEVELOPMENT OF CERVICAL OR ENDOMETRIAL CARCINOMA. The incidence of positive smears (0.06 per cent) in this group was lower than the incidence of carcinoma in situ in well women reported by Kaiser (0.25 per cent) and Boyes (0.56 per cent), respectively. Thus, the incidence of carci-

noma in situ in this study does not differ from that of healthy women and gynecological patients in general.

LONG-TERM FOLLOW-UP

A different perspective is obtained from reviewing other long-term follow-
up studies. Muldon in Dundee, Scotland, studied 374 patients for at least 10 years
after postpartum tubal ligation. He found that 43 per cent of the patients required
further gynecological treatment. Major surgery was needed by 25 per cent (70
patients). When these 70 patients were reviewed separately, it was noted that
50 of them were grand multiparas (gravida 5 or more). Fifteen women had previously been subjected to repeat cesarean section and tubal sterilization at the time
of the last section and three were sterilized at hysterotomy. Of the 22 patients
requiring repair of prolapse, 20 had had four or more confinements. This study
emphasizes that most patients requiring additional major surgery were either grand
multiparas, with five or more pregnancies, or had surgical wounds in the uterus,
either from cesarean section or hysterotomy.[3] The fact that there is a high incidence of subsequent hysterectomy in patients with a previous history of repeat
cesarean section has been noted by many.[16,17,18] Weed (1959) found that 14 per
cent of his patients who had had a cesarean section ultimately underwent hysterectomy.[19] Montague (1959) and Plesch and Sandberg (1963) have suggested
that patients who have had several cesarean sections and now wish to be sterilized
should have elective cesarean hysterectomy in their last pregnancy.[17,18,19] It
would seem reasonable that, in considering sterilization for patients with high
parity, careful evaluation be given to the menstrual history. In patients with a
history of menorrhagia, hysterectomy should be carefully considered as a more
suitable method of sterilization. If there is evidence of prolapse, vaginal hysterectomy with colporrhaphy after the puerperium is the method of choice.

The occurrence of five cases of cervical carcinoma, of which three were
in situ and two were invasive,[3] emphasizes the importance of careful annual
cytologic screening in such patients and the need for cervical cytologic studies
prior to surgery. The hospitalization experience should be used effectively to
educate these patients of the need for a yearly check-up and cytologic screening.

In summary, whenever there is coexistent pelvic pathology, history of
menorrhagia, repeat cesarean section, and high parity, and the patient is over age
35, one ought to consider more extensive surgery, provided that it is safe for the
particular patient being evaluated.

Puerperal Sterilization

TUBAL STERILIZATION—PUERPERAL ABDOMINAL STERILIZATION

This is by far the most widely used, most convenient, and safest method of
puerperal sterilization. It can be done under local or general anesthesia.[20]

Lee and colleagues found that the day on which postpartum sterilization
was carried out had no significant effect on the morbidity rate during the puerperium.[11] The chief advantage of early postpartum ligation is the shortening of
hospitalization time. Nearly all the procedures are performed within the first 24

hours post partum. Although the incidence of failure is slightly higher than in the interval procedure, the convenience of a shorter hospital stay and the avoidance of two hospital admissions far outweigh any gain that might be had through lowering the failure rate.

The most widely used method is the Pomeroy technique. Other operative techniques have been described that attempt to cut down the failure rate. The Irving technique has had no failures, but it requires longer operating time and more attention to detail. Uchida reports a technique bearing his name that has been used in 5000 cases without a failure.[21] By the Uchida technique the serosal surface of the tube is dissected from the body of the tube by injecting a saline-epinephrine solution between the serosa and the tube. This causes a ballooning of the mesosalpinx, which is then incised. The tube is then pulled through the incision and incised; approximately 5 cm. of the proximal limb is excised and ligated with chromic catgut. This remaining proximal limb is allowed to fall back into the balloon. The distal end of the tube is then "purse-stringed" with the serosa so that it projects into the abdominal cavity.

A third method, virtually unknown in this country, is the Oxford technique, described by Stallworthy.[22]

This consists of dividing the tube and mesosalpinx and ligating the cut ends. Number 1 chromic catgut is used on the proximal end of the divided tube and linen thread on the distal end. Both ligatures are left long. The uterine end of the tube is then buried beneath the round ligaments by threading the uncut catgut suture beneath the round ligaments forward from behind. The distal end of the tube, which has been ligated with thread, is then tied with this same catgut in front of the round ligament. The use of catgut on the proximal end of the divided tube is a modification of the technique described earlier. The reason for this is that it has been claimed that if both ends are tied with nonabsorbable sutures, there is an increased danger of recanalization of the tubes. This has been used successfully to support a claim for compensation when pregnancy followed the operation of tubal ligation, though not by the technique described here. The author has no knowledge of pregnancy occurring after this technique has been used. Nonetheless, expert evidence called in support of the plaintiff's claim maintained that most of the recorded instances of pregnancy following tubal ligation had occurred when nonabsorbable sutures were used and for this reason stated that it was negligent for a surgeon to continue to use this type of material. Substantial damages were agreed out of court. The modification of operative technique described above seems wise and removes any possibility of canalization occurring between the two ends of the divided tube.[22]

Whenever the tubal sterilization is performed, the ovaries should be inspected. Several cases of ovarian pathology, dermoids, or other ovarian neoplasms have thus been discovered and treated. There is certainly no justification for the use of the Madlener or cornuectomy procedures, since both are followed by much higher failure rates than the technically easier Pomeroy method.

MORBIDITY AND MORTALITY.   Lu and Chun, studying 5944 cases, reported no mortality directly attributable to the procedure.[13] There were no complications in 96.6 per cent of cases. Pyrexia was noted in 2 per cent, and wound infection in 2.9 per cent.[13]

Lee and associates, in their group of 1169 cases, again noted no deaths attributable directly to the sterilization. The morbidity rate was 9 per cent. However, their reported morbidity involving 430 postpartum patients in a controlled study during the same period was 10.2 per cent.[11] Of a series of 1830 patients studied by Prystowsky and Eastman, two women died of pulmonary embolism, a death rate of 0.3 per cent.[12] These latter two series were done between 1926 and 1950. The morbidity figures now are much lower, as shown by Lu and Chun,[13] owing to advances in surgical sciences.

CESAREAN HYSTERECTOMY

Cesarean section followed by immediate hysterectomy has been advocated as a method of sterilization. In a major report on the subject, encompassing 1000 consecutive operations in patients with one or more cesarean sections, hemorrhage was found to occur in 5.9 per cent of cases, and bladder and ureteral injury were noted in 4.2 per cent and 0.4 per cent, respectively. Miscellaneous complications totaled 1.5 per cent and involved bowel injuries, blood transfusion reactions, and anesthesia complications. Postoperative bleeding, mainly from the ovarian pedicle, which required additional surgery occurred in 1.5 per cent, while 47 patients developed pelvic hematomas or pelvic abscesses requiring vaginal drainage. In the elective group of 600 patients, which included 269 patients who had a cesarean hysterectomy for the purpose of sterilization alone, there were four deaths.[23] The complication rate for the 269 was not listed separately but undoubtedly was lower than in the group; however, one unfortunate death resulted from a transfusion reaction.

Schneider and Tyrone reported 220 cases of cesarean hysterectomy, 191 of which were private patients and 29 nonprivate patients. Their reported morbidity rate was 8.2 per cent in the private patients and 32 per cent in the nonprivate patients. Thirty-two per cent of the private patients and 62 per cent of the ward patients required blood transfusions.[24]

It is difficult to justify cesarean hysterectomy for the sole purpose of sterilization. Certainly the cases must be selected carefully. Undoubtedly on occasion the future welfare of a patient requiring a cesarean section would best be served by immediate hysterectomy.

Elective Interval Sterilization

ABDOMINAL APPROACH

ABDOMINAL TUBAL STERILIZATION.   This is the most commonly used form of interval tubal sterilization, although its preeminence has been challenged by the introduction of various other techniques—e.g., laparoscopy, vaginal tubal ligation, and sterilization through vaginal culdoscopy. Its main advantage is the technical ease with which it can be done and the very small number of complications encountered. The main drawback is that, as in any laparotomy, patients require longer hospitalization than when the vaginal approach is used. The procedures are essentially the same as for puerperal sterilization.

LAPAROSCOPIC CAUTERIZATION.   This method has been given wide publicity recently, perhaps more than is warranted.[25-29] A critical approach to this operation is necessary; in spite of its claimed advantages of having the clinical benefits associated with minor operations, it is not a minor operation. It requires specialized training and, even in more experienced hands, there are still a small number of serious complications. Unrecognized bowel injury is by far the most alarming, other effects being hemorrhage and cauterization of the round ligament. In the Johns Hopkins series, there were five cases of unrecognized bowel injury which were later diagnosed on the fifth postoperative day.[30] Its advocates have stated that an advantage of the procedure is that it can be performed on an ambulatory basis. This is a dangerous misconception, since the procedure should be done in a fully equipped operating room and careful follow-up is essential. There have been several dramatic complications when laparoscopic cauterization was attempted by less experienced operators—e.g., perforation of the external iliac artery and transection of bowel. Laparoscopy is contraindicated in (1) obese women; (2) women with serious cardiac or respiratory problems[31]; (3) patients with acute or chronic pelvic inflammatory disease or in whom there is suspicion of intraperitoneal adhesions.

Another disadvantage is that simple cauterization of the tube is more likely to be followed by recanalization and thus failure to achieve sterility. Gutierrez-Najar reported five failures in eight cases of cauterization through operative culdoscopy.[32] The incidence of failure associated with this procedure will only become clearer after patients treated by this technique have had long-term follow-up.

VAGINAL TUBAL STERILIZATION

INTERVAL VAGINAL TUBAL STERILIZATION.   Von Graff was the first to recommend vaginal tubal sterilization in 1930.[33] The first report on this technique was by Boyson and McRae in 1948; results in 169 patients showed almost no morbidity, and no additional surgical procedure was performed. The reduction in hospital stay was a significant advantage. When the procedure was combined with therapeutic abortion, however, the results were much less favorable.[34] The next report in the literature which involved 100 cases of vaginal tubal ligation, was not published until 1966 (Fort and Alexander).[35] Thus it is apparent that the procedure had not received wide acceptance, in large part because of the unfamiliarity of many gynecologists with the vaginal approach. This is regrettable, since our experiences, as well as those of others, have shown the procedure to be safe and technically easy. This reluctance is more surprising in view of the trend towards advocating vaginal hysterectomy as being safer than abdominal hysterectomy. No published reports have favored abdominal hysterectomy for sterilization, but several have endorsed vaginal hysterectomy for this purpose.[36,37,38]

Recently, several papers have appeared advocating vaginal Pomeroy sterilization. McMaster and Ansari reported 90 cases,[39] and Laufe and Summerson, 263 cases from Pennsylvania.[11] Smith and Symmonds reported on vaginal fimbriectomy; in addition, our experience at Utah involving an unpublished series of 273 cases of vaginal Pomeroy operations is reviewed (see Table 10–2). The higher incidence of technical failure observed in the Utah series occurred because the procedure was performed by a large number of operators, only a few of whom had adequate experience with the vaginal approach.

All of the major complications occurred postoperatively, in the first 48 hours. Patients without complications were safely discharged on the third postoperative day. Vaginal tubal sterilization has also been employed in conjunction

TABLE 10–2. *Complications of Transvaginal Tubal Ligation*

	NUMBER	PER CENT
Pennsylvania series:		
Total number	263	
Technical failure	3	1.1
Minor complications	18	6.8
Febrile response		
Genitourinary infection		
Early P.I.D.		
Major complications	4	1.4
P.I.D. sequelae	3	
Cuff hemorrhage	1	
Utah series:		
Total number	273	
Technical failure	8	2.4
Minor complications	4	1.2
Bleeding from cervix	1	
Bleeding from vaginal edge	2	
Inadvertent opening of rectum	1	
Major complications	4	1.2
Pelvic hematoma	1	
Exacerbation of P.I.D.	3	
Failure (pregnancy)	1	0.3

with early pregnancy termination by suction curettage. In Sogolow's series, there was a 1.1 per cent incidence of technical failure, a 1.4 per cent major complications rate, and an overall morbidity rate of 8.2 per cent.[42] Boyson and McRae's experience with vaginal sterilization at the time of termination of pregnancy showed a much higher number of complications, and these authors advise against it.[34] We concur with Boyson and McRae that there is no need to increase the rates of morbidity and complications by attempting vaginal tubal sterilization in puerperal and postabortal patients.

In our experience, vaginal tubal ligation as an interval method in carefully selected cases is preferable to abdominal interval tubal ligation. This procedure has the following advantages: (1) it is shorter, and hence there is a more economical hospital stay; (2) there is less postoperative pain; (3) there are minimal postanesthetic chest and other complications. The experience gained in this approach is desirable for residents during training because it increases their competence in vaginal surgery. The prerequisites for a safe and successful vaginal tubal ligation are: (1) a free Douglas pouch; (2) a mobile uterus (previous cesarean section does not preclude the vaginal route if the uterus is freely mobile); (3) the absence of evidence of pelvic inflammatory disease. On the average, in less than 3 per cent of cases there is failure to visualize both tubes. This percentage diminishes with increasing experience and proper selection of cases.

OPERATIVE CULDOSCOPY. Clyman[43] has reported on 4000 cases having fewer than 0.1 per cent complications and indicates that the main advantage of this technique is that it can be an office procedure. Among the advantages are: there is no need for an operating room, no abdominal scarring, no need for general anesthesia, no tissue cauterization, and no need for intraperitoneal insufflation. The principal disadvantage of culdoscopic sterilization is that it is technically difficult to learn and carry out. This has been proved by the fact that 50 per cent of Clyman's trainees have discontinued using the procedure. Heavy sedation is used preoperatively, as well as paracervical block plus local anesthetic infiltration of the posterior vaginal fornix. After the culdoscope is introduced, a straight 8 inch hemostat is used to enlarge the opening to approximately 1 inch. Under direct visualization, the fallopian tubes are grasped with the 8 inch hemostat and brought down into the vagina through the culpotomy, and a Pomeroy steriliza- tion is carried out. Further refinement in the technique has been made through the use of tantalum clips to occlude the fallopian tubes without bringing them down. However, the failure rate with the clip method has still to be evaluated by follow-up.[43]

INTERVAL HYSTERECTOMY

It is difficult to support those who recommend and perform hysterectomy as an elective procedure for sterilization. Whether performed abdominally or vaginally, regardless of the surgical skill, the risks to the patient, of both mor- bidity and mortality, are significantly greater with hysterectomy than with tubal ligation. While the average qualified gynecologic surgeon might be prepared to believe he could perform either abdominal or vaginal hysterectomy with little or no operative risk, in reality the procedure must be classified as a major surgical procedure. Moreover, national statistics gathered by the Commission on Profes- sional and Hospital Activities (PAS) reveal a mortality of 0.16 per cent. If it is additionally noted that 33 per cent of the women had postoperative fever, 15 per cent required blood transfusions, 48 per cent were given antibiotics, and that the average hospital stay was 10.3 days, our contention is upheld that hysterec- tomy for the sole purpose of sterilization is rarely justifiable.

It is quite another matter to employ hysterectomy when there is estab- lished pelvic pathology in a multiparous woman, over 35 years of age, who is seeking a permanent method of sterilization. When the woman has vaginal relaxa- tion, incontinence, fibroids, or a history of menorrhagia and repeat cesarean sec- tion, hysterectomy and the assumption of surgical risk by the patient become acceptable.

VAGINAL HYSTERECTOMY

Studies of large series of vaginal hysterectomies in younger women have shown a definitely higher incidence of complications and an increased morbidity rate. Pratt, using his own series of 1000 cases, concluded that vaginal hysterec- tomy produces more complications in younger patients than it usually does in older patients. Postoperative bleeding requiring additional surgery occurred three times as often in younger women compared to older women (3.6 per cent and 1.2 per cent, respectively). Postoperative hematoma occurred in 5.4 per cent in younger women, compared to 2.0 per cent in older women. The need for blood transfusions was also three times greater in younger than in older women, and there were comparable findings for postoperative pyrexia. Two recent reports are available on vaginal hysterectomy employed for elective sterilization. Atkinson and Chappell[37] studied 115 patients whose operations were performed by 9 fully trained gynecologists and reported postoperative pyrexia in 29.6 per cent of cases. Among four patients who required blood transfusions, two pelvic hemotomas

TABLE 10–3.   *Complications of Vaginal Hysterectomy for Elective Sterilization*

COMPLICATION	NUMBER OF PATIENTS
Pelvic hematoma or abscess	7
Vaginal cuff cellulitis	2
Bleeding corpus luteum cyst	1
Pyelonephritis	1
Repaired cystotomy	1
Death (brain stem infarction)	1
Bacteriuria	2
Pneumonia	1

were encountered. One of their patients sustained a bladder injury, which was repaired at the time of surgery. The incidence of major postoperative complications was 11 per cent.

There was one postoperative death, as a result of unrecognized electrolyte imbalance and hypercalcemia in a patient with a parathyroid adenoma.[37] It is pertinent to stress that this paper involved patients who were cared for at a regional Air Force base by fully trained gynecologists. Despite these favorable factors, the morbidity and mortality rates are still very significant. Van Nagell and Roddick[38] reported their experience with 100 patients who underwent vaginal hysterectomy for elective sterilization. The qualifications of those who performed the surgery are not known. In addition, their controls, women who underwent puerperal sterilization, showed a higher incidence of complications than is generally reported in literature. In this series, an overall morbidity of 22 per cent was reported, including two pelvic hematomas, one bladder injury, 11 cases of vaginal cuff cellulitis, and one case of "technical difficulty," in which the patient required two units of blood replacement.[38]

Thus, the cumulative evidence to date indicates that vaginal hysterectomy in women under the age of 35 years, in the absence of pelvic pathology, is not a valid or desirable substitute for tubal sterilization.

Summary and Conclusions

Elective surgical sterilization, as a patient's ultimate choice of a method of family planning, is a relatively simple and safe procedure. If done abdominally post partum, morbidity is minimal and the hospital stay need not be prolonged. Interval elective sterilization is also a safe and simple procedure. Provided that the surgeon has sufficient operative skill, the vaginal approach has advantages over the abdominal laparotomy method. Recent developments include efforts to perform sterilization by either laparoscopic or culdoscopic techniques. These methods require specialized training and experience, and in the series reported to date, significant complications have been encountered. The long-range efficacy and sequelae of these techniques will only be determined with the passage of time.

Hysterectomy has a limited place in gynecology when its primary goal is surgical sterilization. In multiparous patients seeking sterilization, who are 35 years of age or over, whose pregnancies have been terminated by cesarean section, or who have had previous reconstructive uterine surgery, hysterectomy can be the method of choice. This is especially true if the patients have menorrhagia or symptomatic pelvic relaxations. Elective hysterectomy, abdominal or vaginal, solely for sterilization in an otherwise asymptomatic woman is difficult to justify. The morbidity and mortality risks are significant in the best of hands. However, whenever surgical sterilization is being considered, the patient's emotional and psychologic status should be reviewed.

REFERENCES

1. American College of Obstetricians and Gynecologists: Manual of Standards, 1968.
2. American College of Obstetricians and Gynecologists: Manual of Standards. 1968.
3. Muldon, M. J.: Gynecological illness after sterilization. Brit. Med. J. *1*:84, 1972.
4. Lang, L. P., and Richardson, K. D.: The implications of a rising female sterilization rate. J. Obstet. Gynec. Brit. Comm. 75:972, 1968.
5. Campbell, A. A.: The incidence of operations that prevent conception. Amer. J. Obstet Gynec. *89*:694, 1964.
6. Starr, S. H., and Kosasky, H. J.: Puerperal sterilization. Amer. J. Obstet. Gynec. *88*:944, 1964.
7. Moore, J. G., and Russell, K. P.: Maternal medical indications for female sterilization. Clin. Obstet. Gynec. 7:54, 1964.
8. Schulman, H.: Major surgery for abortion and sterilization. Obstet. Gynec. *40*:738, 1972.
9. Wood, C., Leeton, J.: Sterilization by Ovariotexy: A Reversible Technique. Lancet *2*:1213, 1969.
10. Garb, A.: A review of tubal sterilization failures. Obstet. Gynec. Surv. *12*:291, 1957.
11. Lee, J. G., Randall, J. H., and Keetel, W. C.: Tubal sterilization; a review of 1169 cases. Amer. J. Obstet Gynec. *62*:568, 1951.
12. Prystowsky, H., and Eastman, N. J.: Puerperal tubal sterilization; report of 1830 cases. J.A.M.A. *158*:463, 1955.
13. Lu, T., and Chun, D.: A long-term follow-up study of 1055 cases of postpartum tubal ligation. J. Obstet. Gynec. Brit. Comm. 74:875, 1967.
14. Kaiser, R. F., Bouser, M. M., Ingraham, S. C., and Hilberg, A. W.: Uterine cytology. Publ. Health Rep. (Wash.) 75:423, 1960.
15. Boyes, D. A., Fidler, H. K., and Lock, D. R.: Significance of in situ carcinoma of the uterine cervix. Brit. Med. J. *1*:203, 1962.
16. Williams, E. L., Jones, H. E., and Merrill, R. E.: The subsequent course of patients sterilized by tubal ligation. Amer. J. Obstet. Gynec. *61*:423, 1951.
17. Pletsch, D. T., and Sandberg, E. G.: Cesarean hysterectomy for sterilization. Amer. J. Obstet. Gynec. 85:254, 1963.
18. Montague, C. F.: Cesarean hysterectomy: its value as a sterilization procedure. Obstet. Gynec. *14*:28, 1959.
19. Weed, J. C.: The fate of the postcesarean uterus. Obstet. Gynec. *14*:780, 1959.
20. Munson, A. K., and Scott, J. R.: Postpartum tubal ligation under local anesthesia. Obstet. Gynec. *39*:756, 1972.
21. Uchida, H.: Tubal sterilization with technique report (23,000 Cases). Proc. Third World Congr. Obstet. Gynec. *1*:26, 1961.
22. Stallworthy, J.: Abortion. *In* Claye, A., and Bourne, A., eds.: British Obstetrical and Gynaecological Practice. 3rd ed. London, Heinemann, 1963.
23. Barclay, D. L.: Cesarean hysterectomy at The Charity Hospital in New Orleans—1000 consecutive operations. Clin. Obstet. Gynec. *12*:635, 1969.
24. Schneider, G. T., and Tyrone, C. H.: Cesarean hysterectomy. Surg. Gynec. Obstet. *130*:501, 1970.
25. Steptoe, P. C.: Laparoscopy in Gynecology. Edinburgh, E. & S. Livingstone, 1967.
26. Steptoe, P. C.: Recent advances in surgical methods of control of fertility and infertility. Brit. Med. Bull. 26:60, 1970.
27. Cohen, M. R., Taylor, M. B., and Kass, M. B.: Internal tubal sterilization via laparoscopy. Amer. J. Obstet. Gynec. *108*:458, 1970.
28. Black, W. P.: Sterilization by laparoscopic tubal electrocoagulation: an assessment. Amer. J. Obstet. Gynec. *111*:979, 1971.

29. Wheeles, C. R.: An effective, safe, inexpensive method of female sterilization. Reprod. Med. 5:255, 1969.
30. Jones, Howard, W., Jr.: Obstet. Gynec. Surv. 27:384, 1972.
31. Hodgson, C., McClelland, R. M. A., and Newton, J. R.: Some effects of the peritoneal insufflation of carbon dioxide at laparoscopy. Anesthesia 25:382, 1970.
32. Gutierrez-Najar, A. J.: Culdoscopy as an aid to family planning. In Duncan, G. W., ed.: Female Sterilization. New York, Academic Press, 1972.
33. Von Graff, E.: Tubal sterilization by the Madlener technique. Amer. J. Obstet. Gynec. 28:295, 1939.
34. Boyson, H., and McRae, L. A.: Tubal sterilization through the vagina. Amer. J. Obstet. Gynec. 58:488, 1949.
35. Fort, A. T., and Alexander, A. M.: Vaginal Pomeroy sterilization—a description of technique; a review of 100 Cases. Obstet. Gynec. 28:421, 1966.
36. Copenhaver, E. H.: Vaginal hysterectomy. Amer. J. Obstet. Gynec. 84:123, 1962.
37. Atkinson, S. M., and Chappell, S. M.: Vaginal hysterectomy for sterilization. Obstet. Gynec. 39:759, 1972.
38. Van Nagell, J. R., and Roddick, J. W.: Vaginal hysterectomy as a sterilization procedure. Amer. J. Obstet. Gynec. 111:703, 1971.
39. McMaster, R. H., and Ansari, A. H.: Vaginal tubal ligation. Obstet. Gynec. 38:44, 1971.
40. Smith, R. A., and Symmonds, R. F.: Vaginal salpingectomy (fibroidectomy) for sterilization. Obstet. Gynec. 38:400, 1971.
41. Laufe, L. E., and Summerson, S.: Internal vagina tubal ligation. In Duncan, G. W., ed.: Female Sterilization. New York, Academic Press, 1972.
42. Sogolow, S. R.: Vaginal tubal ligation at time of vacuum curettage for abortion. Obstet. Gynec. 38:888, 1971.
43. Clyman, M. J.: Tubal sterilization by operative culdoscopy. In Duncan, G. W., ed.: Female Sterilization. New York, Academic Press, 1972.
44. Pratt, J. H., and Galloway, J. R.: Vaginal hysterectomy in patients less than 36 or more than 60 yrs. of age. Amer. J. Obstet. Gynec. 93:812, 1965.

Preferable Medical and Surgical Methods of Conception Control

Editorial Comment

Despite the phenomenal advances made, the perfect method for conception control remains to be developed. What may be an acceptable and reasonably effective method in an industrialized or so-called developed country may prove unworkable in a less privileged or developing country. Because the undeveloped countries outnumber the developed by a wide margin, we are faced with a dilemma in the problem of restricting the numbers of people that this planet can accommodate. It can be expressed also in the ageless question, "What is the purpose for which humanity lives?" Moreover, in some countries more and more younger women—in their 20's—are requesting permanent sterilization. Thus the physician is confronted with a situation where the old adage applies: whatever else, do no harm.

In determining the methods to be recommended or prescribed for conception control, all the contributors agree that the patient should be treated in a highly individualized manner and subject to follow-up. All too often some form of birth control is dispensed without a history having been taken or a physical examination performed. It has been amply documented that a family history for certain diseases that presumably have a genetic background, such as diabetes mellitus and essential hypertension occurring rather early in life, is a contraindication to oral steroid contraception. Further, it must be recognized that medical methods described here may not be applicable to patients with certain diseases—for example, the patient with cardiac disease. The pill may increase extracellular fluid volume and thus burden the heart, whereas the intrauterine device could invite intrauterine infection, from which might come a bacterial endocarditis. Although much has been learned of their overall metabolic effects on the user, the long-term effects of various steroids contained in the pill have not been fully evaluated.

The intrauterine device appears to be reasonably effective, at least initially, for some 75 to 85 per cent of women. The method has limitations, however, and the complications can be serious. The spontaneous expulsion rate, the therapeutic failure rate, and the patients' common complaints of discomfort and excessive bleeding restrict this method's popular appeal.

A recent experience might serve to indicate the vagaries of the IUD and lend support to some of the statements made here. This concerns a patient with several children who sought help, being about 8 to 10 weeks pregnant despite the presence of an IUD. Pain and bleeding led to examination under anesthesia. The IUD could not be readily removed at the time. However, the threatened abortion was completed surgically. Uterine exploration indicated that the IUD was located in the area of the right cornu of the uterus. It appeared fixed beneath the endometrium, which undoubtedly accounted for its therapeutic failure. An attempt to remove the IUD with reasonable firmness failed and it was elected to permit the patient to have one or more periods and then return for a vaginal hysterectomy and plastic repair. The patient had a first degree procidentia and a history of stress incontinence.

Subsequently, at the time of operation, the appendage of the IUD was not encountered and it was assumed at the moment that the device had been expelled. However, on opening the peritoneum, the IUD was revealed beneath the peritoneal serosa overlying the fundus of the uterus. The uterus revealed no evident area of perforation on either gross or histological examination. In retrospect, we realize that if the IUD had been elsewhere in the abdomen, the assumption undoubtedly would have been made that it had been expelled, an erroneous conclusion. Although it is perhaps impractical in lieu of the numbers that are expelled, it might be suggested that whenever expulsion occurs or is thought to occur, a scout film of the abdomen is indicated.

The question is posed whether the intrauterine device should be removed in the event that pregnancy occurs. Often the appendage is not accessible, and hence the IUD cannot be readily removable. If the pregnancy is free of symptoms and presumably progressing normally, the device is probably best left in situ, depending somewhat on the patient's desires. However, should bleeding and cramps develop, consideration should be given to removing the IUD and terminating the pregnancy. Certainly, the risk of infection is real. It is the opinion of the editors that when fever develops and infection is apparent, it is mandatory that the device be removed. In our experience, intrauterine infection can move rapidly in this circumstance, with the sudden appearance of endotoxic shock and, in the extreme, disseminated intravascular clotting. This seems to be especially true when the intrauterine shield is used, and one wonders whether lethal organisms are being sequestered in the areas covered by the shield. To repeat, in the presence of a threatened abortion, it is recommended that the IUD be removed and the pregnancy terminated forthwith.

The recommendations for hysterectomy as a form of sterilization have been extended beyond its initial restrictions to selected cases at the time of cesarean section. In any series of cesarean hysterectomies a certain percentage of cases fall into this category (see Chapter 11). One of the contributors advocates abdominal hysterectomy in the early postpartum period in lieu of tubal sterilization, which perhaps represents the extreme approach to surgical conception control. The preliminary results compare favorably to those of interval hysterectomy (performed at a later time). Several series have reported vaginal hysterectomy as the preferred method of sterilization. The proponents of hysterectomy reason that patients who have tubal ligation will develop gynecological complaints in a fair percentage of instances, which may eventually require hysterectomy anyway. It may well be that the complication rate of hysterectomy in association with primary cesarean section will not exceed that of hysterectomy in a nonpregnant patient. However, in individuals who had had previous cesarean sections, in which the situation is compounded by extensive adhesions, the operating time is extended, the blood loss is greater, and the urinary tract complication rate is higher compared to results that would be obtained with a subsequent hysterectomy on a nonpregnant organ. Nor is there any question that tubal ligation at the time of cesarean section or immediately following pelvic delivery carries a lower morbidity rate, and the rare death that may occur is unrelated to the tubal procedure per se.

The surgical approach to conception control through sterilization certainly raises controversy and gives rise to sharp differences of opinion. Admittedly there are many women—indeed, the majority—who do not have periodic medical check-ups in accordance with recommended standards. The incidence of carcinoma in situ of the cervix with the threat of invasion and of endometrial cancer may be on the rise. The incidence of these malignancies varies somewhat in different socioeconomic groups, as does the availability of medical care. Such factors must be taken into account and the procedure recommended for conception control tailored to the individual, and this may mean a puerperal hysterectomy in some instances. However, prophylactic procedures must not take precedence, nor should elements within the socioeconomic environment be the deciding factors in patient care. Rather, all patients should have an equal opportunity to receive quality care regardless of any other consideration.

11

The Place of Cesarean Hysterectomy in Current Obstetrical Practice

Alternative Points of View:

By Gail V. Anderson

By David L. Barclay

By Charles Easterday

Editorial Comment

The Place of Cesarean
Hysterectomy in Current Obstetrical Practice

GAIL V. ANDERSON

University of Southern California School of Medicine

Introduction

Cesarean hysterectomy was proposed as a possible solution to the problem of severely infected and complicated obstetrical problems prior to 1800, but not until the latter part of the nineteenth century,[8] or approximately 100 years ago,[3] was the first such operation performed successfully.

The original operation, as described by Porro, involved subtotal hysterectomy, bilateral salpingo-oophorectomy, and attaching of the cervical stump to the abdominal incision so that blood and infected matter could drain to the outside.[8] Prior to this, and even following the introduction of the Porro method, cesarean section was invariably fatal. Often subtotal hysterectomy or various combinations of cesarean hysterectomy and salpingo-oophorectomy are referred to as the "Porro type" of operation. However, only an operation that includes the abdominal drainage aspect can accurately be termed a Porro operation.

A decrease in the number of Porro operations occurred with the introduction of aseptic techniques and modern suturing techniques. A further decrease in the need for cesarean section hysterectomy for grossly infected pregnancies took place with the introduction of blood banks, modern anesthetic techniques, and antimicrobials.

While the initial indications related primarily to obstructed labor with fulminating infection, by 1931 additional indications, such as acute hemorrhage, chronic nephritis, tuberculosis, and sterilization were suggested. By 1948 a significant number of cesarean sections were accompanied by hysterectomy, and hysterectomy was advocated for additional reasons, such as myomata, placenta previa, Couvelaire uterus, placenta accreta, carcinoma of the cervix and sterilization.[8]

In 1951, Davis reported a 19 per cent incidence of hysterectomy following cesarean section and advocated total hysterectomy where uterine pathology was present; he suggested that the procedure be used even when the uterus was otherwise normal in any woman near the end of her reproductive life who requested sterilization. During the past 15 years, there has been an increasing tendency to use this procedure when sterilization is desired following a cesarean section, owing in part to follow-up problems that arise by leaving the uterus in situ.

The highest reported incidence of hysterectomy with cesarean section is 25.9 per cent, and the writers indicate that they have not done a subtotal hysterectomy since 1951.[3] Schneider and Tyrone,[20] also reporting from New Orleans, state that the operation has become more popular because of the incidence of hypermenorrhea, polymenorrhea, pelvic pain, and dysmenorrhea that follow when the uterus is not removed. Others,[5] however, think that tubal ligation following cesarean section is much less of a threat to the patient when the operation is done only for sterilization.

Current Indications

There is little controversy regarding the indications for cesarean hysterectomy in certain emergency and elective situations, which will be examined separately below.

Spontaneous rupture of a previous uterine scar and primary rupture of the uterus are definite indications for the procedure, in spite of the fact that some would argue that repair of the lacerations is possible in some instances. Traumatic or oxytocin induced rupture would be in the same category.

Uterine atony and uncontrolled hemorrhage from the uterus at the time of cesarean section or immediately following, with or without hematoma formation, may require hysterectomy. In these situations, it is important to make the decision before the patient has lost so much blood that impending, irreversible shock is imminent.

Placenta previa in a multiparous patient who desires no further children or in whom postpartum hemorrhage is likely because of continued bleeding from the lower uterine segment, as well as placenta accreta, constitutes a strong indication for hysterectomy. Again the main threat to the patient may be the indecisive action on the part of the obstetrician managing the case.

Abruptio placentae, even with the typical Couvelaire uterus, is not necessarily an indication for such surgery. The coagulation defect that develops in this situation is corrected by fibrinogen or other means, and extensive surgery may compound the problem.

When severe amnionitis from prolonged rupture of the fetal membranes occurs, cesarean section is required as a method of delivery and it should be combined with hysterectomy if the patient is to have the best chance for survival. If the surgeon is experienced in this procedure, extraperitoneal cesarean section may be considered in primigravid patients who desire more children. However, in general, it should be noted that not many surgeons have been trained to do this procedure; consequently, in the face of extensive intrauterine infection it is safest for the mother to have the physician perform a cesarean hysterectomy.

Elective indications include: defective uterine scar formation from previous cesarean section(s), leiomyomas, carcinoma in situ, multiple repeat cesarean sections, vaginal or cervical stenosis, previous Manchester-Fothergill[19] operation, or previous successful anterior and posterior vaginal repairs.

Tubal Ligation vs. Hysterectomy in Elective Indications

Since some reports [2,3,4,16,20] indicate that the morbidity and complication rates in cesarean hysterectomy are no higher than cesarean section and tubal ligation operations, and since there are some problems associated with the retained postcesarean uterus, it seems reasonable to accept cesarean hysterectomy as the preferred operation if the surgeon feels capable and the patient is in no way jeopardized. However, many reports[1,10,12,15,19] indicate that this is a formidable procedure when tubal ligation would just as well solve the basic objective of preventing future pregnancies. However, it seems that efforts should be directed toward improving the operative techniques and reducing the complications, since most of these same complications occur when cesarean section only is performed.

Total vs. Subtotal Hysterectomy

Total cesarean hysterectomy was advocated as the procedure of choice in 1951[7] and since that time several large series have supported this position.[3,16,19,20] Since a retained cervical stump is the main cause of complaint in most postoperative patients who have had this operation[3] and is a possible source of cancer, it should be removed at 6 to 12 months.[19] Therefore, it seems justifiable to spend a little more time, if the patient is not compromised, and remove the cervix at the time of cesarean hysterectomy. The need for additional anesthesia and surgery later may cancel out any advantages gained by not removing the cervix at the time of cesarean hysterectomy.

In addition, second operations for postoperative bleeding and bladder injury are not obviated by not removing the cervix.[17] Indeed, in placenta previa and low-lying placenta accreta, the patient may be in greater jeopardy if the cervix is not removed. With these exceptions, however, if the patient is compromised by shock or a preexisting medical complication which is difficult to control, a subtotal cesarean hysterectomy should be done.

Complications and Prevention

GENITOURINARY TRACT INJURIES

The incidence of inadvertent injury to the bladder or ureter at the time of cesarean hysterectomy has been noted to be significant,[3,16,17] and if unrecognized it may result in a vesicovaginal or ureterovaginal fistula.[16] It has been implied that these are not completely preventable,[3] but it seems all the more important to make every attempt to avoid the injury.

Careful dissection of the bladder flap for the cesarean section and for the subsequent hysterectomy is most important in preventing bladder lacerations. This means sharp dissection for adherent areas, instead of blunt dissection with the sponge attached to the ring forceps, which many surgeons use. If blunt dissection is to be used, the index finger covered with one layer of gauze is safer and more sensitive than a sponge at the end of a long piece of metal (sponge forceps). During this dissection, care must be taken to keep the plane of dissection in the midline so that the "endopelvic fascia" covering the cervix and upper vagina is visible at all times. The dissection should extend no lower than two inches below the vaginal attachment to the cervix, otherwise troublesome venous bleeding will occur.

To avoid unrecognized bladder injury, 500 cc. of normal saline colored with methylene blue dye should be infused into the bladder through a Foley catheter placed prior to surgery. If the bladder is inadvertently entered, the defect should be closed in two layers using 4-0 chromic catgut suture. A continuous first layer avoids the bladder mucosa, and an interrupted suture layer of the Lembert type is placed in the outer layer of the bladder.

Ureteral injuries usually occur at the area of the cardinal ligaments or in the infundibulopelvic ligament area if bilateral or unilateral salpingo-oophorectomy is done. Injuries to the ureter can be avoided by exposing the course of the ureter in the pelvis from the pelvic brim to the cardinal ligament area and its bladder attachment. This can readily be done if there is not extensive extravasation of blood into the broad ligament owing to previous uterine rupture or lateral extension of a transverse uterine incision. This is accomplished by extending the broad ligament incision laterally at the time the round ligament is divided from its uterine attachment. Blunt dissection of the posterior leaf of the broad ligament will permit the ureter to be visualized over its entire course. In addition, special care in placing the hemostats adjacent to the uterus when clamping the uterine artery and the cardinal and uterosacral ligaments will avoid the ureter. If there is any question of ureteral damage, the bladder should be opened at the dome by a transverse incision. After the ureteral orifices have been visualized, ejection of colored urine from previously administered intravenous indigo-carmine dye by both orifices will indicate ureteral integrity or site of injury. If injured or cut, the ureter should be repaired or reimplanted into the bladder at the time of operation.

Hemorrhage

Excessive hemorrhage at the time of cesarean hysterectomy occurs sometimes as a result of choosing the wrong uterine incision. In general, a longitudinal incision into the lower uterine segment is preferred, since lateral extension of a transverse incision into the uterine arteries can complicate the operation. If some extension of the upper part of the incision is necessary, this can be accomplished by using bandage scissors. A low transverse incision should not be performed if the lower uterine segment is poorly developed,[16] since blood loss will be increased and lateral extension through the uterine arteries is more probable.

If the placenta occupies the lower uterine segment, a classical incision will be least likely to cause excessive hemorrhage in the mother or blood loss in the fetus, which may have to be delivered through the placenta. The placenta should be removed and oxytocin administered until the blood supply to the uterus is secured. Instead of closing the uterine incision to decrease blood loss and save operating time, a series of towel clips are used to approximate the edges of the uterine incision (Figure 11–1). Except for a few details, the technique of hysterectomy is similar to hysterectomy in the nonpregnant patient. If the clamps

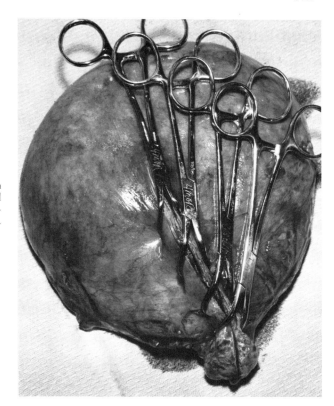

Figure 11-1. Illustration showing manner in which towel clips are used to close the uterine incision instead of suturing.

placed in the uretero-ovarian ligament area are too close to the uterus, the tissue tends to slip out of the clamps and troublesome back bleeding will occur. Dissection of the broad ligament should be kept close to the uterus, otherwise annoying and sometimes heavy bleeding can occur from injury to the venous plexus lateral to the cervix, especially in the area of the cardinal ligaments. When this occurs, the ureter may become compromised while the surgeon is trying to establish hemostasis. Since postoperative bleeding commonly occurs from the utero-ovarian or the infundibulopelvic pedicle when the ovaries are removed, these pedicles should be doubly ligated. The first ligature should be of the "free" type, passed through the avascular space, using the index finger as a guide.

Location of the cervicovaginal junction is sometimes difficult but the junction can be identified either by passing the finger through the cervical canal or extending the longitudinal uterine incision down through the cervix. After the cervix has been detached and removed, a continuous locking suture is placed about the cuff, leaving it open for the later insertion of a medium-sized Penrose drain. After this locking suture is in place, "angle sutures" are placed at the lateral vaginal cuff area, to include the uterosacral and cardinal ligaments. All pedicles should be placed extraperitoneally during the closure of the anterior and posterior leaves of the broad ligament during the peritonealization procedure. With the drain in the "open cuff," blood is less likely to collect and serum hematomas are less likely to form.

MORBIDITY

Appropriate preoperative assessment of the patient's general condition prior to surgery and institution of appropriate corrective measures can do much to reduce the morbidity associated with major operative procedures, especially cesarean hysterectomy.[5,20] The morbidity can vary from 5 to 49 per cent and seems to be uniformly higher in nonprivate patients.[5]

Admittedly, emergency indications for cesarean hysterectomy do not always provide ample time for adequate appraisal of all situations that may contribute to postoperative morbidity. However, on many occasions the "dramatic" and "heroic" nature surrounding the procedure tends to promote undue haste which later good professional judgment will deem to have been without justification.

Since urinary tract infections are a leading cause of postoperative morbidity,[16] preexisting genitourinary tract infections should be diagnosed and treatment instituted during the preoperative or immediate postoperative period. In addition, if any indwelling catheter is to be used more than 24 hours postoperatively, some form of chemotherapy or local antiseptic therapy should be initiated during the immediate postoperative period.

Since aspiration pneumonia from stomach contents is often a serious threat to the patient, the preoperative preparation and selection of anesthesia is highly important.[1] Awareness of this possibility usually is sufficient to enable the surgeon and the anesthesiologist to resolve this problem. If there is extensive uterine infection with or without peritonitis, a stomach or small intestinal tube should be passed during surgery to reduce the possibility of postoperative ileus, which can complicate the postoperative period.

To prevent wound dehiscence and evisceration, some type of retention sutures should be placed in the abdominal incision in all cases in which the postoperative course is likely to be complicated by ileus or when gross infection is present. After closure of the peritoneum and the fascia, the incision should be irrigated copiously with normal saline, to which some may add an antibiotic solution.

Postoperative cellulitis in the operative site (and subsequent abscess formation and peritonitis) is prevented to a large extent by irrigation, exteriorization of pedicles, and keeping the vaginal cuff open as described previously. Irrigation of the pelvic peritoneal area, especially when gross infection is present, will reduce the number of bacteria present and will contribute to morbidity prevention. Leaving the vaginal cuff open with large Penrose drains from the operative site into the vagina prevents the accumulation of blood, serum, and purulent material and reduces the chances of morbidity from pelvic cellulitis, abscess formation, and pelvic peritonitis. The drain should be placed in all patients undergoing cesarean hysterectomy but especially when infection is present. If no infection is thought to be present, the drain may be removed after 1 to 2 days. If infection is present at the time of surgery, the drain should be left in place until all drainage (purulent) has ceased.

Preoperative anemia, prolonged labor, and associated medical diseases contribute to morbidity. Anemia should be corrected prior to surgery in elective procedures and, when possible, before emergency operations. Coagulation defects must be corrected prior to surgery. Preeclampsia, eclampsia, hypertensive vascular disease, and diabetes must be stabilized, especially prior to major obstetrical procedures.

Blood loss at the time of surgery is frequently underestimated. Pritchard has shown the average blood loss at cesarean section to be approximately 1 liter and at cesarean hysterectomy 1.5 liters. However, it has been estimated that the patient can lose up to 1 liter at the time of delivery and cesarean hysterectomy without serious hemodilution. Therefore, single unit transfusion[16] probably is not justified because of the risk of hepatitis. A moment by moment vigilant assessment of the patient will avoid unnecessary blood transfusion. In those instances in which sudden massive infusion of blood is necessary, central venous pressure monitoring will aid in preventing overtransfusion, which would tax the cardiovascular system and precipitate congestive heart failure.

Appendectomy has been shown to increase morbidity and hence, incidental operations should not be done. However, the appendix and ovaries should be examined for pathology; if any disease process is present, appropriate surgery should be performed, since it may be disastrous to leave a diseased appendix or ovary in situ.

Since we can assume that the upper vagina and cervix are not free of bacteria at the time of surgery, it can be assumed that contamination of the operative site in the pelvis always occurs. The healthy patient with adequate nutrition and antibody response can keep this infection localized. However, many socioeconomically deprived patients are not so fortunate. One may assume that infection may be present, though kept at a minimum through good aseptic technique, and administer antibiotics during the postoperative period. These, however, should not be termed "prophylactic" antibiotics since the infection actually is present at the time treatment is instituted.

ANESTHESIA

In all obstetrical surgical procedures close collaboration between the anesthesiologist and surgeon is important for a successful outcome. Moreover, in obstetrics, because life-threatening problems can develop unexpectedly and two lives are threatened, this collaboration is mandatory. This is particularly true of cesarean section and cesarean hysterectomy, in which drugs, anesthetic agents, blood loss, shock, infection, and anoxia can be a threat to mother and fetus.

Since we can assume that most drugs and toxic substances are transmitted directly to the fetus and in general are dose related, it seems reasonable to conclude that the fetus is less likely to be "poisoned" and thus depressed by a conduction or regional type of anesthesia. Consequently, the spinal type of anesthesia appears to be the safest for mother and fetus. The epidural type of conduction anesthesia has certain advantages. With knowledge and skill in management, and ability to anticipate a possible hypotensive episode, these can be handled and avoided without jeopardy to mother and infant.[15] It is recognized that the conduction form may need to be supplemented or replaced on occasion by a general anesthetic.

Inhalation agents are often necessary in emergency surgery, but the halogenated hydrocarbons in general should be avoided in obstetrics. Blood loss is increased with these compounds, and the possibility of liver disease is present in some obstetrical conditions. Cyclopropane seems to be a reasonably safe inhalation agent and very effective when rapid induction is necessary. However, it should be remembered that this agent, as well as others, can affect cardiac rate and rhythm when combined with other drugs necessary in obstetrics, such as oxytocin.

The surgeon should not make the mistake, however, of forcing the anesthesiologist or anesthetist to use an agent, drug, or procedure that he is not accustomed to using. Again, this must be openly discussed between the surgeon and the person responsible for maintaining the patient's physiologic functions during the operative procedure. It will be safest for the patient and less distressful to the surgeon if the anesthesiologist uses those agents, drugs, and anesthesia procedures for which he has most knowledge, experience, competence, and confidence.

Summary

Cesarean hysterectomy, from its inception and even after its general acceptance, has been a controversial procedure. In the beginning, it was inevitably associated with fatal outcome. Porro incorporated exteriorization of the cervix as part of the procedure and achieved the first successful operation. Aseptic technique and suturing advances enabled surgeons to abandon exteriorization of the cervix, with reduction in frequency of this operation for life-threatening obstetrical infections. The introduction of blood banks, anesthesia, and antibiotics further reduced the incidence of this operation.

In modern times, cesarean hysterectomy is performed more frequently and is advocated for elective as well as for emergency obstetrical problems. It is reasonable and safe, provided that constant diligence and effort are exercised to reduce and keep to a minimum the mortality and morbidity associated with the procedure.

Total as opposed to subtotal cesarean hysterectomy has much to recommend it as the procedure of choice. However, surgical expertise should be such that hemorrhage, morbidity, and injury to other structures is no greater than that with the subtotal procedure.

REFERENCES

1. Adraini, J.: Analgesia and anesthesia in cesarean hysterectomy. Clin. Obstet. Gynec. 12:590, 1969.
2. Barclay, D. L.: Cesarean hysterectomy: thirty years' experience. Obstet. Gynec. 35:120, 1970.
3. Barclay, D. L.: Cesarean hysterectomy at the Charity Hospital in New Orleans. Clin. Obstet. Gynec. 12:635, 1969.
4. Bowman, E. A., Barclay, D. L., and White, L. C.: The Bulletin of Tulane University Medical Faculty 23:71, 1964.
5. Brenner, P., Sall, S., and Sonnenblick, B.: Evaluation of cesarean section hysterectomy as a sterilization procedure. Amer. J. Obstet. Gynec. 108:335, 1970.
6. Bradbury, W. C.: Cesarean hysterectomy. West. J. Surg. 63:232, 1955.
7. Davis, M. E.: Complete cesarean section: logical advance in modern obstetric surgery. Amer. J. Obstet. Gynec. 62:838, 1951.
8. Durfee, R. B.: Evolution of cesarean hysterectomy. Clin. Obstet. Gynec. 12:575, 1969.
9. Easterday, C. L.: Cesarean hysterectomy at the Boston Hospital for Women. Clin. Obstet. Gynec. 12:652, 1969.

10. Hayes, D. M., and Andwolfe, W. M.: Tubal sterilization in an indigent population: report of fourteen years' experience. Amer. J. Obstet. Gynec. 106:1044, 1970.

11. Hellman, L. M., and Pritchard, J. A.: Williams Obstetrics. 14th Ed. New York, Appleton-Century-Crofts, 1972.

12. Hofmeister, F. L.: Tubal ligation versus cesarean hysterectomy. Clin. Obstet. Gynec. 12:676, 1969.

13. Howard, P., and Grubbs, T.: Cesarean section and cesarean hysterectomy: a five year evaluation at a non-university teaching hospital. J. Tenn. Med. Assoc. 65:323, 1972.

14. Husbands, M. E., Jr., Pritchard, J. A., and Pritchard, S. A.: Failure of tubal sterilization accompanying cesarean section. Amer. J. Obstet. Gynec. 107:966, 1970.

15. LaPlatney, D. R., and O'Leary, J. A.: Anesthetic considerations in cesarean hysterectomy, anesthesia, and analgesia. Current Researches 49:328, 1970.

16. Mickal, A., Begneaud, W., and Hawes, T., Jr.: Pitfalls and complications of cesarean section hysterectomy. Clin. Obstet. Gynec. 12:660, 1969.

17. Morton, J. H.: Cesarean hysterectomy. Amer. J. Obstet. Gynec. 83:1422, 1962.

18. Pritchard, J. A., Baldwin, R. M., Dickey, J. C., and Wiggins, K. M.: Blood volume changes in pregnancy and the puerperium. II. Red blood cell loss and changes in apparent blood volume during and following vaginal delivery, cesarean section, and cesarean section plus total hysterectomy. Amer. J. Obstet. Gynec. 84:1271, 1962.

19. Riva, H. L.: Indications and techniques for cesarean hysterectomy. Clin. Obstet. Gynec. 12:618, 1969.

20. Schneider, G. T., and Tyrone, C.: Cesarean hysterectomy. Surg. Gynec. Obstet. 130:501, 1970.

The Place of Cesarean
Hysterectomy in Current Obstetrical Practice

DAVID L. BARCLAY

University of Arkansas Medical Center

Introduction

Cesarean hysterectomy was developed as an heroic operation of necessity in an attempt to reduce the exceptional maternal mortality rate of cesarean sections, which until the latter part of the nineteenth century approached 100 per cent in some large maternity hospitals. Cesarean section was an operation of last resort performed under unsterile conditions; the uterus was often infected after protracted labor and prolonged rupture of the fetal membranes. In addition, prior to 1880, it was not customary to close the uterine incision, which predisposed the patient to intraperitoneal hemorrhage and spillage of infected uterine contents.

For about 100 years prior to the first cesarean hysterectomy performed on a woman by Storer, animal experimentation had indicated that the uterus was not essential to life. In 1868 Horatio Robinson Storer performed a cesarean hysterectomy in an attempt to prevent death after cesarean section for obstruction of the birth canal by a uterine tumor in a patient who had been in labor for three days. The patient survived the three hour operation under chloroform anesthesia but died on the third postoperative day.

Edoardo Porro of Pavia, Italy, was convinced, on the basis of animal experimentation, that the uterus was not essential to life. No woman had ever survived a cesarean section in that city. In 1876, therefore, Porro planned for and performed the first successful cesarean hysterectomy. The patient was a dwarf who had obvious pelvic deformity, resulting in absolute cephalopelvic disproportion. The key factor in success appeared to be early operation, after only six to seven hours of labor and rupture of the fetal membranes, a 30 minute operating time, and use of a wire Cintrat's constrictor to secure hemostasis. After incision of the uterus and removal of the infant, the uterus was delivered from the abdominal cavity. The snare was placed over the uterine fundus and both ovaries, snugged securely, and the uterus and adnexae were excised. Peritoneal toilet was accomplished and a drain was placed through the cul-de-sac. The cervical stump was exteriorized through the lower pole of the abdominal incision to prevent intraperitoneal spillage, and the snare was removed with the gangrenous portion of the cervical stump on the fourth postoperative day. The original Porro operation therefore consisted of a subtotal hysterectomy and bilateral salpingo-oophorectomy.

Almost simultaneously, the concepts of infection, cleanliness, and surgical technique were recognized. In addition, in 1880, Max Sanger introduced closure of the uterine incision with multiple sutures to prevent hemorrhage and drainage of lochia into the peritoneal cavity. Therefore, within several years after the performance of the first cesarean hysterectomy the original indications for the operation were no longer being encountered.

Additional information documenting variations in the operative technique and other facts concerning early development of the operation have been thoroughly reviewed by Young.[1]

In the United States, during the first two decades of the twentieth century, the major indication for cesarean hysterectomy was cesarean section performed late in labor and particularly if there were signs of intrauterine infection.[2] Low cervical or extraperitoneal cesarean section subsequently became the procedure of choice in the presence of intrauterine infection.[3]

From 1930 to 1945, major indications were hemorrhage, infection, or uterine pathology, such as uterine fibroids. Little emphasis was placed on elective sterilization. Reis and De Costa summarized the literature from that era and concluded that, in the United States, about 2.54 per cent of cesarean sections were terminated by hysterectomy, with a maternal mortality of 5.2 per cent, in contrast to 3.42 per cent for cesarean section; no attempt was made to separate the results of elective operations from life-saving procedures performed to prevent death from hemorrhage.[4]

With the increased availability of antimicrobial drugs and the introduction of blood banking procedures in the early 1940's, the indications for elective operations were liberalized. In 1951, Davis advocated cesarean hysterectomy for elective sterilization at the time of cesarean section, removal of a diseased uterus, or removal of a uterus no longer functionally useful in a woman near the climacteric.[5] From July 1, 1947, to April 1, 1951, 140 of 700 cesarean sections performed at the Chicago Lying-In Hospital were terminated by hysterectomy.

In 1963, Pletsch and Sandberg reviewed 1819 cesarean hysterectomies reported in the American literature between 1950 and June 1962.[6] The question raised was whether or not cesarean hysterectomy should replace cesarean section and tubal ligation for sterilization. In 1969, Mickal and associates summarized, in tabular form, sixteen reports published between 1951 and 1969; the purpose was to review reported complications.[7]

Definitions

To properly consider the relative safety of cesarean hysterectomy, one must separate and categorize operations on the basis of indications for hysterectomy. In previous publications we have considered only those operations performed after 28 weeks' gestation and following abdominal delivery.[8] Hysterectomies performed after vaginal delivery were excluded from the series. The operations were classified as either elective or emergency; the latter designation included only those operations performed as a life-saving procedure to prevent exsanguination from profuse hemorrhage. Indications for hysterectomy were considered separate and distinct from indications for cesarean section. In the case of uterine rupture with expulsion of the fetus into the abdominal cavity, the case was included as abdominal delivery and emergency hysterectomy.

The suggested classification of cesarean hysterectomies as elective or indicated should be discarded if the implication is that removal of the normal uterus for the sole purpose of sterilization is never indicated.[6] This point is controversial, but on occasion removal of the uterus strictly for sterilization may in fact be more beneficial to the patient than removal of a uterus for extirpation of small uterine leiomyomata.

Indications for Cesarean Hysterectomy

EMERGENCY HYSTERECTOMY

By definition, this is a life-saving procedure performed to control hemorrhage. The noncontractile Couvelaire uterus was, before introduction of fibrinogen in the early 1950's, the chief indication for cesarean hysterectomy.[8] The cesarean section was typically a primary procedure performed to control hemorrhage associated with abruptio placenta in a multiparous patient, prior to term, in the presence of a long and unyielding cervix. Considering the associated hypofibrinogenemia responsible for the extensive myometrial extravasation of blood, one would currently consider this to be a last resort procedure performed after administration of adequate quantities of fibrinogen and oxytocics.

Rupture of a uterine scar or previously intact uterus was the second most common indication for emergency hysterectomy. Spontaneous rupture of the unscarred uterus frequently results from extension of an old cervical laceration; therefore, total hysterectomy is mandatory and one must not overlook an associated vaginal laceration that could result in postoperative hemorrhage (Figure 11–2).

Frank rupture of a prior classical uterine incision is a catastrophic event, often resulting in expulsion of the fetus into the abdominal cavity and near eversion of the uterus (Figure 11–3). Separation of a low segment scar is less dramatic and seldom results in either fetal loss or bleeding. Hysterectomy, because of a defective scar in the lower uterine segment, must, therefore, usually be considered an elective procedure. The exception is the low segment scar that has been penetrated by a low-lying placenta with invasion of the bladder base.

Uterine atony in the absence of uterine fibroids or an anomaly of placental implantation is an uncommon occurrence. Uterine fibroids, particularly the submucous variety, may be unintentionally enucleated, resulting in bleeding, or may interfere with the repair of the uterine incision.

Bleeding from the placental site is usually associated with a low-lying placenta involving the noncontractile lower uterine segment. The result may be placenta accreta, increta, or percreta; the last may result in laceration in the uterine vessels when the placenta is removed.

Extension of a low transverse incision into the uterine vessels is usually the result of injudicious use of a low transverse incision in the presence of a

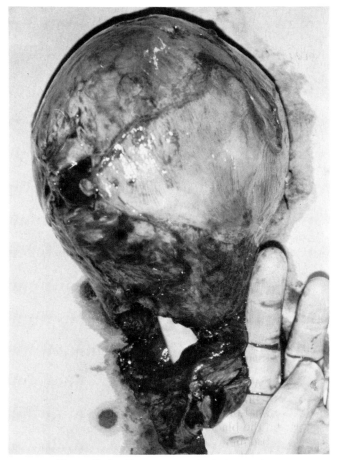

Figure 11-2. Lower segment uterine rupture.

malpresentation. Although hemorrhage may be profuse, the necessity for hyster-ectomy is tempered by the parity and desires of the patient. It has been demonstrated that the uterine vessels or the anterior division of both hypogastric arteries may be ligated and the uterus repaired. The operative procedure, there-fore, depends upon the individual circumstances. The ureter is in close proximity to the uterine vessel laceration and must be identified by palpation prior to placing ligatures.

ELECTIVE HYSTERECTOMY

Whether acknowledged or not, sterilization is the most common reason for elective cesarean hysterectomy. The author's current policy is to offer a choice between hysterectomy or tubal ligation to patients who desire sterilization and who are scheduled to undergo an obstetrically indicated cesarean section. Approx-imately 50 per cent of cesarean sections are repeat operations and one often finds a "defective" uterine scar defined as a thin, avascular, and occasionally trans-parent scar allowing visualization of the infant. It is not surprising that a wound in an involuting organ does not heal well, even in the less muscular, fibrous

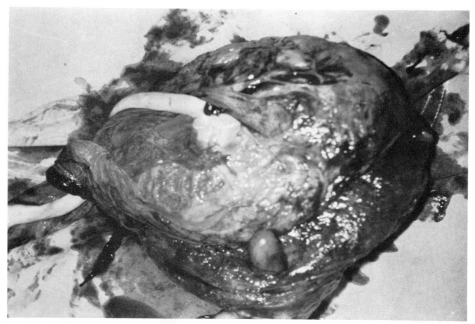

Figure 11-3.   Uterine eversion from rupture of a classical uterine scar.

lower uterine segment. Whether or not this anatomical defect is an indication for sterilization depends upon the extent of the scar dehiscence and the desires of the patient for additional pregnancies. It should be added that there are often dense adhesion between the bladder and lower uterine segment that increase the technical difficulty of subsequent operations.

A poorly healed and transparent classical scar or wide spread uterine damage from extension of the uterine incision is more difficult to repair and potentially more dangerous in subsequent pregnancies; therefore, sterilization is usually indicated.

The means of accomplishing a medically indicated surgical sterilization must be determined on an individual basis.

Uterine fibroids may be removed by cesarean hysterectomy to avoid the necessity for a second operative procedure. Pelvic vascularity and consequent blood loss tend to be somewhat greater than for the usual operation.

Intrauterine infection was one of the original indications for cesarean hysterectomy. Despite the availability of potent broad-spectrum antibiotics, hysterectomy remains a valid procedure for treating infection. Whenever a cesarean section is performed because of prolonged rupture of the membranes and intrauterine infection, particularly in the diabetic patient, hysterectomy should be seriously considered unless preservation of the uterus is essential. Infection remains one of the major causes of maternal mortality.

For intraepithelial carcinoma of the cervix diagnosed during pregnancy, usually by conization, standard management has been observation for the remainder of the pregnancy, vaginal delivery, and reevaluation six to 12 weeks post partum. Currently, however, colposcopic examination and directed biopsy have allowed an accurate diagnosis without conization, and definitive treatment is accomplished by wide cuff cesarean hysterectomy at term if the uterus is not to be preserved. The obvious advantages of administering definitive treatment during one hospitalization have not been overridden by operative or postoperative complications.

In the rare instance of ovarian or breast cancer diagnosed during pregnancy, cesarean hysterectomy and bilateral salpingo-oophorectomy may in some cases be the treatment of choice.

Vaginal and cervical stenosis preventing vaginal delivery may be an indication for hysterectomy, depending upon individual circumstances.

The Surgical Procedure

PREOPERATIVE PREPARATION

During the course of prenatal care of patients scheduled for an elective repeat cesarean section, the possibility of surgical sterilization is discussed. Each patient is allowed to choose either cesarean tubal ligation or cesarean hysterectomy unless uterine pathology exists which should correctly be treated by hysterectomy. Primary counseling is performed by a Community Health Nurse and after a decision is made, appropriate sterilization papers are completed by the patient and her husband. The routine preoperative evaluation consists of urinalysis, complete blood count, fasting blood sugar, blood urea nitrogen, serology, and chest x-ray. The cervix is evaluated for dysplasia or malignancy by means of a Papanicolaou smear and colposcopic examination if indicated. Approximately two weeks prior to term an outpatient amniocentesis is performed for the purpose of determining the lecithin/sphingomyelin ratio. If fetal maturity is demonstrated, the elective operative procedure is scheduled accordingly. Two to four units of whole blood are prepared preoperatively. Vaginal preparation has not been routinely carried out.

OPERATIVE TECHNIQUE

The operation may be performed under either general or spinal anesthesia; preoperative medication consists of atropine administered as a drying agent to avoid excessive respiratory secretions during anesthesia.

The abdomen may be entered through either a vertical or a low transverse incision. A low cervical cesarean section is performed in the usual manner, except that the bladder flap is completely developed prior to incising the uterus; the presence of prior adhesions often requires sharp dissection, which is more easily performed if the fetal head is in the lower uterine segment. The uterus is entered through a low vertical incision that usually extends into the lower portion of the uterine fundus. After delivery of the infant, the uterine incision may or may not be closed with a continuous suture, but more commonly the bleeding edges are grasped with small ring forceps. The placenta may be left in place and the anesthesiologist is asked to add 10 to 20 units of oxytocin to the intravenous infusion. A self-retaining retractor is placed in the abdominal incision, after which the uterine fundus is delivered from the abdominal cavity. The ovaries are inspected, and if oophorectomy is not indicated, the operation is begun by placing a Kocher clamp on the round ligament, which is cut, and the anterior of the leaf of the broad ligament is incised to join the bladder flap incision. The next pedicle to be encountered consists of the utero-ovarian ligament and fallopian tube, which is doubly clamped. If the pedicle is excessively large, the utero-ovarian ligament and the fallopian tube may be clamped and cut separately. The avascular portion of the broad ligament is then incised, and the uterine vessels skeletonized by sharp dissection. Blunt dissection tends to cause tearing of the fragile uterine veins. A retractor can then be placed under the bladder flap, causing sufficient elevation to be certain that the bladder is not in danger at the point at which the uterine vessels will be clamped. The ureter is easily palpated in its course through the cardinal tunnel in the soft, pliable parametrial tissues. The uterine vessels can then be doubly clamped, specifically with Haney clamps, after visualization of the bladder and location of the ureter by palpation. The procedure is then repeated on the opposite side. During the process, exposure is facilitated by traction in the upper pole of the vertical uterine incision. Back bleeding is controlled by a large Kocher clamp on each cornu of the uterus and on the uterine vessels bilaterally.

After all pedicles to the level of the uterine vessels have been clamped and cut, the major blood supply has been controlled and each of the pedicles can be ligated. The utero-ovarian ligament is tied with a free ligature followed by a suture ligature; this pedicle is rather large and if tied too close to the ovary, the ligature tends to cut through the friable ovarian tissues and cause bleeding which may not be apparent at the time of operation. One or two suture ligatures may be placed on the uterine vessels; an adequate pedicle has been provided by double clamping. Here again the ligature must be snug, but if too tight there may be a tendency to place excessive tension on the uterine vein and cause a shearing stress, resulting in bleeding. Usually one more pedicle on the cardinal ligament on either side is necessary before the angle clamps are placed on the vagina and the uterus removed.

Although there has been some discussion about the preferred method for complete removal of the cervix, particularly if it is completely dilated, we have found that compression of the angle of the vagina between the thumb and forefinger forces the lips of the soft cervix upward, allowing identification of the vaginal angle, which is grasped with a large Haney clamp. The uterosacral ligament may or may not be specifically ligated. A similar clamp is placed on the opposite side, and the vagina is incised for removal of the uterus. An angle suture is placed on each side of the vagina and left long for traction, after which the vaginal cuff is closed with figure-eight catgut sutures. Some staff members prefer to leave the vaginal cuff open after placing a continuous locking suture around the edge of the vaginal mucosa. The cuff that is left open will be functionally closed within a matter of hours but is easier to open for drainage.

Hemostasis is secured and the peritoneum is closed with a continuous 2-0 catgut suture. The utero-ovarian ligaments are not sutured to the angle of the vaginal cuff. The ovarian pedicles in particular should be inspected closely for bleeding. Appendectomy may be performed at this time if prior approval has been obtained. After closure of the peritoneum, one may consider performing a Marshall-Marchetti-Krantz procedure if treatment of stress incontinence is indicated. The space of Retzius should be exposed by gentle blunt dissection, and the space drained with a Penrose drain after placement of the sutures. The abdominal incision is closed in the usual manner. A reasonable operating time would be 90 to 120 minutes.

Operative and Postoperative Complications

The primary operative complications are urinary tract injury and excessive blood loss. By definition, an emergency cesarean hysterectomy is performed for hemorrhage, and most operations of this type require administration of whole blood. Although Pritchard has demonstrated that a gravida at term can lose 1 liter of blood with little or no hemodilution in the postpartum period, blood replacement in reported series of elective cesarean hysterectomies has averaged 500 to 1000 cc.[7] However, if replacement of blood loss is done only to improve vital signs or because of a truly excessive blood loss, the number of blood transfusions can be markedly reduced. Using these criteria, there is no doubt that one unit blood transfusions are justified if this amount will stabilize the vital signs. Our experience indicates that currently about 10 per cent of patients undergoing elective cesarean hysterectomy require blood transfusions. The patients are mainly from a clinic population, and the vast majority are operated on by resident physicians.

Urinary tract injuries include recognized bladder injury and repair, postoperative vesicovaginal fistula, or ureteral injuries. In about 2 to 4 per cent of hysterectomies performed after a repeat cesarean section there is injury to the bladder. The key to management is recognition of the injury and two-layer closure, with inversion of the bladder mucosa, followed by continuous bladder drainage for 10 days. Ureteral injuries should by and large be avoidable if the ureter is identified by palpation prior to clamping the uterine vessels. If a ureteral injury is suspected, one can make a longitudinal slit in the ureter at the level of the pelvic brim and insert a ureteral catheter into the bladder. The injury can then be repaired, or the ureter can be reanastomosed, using a minimum number of 4-0 catgut sutures that do not penetrate the ureteral mucosa. Currently a ureteral splint is not used after primary repair of a ureteral injury and a linear ureterostomy at the pelvic brim is used to decompress the ureter during the healing process. A Penrose drain is placed at the site of the ureterostomy and brought out through a flank incision. In the absence of obstruction, the flank drain is usually removed within five days, and ureteral healing progresses uneventfully.

Bladder injury usually occurs at the site of a prior uterine incision or when the bladder is included as the clamp is placed on the uterine vessels. As mentioned previously, there is a distinct advantage to developing the vesicouterine space adequately prior to delivery of the infant. Just prior to clamping the uterine vessels, the bladder should be definitely identified and perhaps elevated out of the field by placing a retractor in the vesicouterine space, and the ureter should be identified by palpation. Only in this way can one be certain that the urinary tract is retracted out of the field of operation.

With few exceptions, recognized and repaired urinary tract injuries will heal primarily. Vesicovaginal fistulae are probably the result of sutures placed through the base of the bladder during closure of the vaginal cuff, resulting in necrosis of the bladder wall and fistula formation within 10 days postoperatively. We have followed the recommendations of Collins and associates, who advocate continuous bladder drainage, hydrocortisone acetate taken by mouth, and repair of the unhealed fistula within 10 days of recognition.[10]

Occasionally the uterine vein is lacerated or the uterine artery slips out of the ligature and retracts laterally in close proximity to the ureter. Under these circumstances, it is best to control bleeding by simple pressure and quickly develop the perivesical and perirectal spaces lateral to the ureter, after which the uterine vessels can be specifically ligated at their origin, or the anterior division of the hypogastric artery can be ligated. Bleeding is then sufficiently controlled to allow identification of the end of the uterine vessel, and another ligature can be secured.

It is commonly stated that morbidity after cesarean hysterectomy is greater than after cesarean section with or without tubal ligation; this has not been our experience. The primary causes of a postoperative febrile course are urinary infection and vaginal cuff infection. It is of interest that in a report of 30 years' experience at the Charity Hospital in New Orleans, postoperative morbidity varied little during the entire period of study.[8]

Postoperative bleeding, consisting of intra-abdominal or vaginal hemorrhage, expanding vaginal cuff or retroperitoneal hematoma, or incisional bleeding that requires suturing, occurs after approximately 3 to 4 per cent of elective operations. Intraperitoneal hemorrhage necessitates secondary surgery in approximately 1 per cent of cases. The site of bleeding is most often the utero-ovarian ligament which may require unilateral salpingo-oophorectomy. Bleeding from the area of the vaginal cuff or uterine vessels is probably best managed by ligation of the anterior division of the hypogastric arteries, which should slow bleeding sufficiently to allow specific identification and ligation of bleeding points. Treatment of large vaginal or retroperitoneal hematomas must be individualized as one would individualize treatment after any other type of hysterectomy.

In the usual uncomplicated case the patient remains in the hospital from six to eight days postoperatively; therefore, removal of the uterus does not unduly prolong hospitalization for the cesarean section patient.

We would expect no greater a postoperative death rate after cesarean hysterectomy than after elective cesarean section alone, or, for that matter, abdominal or vaginal hysterectomy in the nonpregnant patient.

Current Philosophy

Commencing January 1, 1970, patients undergoing cesarean section on the obstetrical service at the University of Arkansas Medical Center were offered a choice of concurrent tubal ligation or hysterectomy if sterilization was desired. During the calendar years 1970 and 1971, there were 5677 deliveries and 398 cesarean sections (7.8 per cent), of which 124 or 31.2 per cent were terminated by hysterectomy. Three of the hysterectomies were classified as emergency and one was a radical operation for cancer of the cervix; therefore, 120 operations were considered to be elective.

Fifty-eight per cent of the hysterectomies were performed after repeat cesarean section. Primary cesarean sections were performed for malpresentations (13), prolonged rupture of the membranes (8), Rh sensitization or diabetes (7), bleeding (5), and miscellaneous reasons (17); nine, or 18 per cent, of the patients were considered to have intrauterine infection associated with prolonged rupture of the fetal membranes.

The vast majority of patients (90.8 per cent) were para 2 or greater prior to the pregnancy under consideration. The age distribution was about as expected in a primarily indigent obstetrical population. Fifty patients (42 per cent) were noted to have had an associated medical illness, such as hypertension with or without toxemia (12), preeclampsia (5), and a variety of other medical disorders.

Indications for elective cesarean hysterectomy are listed in Table 11-1. Ten of the operations were performed to remove a diseased uterus and the remainder were for the primary purpose of sterilization.

During 1970, 14 patients (18.5 per cent) received a blood transfusion during surgery; however, during 1971, only four patients (5.5 per cent) were transfused. During 1970 the resident staff was becoming increasingly familiar with the operation, and not only was the amount of blood loss greater during that year but there was also a greater readiness to transfuse patients to replace blood loss. During 1971, blood replacement was more carefully monitored, and a smaller percentage of patients received transfusions despite the fact that the population served was unchanged. As demonstrated by the studies of Pritchard, the average obstetrical patient can sustain a 1000 to 1500 cc. blood loss without a significant postpartum decrease in the hematocrit.[9] In those patients who were not transfused, the average preoperative hematocrit level was 37 ml./100 ml., decreasing to 31.5 ml./100 ml. postoperatively. The transfused group of patients started with an average preoperative hematocrit level of 31.5 ml./100 ml., averaging 33 ml./100 ml. postoperatively. With few exceptions, transfused patients had a preoperative hematocrit value of between 28 and 30 ml./100 ml.

Unilateral oophorectomy was performed in seven patients either for a benign tumor or more commonly to secure hemostasis in the utero-ovarian pedicle; the reported incidence of oophorectomy is approximately 10 per cent. An appendectomy was performed as an incidental procedure in nine patients. We have no definite views about appendectomy, and if the patient agrees, prophylactic appendectomy can be performed. A wide vaginal cuff was removed in the three patients who had carcinoma in situ of the cervix. If the cervix is removed using the methods described previously, it is possible to excise an adequate vaginal cuff at the time of cesarean hysterectomy.

Two bladder lacerations were recognized and repaired, and both healed primarily. Partial severance of one ureter was recognized and repaired. A linear

TABLE 11–1. *Indications for Hysterectomy*

	1970	1971	TOTAL
Elective Sterilization	38	55	93 (77.5%)
Medical Sterilization			17 (14.2%)
Rh sensitized	3	1*	
Hypertension	0	5	
Orthopedic deformity	0	1	
Sickle cell disease	0	1	
Elderly primipara	0	1	
Diabetes	1	3	
Defective uterine scar	1	0	
Uterine Pathology			10 (8.3%)
Carcinoma in situ	2	1	
Fibroids	1	2	
Intrauterine infection	3	1	
TOTAL	49	71	120 (100%)

* Prior tubal ligation.

ureterostomy at the pelvic brim was performed and a ureteral catheter passed into the bladder, after which the laceration was repaired with three 4-0 chromic catgut sutures that did not penetrate the ureteral mucosa. The ureteral catheter was removed and a flank drain was placed adjacent to the ureterostomy and the area of ureteral repair. The patient was discharged on the eighth postoperative day, and an intravenous pyelogram taken three months postoperatively was normal.

During 1971, a Marshall-Marchetti-Krantz procedure was performed on three patients. The operations were uneventful, and we plan to perform more such procedures for the correction of stress incontinence and to obviate this problem in the patient who has had a cesarean hysterectomy.

The average operating time in 1970 was 110 minutes, and during 1971, after gaining more experience, this was reduced to 93 minutes. Ninety minutes seemed to be a reasonable operating time for the performance of the entire procedure.

Postoperative morbidity, manifested as a temperature of 100.4° F. for two consecutive days beginning on the second postoperative day, was recorded in 35 per cent of the patients in 1970 and in 24 per cent in 1971. The most common complications were urinary tract infections (23 patients) and vaginal cuff infections (18 patients). The most severe complication was a case of suppurative phlebitis and ovarian abscess that required secondary surgery. Postoperative bleeding was recorded in five patients: there was one instance of incisional bleeding and four of vaginal cuff hematoma. In one patient, ligation of a vaginal cuff vessel was necessary. In a large series one can expect approximately a 1 or 2 per cent incidence of reoperation for intra-abdominal bleeding. Despite the 25 to 35 per cent incidence of postoperative morbidity, 55 per cent of patients received antibiotics during the postoperative period, although one must recall that 9 patients were considered to have intrauterine infection prior to cesarean section. Nearly half of the patients received either ampicillin or tetracycline, and five patients were given penicillin for a positive serologic test for syphilis.

Seventy-eight per cent of the patients were discharged on or before the seventh postoperative day. One instance of prolonged hospitalization was necessary because of an ovarian abscess.

Conclusions

In emergency circumstances, a cesarean hysterectomy is life-saving, and the operation has an established place in the practice of obstetrics. On the other hand, removal of the uterus primarily for the purpose of sterilization remains a controversial procedure. From the point of view of the patient, hysterectomy at the time of an obstetrically indicated cesarean section offers the advantages of being convenient and more economical, particularly if hysterectomy has been planned for a later date. The surgeon must be convinced, however, that the risk to the patient is not increased. In addition, the patient and her husband must realize that surgical sterilization is final, regardless of the outcome of the pregnancy.

Our experience to date would indicate that the patient is not being jeopardized at the time of operation or in the immediate postoperative period. The necessity for blood replacement has remained within reasonable limits, as determined by the number of blood transfusions required and the postoperative hematocrit values obtained. Although the incidence of blood transfusions was only 10 per cent during 1971, it is still greater than the number of transfusions usually administered during vaginal hysterectomy in this institution. Studies to determine accurately the amount of blood lost during cesarean hysterectomy are in progress.

The occurrence of only two recognized bladder injuries and no fistulae in a series of 120 patients is not prohibitive and is probably comparable to non-puerperal hysterectomy in a similar group of patients, i.e., those with previous cesarean section.

Finally, it must be decided whether the patient's best interest is better served by hysterectomy or by simple tubal ligation at the time of cesarean section. Although our clinical impression is in agreement with the suggestion of some authors that there is a high incidence of hysterectomy after puerperal tubal ligation, sufficient data are lacking.[11] However, the failure rate of puerperal tubal ligation by itself would not justify hysterectomy. Considering that all of these patients had requested surgical sterilization, the question is whether or not removal of the uterus is more emotionally traumatic to the patient than is tubal ligation. A study to evaluate this problem was attempted, but the mechanics of preoperative evaluation and long-term postoperative follow-up are substantial. The practice of having a preoperative interview of patients scheduled for elective cesarean hysterectomy by a psychiatric nurse practitioner has been started.

Even disregarding the fact that hysterectomy is the most effective means of surgical sterilization, we feel that our patients have positively benefited from this more extensive surgical procedure. The patients in this series were derived primarily from an indigent population considered to be at risk for the development of cervical cancer and pelvic infections. A multitude of problems prevent these patients from receiving a yearly examination and Papanicolaou smear. Many patients scheduled to return for a hysterectomy two to three months post partum have been unable to return. The addition of the Marshall-Marchetti-Krantz urethrovesical suspension procedure to the cesarean hysterectomy operation has obviated the problem of persistent urinary stress incontinence after hysterectomy. Hysterectomy, which originally was only accepted by patients and medical personnel, now is frequently requested in place of tubal ligation. Although occasionally we are requested to perform a primary cesarean section for the sole purpose of removing the uterus, it is only under exceptional circumstances that this would be done.

Prevention of emotional consequences of hysterectomy in the young woman is probably more a matter of preoperative evaluation, selection and counseling of patients than any other factor. It is well documented that ovarian function continues in cyclic fashion and, therefore, physiologically these women should be entirely normal if properly counseled from the psychological point of view.[12]

REFERENCES

1. Young, J. H.: The History of Caesarean Section. London, Lewis, 1944.
2. Williams, J. W.: A critical analysis of twenty-one years' experience with cesarean section. Bull. Johns Hopkins Hosp. 32:173, 1921.

3. Briscoe, C. C.: Cesarean section morbidity and septic mortality in relation to type of operation. Am. J. Obstet. Gynec. *48*:16, 1944.
4. Reis, R. A., and DeCosta, E. J.: Cesarean hysterectomy. J.A.M.A. *134*:775, 1947.
5. Davis, M. E.: Complete cesarean hysterectomy; logical advance in modern obstetric surgery. Am. J. Obstet. Gynec. *62*:838, 1951.
6. Pletsch, T. D., and Sandberg, E. C.: Cesarean hysterectomy for sterilization. Am. J. Obstet. Gynec. *85*:254, 1963.
7. Mickal, A., Begneaud, W. P., and Hawes, T. P., Jr.: Pitfalls and complications of cesarean section hysterectomy. Clin. Obstet. Gynec. *12*:660, 1969.
8. Barclay, D. L.: Cesarean hysterectomy. Thirty years' experience. Obstet. Gynec. *35*:120, 1970.
9. Pritchard, J. A., Baldwin, R. M., Dickey, J. C., and Wiggins, K. M.: Blood volume changes in pregnancy and the puerperium. II. Red blood cell loss and changes in apparent blood volume during and following vaginal delivery, cesarean section, and cesarean section plus total hysterectomy. Am. J. Obstet. Gynec. *84*:1271, 1962.
10. Collins, C. G., Barclay, D. L., and Holmes, J. S.: Total urinary incontinence. Clin. Obstet. Gynec. *6*:236, 1963.
11. Williams, E. L., Jones, H. E., and Merrill, R. D.: Subsequent course of patients sterilized by tubal ligation; consideration of hysterectomy for sterilization. Am. J. Obstet. Gynec. *61*:423, 1951.
12. Doyle, L. L., Barclay, D. L., Duncan, G. W., and Kirton, K. J.: Human luteal function following hysterectomy as assessed by plasma progestin. Am. J. Obstet. Gynec. *110*:92, 1971.

The Place of Cesarean Hysterectomy in Current Obstetrical Practice

CHARLES EASTERDAY

Harvard School of Medicine and Boston Hospital for Women

Controversies of Cesarean Hysterectomy

The controversial aspects of cesarean hysterectomy center on its use for terminal sterilization, especially when the obstetrical indications for primary cesarean section are absent. In life-saving situations, where it is clearly indicated, there can be little question of its value; however, even in such instances, the question of total versus subtotal hysterectomy remains controversial.

The advances in supportive therapy—i.e., anesthesia, blood replacement, antibiotics, and improved surgical technique—have modified the acceptable indications to include many more instances. The risk of sterilization by cesarean hysterectomy in those patients in whom there is no obstetrical indication for a primary cesarean section must be weighed against the risks of sterilization that accompany laparoscopic tubal coagulation or vasectomy.

A review of the literature reveals many reports separating elective and indicated cesarean section, but which, however, fail to list the morbidity, blood loss, or complication rate for the elective group.[1,10,13,15,17,20,22,23,32] The indication for cesarean hysterectomy in the emergency, life-saving situation is undisputed, and blood loss, complications, and prolonged hospital stay are accepted as necessary. The safety of cesarean hysterectomy in elective cases and particularly those in which sterilization is the desired end point, without other pathology being present, is disputed.[4,9,27,31] There have been many questions raised for this selected group. Is the risk low enough to justify the procedure for sterilization alone? Does the choice of total versus subtotal affect the morbidity rate? Does the experience of the operator make a difference in complications and blood loss? Does appendectomy add to morbidity? Should the operation ever be done primarily for sterilization in the absence of gynecological pathology? To what degree is one willing to accept the risks of transfusion, prolonged anesthesia time, and technical complications in view of the lesser procedures available today for sterilization?

Statements have been made that cesarean hysterectomy is far less complicated than the average laparotomy performed in the gynecological service today.[1] Meyer and Countiss,[17] in reporting 101 cesarean hysterectomies, compared them to a similar number of tubal ligations and stated that elective cesarean

367

hysterectomy was relatively safe, although the proper patient selection was important.

Hallatt and Hirsch[13] have expressed the opinion that prophylactic cesarean hysterectomy at the time of cesarean section or sterilization was a logical development in preventive obstetrics and gynecology, and Montague considered it a procedure of choice when both cesarean section and sterilization were required.[19]

A discussion by Von Geary of Patterson's paper[23] emphasized that hysterectomy was frequently inadequate for repair of vaginal relaxation and thus often neglected in the grand multiparous patient.

Durfee[9] has stated that the operation should not be done exclusively for sterilization, and that it carries a higher risk and morbidity rate than tubal ligation for sterilization. He also felt that gynecological indications for removal of the uterus at the time of cesarean section seemed to be the most appropriate reason for electively performing the operation.

Objections to cesarean hysterectomy, as cited by Ward[31] are that it is more difficult, there is a greater operative risk, more morbidity and mortality, greater blood loss, and operative time is increased over that of cesarean section and tubal ligation.

Brenner and associates,[4] in reporting 198 cases, 89 of which were for sterilization, maintain that the risk of morbidity and complications far outweigh the potential benefits, and hold that the desire for sterilization is not an indication for primary cesarean section.

The present state of controversy is best illustrated by the statement by Reis[27]: "For those who believe that hysterectomy in the young woman is not only harmless but also beneficial, when no offspring are desired, it will continue to be a logical development in preventive obstetrics and gynecology. For the less liberal, irreversible annullment of childbearing function, loss of menstruation relatively early, cesarean hysterectomy will not be a rational method of sterilization."

In hopes of helping to resolve some of these questions, a review of the literature and material from the Boston Hospital for Women is presented.

Material

There have been 138 cesarean hysterectomies at the Boston Hospital for Women, Lying-In Division, since the first such procedure was performed in 1933 because of placenta previa with uncontrolled hemorrhage. Of the 13 cases recorded through 1958, 12 were for life-saving indications, and all were subtotal operations. From 1959 through 1972, an additional 125 operations have been performed, 7 of which were subtotal hysterectomies. Ninety-three cases were for elective sterilization, and the remaining hysterectomies were indicated for uncontrolled bleeding—i.e., rupture of the uterus, atony, and placenta accreta or percreta.

The incidence of cesarean section and cesarean hysterectomy related to the total number of deliveries is illustrated in Table 11–2. Although the cesarean section rate has increased in both private and nonprivate patients, the number of cesarean hysterectomies has been reduced, probably because of increasing use of laparoscopic tubal sterilization. The cesarean section rate includes all primary and repeat operations and is higher on the private service, owing to the large

TABLE 11–2. *Incidence of Cesarean Hysterectomy, Boston Hospital for Women*

	CLINIC PATIENTS					PRIVATE PATIENTS*					TOTAL				
Years	Deliv-eries†	Cesarean Section	Per Cent	Cesarean Hyster-ectomy	Per Cent‡	Deliv-eries†	Cesarean Section	Per Cent	Cesarean Hyster-ectomy	Per Cent‡	Deliv-eries†	Cesarean Section	Per Cent	Cesarean Hyster-ectomy	Per Cent‡
1959–63	10,651	494	(4.6)	15	(3)	19,812	1572	(7.9)	19	(1.2)	30,463	2066	(6.7)	34	(1.6)
1964–68	12,181	533	(4.4)	30	(5.6)	20,380	1803	(8.8)	36	(2.0)	32,561	2336	(7.4)	66	(2.8)
1969–72	8821	580	(6.1)	9	(1.5)	15,597	1639	(10.5)	16	(1.0)	24,418	2219	(9.0)	25	(1.1)

* Includes Joslin Diabetic Clinic patients.
† All deliveries.
‡ Per cent of cesarean sections that were cesarean hysterectomies.

TABLE 11–3.   *Parity at Time of Hysterectomy for 138 Patients*

PARITY	NUMBER OF PATIENTS	PER CENT
0	3	2.2
1	19	13.7
2	31	22.4
3	29	21.0
4	25	18.0
5	11	7.9
6	6	4.3
7	8	5.8
8 or more	6	4.3

number of diabetic patients from the Joslin Clinic. The frequency of cesarean hysterectomy does not increase with parity (Table 11–3) as it does with age (Table 11–4). This is a reflection of its use, in the past, for sterilization. The six patients under the age of 24 all had severe obstetrical life-threatening emergencies.

The most frequent indication for hysterectomy other than sterilization was rupture of the uterus or the presence of a placenta accreta (Table 11–5). Myomata uteri and carcinoma in situ of the cervix could be considered as elective indications in that there is very little risk over that of an elective hysterectomy

TABLE 11–4.   *Indications for 138 Cesarean Hysterectomies by Age Distribution, Boston Hospital for Women*

AGE	CESAREAN HYSTERECTOMY	PER CENT OF TOTAL	ELECTIVE FOR STERILIZATION*	PER CENT OF TOTAL	INDICATED CLINICALLY	PER CENT OF TOTAL
20–24	6		0		6	
25–29	20	(14.5)	14	(10.0)	6	(4.3)
30–34	44	(31.9)	29	(21.0)	15	(10.9)
35–39	49	(35.5)	33	(24.0)	16	(11.6)
40–45	19	(13.8)	17	(12.3)	2	(1.4)
TOTAL	138		93	(67.4)	45	(32.6)

* Forty, or 73.5 per cent, of 68 hysterectomies in patients over 35 were for sterilization.

TABLE 11–5.   *Reasons for Performing Cesarean Hysterectomy*

	NUMBER OF CASES
Ruptured uterus	17
Placenta accreta or percreta	15
Sepsis	2
Myomata	2
Carcinoma in situ	4
Uncontrolled bleeding	5
Sterilization*	93
	138

* Prior to 1959, of a total of 13 hysterectomies, 11 were indicated and only two were for sterilization.

for sterilization. They have been included, however, with the clinically indicated cases.

Of the 93 elective sterilizations, 79 patients had had previous cesarean sections, 11 had primary cesarean sections without obstetrical indications and three had valid obstetrical reasons for the primary section.

Blood loss has been reported in terms of transfusions given rather than estimated or measured blood loss. However, the incidence of transfusions in the clinically indicated cesarean hysterectomy is of little clinical importance in evaluating the procedure in that the number given is dictated by the pathology present. In elective cesarean hysterectomies for sterilization, blood loss, measured by replacement, averaged 1040 cc. for 13 patients on the private service (26.5 per cent), and 950 cc. for 22 patients (50 per cent) on the clinic service.

Morbidity, as measured by the standards of the American Committee on Maternal Welfare, was 18 per cent (Table 11–6) for the group of elective cesarean hysterectomies for sterilization. This is in keeping with the lower values reported by other authors (Tables 11–7 and 11–8). The complications that occurred in 14 per cent of the patients (Table 11–9) are of a significant degree of severity—i.e., ureteral damage, pelvic abscesses, and reoperation. Minor complications, undoubtedly, often were not recorded.

Technique

The type of cesarean section incision should be thoughtfully selected and based on specific advantages to be gained in each particular patient, rather than dictated by the habits of the operator. The surgeon should consider whether the lower segment has been thinned by previous labor, the station of the presenting part, and the position of the infant in making his selection. The fetus presenting as a transverse lie with the back down may be difficult to deliver through a transverse lower segment incision. Likewise, the absence of labor may make the lower segment unusually narrow, risking extension of a transverse incision into

TABLE 11–6. *Classification and Results of 138 Cases of Cesarean Hysterectomy at Boston Hospital for Women*

	PRIVATE	CLINIC	TOTAL
Elective for Sterilization	49	44	93 (67 %)
Morbidity	6 (12%)	11 (25%)	17 (18 %)
Complications	4 (8%)	9 (20%)	13 (14 %)
Transfusions*	11 (22%)	20 (45%)	33 (35.5%)
Clinically Indicated	31	14	45 (33 %)
Morbidity	14 (45%)	4 (29%)	18 (40 %)
Complications	6 (19%)	1 (7%)	7 (15 %)
Transfusions*	21 (68%)	11 (80%)	32 (71 %)
		Total	138

* Transfusions
  Elective: Private: 22 units/11 patients; 38 received no blood.
  Clinic: 36 units/20 patients; 24 received no blood.
  Indicated: Private: 64 units/21 patients; 10 received no blood.
  Clinic: 27 units/11 patients; 3 received no blood.

TABLE 11-7. *Morbidity and Mortality Rates for Elective Cesarean Hysterectomy*

NUMBER OF CASES OF TUBAL LIGATION WITH HYSTERECTOMY	MORTALITY	MORBIDITY (PER CENT)	AVERAGE BLOOD REPLACEMENT OR PER CENT REQUIRING TRANSFUSION	COMPLICATIONS (PER CENT)	BLADDER OR URETERAL TRAUMA (PER CENT)	HEMORRHAGE POST-OPERATIVELY (PER CENT)	REOPERATED POST-OPERATIVELY (PER CENT)
Alford (272)	231	0	*	(700 cc)	*	*	*	*
Barclay (866)	689	2	38.8	63%	10.4	5.3 (35 bladder; 2 ureter)	4.5	7.1 secondary closure
Bremner (198)	89	0	29	66%	*	3.3	*	*
Easterday (138)	93	0	18	35.5%	14.0	4.3	4.3	4.3
Montague (103)	75	0	20	58%	29	1.9	3.9	2.6
Patterson (327)	311	0	29	*	*	*	*	*
Pletsch (169)	160	0	18	59% (528 cc)	30	6.8	5.6	*
Powell (6)	69	0	49	62% (784 cc)	*	*	*	*
Sandberg (97)	90	0	14.4	(500 cc)	*	*	3.3	*
Ward (274)	254 Elective 84 Sterilization†	0	*	82%	9.5	*	1.2	1.2

* Data not available.
† Data reported on 84.

TABLE 11–8. *Morbidity and Mortality Rates of Cesarean Section with Tubal Ligation*

	CASES	MORTALITY	PER CENT MORBIDITY	PER CENT OF PATIENTS REQUIRING BLOOD	PER CENT COMPLICATIONS
Meyer	100	0	6	*	14
Montague	369	0	17	21	*
O'Leary	165	0	16	*	*
Powell	112	0	31.5	*	26

* Data not available.

TABLE 11–9. *Complications of Cesarean Hysterectomy in 138 Patients*

ELECTIVE HYSTERECTOMY FOR STERILIZATION (14 PER CENT COMPLICATIONS)

Private Patients	Number	Nonprivate Patients	Number
Hematoma (reoperated)	1	Ureteral damage (nephrostomies)	2
Pulmonary embolus (nonfatal)	1	Postoperative abscesses	2
Ligation of hypogastric artery (at reoperation)	1	Hematomas	2
Severe hemorrhage (bladder flap)	1	Severe hemorrhage (bladder flap)	1
		Cystostomy	2

CLINICALLY INDICATED HYSTERECTOMY (15 PER CENT COMPLICATIONS)

Wound dehiscence	2	Cystostomy	1
Postoperative abscess	1		
Postoperative bleeding	2		
Unrecognized invasive cancer of cervix	1		

the broad ligament and uterine vessels. Whatever incision is chosen should be practically bloodless and permit deliberate, careful dissection and extension if necessary.

The first step is the development of the uterine peritoneal flap, exposing the lower segment of the uterus. This is done by incising the visceral peritoneum (Figure 11–4) transversely 3 cm. above the uterine vesicle fold and retracting it downward. Following exposure of the lower segment, pressure should be applied lateral to the vertical or transverse incision against the underlying presenting part. This compresses the myometrium and minimizes blood loss. Suction enables one to see the line of incision clearly as it is being made. The lateral edge pressure should be maintained during the initial incision until the amniotic sac is entered. Limitation of the opening to 2 cm. with immediate ring clamping of the myometrium minimizes blood loss. As the incision is extended, additional ring clamps are applied. This technique permits a deliberate, controlled, well-visualized entrance to the uterine cavity. Proper timing of the administration of oxytocin will greatly facilitate delivery of the placenta and its separation.

Some surgeons prefer to leave the lower uterine incision open so that they may insert a finger through the canal identifying the cervix. However, the practice of inserting an instrument or a finger through the cervical canal into the

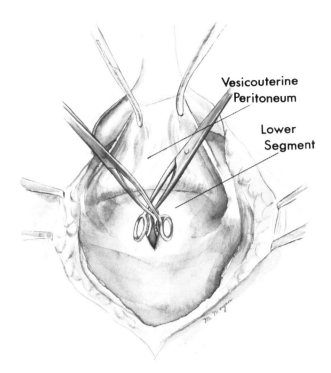

Figure 11-4. Cesarean section, lower segment incision. The visceral peritoneum is incised and together with the bladder is reflected off the lower uterine segment. A vertical (Krönig) or transverse (Kerr) incision is made, with pressure on the presenting fetal part to reduce blood loss. Ring clamps applied as the uterine incision is made reduce blood loss.

vagina readily lends itself to contamination of the abdominal cavity. Following expulsion of the placenta, the incision is rapidly closed with a running suture for hemostasis (Figure 11–5). Some operators have advocated leaving the placenta in situ and quickly clamping the vessels in the broad ligament. This does require, however, controlling blood loss from the cut myometrium of the cesarean incision. The removal of the placenta and quick closure of the uterine incision is preferred.

Increased vascularity, the size of the uterine corpus, the internal bleeding surface of the uterus, and difficulty in identifying the extent of the cervix makes hysterectomy of the gravid uterus considerably different from that in the non-gravid state. Tissue planes are readily developed; however, increased vascularity gives rise to multiple oozing sites if one dissects freely prior to clamping tissue. The practice of skeletonizing the broad ligament prior to clamping the uterine vessels is to be condemned. All tissue in the broad ligament should be clamped prior to dividing. Only in those instances in which time is vital is subtotal hysterectomy justified. Postoperative hemorrhage from the ovarian pedicles has prompted some surgeons to remove the ovaries routinely. Oophorectomy is a simpler operation than leaving the ovaries, but it must be individualized and should not be considered a routine procedure.

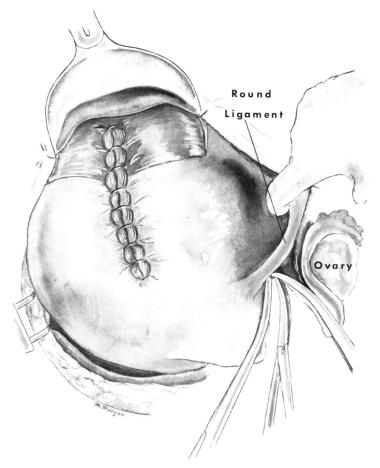

Figure 11-5.   Demonstration of closure of the incision with a running suture for hemostasis prior to the hysterectomy and treatment of the uteroovarian area and round ligament.

When salvaging the ovary (Figure 11–5), the ovarian pedicle, round ligament, and broad ligament should be doubly clamped and divided medial to the ovary, leaving sufficient tissue in the medial clamp to prevent retraction of the uterine pedicle. Close application of the medial instrument puts the grasped tissue under considerable tension, and annoying blood loss results if it slips free. For the operator standing on the patient's left, it is easier to apply the medial clamp first and the lateral clamp second on the right side, reversing the procedure for the left adnexae. Once the supracervical area in the broad ligament is reached (Figure 11–6), it is important to stay close to the cervix, avoiding the ureter. Back bleeding is minimal at this level, and the tissue is less likely to pull out of the clamp. At all times when tissue is divided between hemostats, it is important that the points come together and that the division does not extend beyond the points. Often vessels may bleed between the points at the time of division of the tissue if they are not in close proximity.

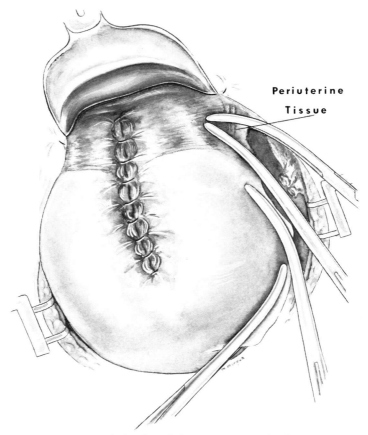

Periuterine
Tissue

Figure 11-6. Division of the broad ligament. Once the lower segment is reached, clamp application is made close to the uterus.

Identification of the cervicovaginal junction, particularly in patients who have been in labor, may be difficult. One author has suggested inserting the finger through the open uterine incision following cesarean section and marking the junction of the cervix and vagina with a suture. We previously marked the junction with a skin clip applied vaginally prior to surgery. Others have suggested extending the uterine incision through the cervix or entering the vagina posteriorly. A simpler technique is that of passing the thumb over the anterior vaginal wall and the remaining fingers of the hand posteriorly and milking the vagina upward toward the corpus. This readily demonstrates the bulk of the cervix and locates the incision site. A closed technique is illustrated in Figure 11–7. This is particularly helpful if one is anxious to avoid contamination of the abdominal cavity with vaginal or uterine contents. Simple applications of a single clamp across both sides of the vagina from side to side is routinely used in most cesarean hysterectomies. Partially closing the clamp and advancing over the vaginal tissue —milking toward the cervix—readily identifies even the dilated cervix, at which point the clamp is closed. The vagina may be sutured prior to removal of the

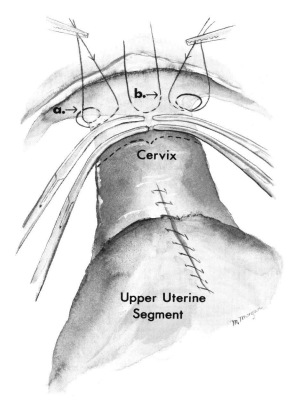

Figure 11-7. Double application of clamps by milking up on the vagina prior to closure. This technique, which leaves no vaginal mucosa on the hysterectomy specimen, is advantageous in avoiding spillage and contamination in septic cases. Routine cesarean hysterectomies
require only the distal clamp. Suture at *a.* overlaps in the outer loop, preventing the loop from
sliding over the divided pedicle. At *b.* is shown closure of the vagina by a mattress suture
(one technique illustrated).

clamps, locking the lateral portion of the suture. This permits closure of the angles
prior to actually opening the vaginal cuff. At this point, one may elect to close
the vagina with a through and through mattress suture in the middle, prior to
removal of the clamps. An alternate method is to remove the instruments and
place interrupted figure-eight sutures in the anterior or posterior cuff, permitting
drainage (Figure 11–8). Such a technique has never resulted in uterine or bladder
damage or subsequent need of surgery for postoperative hemorrhage. Examination of the removed specimen will reveal no more vaginal mucosa attached to the
specimen than obtained by the open technique. A drain may be left in the vagina.

At this point, all tissue having been clamped prior to division and sutured,
there should be little oozing or bleeding from the residual pelvic tissue. The
pedicle of the ovary and round ligament or the pedicle of the infundibulopelvic
vessels is extraperitonealized in closure (Figure 11–8). The ovarian pedicle is not
anchored to the angle of the vagina. This practice may pull loose the ligatures on
the pedicle, in addition to dragging the ovary down over the apex of the vagina.
A drain may be left in the retroperitoneal space and through the vaginal opening
when the cuff has been left open.

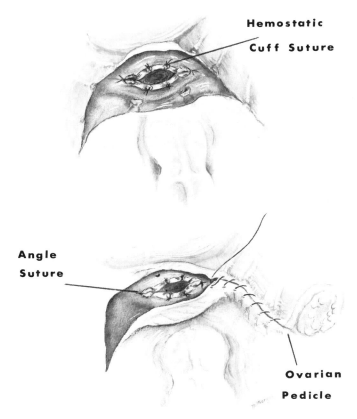

Figure 11-8.   The anterior or posterior cuff may be closed with angle sutures, as illustrated, or as an alternative, left open with interrupted sutures in the remaining cuff. This is preferred to a continuous lock suture.

Conclusion

Careful consideration of the many factors involved indicates that cesarean hysterectomy is not an innocuous procedure; that there is increased technical difficulty, especially following previous cesarean section, in freeing up the bladder; that blood loss is substantially increased over that of cesarean section and tubal ligation; and that morbidity, although of variable degrees, is increased.

The two deaths reported in the literature by Pletsch, one as a result of a pulmonary embolus and the other a patient who would have died as a result of her leukemia, cannot necessarily be attributed to the choice of operation. However, two deaths reported by Barclay in elective cases resulting from transfusion reactions are real factors to be considered. It is the conclusion of the author that primary cesarean section without obstetrical indications should not be done as a step in cesarean hysterectomy for sterilization. Cesarean hysterectomy should be reserved for patients with gynecological or obstetrical pathology, and even the experienced surgeon may encounter unexpected bleeding and technical difficulties. Nonetheless, it is a relatively sound, safe procedure electively when the overall indications justify the risk taken.

Medical judgment must dictate the decision of choice for the individual operator and not what is successful in the hands of a selected few.

REFERENCES

1. Alford, C. D., and Miller, A. C.: Cesarean section hysterectomy: a 10 year review. Amer. J. Obstet. Gynec. 82:664, 1961.
2. Barclay, D. L.: Cesarean hysterectomy at the Charity Hospital in New Orleans—1000 consecutive operations. Clin. Obstet. Gynec. 12:635, 1969.
3. Barclay, D. L.: Cesarean hysterectomy—thirty years' experience. J. Obstet. Gynec. 35:120, 1970.
4. Brenner, P., Sall, S., and Sonnenblick, B.: Evaluation of cesarean section hysterectomy as a sterilization procedure. Amer. J. Obstet. Gynec. 108:335, 1970.
5. Bryant, R. D.: Maternal mortality and morbidity following cesarean section. Clin. Obstet. Gynec. 2:1010, 1959.
6. Crisp, W. E., and Sattenspiel, E.: The morbidity of hysterectomy. Surg. Gynec. Obstet. 120:965, 1965.
7. Davis, M. E.: Complete cesarean hysterectomy. Amer. J. Obstet. Gynec. 62:838, 1951.
8. Dees, D. B.: Should hysterectomy replace routine tubal sterilization? Amer. J. Obstet. Gynec. 82:572, 1961.
9. Durfee, R. B.: Evolution of cesarean hysterectomy. Clin. Obstet. Gynec. 12:575, 1969.
10. Dyer, I.: Total cesarean and puerperal hysterectomy. Obstet. Gynec. 9:696, 1957.
11. Easterday, C. L.: Cesarean hysterectomy at the Boston Hospital for Women. Clin. Obstet. Gynec. 12:652, 1969.
12. Barber, H. R. K., and Graber, E. A.: Surgical Disease in Pregnancy. Philadelphia, W. B. Saunders Co. (in press).
13. Hallatt, J. H., and Hirsch, H.: Total hysterectomy for sterilization following cesarean section. Amer. J. Obstet. Gynec. 75:396, 1958.
14. Hofmeister, F. J.: Tubal ligation versus cesarean hysterectomy. Clin. Obstet. Gynec. 12:677, 1969.
15. Howard, P., and Grubbs, T.: Cesarean section and cesarean hysterectomy—a five year evaluation at a nonuniversity teaching hospital. J. Tenn. Med. Assoc. 65:323, 1972.
16. Lee, J. G., Randall, J., and Keetel, W. C.: Tubal sterilization—a review of 1169 cases. Amer. J. Obstet. Gynec. 62:568, 1951.
17. Meyer, H. and Countiss, E. H.: Cesarean hysterectomy. Amer. J. Obstet. Gynec. 77:1240, 1959.
18. Mickal, A., Begneaud, W. P., and Hawes, T. P.: Pitfalls and complications of cesarean section hysterectomy. Clin. Obstet. Gynec. 12:660, 1969.
19. Montague, C. F.: Cesarean hysterectomy: its value as a sterilization procedure. Obstet. Gynec. 14:28, 1959.
20. Morton, J. H.: Cesarean hysterectomy. Amer. J. Obstet. Gynec. 83:1422, 1962.
21. Nissen, E. D., and Goldstein, A. I.: A prospective investigation of the etiology of febrile morbidity following abdominal hysterectomy. Amer. J. Obstet. Gynec. 113:111, 1972.
22. O'Leary, J. A., and Steer, C. M.: A ten year review of cesarean hysterectomy. Amer. J. Obstet. Gynec. 90:227, 1964.
23. Patterson, S. P.: Cesarean hysterectomy. Amer. J. Obstet. Gynec. 107:729, 1970.
24. Pletsch, T. D., and Sanberg, E. C.: Cesarean hysterectomy for sterilization. Amer. J. Obstet. Gynec. 85:254, 1963.
25. Pritchard, J. A., Baldwin, R. M., Dickey, J. C., and Wiggins, K. M.: Blood volume changes in pregnancy and puerperium. Amer. J. Obstet. Gynec. 84:1271, 1962.
26. Prystowsky, H., and Eastman, N. J.: Puerperal tubal sterilization. J.A.M.A. 158:463, 1955.
27. Reis, R. A.: Cesarean hysterectomy. Clin. Obstet. Gynec. 2:977, 1959.
28. Riva, H. L.: Indications and techniques for cesarean hysterectomy. Clin. Obstet. Gynec. 12:618, 1969.
29. Sandberg, E. C.: Sterilization by cesarean hysterectomy. Obstet. Gynec. 11:59, 1958.
30. Schneider, G. T., and Tyrone, C. H.: Cesarean hysterectomy. Surg. Gynec. Obstet. 130:501, 1970.
31. Ward, S. U., and Smith, A. H.: Cesarean hysterectomy: combined section and sterilization. Obstet. Gynec. 26:858, 1965.
32. Webb, C. F., and Gibbs, J. V.: Preplanned total cesarean hysterectomies. Amer. J. Obstet. Gynec. 101:23, 1968.

The Place of Cesarean
Hysterectomy in Current Obstetrical Practice

Editorial Comment

Admittedly, in this chapter, there is an overlap with material in Chapter 10, but here emphasis is placed on technique. Some differences in operative procedures are readily noted that might prove helpful to the reader in evolving or comparing his own technique with an eye to reducing the complication rate and operating time. Considerable attention is given to the avoidance of ureteral and bladder injury, or—should they occur—how to identify and repair them before the abdomen is closed. Differences in the treatment of vaginal cuff and whether or not to skeletonize the uterine vessels are fully discussed. A closed technique for removal of the cervix is presented to avoid vaginal contamination.

It is properly suggested that these patients be evaluated preoperatively for stress incontinence. Should it exist, the surgeon should consider the Marshall-Marchetti-Krantz procedure to correct this clinical state at the time of cesarean hysterectomy. Hypogastric artery ligation is mentioned, for its value cannot be overemphasized. The procedure is especially indicated when pelvic hematomas are evident and should be carried out before any pelvic manipulation is attempted to locate the site of bleeding. Hypogastric ligation may be life-saving here if local attempts at hemostasis fail or in the rare case of delayed postoperative hemorrhage in vaginal hysterectomy. One may question the wisdom of administering one unit of blood given the risk of hepatitis. If a one unit transfusion is necessary, undoubtedly the giving of two or three units may come even closer to restoring the circulating blood volume to normal.

The question has been raised whether cesarean hysterectomy should be extended to and encouraged for most women having their last cesarean section. Certainly residents in training should be familiar with the operation and should best gain their experience from performing the procedure electively rather than performing it initially under emergency conditions. However, this also implies that the first assistant should be an experienced member of the staff so that the operation is carefully supervised. The policy appears justified when deaths from cesarean section are reviewed. All too often it becomes clear that the patient probably would have survived had the uterus been removed. What does not appear or cannot be determined in such cases is whether or not the operator felt competent to perform a cesarean hysterectomy or perhaps may have reasoned that the patient could be managed by transperitoneal cesarean section with antibiotic coverage and supportive measures. This is especially true in cases of lethal intrauterine infection. The vast majority of these patients have had ruptured membranes for varying periods of time. Although their vital signs can be normal, it is incorrectly assumed that the patient is not infected and can be managed as mentioned above.

Whereas the complications of cesarean hysterectomy by cesarean section with antibiotic coverage were much discussed, the virtues of the operation are rarely mentioned or emphasized. Certainly the pelvis is left in a more "tidy" state than when the uterus is left in situ at cesarean section and there is less chance of adhesion formation, which in turn may encourage intestinal obstruction, immediate or remote. The postoperative course of these patients is usually quite benign, with less distention than in the average cesarean section. Appreciation of the life circumstances of the clientele is necessary, including knowing whether they will be able to return for periodic check-ups required for cancer control. So, it would appear that cesarean hysterectomy deserves wider usage and should be included in the armamentarium of the well-trained obstetrician-gynecologist.

12

Diagnosis and Preferred Management of Urinary Stress Incontinence

Alternative Points of View:

    By R. B. Durfee

    By Thomas H. Green

    By C. Paul Hodgkinson

Editorial Comment

Diagnosis and Preferred Management of Urinary Stress Incontinence

R. B. DURFEE

University of Oregon Medical School

Diagnosis and corrective surgical repair of urinary stress incontinence should be directly related to the etiology of the symptoms. Frequently, the diagnosis and repair are not related, which accounts for many of the conflicting statements and numerous incompetent procedures devoted to management of stress incontinence. The following review may put some of these inaccuracies to rest.

DEFINITION

Stress incontinence is involuntary urine loss under the influence of physical stress, not of one but of several kinds. The condition develops through loss of the anatomical integrity of structures responsible for urinary continence.

NORMAL BLADDER FUNCTION

In order to properly understand these various mechanisms which cause incontinence of urine under stressful conditions, the factors responsible for continence must be examined.

Continence of urine in the female is dependent upon the wholeness of the anatomic components of the pelvis, especially the condition of the supportive tissues of the anterior vaginal wall. This quality is measured by the maturity and thickness of the vaginal mucosa and the ratio of connective tissue to smooth muscle in the supportive layer immediately proximal to the vaginal mucosa.

This sheath of muscle and connective tissue is completely surrounded by the vaginal mucosa and extends from just distal to the hymenal ring cephalad and anterior to the lateral wings of the cardinal ligaments of the uterus. Posteriorly this tissue thins out into the sacrouterine ligaments, and anteriorly it extends cephalad to the under surface of the pubis. The cervix is also enclosed in this condensed sheath of tissue at the level of the anatomic internal os.

The condensation of this tissue in the cardinal ligaments anteriorly from the cervix has been called, among numerous other terms, the "pubocervical-vesical fascia"—which is a misnomer, since histologically it does not resemble "fascia" elsewhere in the body.

Another factor in the maintenance of continence is the length and integrity of the urethra and its relationship to the bladder and the vaginal axis. Normally, the urethra is 3 cm. or more in length. Throughout the entire length of the urethral wall there should be present intact circular muscle fibers. These are the primary forces which completely maintain the continuous existence of urethral tone. The effectiveness of this urethral tone is demonstrated by measuring the intraurethral pressure along its entire length.

The axis of the urethra and the anterior vaginal wall in relation to the other anatomic structures of the pelvis is an essential factor in the preservation of continence. This results, in part, from the intimate relationship between the muscular connective tissue sheath of the anterior vaginal wall and the urethra, especially in the distal third of both organs, where they are inseparable.

The relationship of the urethra and anterior vaginal wall to the neck and floor of the bladder is another factor in the maintainence of continence. The anterior and posterior vesical walls curve away from this area so that a lateral radiographic silhouette of the bladder neck and urethra reveals an angular relationship between these structures. The augmentation or diminution of these angular relationships indicates the presence of proximal supportive tissue structures. The presence of a "posterior urethrovesical angle" as a factor in the preservation of continence depends upon this observation.

The area of the posterior urethrovesical angle represents the point at which the urethral lumen is closed at the moment of maximum vesical pressure against it, which was produced with sudden intra-abdominal stress. This upward rebound or "trampoline effect" of *all the pelvic tissues* to compensate for the sudden excessive downward thrust produces a valve-like closure at the urethrovesical junction which adequately reinforces the continence mechanism. The "pelvic tissues" referred to include the entire levator muscle systems, the perineal muscle systems, and the muscular and connective tissues of the vulva and vagina.

The entirety of the physiologic sphincter mechanism of the bladder is another integral factor responsible for maintaining urinary continence. The capability of the sphincter is related to the shape and size of the internal lumen of the bladder at the vesical neck. This in turn is dependent upon the position of the vesical wall in the region of the vesical neck at the moment of maximum stress.

Mobility of the distal urinary tract is absolutely essential in performance of voiding in women, and it is equally important in maintaining continence with stress.

The general condition of the muscles and connective tissue in the pelvis and the continuity of innervation to *all the pelvic structures* are essential to the correct function and position of the bladder, urethra, and vagina.

Etiology of stress incontinence

It is clear that diagnosis of the causes of stress incontinence depends upon the awareness of the many factors concerned with the maintenance of continence, and that the correction of continence failures is a complicated matter even if the *method* of correction may be simple. The following is a list of causes of stress incontinence:

1. Prolapse of the anterior vaginal wall with formation of a cystocele.

2. Prolapse of the base of the bladder and the posterior urethral wall, with loss of the posterior urethrovesical angle.

3. Alteration of the axis of the vesical floor and the urethra in relation to the vagina and the pelvis.

4. Attenuation or loss of the supportive structures of the vagina, the vaginal mucosa, and the wall of the urethra.

5. Loss of or damage to the circular muscle fibers of the urethra.

6. Fixation of the perivesical and periurethral tissues by fibrosis subsequent to trauma, infection, or surgical procedures in the area.

7. Incompetence of the vesical "sphincter."

8. Urethral shortening.

The causes of pelvic organ prolapse are often subtle. The prolapse frequently is the result of:

1. Loss of resiliency and elasticity in the muscles and connective tissues of the pelvis, owing to genetic background, aging, estrogen lack, or previous trauma.

2. Continued stretching and attenuation of connective tissue support of the anterior vaginal wall.

3. Uterine prolapse with or without relaxation of the posterior vaginal wall or the development of the true pelvic hernia (enterocele).

4. Multiparity or prolonged labors with traumatic instrumental delivery accompanied by vaginal cervical and pelvic floor lacerations, especially the frequently unrecognized rupture of the *deep pelvic supportive structures.*

5. Neurogenic defects secondary to spinal cord disease or related to spina bifida, both obvious and occult.

6. Obesity, increased abdominal girth, and ascites.

7. Chronic constipation, resulting in repeated straining at stool.

8. Chronic pulmonary diseases with constant cough and increased respiratory activity in the struggle for breath.

It must be concluded that ordinarily no single factor alone is the cause of stress incontinence; it is evident that by careful examination and evaluation of symptoms at least two etiologic factors will be found to be involved in almost every case of urine loss owing to stress.

DIAGNOSIS, SYMPTOMS, AND SIGNS

HISTORY OF STRESS INCONTINENCE. Frequently questions regarding the presence of stress incontinence are never asked in a history review.

In this condition, urine may be lost by the following:

1. A sudden increase in intra-abdominal pressure, such as with laughing, coughing, sneezing, and so forth.

2. Stepping up or down on a curb or a flight of stairs.

3. The act of sitting or rising or both.

4. Turning or changing position in bed.

5. The act of kneeling and rising.

6. Multiple body actions involved in sporting activity, such as tennis, golf, and so forth.

7. The act of coitus.

Signs and physical findings

Usually there is evidence of anterior vaginal wall relaxation, with some degree of cystocele. The axis of the urethrovaginal angle may have changed as much as 90 degrees. The urethra has descended and points upward at the urethral meatus. There is an associated loss of the urethrovesical angle posteriorly. Urine or fluid is lost from the bladder upon coughing or straining while the patient is in the lithotomy position. If urine is not lost in this position, it may be observed with the patient standing or squatting. Urine may be lost from the urethra by simple manipulation of the anterior vaginal wall and frequently is lost by downward pressure against the posterior vaginal wall with a Sim's speculum. Urine may escape from the urethra in a constant stream when the bladder is full or on the slightest movement by the patient.

Frequently, none of these losses of urine may be demonstrated until at least 200 ml. of urine or fluid is in the bladder. If there is a large dependent cystocele with a vertical urethra, urine loss with stress may not occur until more than 300 ml. of fluid is in the bladder, and not always then. On the other hand, it may require very little stress and very little fluid in the bladder to demonstrate stress incontinence in the standing position.

Tests

Of the many tests recommended to determine the anterior vaginal wall relaxation or posterior urethrovesical angle loss relationship to the stress, the most effective is placing an opened sponge forceps with each blade in a corner of the anterior vaginal wall at the level of the bladder neck. In the presence of demonstrable urine loss with an obvious anatomical defect or combination of defects, replacement of the tissues upward using this method should produce continence with stress. Direct pressure in the midline with a finger or an instrument which compresses the urethra *is not diagnostic.* What remains to be determined is: *does the elevation of the anterior vaginal wall* at the proper level produce resolution of the stress incontinence or is it the *pressure* against the tissue underlying the urethra and bladder neck (produced by the stretch of the vaginal wall) that results in resolution of the stress incontinence? This is a very important point, for both may be implicated, and, moreover, one does not want to produce an *artificial compression* of the urethra or bladder neck.

To solve this question, the examiner may simply stretch the anterior vaginal wall with the open sponge forceps with minimal upward pressure, or he may use maximum upward pressure with accentuated stretch of the anterior vaginal wall tissue between the blades of the open forceps, or he may use maximum upward pressure with stretch of the anterior vaginal wall. Occasionally, one can accentuate the symptoms of stress incontinence with these manipulations, in which case the presence of fixation owing to a scar is suspected.

X-ray studies

1. Intravenous pyelogram and retrograde studies. These are frequently indicated.

2. Cystoscopic examination using both air and water cystoscopes with urine culture and sensitivity studies.

3. Cystometrogram studies to aid in identifying urge incontinence and chronic interstitial cystitis.

4. Cystograms with or without chain identification of the urethra.

5. Cine voiding cystograms.

6. Catheterization for residual urine after voiding. Essential in eliminating some differential diagnoses.

Various silhouettes of urethrovesical relationships by x-ray methods have been described. Their use in identifying certain types of stress incontinence is fairly accurate, but the applications of a given finding to specific symptoms is far from absolute.

DIFFERENTIAL DIAGNOSIS

A differential diagnosis involves the elimination or identification of other forms of urinary incontinence. These often may be in combination with stress incontinence. These are:

1. Urge incontinence related to spasmodic bladder contractions associated with acute cystitis and more commonly with chronic interstitial cystitis.

2. Neurogenic bladder ranging from total paralysis to various degrees and types of neurologic disease.

3. Incontinence due to fistula (vesicovaginal, urethrovaginal).

4. Involuntary voiding owing to hysteria, emotion, psychosis, enuresis, abnormality of the bladder and urethra, pregnancy, and the pressure of tumors.

5. Incontinence owing to abnormalities of location and function related to previous surgery, such as:

    a. Following vaginal repair of the asymptomatic small cystocele.

    b. After vaginal repair of symptomatic anterior vaginal wall relaxation—especially with vaginal hysterectomy.

    c. Subsequent to removal of a urethral diverticulum.

    d. Following secondary vaginal repairs of failed vaginal surgery for stress incontinence or third, fourth, and even fifth operations.

    e. As a consequence of surgery that shortens the urethra more than 1 to 2 cm. or a repair of a completely incised or lacerated posterior urethral wall.

    f. After simple or radical vulvectomy, total vaginectomy, or posterior exenteration.

    g. As a complication of radical Wertheim hysterectomy.

    h. After failed Marshall-Marchetti-Krantz or anterior vaginal suspension operations.

    i. Subsequent to failed Pereyra or Tauber operations.

    j. Following various sling operations or those using various prosthetic supports.

TREATMENT

Regardless of etiology, it is apparent that in common practice the surgical approach to repair of anterior vaginal wall relaxation stress incontinence, and other forms as well, is primarily vaginal. These may be simple, single, or combination procedures. *The nonsurgical methods are:*

1. Kegel's exercises or muscle training exercises to improve and increase the tonal quality of the pelvic musculature.

2. Vaginal pessaries and other types of intravaginal prostheses to produce continence by pressure against the urethra or urethrovesical junction; some employ low voltage stimulation of the pelvic muscles.

3. Continuous intravesical catheterization, either urethral or suprapubic, in certain operable cases.

SURGICAL METHODS

VAGINAL:

1. Simple Kelly plication and infolding of the bladder wall, posterior urethral wall, and especially the urethrovesical junction, using catgut or Dexon suture in one or more layers. There are approximately 150 variations of this operation.

2. A Kelly-Kennedy operation, with the Kelly portion, as in No. 1, employed first, followed by one or two permanent suture reinforcements with elevation and constriction of the area of the posterior urethrovesical angle or bladder neck. There are also numerous variations of this combined operation.

3. Several operations that recommended incorporating and imbricating tissues *lateral* to the urinary tract and the anterior vaginal wall.

4. Many operations describe the placement of fascial grafts or artificial prostheses vaginally, usually as secondary procedures.

5. Simple lysing of adhesions and freeing of scar vaginally is advocated by Mulvaney and used in combination with above operations as indicated.

ABDOMINAL:

1. Original Marshall-Marchetti-Krantz operation with suture of the urinary tract and anterior bladder wall to the anterior abdominal wall and pubic bone. This procedure has since been modified.

2. Anterior vaginal suspension, with suture of perivaginal connective tissue to the cartilage of the symphysis pubis.

3. Variations of the abdominal approach to repair of anterior vaginal wall prolapse, including those of Burch and Nichols.

4. Urethral "sling" operations performed entirely from above. There are numerous variations of these as well.

COMBINED VAGINAL AND ABDOMINAL:

1. Pererya or Tauber Inco-needle, vaginal-abdominal blind suspension operations.

2. The Ball procedure (combined vaginal and abdominal approach), with some emphasis on re-creation of the anterior vesical angle.

3. The Durfee combined vaginal and abdominal operation, with lysis of vaginal adhesions primarily, followed by abdominal anterior vaginal suspension, which includes anterolateral elevation of the vagina to the obturator membrane bilaterally (Figures 12–1, 12–2, and 12–3).

4. Abdominal-vaginal sling operations (Goebell-Frangenheim-Stoeckel, Aldridge, and others).

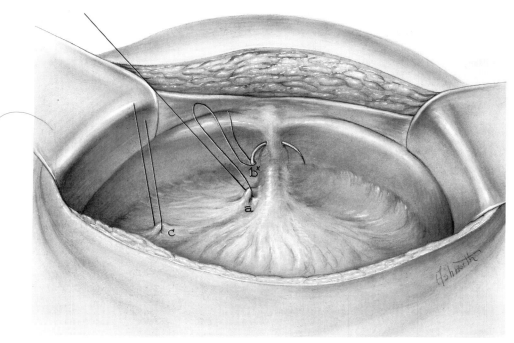

Figure 12-1. Suture placement in anterior vaginal suspension: *a*, single suture or permanent material, preferably Dacron or nylon; this should be placed at right angles to the urethrovesical axis, and often is better with a double throw (not shown); *b*, periurethral suture; placement of this type is rarely done; *c*, suture placement in the superior anterior portion of the vaginal dome in the lateral aspect. The needle placement is in the pubic cartilage in the midline, approximately 1 to 2 cm. from the inferior rim.

5. Zacharin combined repairs.

6. Cantor combined abdominal and vaginal repair.

Based on the following information, what is the most workable approach to stress incontinence and what procedures seem to result in the best results for the longest time?

1. Careful history of urinary tract and voiding problems followed by a clinical examination carefully directed toward eliciting the particular apparent etiologic factors in each case.

2. Look for any other unapparent factors that might contribute to the stress incontinence, for these might become very apparent following a surgical corrective procedure.

3. Do an air cystoscopic examination and a simple cystometrogram as diagnostic procedures in every case of stress incontinence.

4. Include x-ray studies of the bladder with a voiding cystogram in cases of secondary or tertiary repair, iatrogenic stress incontinence, or when there is persistent or early recurrence of symptoms, following any corrective surgery.

PRIMARY REPAIRS

With vaginal hysterectomy, a vaginal approach to repair of anterior vaginal wall prolapse is clearly practical but not predictably good for long-term repair.

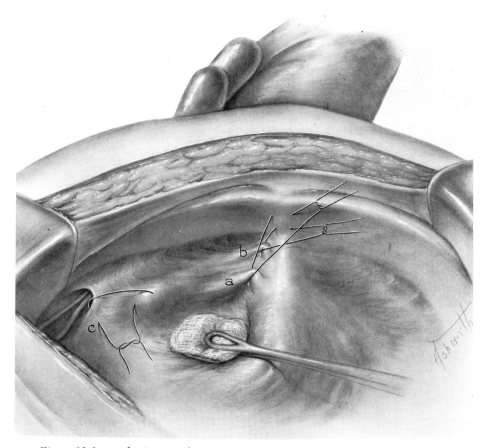

Figure 12-2. a, b, Suture placement and ligation in anterior vaginal suspension. *c,* Suture placement in the obturator membrane with the operator's finger inside the vaginal wall, in order to push the tissues to their point of attachment for the purpose of reducing tension.

The present failure rate or recurrence rate in a 5 to 10 year span is much too high. An abdominal approach to anterior vaginal wall relaxation adds to the surgical manipulation but may produce a better primary cure rate and a lower recurrence rate. The abdominal procedure is more effective when combined with a vaginal dissection, as indicated, with obliteration of a large cystocele, followed by the use of both symphyseal and obturator membrane support, with permanent suture from above. The use of the Pereyra procedure or Tauber's Inco-needle has the risks that are inherent in a blind procedure, with predictable high early failure and recurrence rates related to the absorbable suture.

SECONDARY REPAIR

1. Very few, if any, secondary vaginal repairs are as satisfactory as abdominal operations for previously failed operations or recurrent cases of stress incontinence. The vaginal secondary operation is usually contraindicated.

2. While the anterior vaginal suspension operation, using permanent

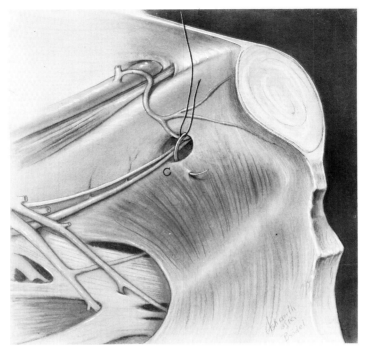

Figure 12-3. Suture placement with needle direction through obturator membrane.

suture, is the preferred repair in secondary or tertiary failed cases, it is not always applicable alone in cases of continued failure or recurrence because of scarring.

3. Indications for a combined vaginal and abdominal operation:

a. In cases of obvious scarring and fixation of the anterior vaginal wall and the urethra and bladder neck.

b. When there is a large recurrent cystocele or a cystocele with a fixed area in the region of the posterior urethrovesical angle.

c. Whenever bladder and urethral function are inhibited by postoperative fibrosis.

d. If the urethra is shorter than 2.5 cm.

e. When the vesical sphincter mechanism fails to close because of scar formation, which is most readily diagnosed by the use of an air cystoscope.

f. When partial or complete vaginal prolapse is present, with or without true enterocele.

g. *All cases* in which there have been two or more postoperative failures or recurrences.

A combined repair, which best restores the anatomic relationships in the sutured area, includes:

1. Lengthening of the urethra.

2. Restoration of the proper urethral axis from vertical to horizontal.

3. Reestablishment of the posterior and anterior urethrovesical angles.

4. Lysing of adhesions, excision of scar, and provision of a proper hammock-like support of the bladder and urethra.

5. The use of *nonreactive permanent suture in the perivaginal and peri-*

urethral connective tissue, but the use of *absorbable suture only in the urinary tract organs.*

In cases of previous multiple surgical procedures with combined failures and a totally scarred area from above and below, in which there is total loss of function of the urethra and vesical neck, it may be necessary to create a new urethra using the bladder wall or the entire vesical neck to make a new urethra (which requires transplantation of the ureters into the posterior vesical wall), or to create an ileal loop bladder as a bypass.

REFERENCES

Ball, T. L.: Gynecologic Surgery and Urology. St. Louis, C. V. Mosby Co., 1963.
Cantor, E. B.: The management of female urinary stress incontinence. Int. Jour. Gynec. Obstet. 11:153, 1973.
Durfee, R. B.: Suspension operations for treatment of pelvic organ prolapse. Clin. Obstet. Gynec. 9:4, 1966.
Pereyra, A. J.: A simplified surgical procedure for the correction of stress incontinence in women. West J. Surg. 67:4, 1959.
Zacharin, R. F.: Stress Incontinence of Urine. New York, Harper & Row, 1972.

Diagnosis and Preferred
Management of Urinary Stress Incontinence

THOMAS H. GREEN, JR.

Harvard Medical School and Massachusetts General Hospital

Until little more than a decade or two ago the diagnosis of urinary stress incontinence in the female was for the most part made casually, primarily on the basis of the history given by the patient. The anatomic abnormality underlying the symptom was not precisely understood at that time. Nor was it appreciated then that there might be individual variations in the underlying abnormal urethrovesical anatomic configuration, and that these variations could have an important bearing on the choice of surgical procedure most likely to completely and permanently correct the stress incontinence in the particular patient being treated. In the ensuing years, there have been important and fundamental additions to our understanding of the etiologic mechanisms involved in this common and troublesome disorder. Both accurate diagnosis and effective management of stress incontinence are dependent on a correct understanding of the characteristic anatomic defect that produces it; hence, a brief introductory section covering this topic is in order.

The Abnormal Anatomy and Pathophysiology of Stress Incontinence

Knowledge of the precise anatomic abnormalities involved in stress incontinence is obviously the key to successful correction of this distressing symptom. It is generally agreed that the basic problem is one of inadequate support to the bladder base, vesical neck, and proximal urethra, with a resulting specific and rather characteristic distortion of the urethrovesical anatomy. However, a few workers in recent years have placed some emphasis on certain other features of the anatomy and physiology of the continence mechanism in an attempt to explain stress incontinence. The following consideration of each of these several interpretations of the basic underlying abnormality should be helpful in presenting our current understanding of stress incontinence.

URETHROVESICAL PRESSURE RELATIONSHIPS

Using direct urethrocystometry, a technique permitting simultaneous recording of the pressures within the bladder and urethra, Hodgkinson and Cobert,[16] Enhorning,[8] Beck and Maughan,[4] and Toews[35] have studied the variations in these pressure relationships in patients with stress incontinence compared to normal continent controls. Their numerous observations indicate clearly that in continent patients with normal urethrovesical anatomy, the pressure at some point in the urethra, invariably in the proximal half, always equals or exceeds that in the bladder. Furthermore, their data revealed that in continent patients, sudden increases in intra-abdominal pressure resulting from cough or similar stresses are transmitted equally to the bladder and the proximal two-thirds of the urethra, maintaining an intraurethral pressure equal to or greater than the intravesical pressure. On the other hand, their studies demonstrated that in patients with stress incontinence, the intrinsic intraurethral pressure at rest tended to be lower (although still greater than resting intravesical pressure), and that coughing reversed the usual pressure differential between the urethra and the bladder, with vesical pressure equalling or exceeding urethral pressure.

Actually, the main conclusion of all these studies seems obvious and hardly necessary to prove, for if a patient has stress incontinence, it follows that during the interval in which the stress is applied the intravesical pressure must necessarily have risen above the intraurethral pressure. Elementary physics, mathematics, and simple logic should render it unnecessary to measure actual pressures to prove this point. However, urethrovesical pressure studies have served to bring into sharper focus one important aspect of the present concept of the pathogenesis of stress incontinence. It is apparent that the normally supported proximal two-thirds of the urethra is basically an intra-abdominal structure. This is why a sudden elevation of intra-abdominal pressure produces the same rise in pressure in the inner two-thirds of the urethra as it does in the bladder. This would seem to be the one really fundamental idea to emerge from the various studies of urethral and vesical pressures, since it clearly relates the disparity in intraurethral pressure in patients with stress incontinence to the fact that the poorly supported proximal urethra has been displaced and now lies outside the intra-abdominal field of force.

URETHRAL LENGTH

A few years ago attention was again focused by some on the potential significance of urethral length to the continence mechanism. Lapides and associates[23] even suggested the possibility that abnormal shortening of the urethra might be an important factor in the development of stress incontinence. He and his co-workers obtained their measurements of urethral length before and after operations for stress incontinence by using a calibrated inlying urethral catheter, exerting downward traction until it was felt that a more auspicious urethral length was indicated by the reading noted on the distal end of the catheter. The accuracy possible with this method seems open to question, since it is well known that the poorly supported urethra is prone to telescope within itself and undergo apparent shortening when placed under artificial tension—i.e., a traction of this sort.

On the other hand, when one employs the metallic bead chain technique of urethrocystography and marks the urethral meatus with a silver dura clip, telescoping never occurs, and it is also a simple matter to obtain extremely precise, undistorted measurements of urethral length both preoperatively and postoperatively. We have now accumulated such measurements in over 300 patients undergoing surgery for stress incontinence. As previously reported,[9] no change whatsoever occurs in urethral length in the majority of patients in whom operative repair has been successful in relieving stress incontinence. Hodgkinson and coworkers,[17] in a study of 105 patients, and Low,[24] in an analysis of 138 patients, made entirely similar observations and reached the same conclusion—that urethral length has no bearing on the problem of stress incontinence.

URETHROVESICAL ANATOMIC RELATIONSHIPS

THE POSTERIOR URETHROVESICAL ANGLE.   Jeffcoate and Roberts[19,20] were among the first to call attention to the importance of the anatomic configuration of the urethrovesical junction and proximal urethra to the continence mechanism. On the basis of their extensive studies using urethrocystography in large numbers of both continent women and patients with stress incontinence, they concluded that the presence of a normal posterior urethrovesical angle was essential to the continence mechanism, and that in patients with stress incontinence it was characteristically absent. Hodgkinson,[15] employing the metallic bead chain technique of urethrocystography in similar studies on continent and incontinent women, reached essentially the same conclusions. It should be pointed out that the location of the bladder neck and urethra with respect to the pubic symphysis is not of direct importance, since many patients with marked bladder descent but with a normal posterior urethrovesical angle are perfectly continent, whereas others, in whom the bladder and urethra remain normally positioned with respect to the symphysis but in whom the posterior urethrovesical angle is obliterated, have severe stress incontinence.

It is therefore not the spatial location of the vesical neck and proximal urethra but the urethrovesical anatomic configuration as specifically manifested by the posterior urethrovesical angle that is involved in the continence mechanism. Urethrocystograms in normal, continent women reveal a flat bladder base and a sharply defined posterior urethrovesical angle (90 to 100 degrees), with at least one-third of the bladder base taking part in the formation of this angle (see Figure 12–4); even on coughing the angle is maintained and there is no funneling or posterior descent of the bladder neck. Patients with stress incontinence, on the other hand, invariably exhibit complete or nearly complete loss of the posterior urethrovesical angle, with resulting funneling and posterior descent of the vesical neck to the most dependent portion of the bladder. Many others, some of whom are cited in the references, have verified this relationship between absence of the posterior urethrovesical angle and the occurrence of stress incontinence. These numerous, well-documented, and convincing urethrocystographic studies demonstrating the loss of the posterior urethrovesical angle as characteristic and of etiologic importance to stress incontinence, together with other evidence, direct and indirect, in support of the validity of this concept can be outlined as follows:

1. When the act of voiding in normal, continent women is studied fluoroscopically, using a radiopaque liquid medium as described by Muellner and Fleischner,[28] obliteration of the normal posterior urethrovesical angle with descent and funneling of the bladder neck immediately prior to detrusor contraction and

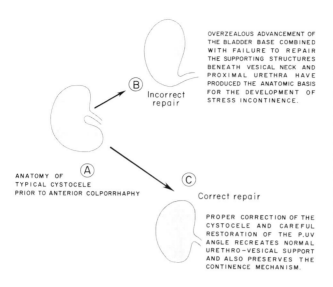

OVERZEALOUS ADVANCEMENT OF THE BLADDER BASE COMBINED WITH FAILURE TO REPAIR THE SUPPORTING STRUCTURES BENEATH VESICAL NECK AND PROXIMAL URETHRA HAVE PRODUCED THE ANATOMIC BASIS FOR THE DEVELOPMENT OF STRESS INCONTINENCE.

B Incorrect repair

ANATOMY OF TYPICAL CYSTOCELE PRIOR TO ANTERIOR COLPORRHAPHY — A

C Correct repair

PROPER CORRECTION OF THE CYSTOCELE AND CAREFUL RESTORATION OF THE P.UV ANGLE RECREATES NORMAL URETHRO-VESICAL SUPPORT AND ALSO PRESERVES THE CONTINENCE MECHANISM.

Figure 12-4. The two basic types of anatomic configuration encountered in patients with stress incontinence, as revealed by the lateral standing-straining view of the urethrocystogram. In both Type I and Type II the posterior urethrovesical angle is lost, but in Type II there is, in addition, an increase in the angle of inclination of the urethral axis, varying from 45 to 120 degrees, depending on the amount of rotational descent of the urethra. The typical lateral straining urethrocystogram found in continent women with normal support is shown for comparison. (From Green, T. H., Jr.: Gynecology—Essentials of Clinical Practice. 2nd Ed. Boston, Little, Brown & Company, 1971.)

actual micturition is observed. In other words, in the normal physiology of micturition, use is made of the potential change in urethrovesical pressure relationships—a change that is favorable to urine flow—which results from loss of the posterior urethrovesical angle, even before the detrusor contraction begins to increase intravesical pressure. Thus, the patient suffering from stress incontinence and exhibiting the characteristic loss of the posterior urethrovesical angle is, anatomically speaking, constantly in the preliminary phase of the voiding act; a sudden increase in intravesical pressure occasioned by cough or similar stress inevitably produces the same result that detrusor contraction achieves during normal micturition.

2. Reference has already been made to the repeated urethrocystographic demonstration, in numerous studies of large numbers of patients, that absence of the posterior urethrovesical angle is the characteristic, essentially universal anatomic abnormality associated with stress incontinence.

3. The vesical neck elevation test of Bonney, Read, and Marchetti, widely and successfully used as an aid in the diagnosis and management of stress incontinence, rests on the fact that one can temporarily prevent stress incontinence by manually restoring and maintaining the normal posterior urethrovesical angle and urethral axis during the course of a pelvic examination.

4. When one considers the nature of the operative procedures for stress incontinence which have been devised over the years, particularly those which have most consistently yielded successful results, it is apparent that the production of a posterior urethrovesical angle is the one important feature common to all. The original "Kelly vesical neck plication stitch" did create this angle, although not nearly so effectively or permanently as do the procedures performed today.[2] A properly performed anterior colporrhaphy has the same effect, but the Marshall-Marchetti urethrovesical suspension and the fascial sling procedures are the most successful of all, reliably creating an adequate posterior urethrovesical angle, as well as restoring a normal urethral axis.

5. Perhaps the most telling evidence is to be found in the many reported studies involving preoperative and postoperative urethrocystograms in patients

undergoing operations to correct stress incontinence.[1,2,3,6,9,14,15,20,21,30,31,32,33] These numerous observations clearly demonstrated that cure of the stress incontinence was always accompanied by restoration of a normal posterior urethrovesical angle and a normal urethral axis. On the other hand, failures or recurrences were just as invariably associated with failure to create or maintain an adequate posterior urethrovesical angle and a normal urethral axis, again as revealed by the post-operative urethrocystograms.

6. Numerous unplanned clinical experiments have occurred in the form of the well-known iatrogenic stress incontinence, which sometimes follows vaginal hysterectomy or anterior colporrhaphy. In a number of such instances, preoperative and postoperative urethrocystograms have clearly shown that a previously adequate posterior urethrovesical angle in a perfectly continent patient had been completely effaced as a result of the vaginal surgery, leading to the immediate development of stress incontinence postoperatively (see Figure 12–5).

THE URETHRAL AXIS. The probable significance of the urethral axis was first brought to light by the classic studies of Bailey in Manchester, England. His continuing observations employing preoperative and postoperative urethrocysto-grams were made and reported during the decade between 1954 and 1964.[1] When

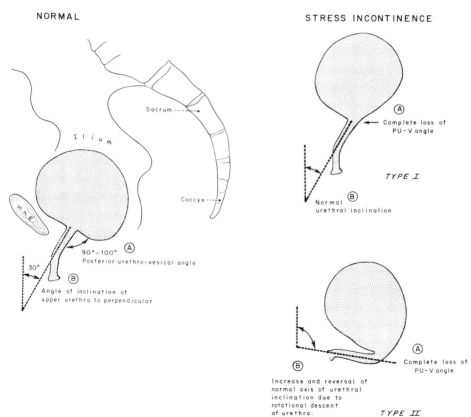

Figure 12-5. Drawings from urethrocystograms illustrating the probable mechanisms involved in the iatrogenic production of stress incontinence following improperly executed anterior colporrhaphy for cystocele. (From Green, T. H., Jr.: Development of a plan for the diagnosis and treatment of urinary stress incontinence. Am. J. Obstet. Gynecol. 83:632–648, 1962).

Bailey's data, together with our own similar observations of a series of 90 patients, were analyzed carefully, it seemed apparent that, in addition to the loss of the posterior urethrovesical angle occurring in all patients with stress incontinence, there was in essence only one other variable feature of basic importance—namely, the urethral axis, or angle of inclination between the proximal two-thirds of the urethra and the bladder base. It therefore seemed possible to define two basic types of anatomy in patients with stress incontinence (see Figure 12–4):

Type I. Type I includes complete or nearly complete loss of the posterior urethrovesical angle, but with the angle of inclination to the vertical of the urethral axis either normal (range, 10 to 30 degrees), or at least less than 45 degrees, as shown on urethrocystograms in the lateral standing-straining view.

Type II. This type is characterized by loss of the posterior urethrovesical angle and, in addition, a definitely abnormal angle of inclination from the vertical of the urethral axis, greater than 45 degrees and often even completely reversed (greater than 90 degrees). Patients with this downward and backward rotational descent of the urethral axis invariably experience the most severe degree of stress incontinence; they are the most difficult to treat effectively and in the past have had the highest failure rates after various operative procedures. Undoubtedly Type II stress incontinence represents the result of a more profound weakening of the supports of the proximal urethra and bladder neck.

This classification of patients with stress incontinence into two separate anatomic categories based on the urethral axis factor (Type I and Type II) has proved to be of great importance to the selection of the proper operative repair for the individual patient. Bailey[1] had found in 1956 that vaginal repair alone, although yielding highly satisfactory results in the Type I patient, produced cure of stress incontinence in no more than 50 per cent of the Type II patients. However, the introduction and subsequent use of his "modified colporrhaphy" in the management of patients with Type II stress incontinence had resulted in a 90 per cent 5 to 10 year cure rate in these cases by the time of his 1963 report. Clinical experience at our institution has been entirely in accord with Bailey's observations. As reported in 1962,[9] retrospective analysis of our material from 5 years previously had revealed that a careful vaginal operation had successfully relieved the stress incontinence in 90 per cent of the patients with the Type I anatomic configuration, but had failed to correct effectively or permanently the abnormal anatomy or relieve the symptom of incontinence in over 50 per cent of the patients with the Type II anatomic defect. However, use of the Marshall-Marchetti suprapubic urethrovesical suspension in the management of 28 women with Type II stress incontinence resulted in a 93 per cent 2 to 5 year cure rate. (The long-term results in a much larger series of patients in whom selection of the operative procedure was based largely on the urethral axis factor are included in the final section of this article, *Treatment and End-Results.*) The significance of the abnormal urethral axis to a better understanding of the pathologic anatomy of stress incontinence, as well as to the selection of the proper operative procedure for a specific patient, has subsequently been confirmed in a number of other reports.[2,3,6,14,30,31,32,33]

The loss of the posterior urethrovesical angle and the downward and backward rotation of the urethral axis which so universally accompany stress incontinence can be interpreted as simply a reflection of poor urethral support, which in turn prevents the normal transmission of sudden intra-abdominal pressure increases to the urethra, thus resulting in stress incontinence. However, since these two specific anatomic changes represent the most objective and essentially universal features of stress incontinence, and since successful operative correction depends on and is invariably accompanied by their restoration to normal, one cannot help concluding that the anatomic configuration of the urethrovesical junction and the proximal urethra is of fundamental importance to a correct understanding of this disorder.

Furthermore, it seems quite likely that absence of the posterior urethrovesical angle is also important of and by itself, not merely as an index of inadequate urethral support. As Hodgkinson, Jeffcoate and Roberts, and other authors have pointed out, loss of the anatomic configuration of the posterior urethrovesical angle results in the displacement of the vesical neck to the most dependent portion of the bladder, thus positioning the internal urinary meatus at the point of maximum hydrostatic pressure. As illustrated in Figure 12–6, this anatomic funneling effect caused by the loss of the posterior urethrovesical angle renders impossible the equal transmission of sudden elevations of intra-abdominal pressure to the lumen of the proximal urethra via its walls and their supports, so that intravesical pressure in the region of the vesical neck rises higher than intraurethral pressure just beyond it, and stress incontinence is the result. This concept of the inherent significance of the posterior urethrovesical angle finds further support in the observation that patients with large cystoceles, in many of whom the vesical neck and proximal urethra have descended markedly and may even lie outside the introitus, never suffer from stress incontinence. Urethrocystograms in such patients demonstrate a normal posterior urethrovesical angle, and, as shown

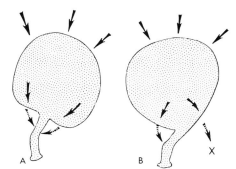

Figure 12-6. Diagrams illustrating the inherent importance of the posterior urethrovesical angle to the continence mechanism. As shown in *A*, the presence of a normal posterior urethrovesical angle permits maximum transmission (indicated by the dashed line arrows) of sudden increases in intra-abdominal pressure on all sides of the proximal urethra. In this way, intraurethral pressure is maintained at a higher level than the simultaneous elevated intravesical pressure, preserving the competency of the vesical neck sphincter mechanism and preventing loss of urine with sudden stress.

In contrast, as shown in *B*, loss of the posterior urethrovesical angle results in displacement of the vesical neck to the most dependent portion of the bladder, the point of maximum hydrostatic pressure. This anatomic funneling effect also renders impossible the equal transmission of sudden elevations in intra-abdominal pressure to the lumen of proximal urethra via its walls and their supports. (The dashed line arrow at *X* serves to indicate the impossibility of any effective transmission of pressure to the posterior aspect of the proximal urethra, as well as the tendency for the "internal urinary meatus" at the level of the vesical neck to be forced open.) Intravesical pressure in the region of the vesical neck thus rises considerably more than intraurethral pressure just beyond it, and stress incontinence occurs. (From Green, T. H., Jr.: The problem of urinary stress incontinence in the female: an appraisal of its current status. Obstet. Gynec. Surv. 23:603, 1968. © 1968, The Williams and Wilkins Co., Baltimore.)

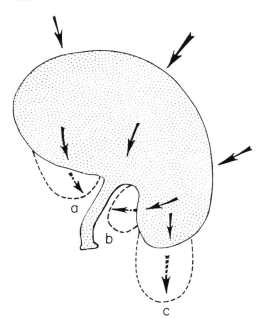

Figure 12-7. Diagram illustrating how the invariable preservation of a normal posterior urethrovesical angle in the presence of even a marked cystocele permits equal transmission of sudden increases in intra-abdominal pressure to the proximal urethra (indicated by the dashed line arrows *a* and *b*). In addition, the simultaneously occurring increase in intravesical pressure may even be rendered somewhat less by virtue of the dissipating effect of the resulting further bulging out of the cystocele (indicated by the arrow at *c*). (From Green, T. H., Jr.: The problem of urinary stress incontinence in the female: an appraisal of its status. Obstet. Gynec. Surv. 23:603, 1968. © 1968, The Williams and Wilkins Co., Baltimore.)

in Figure 12–7, this prevents intravesical pressure from exceeding intraurethral pressure during coughing or similar stresses, despite the fact that the proximal urethra has completely lost its normal "intra-abdominal location."

Similarly, the tendency to rotational downward and backward descent of the urethral axis in patients with stress incontinence would likewise seem to be of importance of and by itself, above and beyond the fact that it is indicative of inadequate urethral support. As illustrated diagrammatically in Figure 12–8, the usual maximal transmission of stress-induced sudden elevations in intra-abdominal pressure to the urethral wall and its surrounding soft tissue supports, which normally produces an increase in intra-urethral pressure equal to the sudden rise in intravesical pressure, no longer occurs. This normal, maximal pressure transmission depends on the urethra remaining in a fixed position and is dissipated and

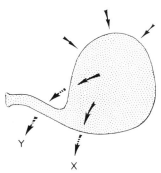

Figure 12-8. Diagram illustrating how, in Type II stress incontinence, transmission to the proximal urethra of sudden increases in intra-abdominal pressure, already impaired by absence of the normal posterior urethrovesical angle (dashed line arrow at *X*), is further reduced by the fact that the pressure being transmitted produces only a dissipating rotational descent of the urethra (dashed line arrow at *Y*), rather than the maximum possible rise in intraluminal pressure within the proximal urethra, which would have occurred had the latter remained in a relatively fixed position. (From Green, T. H., Jr., The problem of urinary stress incontinence in the female: an appraisal of its status. Obstet. Gynec. Surv. 23:603, 1968. © 1968, The Williams and Wilkins Co., Baltimore.)

greatly reduced by the effect of the rotational urethral descent that occurs instead, in response to the sudden stress-induced increase in intra-abdominal pressure. Thus, there is an even greater disparity between the deficiently transmitted rise in intraurethral pressure and the much greater rise in intravesical pressure in patients with both an abnormal urethral axis and an absent posterior urethrovesical angle than in patients in whom loss of the posterior urethrovesical angle is not accompanied by any significant abnormality of the urethral axis.

In summary, the evidence is overwhelming that the specific urethrovesical relationships characterized by the posterior urethrovesical angle and the urethral axis are the crucial factors in the etiology of stress incontinence and in its successful surgical correction. This concept is in no way incompatible with the observed alterations in urethrovesical pressure relationships. It is clear that the latter are in reality secondary to the more fundamental urethrovesical anatomic abnormalities.

Diagnosis

In the management of patients apparently suffering from stress incontinence, the first step is to obtain definite, objective proof of the presence of true, anatomic stress incontinence and to exclude the possibility that some other disorder causing abnormal urinary leakage is merely simulating it. It is obviously of paramount importance not to subject such patients to operations designed to correct true anatomic stress incontinence, since not only can no benefit be expected, but the patient may well be made immeasurably worse, as in the case of a diabetic with bladder neuropathy and secondary overflow and urgency incontinence, in whom complete urinary retention may be the unhappy end-result of the ill-advised surgery.

In addition to a careful history and detailed physical examination, other studies helpful in revealing incontinence resulting from intrinsic pathology of the urinary tract or neurological disturbances affecting bladder function include urinalysis and urine culture, intravenous pyelography, cystoscopy, cystometrograms, and measurement of postvoiding residuals. Invariably all of these studies are normal in the patient with true anatomic stress incontinence.

The so-called vesical neck elevation test, variations of which have been devised independently by Marchetti and by Bonney and Read, is also useful in tentatively establishing that an anatomic abnormality is responsible for the stress incontinence, and that it is potentially correctible by reparative surgery. In Marchetti's extensive experience with this test, as well as that of many institutions, including our own, it has been found to be highly reliable, with occasional exceptions. Low[24] found it to be confirmatory in every case in his analysis of the clinical characteristics of 138 patients with stress incontinence.

However, the most decisive and helpful study of all continues to be the metallic bead chain urethrocystogram, the technique of which has been amply described elsewhere[10] and need not be detailed here. Radiologic study of the urethrovesical relationships not only confirms the presence and precisely demonstrates the extent of the anatomic defect responsible for the symptom in patients with true stress incontinence, but also, when the urethrocystogram is normal, serves to positively exclude those cases in which the abnormal urinary leakage results from some other defect. Routine use of the urethrocystogram makes possible the distinction between the Type I and Type II abnormal urethrovesical anatomic configurations. This additional information enables one to better select the operative procedure most likely to be successful in each case.

There have been only two published reports of difficulties in interpretation and dissatisfaction with chain urethrocystography in the evaluation of patients with stress incontinence.[13,22] Both of these studies suffered from the same serious shortcomings: small numbers of patients were involved in each, and in both the period of postoperative follow-up was far too short to permit any meaningful conclusions regarding correlation of preoperative and postoperative urethrocystograms with the success or failure of the surgery to relieve the stress incontinence. In point of fact, only a small percentage of the patients in these two series failed to exhibit the typical abnormal anatomy in the preoperative urethrocystograms. Furthermore, the initial failure rate during the early postoperative months was much higher than is customary, and the short postoperative follow-up observation periods in these two series varied from only 2 to 18 months. Hence, the inability to completely correlate cure of stress incontinence with the urethrovesical anatomy shown on the postoperative urethrocystograms can hardly invalidate the close correlation between restoration of normal urethrovesical anatomy and permanent cure of stress incontinence observed and reported by so many others. Rather, it suggests that the eventual permanent cure rates in these two exceptional series will decline even further.

Treatment and End Results

A variety of operations to correct stress incontinence have been devised over the years. However, nearly all can be categorized as either basically a vaginal approach (an attempt to reconstruct normal urethrovesical anatomy and support by a dissection and repair from below—e.g., anterior colporrhaphy with vesical neck plication or various modifications of the suburethral myoplasty operation of Ingelman-Sundberg[18]) or a suprapubic approach through the prevesical retropubic space (an effort to restore normal urethrovesical anatomy and support by dissection and resuspension of the involved structures from above—e.g., the Marshall-Marchetti suprapubic urethrovesical suspension[27] and the modification of this developed by Burch,[5] or the various modifications of the fascial sling procedure[34]). A few operative procedures combine elements of both these basic surgical approaches to the problem, examples being the previously cited "modified colporrhaphy" utilized by Bailey,[1] the Ball "combined cystopexy"[3] technique, as well as the more recently devised Pereyra operation,[30] all of which involve a preliminary anterior vaginal paraurethral and vesical neck repair followed by a modified Marshall-Marchetti type of suprapubic urethrovesical suspension.

Probably the most significant advance in the therapeutic approach during the past decade has been the increasing emphasis on precisely defining the anatomic abnormality of the urethrovesical region present in each patient and then selecting the operative procedure of choice for each individual on this basis, wherever possible. The work of Bailey[1] and the studies reported from our hospital in 1962,[9] which defined the two basic types of abnormal urethrovesical anatomic configuration and demonstrated the inability of the standard vaginal procedures to satisfactorily correct the Type II anatomic configuration, have already been presented in detail. Both reports noted that vaginal repair was highly successful in correcting the Type I anatomic defect, but that a suprapubic approach, using the Marshall-Marchetti or fascial sling type of procedure, was necessary to achieve satisfactory cure rates in patients with Type II stress incontinence. Marked improvement in the overall permanent cure rate of stress incontinence was noted when these criteria were used to select the operative procedure of choice. Similar observations and conclusions based on analysis of their own extensive clinical experience have been reported by a number of others,[2,3,6,14,30-33] all of whom employed preoperative and postoperative urethrocystography in the study and management of their patients. Shingleton and associates[32] specifically reemphasized the importance of this, noting that all patients in their series had abnormal chain cystograms preoperatively, whereas their continent controls all had normal urethrocystograms, and that their patients with good operative results all showed restoration of normal urethrovesical anatomy in the postoperative chain cystogram, whereas there was persistence of the typical urethrovesical abnormality in the postoperative urethrocystogram in the patients in whom the operation was not successful. They recorded a marked improvement in their overall results by virtue of selecting the operative procedure in each case on the basis of urethrocystographic demonstration of whether the abnormal urethrovesical anatomy was of the Type I or Type II variety.

It would be appropriate to conclude this section by further documenting the fact that improvement in the permanent operative cure rate of stress incontinence does occur when the operative procedure is selected on the basis of the specific type of urethrovesical anatomic abnormality, revealed by the metallic bead chain urethrocystogram, as follows:

For Type I, the procedure is usually (1) vaginal repair (anterior and posterior colporrhaphy, most often with vaginal hysterectomy), if the overall problem dictates a vaginal approach (see Figure 12–9). (2) In situations in which the overall problem is best handled by an abdominal approach, a Marshall-Marchetti suprapubic urethrovesical suspension is performed, with abdominal hysterectomy and perineorrhaphy when indicated.

For Type II, the procedure is one of the following: (1) If the vaginal approach is believed to be indicated because of associated prolapse and perineal relaxation, vaginal hysterectomy with anterior and posterior colporrhaphy is performed, but in combination with the Marshall-Marchetti suprapubic urethrovesical suspension, which is carried out immediately following completion of the vaginal procedure. (2) If the need for vaginal repair is not evident, a primary Marshall-Marchetti procedure is carried out, with abdominal hysterectomy, if indicated, readily being accomplished first through the same incision (see Figure 12–10). (3) For the occasional failure following the Marshall-Marchetti operation, the rectus fascial sling operation has proved quite effective in ultimately restoring normal urethrovesical anatomy and achieving continence. The rectus fascial sling procedure has in general proved more complicated, and is often attended by significant postoperative voiding difficulties. It has, therefore, been used only infrequently as a primary operation, usually in obese, asthmatic patients with relatively weak, thinned-out tissues available locally, and those in whom severe stresses will be inevitable in the postoperative period. Specific details of operative techniques involved in performing these various surgical procedures have been described elsewhere.[12]

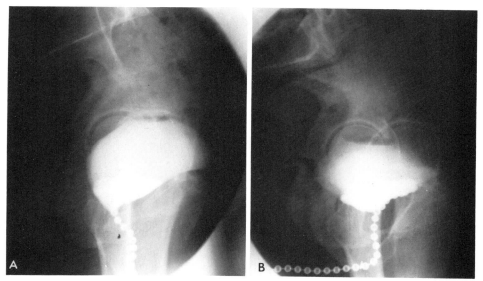

Figure 12-9.   Urethrocystogram in Type I stress incontinence. *A*, Preoperative film; *B*, postoperative film following vaginal hysterectomy and anterior and posterior colporrhaphies. Note restoration of normal posterior urethrovesical angle postoperatively, with relief of stress incontinence. (From Green, T. H., Jr.: Gynecology—Essentials of Clinical Practice. 2nd Ed. Boston, Little, Brown & Company, 1971.)

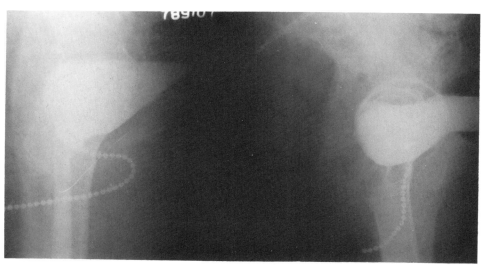

Figure 12-10.   Urethrocystogram in Type II stress incontinence. Preoperative film on the left; on the right, postoperative film following the Marshall-Marchetti suprapubic urethrovesical suspension operation. Note restoration of normal posterior urethrovesical angle and the normal urethral axis of inclination postoperatively, with relief of stress incontinence. (From Green, T. H., Jr.: Gynecology—Essentials of Clinical Practice. 2nd Ed. Boston, Little, Brown & Company, 1971.)

Such a plan of management seems to be providing more logical and effective selection of the particular operation or combination of surgical procedures best suited to correcting the specific type of abnormal urethrovesical anatomic configuration in each individual patient. Although suprapubic operations are frequently called for, this program for selection has the distinct advantage of permitting the retention of the vaginal approach for the many patients in whom this is desirable because of associated uterine prolapse. This procedure may be performed with the confidence that a high rate of cure can be expected in the Type I patients, and with the knowledge that an equally high rate of success can be obtained in the Type II patients by the addition of a supplementary suprapubic urethrovesical suspension to the overall surgical procedure. Among 110 patients undergoing corrective surgery during the period between 1953 and 1957, the overall cure rate was only 80 per cent, but since adoption of this plan of management in 1957, the permanent cure rate in subsequent years has risen to 96 per cent.

We continue to employ this program of management at our institution, and a recent analysis of the end-results reported in 1968[11] offers further convincing evidence for its success. As shown in Table 12–1, 181 patients were treated during the period of 1957 to 1963 and have now been followed for from 8 to 14 years. In addition to the routine preoperative metallic bead chain urethrocystogram, all patients had had one or more postoperative urethrocystograms taken. Without exception, x-ray studies demonstrated the typical abnormal urethrovesical anatomy preoperatively, and, of equal significance, patients cured of stress incontinence presented and continued to retain a normal-appearing urethrocystogram postoperatively, whereas in the operative failures there was reappearance of the characteristic abnormal urethrovesical anatomy on the postoperative films. Type I configuration was present in 35 patients (20 per cent of the total series), and a primary cure rate of 94 per cent was obtained in this group, one additional patient being cured by a second operation, yielding a final cure rate of 97 per cent for the 8 to 14 year follow-up period. Type II abnormal anatomic configuration was present in 146 patients (80 per cent of the total series), and a 90 per cent primary cure rate was achieved by the initial operation; an additional 10 patients in this group were relieved of stress incontinence by a second operation, yielding a final cure rate of 96 per cent over the 8 to 14 year interval of postoperative observation. The final cure rate for the entire group of 181 patients followed 8 to 14 years postoperatively was thus 96 per cent.

As indicated in Table 12–2, the vast majority (26 of 35) of the patients with Type I configuration underwent primary vaginal procedures, with a cure rate of 96 per cent for the vaginal approach. There was also one failure in the group of 9 undergoing a Marshall-Marchetti procedure; this represents an obvious

TABLE 12–1. *Results of Stress Incontinence Treatment Program,*
*Massachusetts General Hospital, 1957–1963**

ANATOMIC TYPE	NUMBER OF PATIENTS	PRIMARY CURE	SECONDARY CURE	FINAL CURE RATE	PERSISTENT FAILURE RATE
Type I	35 (20%)	33 (94%)	1	34 (97%)	1 (3%)
Type II	146 (80%)	131 (90%)	10	141 (96%)	5 (4%)
TOTALS	181	164 (91%)	11	175 (96%)	6 (4%)

* Duration of follow-up: 8 to 14 years.

TABLE 12–2.   *Results of Surgery in 35 Patients with Type I Stress Incontinence*

OPERATION	PRIMARY CURE	SECONDARY CURE	FAILURE	PERSISTENT FAILURE
Vaginal repair, with or without hysterectomy	25	—	1	—
Abdominal hysterectomy and Marshall-Marchetti operation	7	—	1	—
Marshall-Marchetti operation alone	1	—	—	—
Repeat Marshall-Marchetti operation	—	1	—	—
No further surgery	—	—	—	1
TOTAL	33(94%)	1(3%)	2(6%)	1(3%)

TABLE 12–3.   *Results of Surgery in 146 Patients with Type II Stress Incontinence*

OPERATION	CURED	FAILED
Marshall-Marchetti with hysterectomy	73	2
Marshall-Marchetti without hysterectomy	24	5
Marshall-Marchetti with previous hysterectomy	24	2
Vaginal hysterectomy with repairs	3	3
Vaginal hysterectomy with Marshall-Marchetti	4	—
Vaginal repair without hysterectomy	—	2
Fascial sling operation	3	1
TOTAL	131(90%)	15(10%)

technical failure, since this patient was completely cured by a repeat Marshall-Marchetti operation.

Table 12–3 presents the results of the various procedures employed in patients with Type II anatomy. It is of considerable interest from the standpoint of one particular technical question (should hysterectomy usually accompany a Marshall-Marchetti operation?), and it also emphasizes once more the relative inability of the standard vaginal approach alone to correct stress incontinence of the Type II anatomic variety. Seventy-three of 75 patients undergoing the Marshall-Marchetti procedure with concomitant abdominal hysterectomy were cured (97 per cent), and 24 of 26 patients who had undergone prior hysterectomy for other causes and who were then treated by us for stress incontinence by the Marshall-Marchetti operation were cured (92 per cent). On the other hand, in 29 patients in this series, the uterus was left in place at the time the Marshall-Marchetti operation was done, and the cure rate was only 83 per cent. This experience strongly suggests, and in fact has led us to adopt, a policy of concomitant hysterectomy whenever a Marshall-Marchetti operation is performed for Type II stress incontinence, unless there is a good reason to avoid removal of the uterus—e.g., occasionally in younger patients in whom preservation of child-bearing function is desired, or in an elderly patient for whom the addition of hysterectomy might unnecessarily increase the operative risk or morbidity. That concomitant hysterectomy need not be mandatory is obvious from the reasonably satisfactory cure rate of 83 per cent observed in this series when the Marshall-Marchetti procedure alone was done, and also from Marchetti's report[26] of having done the procedure in a number of young women who later conceived and underwent vaginal delivery without subsequent recurrence of their stress incontinence. Nevertheless, it seems apparent that if conditions are favorable and there is no valid reason to preserve the uterus, concomitant hysterectomy will increase the permanent, long-term cure rate of the Marshall-Marchetti suprapubic urethrovesical suspension.

That the standard vaginal approach is relatively ineffective in correcting Type II stress incontinence is also emphasized in Table 12–3. A small number of patients were selected for vaginal procedures because they were relatively poor candidates for abdominal surgery, in spite of the knowledge that their urethrovesical anatomic abnormality was of the Type II configuration. Six underwent vaginal hysterectomy with anterior and posterior colporrhaphies, and, as expected, only three were cured, the 50 per cent cure rate being identical to that noted by Bailey and also reported in our own previous series. Two patients underwent anterior and posterior colporrhaphies alone, without hysterectomy, and neither was relieved of her stress incontinence. It is of further interest to note, in Table 12–4, that all five of these initial failures to cure Type II stress incontinence by a vaginal approach were later cured by a properly selected second operation—a Marshall-Marchetti in two patients and a fascial sling in the third patient of the three failures following vaginal hysterectomy and repairs; and hysterectomy plus a Marshall-Marchetti in the two failures following vaginal repairs alone. In contrast (see Table 12–3), four patients with uterine prolapse accompanying their Type II stress incontinence underwent vaginal hysterectomy with concomitant Marshall-Marchetti urethrovesical suspension as their primary operation, and all four were completely cured of their stress incontinence.

As noted in Tables 12–3 and 12–4, the fascial sling operation was used only 11 times in this series of 181 patients. It was employed as the primary operation in four patients who were obese and asthmatic, with three cures (75 per cent), and as the second operation on seven occasions following an initial failure, with cure occurring in six patients (86 per cent). A number of these patients experienced prolonged voiding difficulties, a few requiring catheter drainage for 3 to 6 months. Thus, the fascial sling procedure, though a somewhat more complicated and extensive procedure than the Marshall-Marchetti operation, has yielded very

TABLE 12–4. *Results of Secondary Surgery in 15 Patients with Type II Stress Incontinence and Failure of Primary Operation*

PATIENTS CURED BY REPEAT OPERATIONS (10 PATIENTS)			
Failed Primary Procedure	*No.*	*Successful Secondary Procedure*	*No.*
Vaginal hysterectomy and repairs	1		
Marshall-Marchetti and hysterectomy	1	Fascial sling operation (2 with	
Marshall-Marchetti without hysterectomy	2	hysterectomy)	6
Marshall-Marchetti with previous hysterectomy	2		
Vaginal repairs without hysterectomy	2	Marshall-Marchetti with hysterectomy	2
Vaginal hysterectomy and repairs	2	Marshall-Marchetti alone	2
UNSUCCESSFUL MULTIPLE SECONDARY SURGERY (2 PATIENTS)			
Marshall-Marchetti without hysterectomy	1	Vaginal repairs; fascial sling	1
Fascial sling	1	Marshall-Marchetti; vaginal repairs; vaginal sling	1
PERSISTENT FAILURE (3 PATIENTS)			
Marshall-Marchetti with hysterectomy	1	No further surgery	3
Marshall-Marchetti without hysterectomy	2		

satisfactory results when used selectively in situations in which the Marshall-Marchetti procedure either has already failed or seems less likely to be effective.

REFERENCES

1. Bailey, K. V.: A clinical investigation into uterine prolapse with stress incontinence. Treatment by modified Manchester colporrhaphy. J. Obstet. Gynec. Brit. Emp. Part I, 61:291, 1954; Part II, 63:663, 1956; and Part III, 79:947, 1963.
2. Barnett, R. M.: The modern Kelly plication. Obstet. Gynec. 34:667, 1969.
3. Barnett, R. M.: Ball combined cystopexy. Obstet. Gynec. 36:547, 1970.
4. Beck, R. P., and Maughan, G. B.: Simultaneous intraurethral and intravesical pressure studies in normal women and those with stress incontinence. Am. J. Obstet. Gynec. 89:746, 1964.
5. Burch, J. C.: Cooper's ligament urethrovesical suspension for stress incontinence. Am. J. Obstet. Gynec. 100:764, 1968.
6. Crist, T., Shingleton, H. M., and Roberson, W. E.: Urethrovesical needle suspension: postoperative loss of vesical neck support demonstrated by chain cystography. Obstet. Gynec. 34:489, 1969.
7. Dutton, W. A.: The urethrovesical angle and stress incontinence. Canad. Med. Ass. J. 83:1242, 1960.
8. Enhorning, G.: Simultaneous recording of intravesical and intraurethral pressure; a study on urethral closure in normal and stress incontinent women. Acta Chir. Scand. (Suppl.) 276:1, 1961.
9. Green, T. H., Jr.: Development of a plan for the diagnosis and treatment of urinary stress incontinence. Am. J. Obstet. Gynec. 83:632, 1962.
10. Green, T. H., Jr.: Urinary stress incontinence. In Meigs, J. V., and Sturgis, S. H. (eds.): Progress in Gynecology. Vol. IV. New York, Grune and Stratton, Inc., 1963.
11. Green, T. H., Jr.: The problem of urinary stress incontinence in the female: an appraisal of its current status. Obstet. Gynec. Surv. 23:603, 1968.
12. Green, T. H., Jr.: Operative management of urinary stress incontinence. Cooper, P. (ed.): The Craft of Surgery. Boston, Little, Brown & Co., 1971.
13. Greenwald, S. W., Thornbury, J. R., and Dunn, L. J.: Cystourethrography as a diagnostic aid in stress incontinence. Obstet. Gynec. 29:324, 1967.
14. Harer, W. B., Jr., and Gunther, R. E.: Simplified urethrovesical suspension and urethroplasty. Am. J. Obstet. Gynec. 91:1017, 1965.
15. Hodgkinson, C. P.: Relationships of the female urethra and bladder in urinary stress incontinence. Am. J. Obstet. Gynec. 65:560, 1953.
16. Hodgkinson, C. P., and Cobert, N.: Direct urethrocystometry. Am. J. Obstet. Gynec. 79:648, 1960.
17. Hodgkinson, C. P., Drukker, B. H., and Hershey, G. J. G.: Stress urinary incontinence in the female. VIII. Etiology, significance of the short urethra. Am. J. Obstet. Gynec. 86:16, 1963.
18. Ingelman-Sundberg, A.: Plastic repair of the pelvic floor with a report of 31 cases of stress incontinence. Acta Obstet. Gynec. Scand. 30:318, 1950.
19. Jeffcoate, T. N. A., and Roberts, H.: Observations on stress incontinence of urine. Am. J. Obstet. Gynec. 64:721, 1952.
20. Jeffcoate, T. N. A., and Roberts, H.: Stress incontinence of urine. J. Obstet. Gynec. Brit. Emp. 59:685, 1952.
21. Jeffcoate, T. N. A., and Roberts, H.: Effects of urethrocystopexy for stress incontinence. Surg. Gynec. Obstet. 98:743, 1954.
22. Kitzmiller, J. L., Manzer, G. A., Nebel, W. A., and Lucas, W. E.: Chain cystourethrogram and stress incontinence. Obstet. Gynec. 39:333, 1972.
23. Lapides, J., Ajemian, E. P., Stewart, B. H., Lichtwardt, J. R., and Breakey, B. A.: Physiopathology of stress incontinence. Surg. Gynec. Obstet. 111:224, 1960.
24. Low, J. A.: Clinical characteristics of patients with demonstrable urinary incontinence. Am. J. Obstet. Gynec. 88:322, 1964.
25. Marchetti, A. A.: The female bladder and urethra before and after correction for stress incontinence. Am. J. Obstet. Gynec. 58:1145, 1949.
26. Marchetti, A. A.: Urinary incontinence. J.A.M.A. 162:1366, 1956.
27. Marchetti, A. A., Marshall, V. F., and Shultis, L. D.: Simple vesicourethral suspension for stress incontinence of urine. Am. J. Obstet. Gynec. 74:57, 1957.
28. Muellner, S. R., and Fleischner, F. G.: Normal and abnormal micturition; study of bladder behavior by means of the fluoroscope. J. Urol. 61:233, 1949.

29. Pereyra, A. J.: A simplified surgical procedure for the correction of stress incontinence in women. West. J. Surg. 67:223, 1959.
30. Pereyra, A. J., and Labherz, T. B.: Combined urethrovesical suspension and vaginourethroplasty for correction of stress incontinence. Obstet. Gynec. 30:537, 1967.
31. Schonberg, L. A., Wentzel, G. M., and Higgins, L. W.: Urethrocystography, a practical office procedure in the evaluation and treatment of stress incontinence. Am. J. Obstet. Gynec. 86:995, 1963.
32. Shingleton, H. M., Barkley, K. L., and Talbert, L. M.: Management of stress urinary incontinence in the female. Use of the chain cystogram. South. Med. J. 59:547, 1966.
33. Steinhausen, T. B., Kariher, D. H., Sherwood, C. E., and Erdman, F. S.: Chain urethrocystography before and after urethrovesical suspension for stress incontinence. Obstet. Gynec. 35:405, 1970.
34. TeLinde, R. W.: The urethral sling operation. Clin. Obstet. Gynec. 6:206, 1963.
35. Toews, H. A.: Intraurethral and intravesical pressures in normal and stress-incontinent women. Obstet. Gynec. 29:613, 1967.

Diagnosis and Preferred
Management of Urinary Stress Incontinence

What is the Best Means to Diagnose and Treat Stress Urinary Incontinence?

C. PAUL HODGKINSON

Henry Ford Hospital

INTRODUCTION

In the previous volume of *Controversy in Obstetrics and Gynecology* the Editors stated that their objectives were to challenge well established medical dogmas in the light of recently developed diagnostic techniques and therapeutic advances to determine if there were a better way or ways for patients to be managed. This is a bold undertaking because to deviate from traditional views may lead to an incendiary venture of controversy and conflict. Yet, medical progress depends upon those who are brash enough to say that the old way is no longer good enough and that their way is better. But, if the opinions stated in this volume are challenges to the authors, they are greater challenges to the readers, because, in the end, it is the readers who must weigh, compare, and select the ideas and techniques which seem best.

In these respects there is no better subject of controversy than stress urinary incontinence (SUI). Thirty years ago, tradition dictated the management and expected "cure" rate: "Do a vaginal plastic first and if this fails go above" because "85 per cent of operations succeed and 15 per cent fail." Empiricism ruled the day and why an operation succeeded or failed was merely a matter of conjecture. Over the past 20 years, objective techniques of diagnosis have been introduced and surgical procedures have been proposed, which, of course, their proponents claim to be rational. Enthusiasts now make pleas to individualize the treatment of each patient, based on objective study techniques, and claim that the failure rate should be less than 5 per cent.

The opinions stated in this chapter reflect efforts made over the past 20 years to treat SUI objectively. At the outset, it should be clearly stated that objective techniques of study were never intended to replace clinical judgment;

412

SUI then, as now, is a clinical problem that cannot be reduced to the finite measurement of angles and curves. However, these objective techniques of study *have* been intended to provide the clinician with valuable information which cannot be obtained by clinical means alone, and this information can supplement and reinforce clinical evaluation of a patient and make it possible to render better and more reliable, successful treatment.

Modern objective investigative studies for SUI were begun in the early 1950's with reports by Jeffcoate and Roberts[1] in England and by Hodgkinson[2] in the United States. In both studies the bladder silhouette was demonstrated by instillation of a radiopaque dye into the bladder. Anteroposterior and lateral radiograms were taken with the patients erect, during rest and straining. Jeffcoate and Roberts demonstrated urethral configuration by means of a soft rubber catheter, and Hodgkinson employed a metallic bead chain. With the Jeffcoate-Roberts technique the urethra appeared to be straight, which made its junction with the bladder base angular. With the metallic bead chain technique, the delicate configuration and mobility of the urethra were undistorted and uninhibited, and the configuration was one of curves rather than angles. Jeffcoate and Roberts equated the diagnosis of SUI with "loss of the posterior urethrovesical angle," while Hodgkinson stated that displacement of the urethrovesical junction during the straining effort to the lowest level of the bladder, without posterior rotation of the bladder, was consistent with the diagnosis of SUI. Jeffcoate and Roberts emphasized that "loss of the posterior urethrovesical angle" was simply a radiographic sign and that the important feature was the general configuration of the urethrovesical junction and not the degree of angulation.

In 1963, Hodgkinson and associates[3] compared radiograms using both the metallic bead chain and the catheter techniques in the same patient. This study showed most effectively that the catheter not only caused a straightening of the urethra but also limited its downward mobility during the straining effort. Urethrovesical angulation was, as shown by this study, largely an artifact of the catheter technique.

An important milestone in the objective study of SUI was made apparent following the report by Marshall, Marchetti, and Krantz[4] on the technique of a "simple" retropubic operation for SUI. Prior to this report, most of the operations devised for SUI had as their major objectives a tightening or a reinforcement of the urethral sphincter as the means of curing SUI. In the Marshall-Marchetti technique, no effort was made to plicate or narrow the urethra. Using metallic bead chain urethrocystography, it soon became apparent that success of the procedure could be directly correlated with retropubic elevation of the urethrovesical junction to a level above the base of the bladder during the straining effort. From these observations, it was deducted that in SUI the urethral closing mechanism was not pathologically injured, but simply under stress; that, if stress was removed from the urethra by supporting it from below, the closing mechanism of the urethra could regain its normal tonus and again function effectively. The soundness of this observation has been proved on comparison of pre- and postoperative metallic bead urethrocystograms for hundreds of patients, with various types of operations for SUI. Regardless of the operative procedure used, durable success of the procedure can be equated with secure elevation of the urethrovesical junction above the lowest level of the base of the bladder during the straining effort.

Likewise, metallic bead urethrocystograms have decisively shown that neither the degree nor incidence of SUI can be directly correlated with the clinical estimation of relaxation of the vaginal wall supporting tissues. The most severe type of SUI may occur in patients whose bladders are located at a high retropubic level with no descensus during straining. Also, in patients with severe uterovaginal prolapse from maximum relaxation of supporting tissues, continence is the rule. In patients with SUI, metallic bead chain urethrocystography provides objective information which cannot be obtained by clinical evaluation alone. With the slight expense and little technical bother involved, plus the additional objective knowledge provided, there is little reason for not performing both pre- and postoperative metallic bead chain urethrocystograms on all patients operated upon for SUI. If for no other reason, comparison of the radiograms should be made in order to obtain objective evidence of what anatomic changes were effected by the operative procedure, as well as evidence as to why the operation succeeded or failed.

The thesis that urethrovesical radiograms are not dissimilar in so called normal subjects and in patients with SUI, which derived from comparative observations, is not valid. When man assumed upright posture, the urethrovesical relationships to each associated structure and to the surrounding tissues were vastly altered. Compared to structural configurations in the quadruped, in the erect position the junction of the female bladder with the urethra was changed from a lateral to an inferior position, and the inferior support to the longitudinal urethra afforded by the symphysis was lost. Thus, the stage was laid for the development of SUI. Questionnaire studies of nulliparous subjects are all in agreement that the human female is not a very continent individual. Well over 50 per cent of subjects admit to having some degree of SUI on extreme stress, and after childbirth the incidence is considerably higher.

Sufficient anatomic studies have been performed on human urethrovesical structures to decisively state that there is neither an anatomic nor a functional sphincter in the female urethra. Voluntary control depends upon smooth muscle tonus of the urethra plus reinforcement from ancillary fibromuscular supporting tissue. Given maximum weakness of the supporting structures at the point of the urethrovesical junction, the downward thrust incidental to a sudden increase in intra-abdominal pressure will cause vertical descent of the urethrovesical junction and a concomitant dilating influence on the inner urethra from the increased pressure transmitted to the urine contained in the bladder. On the other hand, if the infraurethrovesical junction supporting tissues are relatively strong, and the posterior bladder supporting tissues are weak, the downward thrust from sudden increased intra-abdominal pressure will cause the posterior bladder to descend, while the urethrovesical junction will remain relatively fixed. Analyzed from the standpoint of hydrodynamics, this means that the increased intravesical pressure transmitted from the abdomen is dissipated in the weakness of the posterior bladder, while the relatively well supported urethra is compressed from above downward. Thus, in the SUI configuration, the downward thrust of increased intra-abdominal pressure tends to open the urethra from within, while the configuration of posterior uterovaginal prolapse tends to compress the urethra externally from above. The same hydrostatic effects apply to successful urethropexy operations, whether performed abdominally or vaginally. This also explains why SUI develops after overzealous repair of a cystocele when it was not present before operation.

Because the human female has a natural propensity to lose urine on occasions of severe intra-abdominal stress, it is most important that baselines be established for definition of what constitutes normal urinary control for the human female. In the human male, normal urinary continence is under absolute voluntary control; in men, urinary dribbling or accidental urine loss calls for immediate urologic consultation. In the human female, on the other hand, such is not the case. Most women are accustomed to losing small amounts of urine on sudden intra-abdominal stress, particularly if their bladders are full or if they are caught unawares. However, in the majority of normal women, the incidence of urine loss is infrequent and the volume small, and they have no difficulty handling their social life without fear of embarrassment. This degree of loss of urinary control can be recognized to fall within the normal category and both pre- and postoperative judgments should be made on this basis.

Clinical SUI, therefore, is a matter of increased frequency of incontinence and increased volume of urine loss. Clinical SUI may be defined as the uncontrollable loss of urine through the intact urethra incidental to sudden increased intra-abdominal pressure, occurring sufficiently frequently and in sufficient volume as to limit social activity and cause embarrassment. This definition should be kept in mind, particularly by younger gynecologists, in contemplating the recommendation of an operation for correcting anatomic relaxation of the vaginal wall. Repairing vaginal wall relaxation in asymptomatic patients simply for aesthetic purposes may precipitate disastrous SUI.

DIFFERENTIAL DIAGNOSIS

Clinical SUI must be differentiated from all other forms of incontinence, including detrusor dyssynergia, urgency incontinence, and psychogenic incontinence.

In *clinical SUI* urine is lost as a spurt through the external urinary meatus precisely at the time of a peak of increased intra-abdominal pressure. The pressure motivating urine loss in SUI is always transmitted pressure from an extravesical source and it never occurs as the result of increased intrinsic pressure from detrusor contraction. The urine loss occurs most frequently when the patient has a moderately full bladder and when she is in the erect position, and there is never a sense of demanding urgency. The urine loss promptly ceases when the pressure falls.

This is in contrast to urine loss from *detrusor dyssynergia*. In this condition urine is lost as the result of increased intrinsic bladder pressure from contraction of the detrusor muscle. Except for mild cramping sensations, patients generally have no awareness of impending urine loss. Two types of detrusor dyssynergia have been recognized: *Type I* detrusor contraction occurs as the result of some physical effort, such as changing from a horizontal to an erect position, coughing, sneezing, and so forth; and *Type II* occurs spontaneously when the patient is quietly at rest and the detrusor contraction is apparently stimulated by a certain degree of bladder fullness. Type II is not likely to be confused with SUI because there is no physical effort involved. Type I, on the other hand, may be confused with SUI because the detrusor contraction is set off as the result of skeletal muscle activity, which is similar to that which causes SUI. In Type I detrusor dyssynergia, however, there is a time-relation difference: the urine loss does not occur precisely at the time of increased intra-abdominal pressure, as in SUI, but at a delayed interval of 10 to 20 seconds after the peak of increased intra-abdominal pressure has subsided. In Type I, urine is not lost as a spurt but rather as a continuous flow of urine extending over a period of about 10 seconds. The pattern of urine flow in detrusor dyssynergia of either type occurs because smooth muscle of all types responds to a stimulus in a slow, undulating peristaltic cycle, which cannot be interrupted until the cycle is complete. Skeletal muscle responds to a stimulus with an all-or-none reaction, which can be inhibited or continued at will.

In *urgency incontinence* urine is always lost as the result of a painful sense of urinary urgency. It may occur as the result of either, or both, intrinsic and extrinsic bladder pressures, and the urine loss may be provoked by physical, chemical, or bacterial stimuli. Usually there is associated intrinsic bladder pathology.

Psychogenic urinary incontinence, fortunately, is a relatively rare type of accidental urine loss which is always initiated by voluntary effort. Detection is extremely difficult, if not impossible, by clinical means. Usually the condition is of long standing and the patient herself may not recognize that her loss of urine is the result of an effort habit. Psychogenic urinary incontinence can be recognized easily with direct electrourethrocystometry if a rectal pressure lead is incorporated into the system. With this technique the loss of urine can be correlated precisely with voluntary efforts, and there is never evidence of initiation of voiding by involuntary detrusor contraction.

All forms of vesicourethral pressure dysfunctions are best studied by direct electrourethrocystometry, a technique first described by Hodgkinson and Cobert[5] in 1960. With this technique, the vesical and urethral pressures are continuously monitored as the bladder naturally fills with urine, from the time the bladder is empty until it becomes oppressively full. Because no other fluid is instilled into the bladder by catheter, subjective influences are reduced to a minimum, and delicate pressure changes in the bladder and urethra are detected easily. With a rectal pressure lead incorporated into the system, the spontaneous pressure curves of detrusor dyssynergia are distinguished easily from rises in pressure incidental to voluntary efforts involving the Valsalva maneuver. Direct electrourethrocystometry has provided valuable objective basic data for the study of the various dysfunctions of the female bladder and urethra.

TREATMENT

While the treatment of clinical SUI is always surgical, operation should be avoided in patients with detrusor dyssynergia because the severity of their difficulty may be aggravated. Some patients with detrusor dyssynergia respond favorably to anticholinergic drugs. However, for unknown reasons, all patients with this condition do not respond predictably to anticholinergic drugs and, for them, there is no satisfactory treatment. Because such patients generally lose urine when their bladders reach a certain degree of critical fullness, they should avoid excessive ingestion of fluid, diuretic drugs, and urinary stimulants. They should be taught to empty their bladders on a timed schedule rather than waiting until they acquire a sense of urgency. Patients with detrusor dyssynergia generally carry rather high residual urine volumes, and they are subject to recurring bladder infections. Every effort should be made to avoid urethrovesical instrumentation.

Patients with urgency incontinence generally have intrinsic bladder pathology and should receive urologic treatment. Trigonitis and chronic bacteriuria are common in patients with urgency incontinence. Proper toilet habits should be taught, and they should be instructed to void promptly when they experience a sense of urgency and not to try to hold back their urine flow. Cineradiography of voiding has shown that when the stream is voluntarily cut off, the urine in the medial two-thirds of the urethra is returned to the bladder. Culture studies have shown that the distal half of the urethra frequently harbors pathogenic bacteria and stopping the urinary stream may flush contaminated urine back into the bladder. Once the voiding process is started, women should void to completion and not intermittently try to interrupt the urine stream. Bacterial infections of the vagina and cervix should be eradicated. Proper dietary control should be advised to prevent chemical cystitis from ingesting acid-excreting foods, such as tomatoes.

Patients with SUI often have an associated urgency incontinence which develops from their constantly trying to inhibit the urinary stream to avoid wetting their clothing. Studies have shown that about 17 per cent of patients with SUI had primary chronic bacteriuria on admission to the hospital, compared to 10 per cent for other patients entering the hospital for gynecologic surgery.

Psychogenic urinary incontinence is difficult to treat, and the results are unpredictable. Generally, long-term psychotherapy is necessary. Great value has been achieved by demonstrating to the patient, from a direct electrourethrocystometric tracing, precisely the cause of her difficulty. Not infrequently, the etiology dates back to early childhood and it may stem from anxiety and resentment incidental to toilet training. All who work in obstetrics are aware of the mother who complains that her well-trained 3 year old started wetting his or her pants after a new baby was taken home!

Direct electrourethrocystometry has shown that mature domination over bladder control occurs only after detrusor autocontractility has been completely suppressed. Apparently this is a learned function achieved by childhood toilet training. In psychogenic urinary incontinence, mature domination over detrusor autocontractility either has not been achieved or has subsequently been lost. Since mature detrusor control is a learned function, apparently it can be unlearned also. Patients with long-standing vesicovaginal fistulae often lose urine from detrusor dyssynergia after successful repair of the fistula. Rehabilitation may be tedious and not entirely successful.

Treatment of clinical SUI requires surgical correction of the disturbed urethrovesical relationships. The crux of any successful operation for SUI is maintained elevation of the urethrovesical junction above the lowest level of the bladder during the straining effort. The best technique for achieving this objective depends upon the anatomic relationships of each individual patient. If there is distressing vaginal wall relaxation, and if the SUI is not too severe, generally this objective can be accomplished by a vaginal plastic procedure, provided that over-zealous repair of the cystocele is not done. However, in patients with bladders already located at relatively high retropubic levels, vaginal plastic procedures to relieve SUI are uncertain and frequently short-lived. Retropubic urethropexy by elevating and fixing the paravaginal fascia to the ileopectineal line at the brim of the bony pelvis, accomplished through a lower abdominal incision, has given the most dependable and durable results.

Unfortunately, the anterior vaginal wall fascia and other pelvic supporting tissues, which were weakened, stretched, and torn during previous vaginal deliveries, and which were further attenuated by estrogen deprivation in postmenopausal patients, are ill suited to withstand the continual downward thrusts of increased intra-abdominal pressure and the unremitting pull of the force of gravity. No tissue included in a vaginal plastic procedure, including the recently rediscovered pubo-urethral ligaments,[7,8] can be depended upon to permanently maintain the urethrovesical junction at the high level at which it apparently was placed at the time of operation. The so-called "85 per cent cure rate" once claimed for vaginal plastic operations has not been substantiated by recent studies. Low[9] found the failure rate of vaginal plastic operations to be as high as 50 per cent. Because postoperative attenuation of pelvic fasciae is a progressive process, recurrence of SUI occurs gradually, and operative results should be appraised at six, 12 and 24 month intervals for all types of operations.

In the moderately thin patient with a relaxed anterior vaginal wall, retropubic urethropexy by the vaginal wall technique is performed easily and the complication rate is low. However, this does not hold true for patients with recurrent SUI after previous vaginal plastic or suprapubic operations. In such patients, the vaginal wall may be too taut and too scarred to permit its elevation to the ileopectineal line. Dissection is difficult and complicated. Perforations of the bladder and urethra are common and often compounded. In such patients, other means to support the urethrovesical junction are necessary. I have found the use of suburethral slings devised from crossing the uterine ends of the round ligaments beneath the urethrovesical junction to be an effective means of elevating the urethrovesical junction. Recently, various forms of plastic mesh have been advocated for suburethral slings. Although Nichols[10] recently reported favorable results with Mersilene, Williams and TeLinde[11] and Ridley[12] found Mersilene unsatisfactory because of a high incidence of retropubic infection and a tendency for it to cut through the urethra. Morgan reported favorable results with Marlex.[13] The effectiveness of plastics as suburethral slings for the treatment of SUI probably has not been fully established.

Postoperative bladder drainage

As first reported in 1966 by Hodgkinson and Hodari,[14] suprapubic catheter cystostomy has continued to be a satisfactory means of draining the bladder following all types of operations for SUI. As compared to the use of a transurethral Foley catheter, many reports have confirmed the major attributes of the method: increased comfort to the patient, reduced nursing care, and a reduced incidence of bladder infection. With this technique, transurethral catheterization may be entirely eliminated, regardless of how long it takes for the patient to reestablish voluntary voiding.

"The Foley catheter syndrome"

The overall spectrum of side-effects that result from removing a transurethral Foley catheter too soon are not generally appreciated. Over the past several years, in some patients referred for consultation because of continued bladder dysfunction, electronic direct urethrocystometry has demonstrated high residual urine volumes and incomplete detrusor contractions on voluntary voiding. Significant bacteriuria of bladder urine was usually present. Each of the patients gave similar histories of previously having been operated on for some gynecologic condition which required bladder drainage postoperatively; each had had difficulty in reaching a satisfactory voiding pattern. Usually the patients were sent home with a Foley catheter and returned to the doctor's office to have it removed a week or so later. If spontaneous voiding followed removal of the catheter, no further bladder studies were done until the patient complained of being unable to empty the bladder or because of repeated bouts of urinary tract infection. I have designated the condition (for lack of a better name) the "iatrogenic retention syndrome," colloquially called the "Foley catheter syndrome," to signify that the condition possibly resulted from removing the Foley catheter too soon and to indicate that the condition was on a functional rather than a pathogenic basis. Tentatively, it is speculated that the condition developed because the detrusor muscle, as a smooth muscle, has the capability of adapting to various degrees of bladder fullness without losing tonus. I have visualized the patients involved as having had rather large residual urine volumes when the catheters were removed. As the result, when they developed a sense of urinary urgency, they were able to void only partially because the detrusor muscle did not completely contract. Gradually, in voiding, the detrusor muscle became conditioned to contracting down to the space occupied by the large residual urine volume, and then detrusor contractions ceased. As time went on, this conditioned reflex became more firmly established, and these patients' bladders never became completely empty.

From experience with this condition, the following treatment program has proved to be reasonably satisfactory. First, the patient's urethra and bladder have been urologically examined to rule out mechanical obstruction. Second, the urethra has been dilated once weekly with Hegar dilators to as high a caliber as possible without excessive discomfort. Third, a suprapubic cystostomy catheter has been installed into the bladder. The patient has been instructed to void at four-hour intervals and, after voiding, to completely empty her bladder by opening the suprapubic catheter. Also, she has been instructed to record both the amount of urine she voids and the amount of urine drained from the suprapubic catheter. She has been informed that the success of her treatment depends upon close adherence to the schedule outlined for her, and that she should not expect her bladder muscle to regain full function for several days or weeks. When the volume of residual urine has been reduced by about 50 per cent, the voiding interval is increased to six hours, and later the patient is instructed to void according to her sensation of urgency. The suprapubic catheter has not been removed until the residual urine volume has constantly remained below 30 cc. after the catheter has been clamped continually for 24 hours. The duration of treatment for some patients with well ingrained "iatrogenic detrusor dysfunction" has been as long as two months. It has been assumed that by this program the detrusor muscle gradually has become conditioned to adapting to the space occupied by smaller and smaller residual urine volumes, and when voiding occurred, the muscle contraction now did not stop at the large residual urine volume which was present when the treatment was begun.

SUPRAPUBIC CYSTOSTOMY APPARATUS

Finally, comment should be made upon the suprapubic cystostomy apparatus. In the original report,[14] straight plastic catheters were stated to be unsatisfactory because the bladder end of the catheter frequently passed into the urethra and produced obstruction to urine outflow. In experience with balloon-type catheters, such as the Foley catheter, unsatisfactory bladder drainage was experienced in over 15 per cent of patients. Apparently, with the Foley catheter, when the bladder was collapsed, the end of the catheter distal to the balloon passed into the internal urethra and caused the catheter to be nonfunctional. Efforts to modify the Foley catheter by placing holes above the balloon were not entirely satisfactory. Also, it was noted that catheters of the Foley type had the additional disadvantage of possessing a smaller functional lumen, as a consequence of which urine drainage was less efficient.

Of all the catheters we have used, none has been superior to the No. 12 Malecot soft rubber catheter. The mushroom-like flared tip of the catheter is sufficiently bulbous to prevent its being passed into the inner urethra, and the four openings in the distal end are sufficiently large to prevent easy obstruction. Also, this catheter is readily available as a standard hospital item, and it is far less expensive than the kits introduced recently. The only inconvenience to the Malecot catheter is that it must be stretched over a metal stylet to permit its introduction through the cannula of the trochar used for inserting it into the bladder.

Recently, the Bonanno catheter*[15] has been tested. This unique Teflon catheter has a "memory" curve built into the distal end which has effectively prevented its being passed into the distal urethra. For insertion, the catheter is straightened over a metal stylet and insertion is made by the "intra-cath" technique. The only disadvantage noted at this time has been a few instances of obstruction from calcareous incrustation in catheters installed for long periods of time. Compared to the Malecot, the Bonnano catheter is expensive, and from a functional standpoint, it is only slightly inferior.

CONCLUSIONS

1. Although controversy over all aspects of SUI is present today, as it has been in the past, advances in objective techniques for study of the condition have improved the diagnosis and results of treatment.

2. The empiric treatment of SUI at this time in history is no longer justified, and the "85 per cent cure rate and 15 per cent failure rate" is no longer an acceptable dictum.

3. The premium operation for SUI is the first operation, and, after this, the success rate decreases directly according to the number of previous operations.

4. Objective study techniques have made it possible to individualize operative objectives; operative plans should be devised to correct specific defective anatomy.

5. With accurate preoperative diagnosis, the immediate failure rate for primary operations for SUI should be no greater than 2 per cent and for late recurrence no more than 5 per cent.

---

* Available from Becton, Dickinson & Co., Rutherford, New Jersey.

6. For patients with recurrent SUI who have had multiple operations, the results to be expected are somewhat unpredictable, but satisfactory results usually are possible in over 95 per cent of patients.

7. Postoperative bladder drainage is best accomplished by suprapubic cystostomy, provided the proper equipment is used.

REFERENCES

1. Jeffcoate, T. N. A., and Roberts, H.: Observations on stress urinary incontinence of urine. Am. J. Obstet. Gynec. 64:721, 1952.
2. Hodgkinson, C. P.: Relationship of the female urethra and bladder in urinary stress incontinence. Am. J. Obstet. Gynec. 65:560, 1953.
3. Hodgkinson, C. P., Drukker, B. H., and Hershey, G. J. C.: Stress urinary incontinence in the female. VIII. Etiology, significance of the short urethra. Am. J. Obstet. Gynec. 86:16, 1963.
4. Marshall, V. F., Marchetti, A. A., and Krantz, K. E.: Correction of stress incontinence by simple vesicourethral suspension. Surg. Gynec. Obstet. 88:509, 1949.
5. Hodgkinson, C. P., and Cobert, N.: Direct urethrocystometry. Am. J. Obstet. Gynec. 79:648, 1960.
6. Hodari, A. A., and Hodgkinson, C. P.: Iatrogenic bacteriuria and gynecologic surgery. Am. J. Obstet. Gynec. 95:153, 1966.
7. Zacharin, R. F.: The suspensory mechanism of the female urethra. J. Anat. 97:423, 1963.
8. Miley, P. S., and Nichols, D. H.: The relationship between the pubo-urethral ligaments and the urogenital diaphragm in the human female. Anat. Record 170:281, 1971.
9. Low, J. A.: Management of anatomic urinary incontinence by vaginal repair. Am. J. Obstet. Gynec. 97:308, 1967.
10. Nichols, D. H.: The Mersilene mesh gauze-hammock for severe urinary stress incontinence. Obstet. Gynec. 41:1, 1973.
11. Williams, T. J., and TeLinde, R. W.: The sling operation for urinary incontinence using Mersilene ribbon. Obstet. Gynec. 23:92, 1964.
12. Ridley, J. H.: Appraisal of Goebell-Frangenheim-Stoeckel sling operation. Am. J. Obstet. Gynec. 95:714, 1966.
13. Morgan, J. E.: The suprapubic approach to primary stress urinary incontinence. Am. J. Obstet. Gynec. 115:316, 1973.
14. Hodgkinson, C. P., and Hodari, A. A.: Trochar suprapubic cystostomy for postoperative bladder drainage in the female. Am. J. Obstet. Gynec. 96:773, 1966.
15. Bonanno, P. J., Landers, D. E., and Rock, D. E.: Bladder drainage with the suprapubic catheter needle. Obstet. Gynec. 35:807, 1970.

Diagnosis and Preferred
Management of Urinary Stress Incontinence

Editorial Comment

It is apparent that there is a degree of preventability of stress incontinence if well established obstetrical principles are strictly adhered to in the conduct of delivery. These involve the avoidance of trauma through ineptly performed or ill advised forceps operations or by uncontrolled deliveries. Rather, the objective is to allow the fetal occiput to bypass the inferior margin of the maternal symphysis without pressure being exerted against the urethra and bladder neck, thus preventing the disruption of the underlying supporting tissue of these structures. This calls for controlled delivery by outlet forceps if need be and a properly timed episiotomy in order to permit the fetal occiput to recede posteriorly and not cause pressure against these vital structures.

It should be an obstetrical axiom that, barring unavoidable emergency situations, "no woman who is continent prior to delivery should develop stress incontinence, provided delivery is conducted properly in accordance with the above principles."

It will be of more than morbid interest to observe whether patients who are delivered by the so-called "natural childbirth" methods will develop urinary stress incontinence to any degree when they reach 40 years of age and beyond. If this occurs, it will be an unnecessary price for the mother to pay for a spontaneous delivery, and certainly the delay in the delivery of the fetus as it becomes arrested on the perineum can also lead to both immediate and remote damage to the newborn.

It is no longer acceptable to plan therapy simply on the patient's statement that she loses "her water." As emphasized by the contributors to this chapter, there should be no question that a careful and detailed history is basic in determining the diagnosis and treatment to be pursued in the patients whose complaint is urinary incontinence. All writers agree that this must be followed and confirmed by a cystourethrogram study to determine without doubt that the patient does indeed have stress incontinence, not some other form of incontinence, also to determine the type that is present. It is only after these studies have been performed that conclusions can be drawn and recommendations made to the patient regarding the type of surgical treatment indicated, if any.

There appears to be general agreement by the writers that stress incontinence occurs when the urethrovesical junction is depressed to the lowest level or base of the bladder, when the patient strains. This phenomenon is described as resulting from the loss of the angle formed by the posterior surface of the urethra and the bladder. Where the posterior urethrovesical angle is thus obliterated, Green chooses to designate it a Type I lesion. Green also describes a Type II lesion in which the Type I changes occur and in addition there is a downward and backward rotational descent of the urethral axis. It is the latter group in which he believes the failure rate has and probably will continue to be the highest. It is here also that the various suprapubic urethrovesical suspension procedures have added immeasurably to increasing the cure rate.

There are some who might regard the many definitions and interpretations of cystourethrograms as reflecting differences of opinion, but, as one writer states, it may well be more a matter of semantics. The basic issue, which has been clearly stated, is that no patient should be subjected to surgery prior to cystourethrogram studies—small series to the contrary—and that the operation selected should be tailored to the type of lesion accountable for the stress incontinence. Such an approach also will eliminate iatrogenic incontinence, as Hodgkinson has so vividly described, and avoid surgery in those patients who have what might be designated functional incontinence.

13

Gynecologic Surgery in Women Desirous of Further Childbearing

Alternative Points of View:

    By Clayton T. Beecham and Jackson B. Beecham

    By R. Clay Burchell

    By T. N. Evans and H. Amirikia

    By Tiffany J. Williams and Richard S. Sheldon

Editorial Comment

Gynecologic Surgery
in Women Desirous of Further Childbearing

CLAYTON T. BEECHAM

Geisinger Medical Center

JACKSON B. BEECHAM

University of Vermont Medical Center

Surgical treatment of various gynecologic conditions, with its immediate therapeutic results, adds considerable depth to the specialty of gynecology. When to operate and what type of procedure to perform is not always easy to decide. Built into a surgeon's judgment must be one straightforward question: "Does this problem justify the risk of a trip to the operating room?"

The very nature of gynecologic pathology, when considered for patients who desire additional childbearing, precludes hard and fast rules, and serious arguments for or against various operative procedures may be found. Not infrequently they are based on emotional factors rather than on actual clinical experience; how the unwary can detect these pronouncements is an elusive issue.

Sound judgment backed by understanding of pathophysiology is necessary to maintain childbearing capacity in women undergoing pelvic surgery. Fortunately, most clinical problems are best treated by conservative procedures; however, life-threatening diseases may be encountered in women's reproductive years, and serious decisions are called for. Proper surgical therapy requires a prior discussion with the patient and her husband whenever possible, in order that the physician be fully cognizant of their wishes.

Gynecologic Considerations

BENIGN UTERINE ENLARGEMENT

Leiomyomas are found often enough in the reproductive years to make myomectomy a more common procedure than it may appear to be. Enthusiasm seems low for this restorative operation, presumably because fertility rates after myomectomy are not encouraging. In addition, the recurrence of myomas is said to be high enough to usually warrant hysterectomy in the first place.

Neither of these arguments is powerful. While fertility in women who develop leiomyomas is below normal, a high enough success rate follows surgery to support such effort. On the other hand, one can vigorously refute the statements on recurrence—as a matter of fact, they are exceedingly rare. In general, conservative surgery for leiomyomas is indicated in those women under 35 years of age who desire more children.

Benign ovarian enlargement

Familiar to all is the non-specific "slightly" enlarged ovary. Happily, however, in most cases, the enlargement disappears with the next menstrual period after two cleansing enemas; when the ovary remains at 5 to 6 cm., an exploratory laparotomy is necessary. In order of decreasing frequency, one encounters endometriomas, benign cystic teratomas, serous cystadenomas, and mucinous cystadenomas, as well as more bewildering lesions from secondary Müllerian epithelium. Casting a shadow over this array of pathologic conditions is a potential for malignant change. To balance an actual or latent threat to life with desire to leave the reproductive capacity intact requires prudent assessment. This very fact sets the stage for controversy.

Specific ground rules for ovarian resection or oophorectomy are self-evident to many gynecologic surgeons and perplexing to others. It is well to reflect upon these points:

1. Malignant change may come to any body tissue.
2. The talent to predict what will happen to normal ovarian tissue, or to a benign ovarian lesion, is not part of any surgeon's endowment.
3. Prophylactic surgical extirpation of the ovary requires careful individualization to each patient.
4. Viewing all benign ovarian enlargements as villainous processes that will surely destroy the patient is unsound.
5. The ovary is essential to femininity in the young female.

Few dispute the applicability of ovarian salvage through the local resection of ovarian endometriomas. Yet controversy may arise in the handling of a large (8 to 10 cm.) endometriotic ovarian process. The contention is based on a presumed lack of normal ovarian tissue for reconstruction. If an endometrioma is part of a widespread disease, suppressive therapy should be instituted with surgery and continued until decidual necrosis with atrophy takes place. Such a plan is preferable to advising a postoperative crash course in conception.

Benign cystic teratomas lend themselves particularly well to resection and preservation of the unresected portion. Regardless of the patient's wishes for or against having other children, the preferable treatment in women under 40 years of age is resection, not oophorectomy.

Ovarian carcinoma

Selective conservative therapy in the presence of ovarian malignancy has gained support largely through the work of Moench[1] and Munnell.[2] Preservation of the contralateral ovary is suitable in stage Ia malignancies if the ovarian capsule is intact, if peritoneal fluid or washings are free of tumor cells, and if the second ovary is free of disease, as proved by biopsy.

Forty years ago, Moench reported a 5 year survival rate of 82 per cent in 72 patients on whom he had performed unilateral oophorectomy for adeno-carcinoma. In 67 women on whom he had performed bilateral oophorectomy, the salvage rate of 79 per cent was not significantly different. When we have had the opportunity as well as the desire to preserve childbearing function under these circumstances, there have been no deaths from the malignant process.

CARCINOMA IN SITU OF THE CERVIX

Polemics involving the management of noninvasive cervical carcinoma often reflect more emotional heat than intellectual light.

Few will dispute that carcinoma in situ is the tissue state immediately preceding invasive cancer. Eager optimism for minimal treatment in management of this lesion is not supported by facts or by experience. Four per cent of 150 stage V cervical carcinomas referred to us for therapy (previously treated else-where) are the result of less than optimal treatment of noninvasive disease.

Recognition of that simple clinical fact must be accepted by the gyne-cologist when he treats an in situ carcinoma by conization, in order to preserve childbearing function. Further, a clinician who initiates minor therapy for a major lesion is *totally responsible* for the patient's follow-up study and care. If the patient is lost to follow-up, or is immune to appropriate follow-up observa-tions, the gynecologist is responsible for the subsequent development of an inva-sive cancer because he initiated therapy. In no sense can the physician absolve himself by washing his hands of the situation and saying, "but she didn't return for her checkups." When a patient insists on treatment by uterine salvage, she must be fully informed concerning the operation. With this proviso, conservation may be warranted in carefully selected patients who are under 30 years of age and who have two children or fewer.

ADENOCARCINOMA OF THE VAGINA

This recently reported lesion,[3,4] if not fatal, is cured only by radical pelvic surgery. The necessity of such extirpative treatment is particularly unfortunate, since this clear cell carcinoma occurs almost exclusively in girls or young women who were in utero when their mothers received stilbestrol as therapy for threat-ened abortion.

Vaginal adenosis and adenocarcinoma of the vagina frequently coexist; such a relationship suggests that adenosis is a precursor of the malignancy.[5] Local excision with skin grafting, or cryosurgical obliteration of this benign lesion, may preserve reproductive function in these patients by preventing the development of cancer and the consequent necessity of radical therapy.

HODGKIN'S DISEASE

Women of reproductive age are frequently encountered among those patients who develop Hodgkin's disease. This malignancy, depending on its stage, is frequently curable with radiotherapy. The sterility caused by pelvic nodal irradiation is usually considered a modest price to pay for remission.

Ovarian castration can be avoided, however, if the ovaries are transposed either to a midline position[6,7] or to the lateral parietal peritoneum near the iliac crest.[8] Such lateral translocation exposes the ovaries only to radiation scatter. Midline oophoropexy allows the ovaries to be shielded with lead blocks during irradiation without interfering with cancericidal doses to the external iliac, hypogastric, or obturator nodes. Such prophylactic surgery is particularly appropriate in those hospitals in which laparotomy is used for accurate staging of Hodgkin's disease.

If their ovaries are exposed only to small doses of gamma rays, these women ovulate and several normal pregnancies have occurred. The small potential for radiation-induced genetic or malignant change in future generations must be weighed against the woman's desire for children (or for other children). The prognosis for survival in Hodgkin's disease is good if there is a two year disease-free period following irradiation. It is logical, therefore, to forbid pregnancy during this interval.

VAGINAL RELAXATION

One of the most distressing symptoms resulting from loss of muscular function and faulty organ position is stress urinary incontinence. Soiling and wetness are an annoyance of major proportions. Fortunately this is not usually a problem with young women but may manifest itself in the middle reproductive years, at a time when a patient may hope for one more pregnancy.

Most gynecologists like to defer surgical therapy until a woman has had her family and then do a vaginal hysterectomy with both anterior and posterior vaginal plastic repair. For the occasional woman who backs away from this "end of the road" therapy, a Manchester procedure may be performed. Aside from the steps in anterior parametrial fixation, careful deep dissection to the urogenital diaphragm and Kelly plication sutures to correct the funnel and loss of ure-throvesical angle usually are rewarding. Obviously a cesarean section will be required if the patient conceives and if the operation was successful in curing the stress incontinence.

Minor degrees of uterine prolapse may occur in women during their reproductive years. Most are unaware of their anatomical defect until it is pointed out by a gynecologist. Extreme prolapse may be an important feature in infertility; if so, a Manchester operation could be carried out. Let us hasten to add that our remarks are not meant as an enthusiastic endorsement of the Manchester procedure; we regard it as a stop-gap therapy to be employed in very rare and special instances.

Uterine prolapse during pregnancy is another uncommon lesion. Any type of round pessary, large enough to rest on the levator sling, will hold the uterus in position until its enlargement precludes prolapse (14 to 16 weeks), after which the ring should be removed. Following delivery, surgical correction can be tailored to each case.

Obstetrical Considerations

ECTOPIC PREGNANCY

Tubal pregnancies are a common cause of infertility. Nearly 25 per cent of patients are childless at the time of their first ectopic gestation[9] and only 50 per cent of all women treated for this disease will conceive in the future. Unfortunately, in 10 per cent of these women a zygote will again implant outside the uterus.

Salpingoplasty neither increases nor decreases the chance of subsequent gestation,[10] although it probably does not increase the rate of recurrent ectopic gestation either. Unfortunately, polyethylene stents used to irrigate the tubes with antibiotics and steroids have not fulfilled their promise.[9] Only if a woman has had one tube previously removed is conservative tubal surgery generally considered worthwhile. In such an otherwise hopeless situation, tuboplasties have occasionally resulted in the transmission of a fertilized ova to a normal intrauterine implantation site.[11]

Perhaps more important than the management of the tubes themselves is careful control of the operative site.[12] All blood should be removed from the peritoneal cavity before closure, and prophylactic antibiotics should be instituted. Careful postoperative follow-up for patency of the remaining tube may relieve early blockage with insufflation or hydrotubation.

There are some clinical data to support the removal of the ovary along with the involved tube. Even though the number of fetuses coming to term may not be significantly increased, the overall pregnancy rate is improved 14 per cent[13] without any increase in recurrent ectopic pregnancies. Since newborn intensive care nurseries are currently retrieving a significant proportion of premature infants weighing over 1500 grams, salpingo-oophorectomy is a rational form of treatment in tubal pregnancy.

A second reason for this surgical procedure should be considered. External migration of the unfertilized egg is probably quite common,[14] and in at least 15 per cent of ectopic pregnancies the corpus luteum of pregnancy is found on the contralateral side from the site of gestation.[15] Salpingo-oophorectomy rather than mere salpingectomy eliminates external migration as a mechanism in future ectopic pregnancies, and thus enhances childbearing potential.

POSTPARTUM HEMORRHAGE

Most postpartum bleeding is uterine. Retained secundines are usually recognized from examining the placenta or exploring the uterus. Uterine rupture may be hard to palpate, but should be suspected if the uterus is boggy and the abdomen distended while the blood pressure and hematocrit are dropping. If the uterus is not boggy, the same clinical picture can occur with liver rupture in severe toxemia; many cases of hepatic hemorrhage in pregnancy have been encountered with preoperative diagnosis of uterine rupture,[16] and in some cases hysterectomies were performed unnecessarily. Hepatic rupture, usually related to severe preeclampsia or eclampsia, is caused by an associated disseminated intravascular coagulation (DIC).[17] Any postpartum hemorrhage in a patient with toxemia of pregnancy must have a clotting deficiency excluded, particularly before surgery is performed.

The extent of vaginal lacerations may be difficult to evaluate, especially if they involve the fornix or cervix, for these can extend into the broad ligament, with massive blood accumulation. The typical picture is, therefore, shock out of proportion to blood loss.[18]

The basic principles of managing postpartum hemorrhage are not new and will not be extensively covered here. Nevertheless, hysterectomy is often employed by the inexperienced obstetrician in the absence of sound principles of management or knowledge of pathophysiologic processes in the puerperium. Preservation of life far outweighs any considerations of future childbearing, but in many instances, both goals can be realized if some of the following points are considered.

Cervical and vaginal lacerations may require up to three assistants for adequate, atraumatic retraction and exposure; poor exposure is the single most important cause of prolonged bleeding, tissue trauma, and edema. If external and occult (intra-abdominal) blood loss continues, laparotomy is indicated. While hysterectomy is usually necessary when uterine rupture occurs, it is doubtful whether removal of the uterus is always the easiest or wisest method of stemming other sources of pelvic hemorrhage. Hypogastric artery ligation without hysterectomy is usually successful in stopping postpartum bleeding from the uterus, broad ligament, or upper vagina. It does not stop flow through the uterine arteries, however[19]; these patients menstruate regularly and can become pregnant again.[20] The primary effect of hypogastric artery ligation is the significant drop produced in arterial pulse pressure. This means that in those occasional cases in which hypogastric artery ligation itself is unsuccessful, further bleeding can be stopped by uterine packing, since pressure will be applied against a venous-like system.

The rarity of placenta accreta should not prevent any physician from developing a thorough plan of management for this obstetrical complication, which in earlier years was accompanied by a serious mortality rate. Conservative management today can be consistent with 100 per cent survival.[21,22,23] Postpartum hemorrhage may not even be a problem, particularly if the placenta accreta is complete. Partial placenta accreta, however, requires manual extraction, curettage, oxytocics, and vigilant monitoring of blood loss.

The necessity of preserving childbearing function in women with placenta accreta is minimized by the fact that it occurs almost exclusively in multigravidas. Nevertheless, a trial of conservative therapy prior to hysterectomy is often justified, provided that preparations are made for vigorous replacement of blood on the basis of amount of blood loss, pulse, blood, and central venous pressures, serial hematocrits, urine output, and urine specific gravity.

Delayed postpartum hemorrhage most frequently occurs eight to 14 days after delivery.[24,25] Since hemorrhage is usually massive, a curettage may be performed with excessive vigor, denuding the endometrium and predisposing the patient to Ascherman's syndrome or placenta accreta. If initial sharp and suction curettages do not control bleeding, a uterine umbrella pack is appropriate. Occasionally, laparotomy is necessary; hypogastric ligation again is the first indicated procedure. Persistent bleeding from subinvolution of the placental site can be arrested by hysterotomy and excision of this area[26] if uterine preservation is warranted. In other instances, hysterectomy should not be deferred.

GESTATIONAL TROPHOBLASTIC DISEASE

The management of noninvasive hydatidiform mole has never posed a particular threat to a woman's reproductive function. The traditional therapy of those trophoblastic neoplasms with invasive or metastatic potential, however, usually involved hysterectomy.

A small breakthrough in maintaining childbearing capacity in those women with locally invasive moles occurred when several cases of chorioadenoma destruens were successfully cured after hysterotomy and local excision of the tumor.[27]

With the advent of chemotherapy, survival statistics for malignant trophoblastic neoplasm dramatically improved.[28] In addition, reproductive function could be maintained. So far, offspring have had no associated genetic or malignant transformations. Hysterectomy is only necessary with intractable bleeding or persistently elevated gonadotropin titers following appropriate chemotherapy. Surgery is usually not required for the associated theca lutein cysts, since the ovaries usually return to normal size in one to three months after institution of therapy.[29]

PELVIC NEOPLASMS COMPLICATING PREGNANCY

Occasionally benign pelvic tumors threaten childbearing by complicating pregnancy. Even though 75 per cent of adnexal masses are found on the first prenatal visit,[30] many surgeons defer ovarian cystectomy until after the first trimester in hopes of decreasing the risk of abortion. There are few if any clinical data supporting this concept, however.

The real risk of premature labor comes from, among other things, pelvic inflammation; such a complication is frequent, with torsion or rupture of an adnexal mass. Rupture of a common tumor, such as a benign cystic teratoma, almost always occurs in pregnancy.[31] Therefore, if an adnexal mass is larger than 5 to 6 cm. on the first prenatal visit, it may be advisable not to delay surgery, particularly in a "premium" pregnancy. Appropriate intervention may in fact decrease first and second trimester fetal wastage, and should reduce prolonged labor at term from soft tissue dystocia. It is wise to bisect the contralateral ovary in all instances, not only when there are dermoid cysts.

As with nonpregnant women, frozen section should be employed, particularly if papillations or other signs of malignancy are encountered. Most benign ovarian lesions should undergo local excision rather than oophorectomy; needless ovarian sacrifice can inhibit future fertility.

Although luteomas of pregnancy apparently represent an exaggerated physiological response to the increased endocrine stimulus of gestation,[32] they should not be left to regress following delivery, since they closely resemble hilus cell tumors, and the differentiation can only be made microscopically.

Uterine leiomyomas often hypertrophy in the prenatal period. Unless they are pedunculated, these are best left undisturbed at cesarean section, since the usual indication for myomectomy (infertility) is obviously absent, and excision will be bloody. There will be, in addition, a second uterine scar to be concerned about in future gestations.

PELVIC THROMBOPHLEBITIS

Hysterectomy has no role in the usual management of this disease; it is unnecessary and hazardous. Intravenous anticoagulation is the therapy of choice.

Inferior vena cava and ovarian vein ligation are indicated if a pulmonary embolus develops after medical management. Surgery is not interdicted antepartum, since live births can occur.[33-37] Similarly, women can conceive after venous interruption;[38,39] this should be considered if the patient strongly requests a second pregnancy. Postoperative edema and other sequelae should be minimal in the otherwise healthy young woman.[39,40] If sterilization is indicated, the less manipulative tubal ligation is preferred over hysterectomy. Ovaries need not be removed, since their function will be maintained after pelvic vein ligation.

Summary

A true gynecologic surgeon, while appreciating areas of controversy, understands and generally accepts the need of conservation. When operating upon women who specifically request the preservation of childbearing capability, he must be informed in matters of pathology and pathophysiology. In emergency circumstances when conference with the patient or husband is not possible, the obstetrician-gynecologist must rely on preconceived plans of management that incorporate an appropriate (but not zealous) concern for the woman's reproductive capacity. "Radical" conservatism has a place in the treatment of a woman who is hemorrhaging, provided that blood volume is scrupulously monitored.

REFERENCES

1. Moench, L. M.: A clinical study of 403 cases of adenocarcinoma of the ovary: papillary cystadenoma, carcinomatous cystadenoma, and solid adenocarcinoma of the ovary. Amer. J. Obstet. Gynec. 26:22, 1933.
2. Munnell, E. W.: Is conservative therapy ever justified in stage Ia cancer of the ovary? Amer. J. Obstet. Gynec. 103:641, 1969.
3. Herbst, A. L., Ulfelder, H., and Poskanzer, D. C.: Adenocarcinoma of the vagina. New Eng. J. Med. 284:878, 1971.
4. Greenwald, P., Barlow, J. J., Nasca, P. C., Burnett, W. S.: Vaginal cancer after maternal treatment with synthetic estrogens. New Eng. J. Med. 285:390, 1971.
5. Blaikley, J. B., Dewhurst, J. B., Ferrcira, H. P., and Lewis, T. L. T.: Vaginal adenosis: clinical and pathological features with special reference to malignant change. J. Obstet. Gynaec. Brit. Comm. 78:1115, 1971.
6. Baker, J. W., Peckham, M. J., Morgan, R. L., and Smithers, D. W.: Preservation of ovarian function in patients requiring radiotherapy for para-aortic and pelvic Hodgkin's disease. Lancet 1:1307, 1972.
7. Ray, G. R., Trueblood, H. W., Enright, L. P., Kaplan, H. S., and Nelson, T. S.: Oophoropexy: a means of preserving ovarian function following pelvic megavoltage radiotherapy for Hodgkin's disease. Radiology 96:175, 1970.
8. Nahhas, W. A., Nisce, L. Z., D'Angio, G. J., and Lewis, J. L., Jr.: Lateral ovarian transposition. Obstet. Gynec. 38:785, 1971.
9. Timonen, S., and Nieminen, U.: Tubal pregnancy, choice of operative method of treatment. Acta Obstet. Gynec. Scand. 46:327, 1967.
10. Abrams, J., and Farell, D. M.: Salpingectomy and salpingoplasty for tubal pregnancy: survey of the literature. Obstet. Gynec. 24:281, 1964.
11. Stromme, W. B., McKelvey, J. L., and Adkins, C. D.: Conservative surgery for ectopic pregnancy. Obstet. Gynec. 19:294, 1962.
12. Grant, A.: The effect of ectopic pregnancy on fertility. J. Clin. Obstet. Gynec. 5:861, 1962.
13. Bender, S.: Fertility after tubal pregnancy. J. Obstet. Gynec. Brit. Emp. 62:400, 1956.
14. Eastman, N. J.: Editorial comment. Obstet. Gynec. Surv. 13:817, 1958.
15. TeLinde, R. W., and Mattingly, R. F.: Operative Gynecology. 4th Ed. Philadelphia, J. B. Lippincott, 1970.

16. Watson, W. J., Pilcher, D., Beecham, J. B., and Clapp, J. F.: Liver rupture in pregnancy. Surg. Gynec. Obstet. (in press).
17. Beecham, J. B., Watson, W. J., and Clapp, J. F.: Preeclampsia, eclampsia and disseminated intravascular coagulation. Amer. J. Obstet. Gynec. (in press).
18. Fliegner, J. R. H.: Postpartum broad ligament hematomas. J. Obstet. Gynaec. Brit. Comm. 78:184, 1971.
19. Burchall, R. C.: Physiology of internal iliac artery ligation. J. Obstet. Gynaec. Brit. Comm. 75:642, 1968.
20. Shinagawa, S.: J. Jap. Obstet. Gynec. Soc. 9:19, 1962. Quoted by Le Cocq, F.: Internal iliac artery ligation. Amer. J. Obstet. Gynec. 95:320, 1966.
21. McKeogh, R. P., and D'Errico, E.: Placenta accreta: clinical manifestations and conservative management. New Eng. J. Med. 245:159, 1951.
22. Brody, H.: Placenta accreta: report of five cases and a plan of management. Canad. Med. Ass. J. 89:499, 1963.
23. Torbet, T. E., and Tsoutsoplides, G. C.: Placenta previa accreta: conservative management. J. Obstet. Gynec. Brit. Comm. 75:737, 1968.
24. Dewhurst, C. J.: Secondary post partum hemorrhage. J. Obstet. Gynaec. Brit. Comm. 73:53, 1966.
25. Thorsteinsson, V. T., and Kempers, R. D.: Delayed postpartum bleeding. Amer. J. Obstet. Gynec. 107:565, 1970.
26. Beecham, C. T., and Rohrbeck, C. W.: Exploratory hysterotomy in the treatment of chorioadenoma destruens and postpartum hemorrhage. Obstet. Gynec. 23:160, 1964.
27. Wilson, R. B., Beecham, C. T., and Symmonds, R. E.: Conservative surgical management of chorioadenoma destruens. Obstet. Gynec. 26:814, 1965.
28. Lewis, J. L., Jr., Ketcham, A. S., and Hertz, R.: Surgical intervention during chemotherapy of gestational trophoblastic neoplasms. Cancer 19:1517, 1966.
29. Goldstein, D. P.: In Kistner, R. W., Gynecology: Principles and Practice. 2nd Ed. Chicago, Year Book Medical Publishers, 1971.
30. Booth, R. T.: Ovarian tumors in pregnancy. Obstet. Gynec. 21:189, 1963.
31. Malkasian, G. D., Dockerty, M. B., and Symmonds, R. E.: Benign cystic teratomas. Obstet. Gynec. 29:719, 1967.
32. Novak, E. R., Jones, G. S., and Jones, H. W.: Novak's Textbook of Gynecology. 8th Ed. Baltimore, Williams & Wilkins, 1970.
33. Pizarro, A. R., and Roth, O.: Inferior vena cava ligation in early pregnancy. Amer. J. Obstet. Gynec. 101:265, 1968.
34. Rubin, H.: Ligation of the inferior vena cava in early pregnancy. Amer. J. Obstet. Gynec. 80:542, 1960.
35. Sautter, R. D., Fletcher, F. W., and Lewis, R. F.: Inferior vena cava and ovarian vein ligation during late pregnancy. Obstet. Gynec. 32:267, 1968.
36. Stone, S. R., Whalley, P. J., and Pritchard, J. A.: Inferior vena cava and ovarian vein ligation during late pregnancy. Obstet. Gynec. 32:267, 1968.
37. Young, R. L., and Derbyshire, R. C.: Ligation of the inferior vena cava during pregnancy. Ann. Surg. 131:252, 1950.
38. Collins, C. G., Weinstein, B. B., Norton, R. O., and Webster, H. D.: The effects of ligation of the inferior vena cava and ovarian vessels on ovulation and pregnancy in the human being. Amer. J. Obstet. Gynec. 63:351, 1952.
39. Collins, J. H., Bosco, J. A. S., and Cohen, C. J.: Pregnancy subsequent to ligation of the inferior vena cava and ovarian vessels. Amer. J. Obstet. Gynec. 77:760, 1959.
40. Ochsner, A., Ochsner, J. L., and Sanders, H. S.: Prevention of pulmonary embolism by caval ligation. Ann. Surg. 171:923, 1970.

Gynecologic Surgery
in Women Desirous of Further Childbearing

R. CLAY BURCHELL

Hartford Hospital

Indications for gynecologic surgery have undergone a revolution during the last 50 years. Although the transition is incomplete, there is sufficient information to predict the end result. Basically, the emphasis has shifted from anatomy to physiology, and from anatomic restoration to improvement of function. Reproductive, endocrine, and sexual function are primary considerations today, and few gynecologic procedures are contemplated without considering the subsequent effect upon function.

Moreover, this changing emphasis has had another profound effect: the patient's desires are now viewed as important. The physician cannot make a valid decision about function without the patient's cooperation. The functional approach necessitates a partnership.

To understand how preservation of reproductive function affects indications for operation, one must consider this transition; why it occurred, what has happened, where it is leading, and the responsibility it places on physicians and patients.

Operative indications over the years have been affected by several factors, of which increasing knowledge has been one of the most important. The emphasis was on anatomy 50 years ago because anatomy and pathology were better understood than physiology. There were adequate gross and microscopic descriptions of normal and abnormal pelvic tissues. It was logical to think in terms of removal of abnormal organs if anatomic restoration was impossible. So little was understood about function that it was considered secondary. But as knowledge increased and was applied, function became more important.

The tremendous increase in operative safety has been another factor in making the transition possible. Minor gynecologic procedures in 1920 were dangerous; major procedures in 1970 are relatively safe. Increased safety has allowed the emphasis to be placed on what is best for the patient rather than whether or not she will survive the operation that is indicated.

Operative indications have also changed as a result of patient expectations. Today, many women demand a share in any decision affecting their lives rather

436

than simply assuming the "doctor knows best." In this respect, reproductive, endocrine, and sexual function are central issues. For example, there has been almost a total change in professional attitude toward elective sterilization during the last decade, primarily generated by patients.

The significant difference between the anatomic and functional approaches lies in the *thinking used to make the decision.* In some cases, the final decision will be the same, but it will be arrived at from opposite points of view. The treatment of uterine myomas illustrates the change in thinking.

Sixty years ago, Kelly[1] recommended that myomectomy be performed in younger women to preserve the uterus and hysterectomy in older women if an operation were necessary. He was considering supracervical hysterectomy because total hysterectomy was too dangerous to employ for benign conditions. The anatomic emphasis associated with age rather than function was also evident, even though myomectomy was more dangerous than hysterectomy. Approximate mortality at the time was 3 to 5 per cent for myomectomy, 2 to 4 per cent for supracervical hysterectomy, and 6 to 10 per cent for total hysterectomy.

Thirty years later, in 1942, Curtis[2] shifted emphasis and recommended myomectomy during the childbearing period. He did note that preservation of function in this manner was more dangerous than performing hysterectomy. Total hysterectomy was suggested if the cervix was diseased, but this recommendation was invalidated to some extent by references to several patients who died after total hysterectomy.

Brewer[3] recommends hysterectomy (total) as the treatment of choice for myomas unless further childbearing is desired. In that case, myomectomy is used. This constitutes the functional approach. When treatment is indicated, restore function if desired, or remove the uterus if function is unnecessary.

The crux of this transition, and the aspect that causes confusion, is that the same operation has been performed for opposite reasons at different times. Myomectomy was used to restore normal anatomy at one time without regard to childbearing desire. Now reproductive function is paramount, and myomectomy is virtually never used simply to restore anatomy.

Sharing of responsibility for decision making with the patient has been an increasing trend over the years. This is important, but it would be unfortunate if it were carried too far. Elective sterilization is pretty well accepted, and sometimes hysterectomy is employed to sterilize the patient. Although this may need to be a joint decision, patients would suffer if the physician were to inadvertently shed all responsibility and caution in order to give the patient "hysterectomy on demand." A balance between authority and responsibility within the professional relationship needs to be carefully worked out.

In utilizing functional rather than absolute indications for gynecologic surgery, selected clinical problems can be used for illustration. They are grouped on the basis of how the desire for reproductive function affects indications for operation or the operative procedure itself (Table 13–1).

The first group comprises problems that are either life-threatening, incapacitating, or so damaging to the reproductive tract that subsequent childbearing is known to be impossible. Included would be virtually all invasive carcinomas. The standard curative treatment is indicated. In this situation the patient's desire for children should not compromise her chances for cure. Life-threatening infections are also included in this group. Hysterectomy may be mandatory to save the

TABLE 13–1.   *Selected Gynecologic Problems in Patients Desiring More Children*

FIXED INDICATION, FIXED PROCEDURE	FIXED INDICATION, MODIFIED PROCEDURE	MODIFIED INDICATION, FIXED PROCEDURE
Invasive carcinoma	Benign ovarian cyst	Stress incontinence
Septic abortion	Uterine myoma	Uterine prolapse
Incapacitating pelvic inflammatory disease	Ectopic pregnancy	Cystocele
	Carcinoma in situ of cervix	Rectocele
	Adolescent menorrhagia	
	Pregnancy hemorrhage	

patient's life in cases of septic abortion. Severe pelvic inflammatory disease would be placed in this group when the patient had *incapacitating* pain or recurrent abscesses. Although the infection might not be life-threatening, there would probably be sufficient damage to the tubes and ovaries to preclude reproductive function.

The operative procedure rather than the surgical indication is modified with the second group of problems. Benign tumors, certain pregnancy states, and serious hemorrhage compose this group. Operation is necessary, and sometimes life-saving, but an alternate procedure can be utilized to preserve function.

With benign tumors, the tumor alone, rather than the whole organ including tumor, is removed when the patient wants more children (Table 13–2). Two examples are myomectomy and cystectomy. Myomectomy is performed instead of hysterectomy for uterine myomas. With dermoid or simple cysts of the ovary, cystectomy may be utilized instead of oophorectomy.

Treatment for ectopic pregnancy is modified under certain circumstances. Normally a salpingectomy is done. If the patient wants more children and the last remaining tube is involved, the pregnancy alone may be removed, with an attempt at tubal reconstruction.

Hysterectomy is the standard treatment for carcinoma in situ. Actually this procedure probably overtreats the condition so that when more children are desired a large cervical cone is considered sufficient therapy.

Finally, the treatment of uterine hemorrhage may be affected by the desire for more children. There are two different situations possible, depending upon whether bleeding is associated with pregnancy or not. In the non-pregnant patient, dilatation and curettage or hormone therapy should be used instead of hysterectomy. Adolescent menorrhagia is an example. Hysterectomy should not be used except as a last resort to save the patient's life. A different situation occurs when uterine hemorrhage is associated with a pregnancy episode (abruptio placentae, postpartum bleeding). Hysterectomy might be the treatment of choice for

TABLE 13–2.   *Operative Procedures and Reproductive Function*

CLINICAL PROBLEM	FAMILY COMPLETED	CHILDREN DESIRED
Ovarian cyst	Oophorectomy	Cystectomy
Uterine myoma	Hysterectomy	Myomectomy
Ectopic pregnancy	Salpingectomy	Salpingoplasty
Carcinoma in situ	Hysterectomy	Therapeutic cone
Severe menorrhagia	Hysterectomy	Dilatation and curettage, hormone therapy
Pregnancy hemorrhage	Cesarean hysterectomy	Internal iliac artery ligation

a woman who has completed her family. Other methods of treatment, such as internal iliac artery ligation, should be employed when more children are desired. Nothing is more tragic for a woman wanting children than to have a hysterectomy that was not absolutely mandatory.

In the second group, the desire for children modified the *operation* rather than the indications for it. In the third group, the opposite situation holds—the *indications* rather than the procedures are altered. Operations for these clinical problems are elective and complicate further childbearing, so that the procedure is frequently postponed until the family is completed. Typical examples are stress incontinence, uterine prolapse, and vaginal relaxation. The physician and patient balance the symptoms against the complications of childbearing after operation.

This functional approach to gynecologic surgery demands increased knowledge and wisdom from the physician. The difficulty is that he must help the patient choose the best option for care rather than simply deciding for himself what she should do. On the other hand, he cannot abdicate from the decision-making process and let her make the decision alone.

Both physician and patient need to understand each other regarding the patient's desire for children and the strength of this desire. If the planned course of action is altered as a result of operative findings, the physician will have to decide alone what to do. When the unexpected possibility of hysterectomy arises at operation, the first questions are: Does the patient want more children? and How does she feel about hysterectomy? The gynecologist should know these answers *before* he operates.

A difficult situation arises when the patient and physician disagree. What is the physician to do when she wants more children and there is a real medical contraindication? Counseling is important in this situation to explore options. Exactly how the decision was made should be discussed. Was it made alone or with her husband? How did he affect the decision? Does she really understand the medical consequences of having more children? Does he? Are the consequences really as serious as the physician first thought, or was he inadvertently pressing his own value position?

If there is still disagreement, the physician and patient should review the decision-making process in view of the past. Have the patient's previous important decisions turned out well? If so, they may want to give more weight to her views in this matter. If past decisions have been unfortunate, she may wish to think further. In the final analysis it may come down to deciding how many children would be best for a woman in her situation.

My personal feelings were developed over a 15 year period. I would do everything possible, even at increased risk, to help a woman have one or two children that she badly wanted. With significant risk, I would discourage the same patient from having more than two children. The number two was chosen because the differences between having two, one, or no children are qualitative as far as parents and siblings are concerned. The differences between two or more children are quantitative. It seems to me to be as tragic for a woman to be denied the second child she wants as it is for a mother of five to have a life-threatening sixth pregnancy. Obviously, personal feelings should not be imposed but can serve as a possible guideline for reviewing the final decision.

In summary, treat the uterus as a functional organ. When there are problems, preserve and restore it if function is desirable, and remove it if function is no longer necessary. Obviously, the uterus should not be removed simply because function is completed and it is there!

REFERENCES

1. Kelly, H. A.: Medical Gynecology. New York, D. Appleton & Company, 1911.
2. Curtis, A. H.: A Textbook of Gynecology. 4th Ed. Philadelphia, W. B. Saunders Co., 1942.
3. Brewer, J. I.: Textbook of Gynecology. 3rd Ed. Baltimore, Williams & Wilkins Co., 1961.

Gynecologic Surgery
in Women Desirous of Further Childbearing

T. N. Evans and H. Amirikia

Surgical attempts to restore fertility in women have often been based more on sophistry than on science. Operative design and indications not infrequently have resulted from fallacious reasoning related more to fiction than to fact. Nevertheless, a recrudescence of interest in operative correction of female infertility seems justified considering the improved understanding of the physiology and pathology of human reproduction. In the past, most such operations have been unsuccessful. However, the future success rate should increase because of improved diagnostic methods and surgical techniques.

Cohen[1] indicated that 10 to 15 per cent of human beings are infertile. In approximately 40 per cent of infertile women, sterility results from obstruction of the fallopian tubes.[2] The most common factor in tubal obstruction is infection. If left untreated, only a small proportion of patients with obstructed oviducts will conceive. However, nonoperative treatment may result in a 23 per cent pregnancy rate.[3]

Less common causes of infertility and unsuccessful pregnancies relate to congenital anomalies of the uterus which are usually variants of the bifid uterus. Strassmann[4] in 1907 was the first to perform unification of a double uterus. Approximately one in every four women with a double uterus will have serious reproductive problems and no living children.[5] These patients may present with premature labor, repeated abortion, or primary infertility.

Success in the surgical treatment of infertility is related more to careful patient selection than to any other factor. Complete evaluation of both partners is essential. Too often the male partner is inadequately examined before surgery for correction of female infertility is performed. Evaluation of the ages and general health of the couple, as well as of their reproductive organs, is important. Previous pelvic surgery warrants thorough investigation.

Sterility alone is never an indication for surgery until all other possibilities have been excluded. Surgery should be considered only after ovulation has been confirmed or induced, repeat semen analysis has been found to be normal, and all other causes of infertility have been eliminated—and the prospects of the couple as good parents have been assessed. Elective surgery should be reserved for those couples who desperately want a successful pregnancy after all other causes of infertility have been eliminated except for the one for which surgery is designed. Such patients should be not only good surgical risks but also good psychiatric risks. Prognosis should be presented with candor, for surgical failures often result in disheartened, discouraged, and depressed patients.

Evolution of the surgical approach to infertility began in 1884 when Ruge[6] first reported the excision of a uterine septum in a woman who had had two abortions. This patient subsequently had a term pregnancy. The first operation on diseased fallopian tubes for the relief of infertility was performed by Martin[7] in 1885. Nine years later, Mackenrodt[8] described the first two successful cases. In 1896, Watkins[9] performed the first operation for tubal implantation; a subsequent pregnancy in this patient ended in abortion. Estes[10] in 1909 and Tuffier and Letulle[11] in 1924 reported their operations for transplantation of the ovary following salpingectomy. These procedures have proved to be of little use and are performed infrequently today. Since these pioneering steps, numerous other procedures have been devised. Poor or equivocal results found in surveys by Greenhill[12] and by Siegler and Hellman[13] of the earlier part of the twentieth century suggested that any real benefit may have occurred by chance.

New wrinkles added to old operations previously discarded serve to give them approbation. There have been appreciable improvements in operative techniques, availability of antibiotics, and polyethylene and silicone splints and prostheses, as well as improvements in preoperative diagnostic techniques, especially endoscopy, to refine patient selection.

Prevention of infertility is a major consideration in view of the rapid expansion of the number of gynecological operations. Mutilating operations should be avoided whenever possible in women whose reproductive potential should not be terminated because of age or other valid reasons.

Numerous factors may be involved, including congenital anomalies of the Müllerian ducts involving vagina, uterus, and fallopian tubes. Other significant factors are infection, tumors such as uterine fibroids, ovarian cysts, and endometriosis. Although the Stein-Leventhal syndrome is now largely treated medically, ovarian wedge resections are still required on rare occasions. Causes of unsuccessful pregnancies are just as significant as causes of conception failures. An incompetent cervix may be amenable to surgery. Other factors include endometrial polyps, fixed retrodisplacement of the uterus owing to inflammatory adhesions or endometriosis, and endometrial synechiae (Asherman's syndrome).[14]

Tuboplastic surgery may be carried out at the time of operation for ectopic pregnancy. If there is an underlying inflammatory factor, another ectopic pregnancy may occur. However, salpingostomy at the time of such surgery may result in a subsequent intrauterine pregnancy.[15]

Previous tubal sterilization operations may be an iatrogenic cause of infertility. Several types of uterine anomalies may lead to habitual abortion or premature labor (Figure 13–1). Rarely, hematometra in a noncommunicating horn of the uterus may serve as an indication for metroplasty. Different operative procedures have been designed for correction of these defects (Figure 13-2). Those with septate uteri seem to be more likely to have reproductive problems than those with a bicornuate uterus.[16]

Palmer[17] set forth some absolute contraindications to surgery: (1) any other obvious cause of sterility in the husband or wife if not cured, (2) women

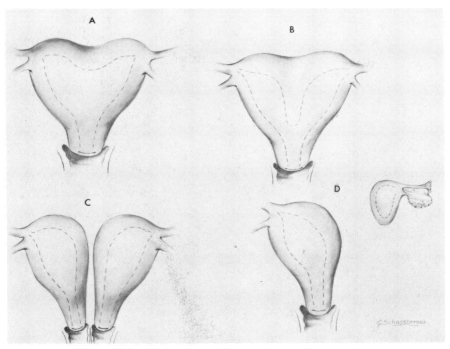

Figure 13-1.   Various types of congenital uterine anomalies.

over 37 years of age, (3) recent acute or subacute inflammation, and (4) the probability of tuberculosis as the cause of tubal occlusion.

One of the principal functions of the oviducts is to transmit ova from the ovary to the site of fertilization in the fallopian tube and then on to the uterus to the site of implantation. Although human capacitation of spermatozoa has not been established, the oviduct may well serve as a conditioning chamber as well as a conduit for spermatozoa. It would appear that minimal essentials for successful pregnancy would be oviducts with two ostia and patency of the canal. However, in the presence of tubal dysfunction or inflammatory damage of the endosalpinx, these "minimal essentials" are not adequate.

The frequency of uterine anomalies seems to be increasing. These data may be deceptive, however, since more anomalies may be recognized because of the increased frequency of hysterosalpingography. Uterine anomalies of all degrees may occur in as many as 1 per cent of women.[18] An externally divided uterus with two separate uterine bodies may be classified by the degree of bifurcation into uterus arcuatus, uterus bicornis unicollis (bicornuate uterus), and uterus bicornis bicollis or uterus didelphys (two corpora and two cervices). An externally unified uterus may have two endometrial cavities: uterus septus (septum reaches the internal os) or uterus subseptus (septum does not reach the internal os). One group may have an asymmetric configuration consisting of a double uterus with one rudimentary horn or a hemiuterus with only one horn developed, sometimes associated with a tiny rudimentary uterus adjacent to the opposite ovary (Figure 13-2). With the hemiuterus, pregnancy can reach a point beyond which it cannot progress; and either abortion or premature labor results.

Such anomalous uteri are associated with an increase in pregnancy compli-

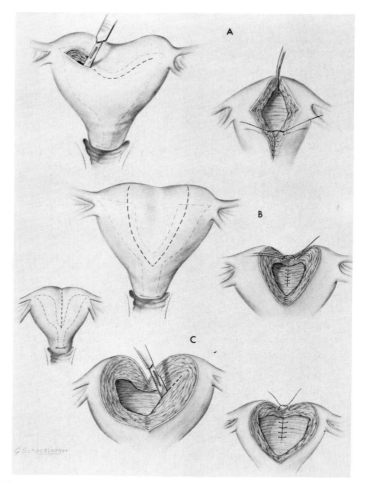

Figure 13-2.   Operations designed to correct congenital uterine defects.

cations: breech presentation (20 per cent), transverse lie (5.2 per cent, compared to the usual incidence of 0.2 per cent), and retained placenta (15 per cent, compared to the usual 1 per cent).[18] Occasionally, there may be associated dysmenorrhea and dyspareunia because of cryptomenorrhea or a vaginal septum.

All uteri are bicornuate in the early stages of embryologic development. Complete lack of fusion leads to uterus didelphys, whereas simple failure of the midline structures to regress results in a uterus septus. Confirmation of the type of uterine anomaly is usually established by hysterosalpingography.

Other lesser defects, such as a fibrotic hymen, transverse vaginal septum, or partial or complete vaginal agenesis, may prevent introition. Conception will occur after these defects are corrected only if the upper Müllerian system is intact.

Vaginal and cervical obstructive lesions may result from strictures or synechiae owing to chemicals inserted to accomplish abortion, or from cautery infection, or poor healing after surgery. Cervical polyps, severe erosion, or eversion of the cervix, as well as cervical fibroids or prolapsed submucous fibroids, may require surgical intervention. Although in most cases incompetence of the cervix appears to result from congenital factors, lacerations of the cervical wall or repeated cervical dilatations and uterine curettages may be causative factors.

Conservative operation for uterine fibroids consisting of myomectomy is warranted in any patient who is desirous of future pregnancy, provided there are no other contraindications. The means by which a fibroid interferes with conception depends on its size, location, and the extent to which it competes with a developing fetus for blood supply. Nidation may be prevented mechanically by a fibroid which distorts the endometrial cavity. Very large fibroids may also prevent sperm migration because of the long distance spermatozoa must travel to reach the fallopian tubes or as a result of partially obliterating the cornual portion of the tube. Indications for myomectomy usually include both infertility and symptoms caused by the fibroids themselves.

Asherman's syndrome must be considered in any patient who has hypomenorrhea or amenorrhea and infertility following uterine curettage, especially post partum or following abortion.

Preoperative Selection

Diagnostic studies should be deferred in any patient with active or recently active pelvic inflammatory disease. Endometrial biopsy helps in excluding chronic endometritis, which is of major prognostic significance, especially if of tuberculous origin. Curettage or endometrial biopsy may also provide confirmatory evidence of ovulation.

Hysterosalpingography is the best screening procedure to detect abnormalities of the uterus and fallopian tubes, such as anomalies, dilatation, constriction, or obstruction, as well as thickening or atrophy of the tubal mucosa and failure of peritoneal spill. However, these radiologic findings can be deceptive. Ozaras[19] suggests that presence or absence of tubal rugae markings on preoperative tubograms may be helpful in improving patient selection since the rugal pattern is a reflection of whether or not inflammatory damage is too great for a successful result.

Introduction of fiberoptic endoscopy has been a major advance in that it has proved to be of great value in patient selection. Injection of an indigo carmine solution at the time of either culdoscopy or laparoscopy helps to localize the site of tubal obstruction and also aids in assessment of the extent of adnexal disease. Laparotomy to restore fertility in women should be preceded by laparoscopy and tubal perfusion studies. If the ampulla is threadlike or without longitudinal plicae, the prognosis is poor.[17] A nodular block at the cornua may result from infection. However, if the distal two-thirds of the tubes are healthy, without kinking or adhesions, and the fimbriae and ovaries appear to be normal, reimplantation may be successful.

Jones and associates[16] emphasized that luteal phase deficiencies may occur in patients with uterine anomalies. Endocrine studies should be initiated in such patients and the defects corrected before surgery. Incredibly, on rare occasions one may still see a patient with primary sterility who has no other problem except a uterine malformation, in whom unification leads to full-term pregnancy. Buccal smears and karyograms in nearly all patients with Müllerian duct defects are normal.

Types of Operations

Conservative surgery in dealing with endometriosis, uterine fibroids, pelvic inflammatory disease, and benign ovarian neoplasms may result in preservation of fertility. Age of the patient, extent of her disease, and the experience of the gynecologic surgeon are major considerations.

Operations performed most commonly to restore fertility in women are salpingolysis, salpingostomy, tubal reimplantation, and tubal anastomosis (Figures 13-3 and 13-4). Less commonly, myomectomies and plastic surgical reconstructions of congenital Müllerian defects are carried out. Even more rarely and with almost uniform failure, a new salpinx is constructed or bilateral homeoplastic transplantation carried out. Transplantation of the ovaries into the uterus has almost always failed; and when pregnancy does occur, serious complications may result—e.g., uterine rupture.

Using delicate surgical instruments specifically designed for fine plastic work, along with the use of inert suture and splinting material, may determine success or failure. In 1921, Bonney[20] devised a method of tubal implantation for cornual obstruction by passing a piece of silkworm gut through the fimbriated end of the tube into the uterus and out through the cervix. More recently, a similar technique has been employed using polyethylene tubing. In 1939, Gepfert[21] described a method of maintaining tubal patency after salpingostomy by implanting allantoin membrane into the tubal lumen. Even the use of a ring of cartilage has been used in an attempt to preserve patency of a newly created ostium.[22] In 1949,

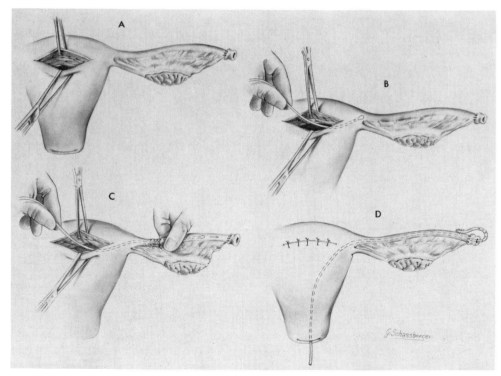

Figure 13-3.   Salpingostomy and tuboplasty.

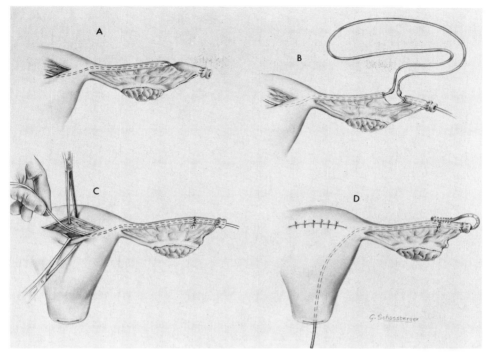

Figure 13-4. Tuboplasty after partial tubal resection.

Castello[23] demonstrated the effects of steel wire, silver wire, whalebone filament, and polyethylene tubing on tubal reconstruction in monkeys. Use of biologically inert polyethylene tubing as a splint over which endosalpinx can grow has been a significant improvement. Ends of these splints may be brought out at the angles of an abdominal wound or through the cervix for removal three to six months later, depending on the extent of damage observed at the time of surgery (Figure 13-4).

Mulligan-Rock[24] silastic hoods maintain patency of the reconstructed fimbriae but require repeat laparotomy in most instances (Figure 13-5). Clyman[25] describes a method for removal of the hoods via the usual culdoscopy approach under local anesthesia. Roland's spiral Teflon stents have an advantage in that they can be removed without repeat operation.[26] Others have attempted to prevent adhesions by completely sealing the tube in a hood formed from a film of amnion-chorionic membrane.[27] No pregnancies after this procedure have been reported as yet. Even omentum has been used to cover uterine scars and raw areas of the pelvic floor after freeing endometriosis or tubo-ovarian masses.[28]

At time of tubal surgery, it is often helpful to distend the uterus with saline after obstructing the isthmus with a clamp, so that the uterus and tubes proximal to obstruction are distended (Figure 13-6).[29] Instillation of dilute indigo carmine solution may help in delineating the extent of obstruction and its location.

Metroplasty for the various bifid anomalies of the uterus (Figure 13-1) was first described by Paul Strassmann[1] and popularized by his son.[30] The operation is designed to unite what nature did not. Variations of this procedure have been described (Figure 13-2). We have found the original operation to be quite satis-

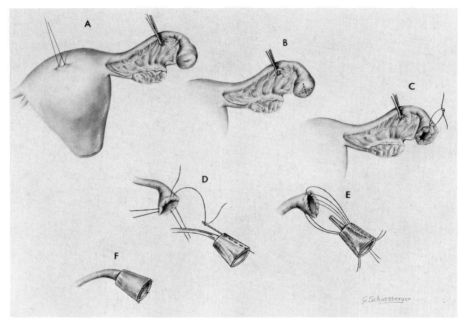

Figure 13-5.   Tuboplasty utilizing silastic hoods.

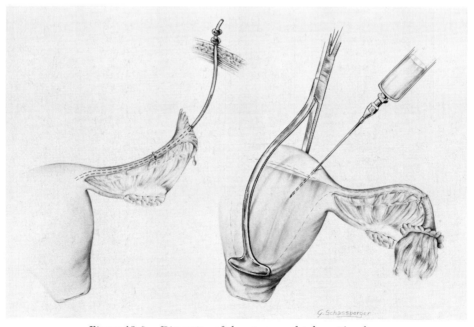

Figure 13-6.   Distention of the uterus and tube with saline.

factory. A transverse incision into the uterus seems preferable in order to preserve tissue, resulting in a relatively normal sized uterine cavity. When the transverse incision is closed with an anteroposterior suture line, the raw edges are generally held apart. In some instances, an intrauterine contraceptive device may be left in the uterus during the healing stages. Instillation of a dye into the uterine cavity before surgery may help delineate the two endometrial cavities. Care must be taken to place the initial transverse incision into the uterus between the insertions of the round ligaments to avoid tubal damage. Tubal patency must always be assessed before and after such an operation. Although a septum of the uterus may be removed with the vaginal approach,[31] laparotomy generally permits a more careful dissection.

About 5 per cent of infertile patients have uterine fibroids.[33] Presence of fibroids in an infertile patient does not necessarily imply a causative relationship. All other contributing factors must be considered before myomectomy. Sterility may be caused by obstruction from uterine fibroids, distortion of the uterine cavity, associated hyperplasia of the endometrium, or alteration of the blood supply to the endometrium at the site of attempted nidation. Hysterosalpingography is essential in determining to what extent fibroids encroach on the endometrial cavity. Before myomectomy is attempted, the patient must be prepared for a possible hysterectomy. Remarkable results can be obtained with careful dissection in removing numerous myomata, with preservation of as much myometrium as possible and meticulous reconstruction of the uterus.

Synechiae within the uterus (Asherman's syndrome) may be removed by curettage when they cause minimal distortion of the endometrial cavity. Extensive obliteration with almost complete atresia of the uterine cavity cannot be corrected by curettage. In three instances, we have performed abdominal hysterotomy with extensive excision of scar tissue and reconstruction of a normal sized uterine cavity, in which an intrauterine contraceptive device was placed for 6 months before removal. In all three instances the previous amenorrhea was replaced by normal menstruation, and two of these patients became pregnant. One has just been delivered following premature labor at 7 months' gestation, with the infant dying neonatally. The obstetric sequence in this patient suggests an incompetent cervix.

Transplantation of endometrial tissue has been described.[34] Even a small patch of remaining endometrial tissue may result in spontaneous regeneration of the mucosa. Strassmann[35] described six patients with complete atresia in whom a similar procedure was done, but in addition a fallopian tube was partially brought down through a tunnel into the endometrial cavity. Strassmann suggested that the tubal epithelium was the source of mucosal regeneration, but the excised scar tissue did contain endometrial remnants.

Postoperative hydrotubations between menstruation and ovulation may be important in preserving tubal patency both following removal of splints and, especially, when splints are not used. Such tubal perfusions are continued before ovulation in each cycle until there is assurance of a free flow. All sorts of drug combinations have been used. We use a corticosteroid solution—50 mg. of cortisone acetate in 20 cc. of physiologic saline.

Conservative surgery in dealing with endometriosis, uterine fibroids, pelvic inflammatory disease, benign ovarian neoplasms, preinvasive carcinoma of the cervix, relaxation of the pelvic floor, and urinary incontinence may result in preservation of fertility. Age of the patient, extent of her disease, and experience of the gynecologic surgeon are major considerations. Surgical castration of any young woman should be preceded by a critical appraisal of the indications.

Even extensive pelvic endometriosis may be amenable to conservative surgery with preservation of reproductive function. Initially, seemingly impossible situations may be dealt with successfully after prolonged and careful dissection. In each instance, the desire for pregnancy must be weighed against the risks of recurrent disease and operative complications.

Preservation of fertility is often a major consideration when surgical intervention is required because of pelvic infections in young women. Extensive inflammatory damage usually offers a poor prognosis for future pregnancy. However, pregnancy has followed even drainage of a tubo-ovarian abscess or unilateral adnexectomy.

Cystic teratoma or dermoid tumors of the ovary are frequently encountered in young women. They are rarely malignant (1 per cent) and are bilateral in about 20 per cent of patients. Meticulous excision of these tumors may permit preservation of normal ovarian tissue sufficient for subsequent pregnancy.

Preinvasive cancer of the cervix may be overtreated. Conization of the cervix for this disease has been followed by successful pregnancy in many instances. This sequence seems to be safe and appropriate provided that periodic postoperative cytologic studies are carried out.

Conservative treatment of a relaxed pelvic floor and uterine prolapse, with or without stress urinary incontinence, may be followed by pregnancy. Cystoceles and rectoceles do not necessarily recur as a result of vaginal delivery following surgical repair. Coexistent uterine prolapse may be treated by performing partial amputation of the cervix (Manchester operation). Although fraught with increased obstetric complications (e.g., premature labor), this operation should remain in our armamentarium in dealing with the very young.

Experimental Operations

Previous poor results or almost hopeless operative findings, such as previous excision or total damage to the fallopian tubes, have led to a search for newer operative approaches. Castallo[23] encouraged more extensive tubal reconstructions by demonstrating that the resected fallopian tube of the monkey would regenerate across a bridge of polyethylene tubing. Vein and arterial grafts,[36] the vermiform appendix,[37,38] and artificial tubing have been used to replace the oviducts. Reversed seromuscular ileal grafts have been used to replace the uterine cornua.[40] It seems that such attempts are doomed to failure and moreover that they ignore the important physiologic functions of the fallopian tubes and their highly specialized ciliated cells. One of the more intriguing experimental operations has involved the use of tissue adhesive (methyl-2-cyanoacrylate monomer) to stick transected tubes back together over a No. 1 plain catgut suture splint.[41]

Results

Review of results of operations to correct infertility in women during the past 10 years is a frustrating experience, since many reports are not comparable. Numerous variations of operative procedures are carried out unilaterally or bilaterally, with wide variation in the methods of patient selection. There does appear to be improvement in success rates since the earlier reports[12,13] (Table 13–3). One of the difficulties in assessing results lies in the fact that many operations carried out for correction of infertility are never reported. Furthermore, celiotomy may be undertaken but the intended operation may not be carried through because of discouraging findings. Such exclusions in reports of results are misleading. Many details necessary for a valid comparative analysis are omitted. Specific ground rules must be established in compiling surveys of experience in this field if significant data are to be obtained. It is not possible to compare unilateral with bilateral operations. Pregnancy rates alone do not provide as important information as the percentage of successful pregnancies. One report involves 300 patients who had tuboplasty operations with a 10.3 per cent conception rate postoperatively. However, critical review of the hysterosalpingograms and the records of these patients show that success was unquestionably the result of the operation in only 2.7 per cent.[19] Pregnancy following a tubal sterilization operation is almost as frequent. Pre- and postoperative hysterosalpingograms would help in evaluating results. Siegler[47] suggests a new category, combined tuboplasty, useful in evaluating results when different procedures are used on each side. Errors may also occur from false negative tubal patency tests when tubal patency may be demonstrated at operation after the tubes were thought to be closed. Polemics about the duration of follow-up required for inclusion of a given case have not been resolved. Although there are exceptions, patients who have not become pregnant within two years after surgery might be considered to have had operative failures. Therapeutic effects of individual plastic operations on the tubes cannot be properly assessed unless there is positive proof that both tubes were occluded prior to operation.

Whereas polyethylene splints are advocated by most, others[17] have regarded them as unnecessary, attributing successes largely to the postoperative administration of corticosteroids.

Metroplasties because of infertility have been far more successful than operations on the oviduct.[18,48] A combination of a Strassmann metroplasty and bilateral tuboplasty has resulted in a normal pregnancy.[18]

TABLE 13–3. *Results of Operations to Restore Fertility in Women*

SERIES	YEAR	NUMBER	OPERATION	PER CENT PREGNANCIES
Greenhill[12]	1937	818	Tuboplasty	6.6
Rutherford *et al.*[42]	1939	43	Tuboplasty	48.8
Green-Armytage[43]	1957	38	Tuboplasty	42.2
Mutch[44]	1959	42	Tuboplasty	11.0
Mroeh *et al.*[45]	1967	23	Tuboplasty	8.7
Ozaras[19]	1968	300	Tuboplasty	10.3
O'Brien *et al.*[3]	1969	173	Tuboplasty	35.3
Roland and Leisten[26]	1972	130	Tuboplasty	25.0
Young *et al.*[46]	1970	114	Multiple operations	32.5
Strassmann[18]	1966	263	Metroplasty	67.2
Ingersoll[52]	1963	139	Myomectomy	85.0

When the fimbriae have been occluded by previous pelvic inflammatory disease or when a hydrosalpinx is present, patency of the tubes can be established in most patients. However, few pregnancies result. We reviewed the last 30 patients in whom we carried out bilateral tuboplasty, for whom postoperative tests indicated a tubal patency rate of 93 per cent. However, pregnancies have occurred in only 40 per cent.

Pelvic tuberculosis remains a serious problem, with a poor prognosis for future pregnancies. Varela-Nuñez[49] reviewed numerous reports of genital tuberculosis and found only 53 pregnancies after surgery, and 55 per cent of these were tubal pregnancies. This high incidence of ectopic pregnancy may be attributable to the extensive fibrosis and calcification that occur in tuberculous salpingitis, with obvious interference with tubal function.

Dunselman[50] collected from the literature 290 cases of metroplasty and found 87 per cent pregnancy wastage prior to surgical correction of the defect. This was almost completely reversed afterwards. An improvement of fetal salvage rate from 21 to 82 per cent has been reported by others.[51]

Women who have had multiple myomectomies and are carefully selected for surgery have an approximately 30 per cent chance of having a successful pregnancy after operation. Approximately 10 to 15 per cent will have recurrent symptoms severe enough for hysterectomy within 5 years.[52,53]

Forty to 50 per cent of patients should become pregnant after conservative operation for endometriosis, which generally consists of partial resection of the ovaries, destruction or removal of implants on the pelvic peritoneum, and in some instances presacral neurectomy.[33]

Complications

In most series of tuboplasty operations, there is about a 10 per cent incidence of subsequent ectopic pregnancy.[54] If abortions are included, pregnancy wastage increases to 15 to 20 per cent. Psychiatric complications may be serious, and their frequency again relates to patient selection.

Cornual rupture at the site of tubal implantation may occur, and four previous cornual ruptures after salpingectomy with cornual excision of the tube have been reported.[55] Foreign body reaction to polyethylene tubing used as a splint, with formation of a sterile abscess, has been reported.[56]

Discussion

It is clear that more than tubal patency must be considered in assessing the success of tubal operations. Better patient selection and the use of stents have improved results. However, the only successful result is a pregnancy which produces a normal infant. Results are notoriously poor when inflammatory disease has been the basis of obstruction leading to tuboplasty. Obviously, the highly specialized ciliated epithelium of the endosalpinx is of critical importance. Patency is not a sure index of tubal function, since it is only an anatomical description that does not guarantee adequacy of physiologic activities. The mammalian oviduct must perform a variety of functions in the transport and development of gametes. Adhesions around the fimbriae may interfere with ovum pickup and with tubal peristalsis. Occlusions associated with relatively normal tubal epithelium are quite amenable to successful surgery. When not associated with intrinsic tubal disease, a high success rate is associated with lysis of adhesions. Ovum pickup is dependent on the functioning of the fimbriae. Extensive scars from chronic infection possibly should be viewed as a contraindication to tuboplastic surgery. Nevertheless, it is easy to be tempted by the imploring infertile woman during her stubborn quest for pregnancy. Patients who are operated on for pelvic inflammatory disease usually return to the same environment in which they originally contracted the infection.

Other factors affecting the results of surgery are the experience and skill of the operator and the delicacy with which he handles tissues. Results of surgical efforts to restore fertility are least rewarding when carried out at the site most frequently involved in the etiology, the fallopian tubes.

Rigid indications for surgery of this sort should be maintained if we are ever to establish its real worth. In this era of a burgeoning population and a shortage of physicians, justification for many of the operative procedures currently carried out may be increasingly difficult to find.

A fresh look, ameliorated by healthy skepticism, may result in better results in the future, even though past results have been discouraging. Candor in assessing the prognosis of a procedure is of critical importance. When confronted with a poor prognosis for operation, the couple may well abandon their attempts for surgery and initiate adoption. It is critical to exercise good judgment in the preoperative evaluation, with careful patient selection. These considerations are at least as important as the surgical technique. In major surgery there is the omnipresent hazard of overenthusiasm and distortion of judgment.

It seems certain that future improvements will depend on better understanding of the physiology and pathology of the human reproductive system. Increased knowledge of uterine and tubal function should lead to more rational selection of cases for surgery.

REFERENCES

1. Cohen, M. R.: A simplified plan for the infertile couple. Postgrad. Med. 36:337, 1964.
2. Rubin, I. C.: Uterotubal insufflation as a test for tubal patency, 1920–1940. Am. J. Obstet. Gynec. 40:628, 1940.
3. O'Brien, J. R., Arronet, G. H., and Eduljee, S. Y.: Operative treatment of fallopian tube pathology in human fertility. Am. J. Obstet. Gynec. 103:520, 1969.
4. Strassmann, P.: Die operative Vereinigung eines doppelten uterus; nebst Bemerkungen uber die Korrektur der sogenannten Verdoppelung des Genitalkanales. Zentralbl. Gynak. 31:1322, 1907.
5. Jones, H. W., Jr., and Jones, G. E. S.: Double uterus as an etiological factor in repeated abortion: indications for surgical repair. Am. J. Obstet. Gynec. 65:325, 1953.
6. Ruge, P.: Bericht uber die Verhandlungen der Geselleschaft fur Geburtshilfe und Gynakologie zu Berlin. Sitzung vom 3. Juni 1883. Ztschr. f. Geburtsh. u. Gynak. 10:141, 1884.
7. Martin, A.: Handbuch der Krankheiten der Weiblichen Adnexorgane. Band I. Die Kronkeit der Eiliter. Leipzig, Germany, Karger, 1885.
8. Mackenrodt, A.: Berichte aus gynakol. Gesellschatten u. Krankenhausern. I. Demonstration von Praporaten. Zentralbl. Gynak. 18:826, 1894.
9. Watkins, T. J.: Salpingostomy and pregnancy. Discussion. Am. J. Obstet. Gynec. 64:134, 1911.

10. Estes, W. L.: A method of implanting ovarian tissue in order to maintain ovarian function. Pennsylvania Med. J. 13:610, 1909.
11. Tuffier, M., and Letulle, M.: Transposition de l'ovaire pourvu de son pédicule vasculaire dans l'utérus après ablation des salpingites (29 opérations). Presse Méd. 32:465, 1924.
12. Greenhill, J. P.: Evaluation of salpingostomy and tubal implantation for treatment of sterility. Am. J. Obstet. Gynec. 33:39, 1937.
13. Siegler, A. M., and Hellman, L. M.: Tubal plastic surgery. Fertil. Steril. 7:170, 1956.
14. Asherman, J. G.: Amenorrhoea traumatica (atretica). J. Obstet. Gynaec. Brit. Comm. 55:23, 1948.
15. McEwen, D. C.: Reconstructive tubal surgery. Fertil. Steril. 17:39, 1966.
16. Jones, H. W., Jr., Delfs, E., and Jones, G. E. S.: Reproductive difficulties in double uterus. Am. J. Obstet. Gynec. 72:865, 1956.
17. Palmer, R.: Salpingostomy—a critical study of 396 personal cases operated upon without polyethylene tubing. Proc. Roy. Soc. Med. 53:357, 1960.
18. Strassmann, E. O.: Fertility and unification of double uterus. Fertil. Steril. 17:165, 1966.
19. Ozaras, H.: The value of plastic operations on the fallopian tubes in the treatment of female infertility. Acta Obstet. Gynec. Scand. 47:489, 1968.
20. Bonney, V.: Fruits of conservation. J. Obstet. Gynaec. Brit. Emp. 44:1, 1937.
21. Gepfert, J. R.: Studies on reconstruction of fallopian tube: preliminary report of original technique. Am. J. Obstet. Gynec. 38:256, 1939.
22. Barsky, A. J., and Blinick, G.: The use of cartilage grafts to maintain patency of the fallopian tubes. Plast. Reconst. Surg. 11:87, 1953.
23. Castallo, M. A.: Experimental recanalization of fallopian tubes in Macacus rhesus monkey. Fertil. Steril. 1:435, 1950.
24. Mulligan, W. J., Rock, J., and Easterday, C. L.: Use of polyethylene in tuboplasty. Fertil. Steril. 4:428, 1954.
25. Clyman, M. J.: Silastic hoods in tuboplasty: a new approach to their removal. Fertil. Steril. 19:537, 1968.
26. Roland, M., and Leisten, D.: Tuboplasty in 130 patients. Improved results due to stents and preoperative endoscopy. Obstet. Gynec. 39:57, 1972.
27. TenBerge, B. S., and Lok, T. T.: Plastic surgery of closed tubes with chorion-amnion. Fertil. Steril. 5:339, 1954.
28. White, M. M.: The use of omental patches in the surgery of subfertility. Internat. J. Fertil. 7:163, 1962.
29. Shirodkar, V. N.: Factors influencing the results of salpingostomy. Internat. J. Fertil. 11:361, 1966.
30. Strassmann, E. O.: The Strassmann operation for double uterus. A fifty year experience. Obstet. Gynec. 10:701, 1957.
31. Mossop, R. T.: Per-vaginal correction of the septate uterus. Central African J. Med. 15:284, 1969.
32. Marshall, B. R., and Evans, T. N.: Cerclage for cervical incompetence. Obstet. Gynec. 29:759, 1967.
33. Lash, A. F.: Surgery in infertility. Illinois Med. J. 134:283, 1968.
34. Westman, A.: Pregnancy following endometrial homotransplantation. Am. J. Obstet. Gynec. (Supp.) 61A:15, 1951.
35. Strassmann, E. O.: Surgical reconstruction of a functioning uterine cavity in six patients having complete atresia. South. Med. J. 49:458, 1956.
36. Davids, A. M., and Bellwin, A.: Reconstruction of fallopian tubes by vein and artery transplants. Fertil. Steril. 5:339, 1954.
37. O'Neill, J. J.: The use of the vermiform appendix as a fallopian tube. Am. J. Obstet. Gynec. 95:219, 1966.
38. Halelamira, S., Thumaporn, M., and Buranavithayanon, H.: The use of the vermiform appendix as a fallopian tube. Internat. Surg. 49:162, 1968.
39. Hayashi, M.: Surgical procedures for establishing tubal patency (salpingoplasty). Am. J. Obstet. Gynec. 84:79, 1962.
40. Charles, A. G., Labes, J. E., Cohen, M., Fitch, L. B., and Shoemaker, W. C.: Technique for substitution of the uterine tube. Obstet. Gynec. 20:174, 1962.
41. Harrell, W. B., Dugan, G. T., Chappell, R. H., and Farris, H.: Simulated tuboplasty using tissue adhesive on uterine horn in canines. J. Arkansas Med. Soc. 65:433, 1969.
42. Rutherford, R. N., Lamborn, H. M., and Banks, L. A.: Surgical treatment of sterility. Am. J. Obstet. Gynec. 58:673, 1949.
43. Green-Armytage, V. B.: Tubo-uterine implantation. J. Obstet. Gynec. Brit. Emp. 64:47, 1957.
44. Mutch, M. G.: Sterility and tuboplasties. Fertil. Steril. 10:240, 1959.

45. Mroeh, A., Glass, R. H., and Buxton, C. L.: Tubal plastic surgery. Fertil. Steril. *18*:80, 1967.
46. Young, P. E., Egan, J. E., Barlow, J. J., and Mulligan, W. J.: Reconstructive surgery for infertility at the Boston Hospital for Women. Am. J. Obstet. Gynec. *108*:1092, 1970.
47. Siegler, A. M.: Comments on tubal plastic operations. Internat. J. Fertil. *9*:561, 1964.
48. White, M. M.: Uteroplasty in infertility. Proc. Roy. Soc. Med. *53*:1006, 1960.
49. Varela-Nuñez, A.: Tubal pregnancy following treated genital tuberculosis. Report of two cases and review of the literature. Am. J. Obstet. Gynec. *82*:1162, 1961.
50. Duselman, G. A. J. (quoted by Genelland Sjövall): The Strassmann operation: results obtained in 58 cases. Acta Obstet. Gynec. Scand. *38*:477, 1959.
51. Capraro, V. J., Chuang, J. T., and Randall, C. L.: Improved fetal salvage after metroplasty. Obstet. Gynec. *31*:97, 1968.
52. Ingersoll, F. M.: Fertility following myomectomy. Fertil. Steril. *14*:596, 1963.
53. Wiener, W. B., and Head, C. M.: Abdominal myomectomy: a surgical procedure in infertility patients. J. Mississippi Med. J. *5*:261, 1964.
54. Wainer, A. S., and Castallo, M. A.: Surgical treatment of tubal occlusion. Clinical Obstet. Gynec. *2*:789, 1959.
55. Whitney, D. J., and Rivlin, M. E.: A case of rupture of the uterus at the site of tubal implantation. J. Obstet. Gynaec. Brit. Comm. *73*:858, 1966.
56. Kantor, H. I., and Kamholz, J. H.: Complication of tubal reimplantation. Fertil. Steril. *8*:438, 1957.

Gynecologic Surgery
in Women Desirous of Further Childbearing

Management of Ovarian Neoplasia in Pregnancy

Tiffany J. Williams and Richard S. Sheldon

Mayo Clinic and Mayo Foundation

Because of widely diverging methods of reporting, it is difficult to determine the incidence of ovarian enlargement, ovarian neoplasm, or ovarian malignancy in pregnancy.[4,12] Certain reviews relate specifically to malignant ovarian neoplasm; however, most of the malignancies are recorded as reports of an individual case.[2,5] Hence, few physicians have an opportunity in their lifetime to form an adequate opinion, based on personal experience, as to the proper management of such ovarian neoplasms in pregnancy.

Ovarian Enlargement or Neoplasm

The management of ovarian neoplasm or enlargement during pregnancy may be predicated on two factors—the size of the ovarian enlargement and its consistency. Even though the pregnant patient tends to be somewhat younger than those patients who are subject to ovarian carcinoma, the possibility of malignancy must be considered and is the specific subject of this discussion. In fact, ovarian cancer has been recorded in pregnant women as young as 20 years.

There would seem to be little reason to change the criteria for evaluation of ovarian enlargement in the pregnant and nonpregnant female. The ovarian enlargements may be divided further into two categories—cystic and solid. The decision that must be reached is whether or not the enlargement is physiologic or neoplastic. Inasmuch as there are no physiologic solid ovarian enlargements, any solid ovarian growth requires exploration, regardless of its size, as it must be neoplastic and may possibly be malignant.

On the other hand, an ovarian *cyst* may be either physiologic or neoplastic. During the early months of pregnancy, the presence of a corpus luteum may be anticipated but this is physiologic, not requiring surgical intervention. A neoplastic cyst, on the other hand, will persist and may increase in size.

It has been found from experience that physiologic ovarian cysts smaller

456

than 5 to 6 cm. are likely to regress. Conversely, a physiologic ovarian cyst larger than 6 cm. is less likely to regress and, indeed, has an increased likelihood of presenting as a surgical emergency, with torsion, infarction, hemorrhage, and infection, or it may cause mechanical dystocia in the event of labor.

In view of this experience, follow-up examination of ovarian cysts that are less than 5 to 6 cm. in size is accepted practice. If they regress, nothing further is required; if they persist or enlarge, definitive diagnosis is necessary and exploration and histologic evaluation are required. An ovarian cyst larger than 6 cm., even if physiologic, is prone to cause complications and should be investigated surgically. These criteria are valid in the pregnant as well as in the nonpregnant patient.

In recent years, ovarian enlargements have been diagnosed more frequently as a result of earlier examinations during gestation. Follow-up of ovarian enlargement is indicated and, if the enlargement persists after 4 to 6 weeks, definitive steps are indicated regardless of the duration of pregnancy. As is the case with all ovarian enlargements, the primary method of diagnosis is usually bimanual examination. Earlier reports suggested the use of roentgenography in diagnosing such special tumors as dermoids; however, this method is contraindicated during pregnancy. The use of ultrasound as a diagnostic method is helpful in recognizing ovarian tumors without causing risk to the mother or fetus.

It has been stated that the ideal time for surgical treatment of an ovarian tumor in a pregnant woman is in the middle trimester. Usually by the time the follow-up examination of a smaller tumor, discovered in early pregnancy, is terminated, the patient will already be in the middle trimester. By this time the placenta has supplanted the corpus luteum in maintaining the pregnancy. Numerous reports show that early removal of the corpus luteum will not affect the pregnancy and, accordingly, it would seem to make little difference when an indicated operation is performed in the first half of gestation. However, premature labor may be precipitated when an operation is performed in the latter part of pregnancy. Hence, if ovarian tumor is not diagnosed until late in pregnancy, there may be some justification in delaying exploration until the fetus is viable and can be delivered safely by cesarean section.

The earlier literature on ovarian tumors and pregnancy specifically points out the dangers of torsion, rupture, hemorrhage, and infection when ovarian tumors are allowed to exist throughout labor and into the puerperium.[7,8,13] Consequently, it is recommended that a tumor diagnosed at labor should not be subjected to the stresses of labor and delivery, with their subsequent complications. Ovarian tumors diagnosed immediately before or during labor should be explored at that time. One additional complication in the pregnant woman that might be anticipated is blockage of the birth canal by the tumor. Examination at the time of onset of labor will make such a dystocia problem obvious, and surgical treatment is indicated. Culdocentesis and aspiration of the tumor have been mentioned, particularly in the older literature, but these are contraindicated in the modern practice of obstetrics.

Torsion of ovarian tumors, with subsequent infarction, rupture, or hemorrhage presenting as acute abdominal emergencies, should be explored immediately, regardless of the stage or duration of pregnancy.

Of importance in the management of the ovarian tumor at the time of operation are: (1) the gross appearance of the tumor and (2) the histologic diagnosis. The surgeon must be familiar with the gross pathology of the ovary, and either cryostat or frozen section diagnosis also should be available to him. The management of the patient is dependent on the information gained by these two diagnostic methods.

When the condition of the abdomen is acute, owing to torsion, rupture, or hemorrhage, extirpation of the involved adnexa is required. If the tumor is benign, unilateral salpingo-oophorectomy suffices as adequate treatment, whether the tumor is physiologic or neoplastic.

A common neoplasm that appears in association with pregnancy is the dermoid cyst. If this diagnosis can be made grossly, resection is indicated rather than salpingo-oophorectomy, provided that the tissue is normal-appearing, viable ovarian tissue. Because of the high incidence of bilaterality, adequate evaluation of the opposite ovary is important and bisection is recommended. Microscopic confirmation is all that is otherwise required. Any benign ovarian neoplasm may be resected, provided that rupture does not occur. If such a course is undertaken and the malignant cyst ruptures, the survival of the patient may be jeopardized.[14]

Ovarian Malignancy

The controversy that arises in the management of ovarian neoplasm in pregnancy deals specifically with malignancy. The accepted treatment of choice for ovarian cancer is total abdominal hysterectomy, bilateral salpingo-oophorectomy, and omentectomy with or without subsequent radiotherapy or chemotherapy.[14] Such treatment in the instance of the pregnant female would obviously sacrifice the pregnancy. If the patient is older and has living children, it would seem unwise to accept anything but the treatment of choice, regardless of the grade or stage of the malignancy. The most recent reports in the literature by Creasman and associates,[1] Tawa,[11] and others have indeed urged this management for all patients with ovarian cancer, even if they are pregnant.

Some controversy, however, exists in the case of a young patient with intracystic grade 1 malignancy (unilateral) who is in her first pregnancy or who is strongly desirous of continuing the pregnancy. Falk and Bunkin,[6] Jubb,[9] and others[10] suggest that unilateral salpingo-oophorectomy is satisfactory treatment when only one ovary is involved. Scattered reports in the literature would seem to show that this is feasible despite the recommendations to the contrary.

A study of a large number of ovarian malignancies, categorized by grade and stage as well as by histologic type, shows that the grade and the stage of the tumor are the most significant factors in the patient's survival.[14] It would seem reasonable, then, to apply these criteria to ovarian malignancies in the young pregnant woman as well. Studies show that survival with a stage I, grade 1 carcinoma of the ovary after complete operation approximates 90 per cent regardless of histologic type.[3,14]

Indeed, a further study carried out among young women under 30 years of age shows that when an ovarian malignancy is grade 1, unilateral, encapsulated, nonruptured, and nonadherent, there is 100 per cent survival at 5 years provided that the opposite ovary is normal.[15]

Such information is available specifically in the studies by Munnell and co-workers[10] and by Jubb,[9] and these authors refer to the possibility of such conservative therapy. It is reasonable, then, in the instance of a pregnant woman, to perform only unilateral salpingo-oophorectomy even for a malignant tumor if it is low-grade, unilateral, encapsulated, nonruptured, and nonadherent. Bisection of the opposite ovary is necessary to confirm this belief. If the tumor is of a high grade or stage, total abdominal hysterectomy and bilateral salpingo-oophorectomy are indicated, without regard for the fetus.

If the tumor is discovered at 32 weeks or beyond, it is feasible to defer surgery until maturity is determined or assumed at 36 to 37 weeks' gestation, unless there is an acute problem. One could then do the necessary cesarean hysterectomy and bilateral salpingo-oophorectomy as required. One would hope that the benefits derived by the fetus outweigh the risks involved for the mother in delaying surgical treatment of the tumor.

Summary

The management of a symptomatic ovarian neoplasm in pregnancy requires immediate operation, usually because of an intra-abdominal catastrophe, such as torsion, infarction, hemorrhage, rupture, or suppuration.

The treatment for an asymptomatic ovarian neoplasm is predicated on the size and consistency of the tumor. If the tumor is solid, exploration is required, as the tumor has the potentiality of being malignant. If the tumor is cystic, it may be either physiologic or neoplastic. A cyst smaller than 5 to 6 cm. in diameter has a significant chance of being physiologic and of undergoing spontaneous regression. Observation to confirm such regression is required. If, however, the cyst persists or enlarges, or if it is larger than 6 cm., surgical treatment is indicated.

The management at the time of operation is dictated by the gross and microscopic picture of the ovarian tumor. If gross and microscopic evidence indicates that the tumor is benign, unilateral salpingo-oophorectomy is satisfactory treatment. In the case of a dermoid cyst, resection is recommended.

If the tumor is grossly malignant, the age and parity of the patient and the duration of pregnancy become factors in making the appropriate decision. If the patient is older or has living children, total abdominal hysterectomy, bilateral salpingo-oophorectomy, and omentectomy are the treatment of choice. If the patient is young and does not have a family, however, then the grade and stage of the tumor are significant. A unilateral, stage I, encapsulated, nonadherent, nonruptured, grade 1 malignant lesion may be managed by unilateral salpingo-oophorectomy. Tumors of higher grade or stage are managed best by abdominal hysterectomy and bilateral salpingo-oophorectomy.

REFERENCES

1. Creasman, W. T., Rutledge, F., and Smith, J. P.: Carcinoma of the ovary associated with pregnancy. Obstet. Gynec. 38:111, 1971.
2. David, M. P., Cohen, E., Soferman, N., et al.: Adénocarcinome de l'ovaire bilatéral et grossesse extra-utérine: à propos d'une observation. Gynec. Obstet. (Paris) 68:65, 1969.
3. Decker, D. G., Mussey, E., Williams, T. J., et al.: Grading of gynecologic malignancy: epithelial ovarian cancer. In Proceedings of the Seventh National Cancer Conference. Philadelphia, J. B. Lippincott, 1973, pp. 223–231.

4. Divino, L. E., Jr., and Hoskins, B. L.: Masculinization in pregnancy. Obstet. Gynec. 28:842, 1966.

5. Dougherty, C. M., and Lund, C. J.: Solid ovarian tumors complicating pregnancy: a clinical-pathological study. Am. J. Obstet. Gynec. 60:261, 1950.

6. Falk, H. C., and Bunkin, I. A.: The management of ovarian tumors complicating pregnancy. Am. J. Obstet. Gynec. 54:82, 1947.

7. Freeth, D.: Primary carcinoma of the ovaries causing obstructed labour. J. Obstet. Gynaec. Brit. Comm. 57:232, 1950.

8. Grimes, W. H., Jr., Bartholomew, R. A., Colvin, E. D., et al.: Ovarian cyst complicating pregnancy. Am. J. Obstet. Gynec. 68:594, 1954.

9. Jubb, E. D.: Primary ovarian carcinoma in pregnancy. Am. J. Obstet. Gynec. 85:345, 1963.

10. Munnell, E. W., and Taylor, H. C., Jr.: Ovarian carcinoma: a review of 200 primary and 51 secondary cases. Am. J. Obstet. Gynec. 58:943, 1949.

11. Tawa, K.: Ovarian tumors in pregnancy. Am. J. Obstet. Gynec. 90:511, 1964.

12. Thomas, E., Mestman, J., Henneman, C., et al.: Bilateral luteomas of pregnancy with virilization: a case report. Obstet. Gynec. 39:577, 1972.

13. Traut, H. F., and Kuder, A.: Pelvic tumors complicating pregnancy. Int. Clin. 3:285, 1940.

14. Webb, M. J., Decker, D. G., Mussey, E., et al.: Factors influencing survival in stage I ovarian cancer. Am. J. Obstet. Gynec. 116:222, 1973.

15. Williams, T. J., Symmonds, R. E., and Litwak, O.: Management of unilateral and encapsulated ovarian cancer in young women. Gynec. Oncol. 1:143, 1973.

Gynecologic Surgery
in Women Desirous of Further Childbearing

Editorial Comment

The maintenance of function of the female reproductive organs or their restitution to function is the hallmark of a conscientious and conservative gynecologist. It is this attitude and philosophy that separates gynecologic operation from the overall field of general surgery. The truth of this statement is amply demonstrated in this chapter, since many conditions listed might well be treated surgically at the time of diagnosis. Emphasis on maintenance of function, however, has led to some controversies, as indicated by the procedure of myomectomy. If there is any indication for this operation it is in the patient with an infertility problem and when the hysterogram suggests that the tumor might encroach on the uterine cavity and cause the patient to abort in the event of pregnancy. It is reassuring but somewhat puzzling to be informed that recurrence of tumors is rare following myomectomy, but this presupposes that all of the myomas have been removed, even those that are seedling in character. If there is any general advocacy of this operation the physician should certainly be familiar with the natural history of leiomyomas during the course of pregnancy. Even patients with leiomyomas large enough to occupy the pelvis and surrounding areas usually do well, should they become pregnant. To be sure, tumor(s) may effect a disturbance in blood supply, with possible necrosis, which is usually managed by medical means and observation. Also, early in pregnancy a leiomyoma may enlarge at a greater rate than the uterus does. However, the tumor will cease to grow by the end of the first trimester, and although its presence is of some annoyance, it will rarely be of any medical consequence. Following labor and delivery, the tumor recedes, usually to its original size, and remains quiescent. Moreover, the leiomyoma may not enlarge in a subsequent pregnancy, presumably because its blood supply has been impeded in some way in the previous pregnancy. The tumor has usually developed some degree of calcification, and the musculature fails to respond and increase in size.

Should the tumor be located on the lower portion of the uterus and obstruct the birth canal, the condition may correct itself spontaneously, for as the uterus enlarges, the tumor moves out of the pelvis and becomes an abdominal organ. An intramural fibroid occurring in pregnancy tends to be extruded from the uterus and to become pedunculated. It is this type of tumor that may need removal because of torsion.

But, to return to myomectomy, anyone who has observed the state of the abdomen at cesarean section in women with previous myomectomies can attest to the extensiveness of the adhesions that are commonly encountered. In fact, in some instances it is well to dissect the adhesions from the uterus prior to delivery if by chance there is need to perform a cesarean hysterectomy, so that time will not be lost in freeing the uterus from its iatrogenic impediments. Certainly intestinal obstruction is a greater hazard for patients who have been subjected to a multiple myomectomy than for almost any other abdominal procedure. Definitive therapy for uterine myomata—i.e., hysterectomy—is best postponed, if it is possible, until after childbearing.

Uterine prolapse is being seen less frequently in current practice. However, when it occurs it can usually be managed conservatively until after childbearing by the use of a pessary. A definitive procedure of vaginal hysterectomy and plastic repair can then be performed. The Fothergill-Manchester procedure apparently is still being used, and undoubtedly in the very rare patient it is necessary to preserve childbearing when a pessary fails to reduce the prolapse. However, there are many who feel that this operation is at best a compromise. The shortening of the cervix encourages pregnancy loss, either by miscarriage or from premature rupture of the fetal membranes.

The treatment of stress incontinence in women desiring other children is dependent primarily on the extent of the symptoms and the number of children contemplated. The fact that the patient is incontinent indicates that she has received less than optimal obstetrical care previously and undoubtedly should have been delivered by methods other than the one selected. Hence, most of these patients—if not all—should be delivered by cesarean section if the continence has been alleviated surgically.

The discourse on the surgical management of the infertile patient speaks for itself, for the results are impressive. The infertile patient, who after careful evaluation might benefit by tubal surgery, should be managed by those with judgment gained mainly through experience and who are familiar with all of the operative techniques. These patients should not be placed in the hands of the gynecologist who only occasionally treats such cases.

Finally, in the event of pregnancy, complications can arise over which there may be controversy as to whether or not the reproductive organs should be preserved in the overall management of the complication. This is illustrated in the case of placenta accreta. Undoubtedly, nonoperative management has a greater chance of success when the placenta accreta is total. The placenta eventually sloughs away over a period of weeks or months. However, this is somewhat at variance with the experience of many obstetricians, especially with the partial or focal type of placenta accreta, for this method of management—whatever else it does—presupposes that there is a highly efficient blood bank close at hand. Rather, placenta accreta of whatever degree is more safely treated by hysterectomy when the diagnosis is initially established, and even here supportive measures may well include several transfusions.

The ultimate in conservation of the reproductive system is represented by the local incision of a chorioadenoma destruens. With the introduction of chemotherapeutic agents this procedure may no longer be necessary. However, patients with this condition are often nulliparas and hence preservation of the uterus is desirable. Drs. Beecham and Beecham and others have successfully treated such patients by local excision and thereby retained the childbearing function for the patient. Indeed there are patients who have subsequently become pregnant and been delivered successfully following what appears to be a somewhat radical approach to patient management.

The surgical treatment of vaginal adenosis is controversial and each patient's treatment must be individualized. In general, local incision appears to be adequate and certainly in these young women would be preferable. This is a subject which is open to controversy, although it will eventually be resolved.

Ovarian malignancy in pregnancy is given special consideration in this chapter despite its infrequency. Whenever the condition is encountered there is often considerable controversy over whether or not the patient should be reoperated on immediately and the pregnancy sacrificed, once the diagnosis is established by histological section. It frequently happens that the ovarian tumor was not considered malignant at the time laparotomy was performed for its removal. Further questions include whether the patient should be reoperated on following delivery or simply followed up without further surgery.

Most papers—and presumably most physicians—tend to take the more radical approach but there are exceptions. The world literature tends to support the Mayo Clinic experience, which is to treat the patient in accordance with the type of malignancy present. When the malignancy is of low grade, the patient may well be followed up, with survival being anticipated. If reoperation is indicated, as it is in the more malignant types, the patient's wishes must be given consideration. This is exemplified by the case of dysgerminoma. In the pure type, the outlook is highly favorable, whereas in the mixed type, the outlook is bleak regardless of treatment. In this case the patient may wish to decide what course of action to pursue with respect to her present pregnancy.

14

Management of Benign Lesions Related to the Diagnosis of Early Breast Cancer

Alternative Points of View:

    By C. D. Haagensen

    By Erle E. Peacock

    By George V. Smith and Robert L. Shirley

Editorial Comment

Management of Benign Lesions Related to the Diagnosis of Early Breast Cancer

The Role of the Gynecologist in the Differential Diagnosis of Benign Abnormalities of the Breast and Early Breast Carcinoma

C. D. Haagensen

Columbia-Presbyterian Medical Center

Gynecologists can make an important contribution to the early diagnosis of breast carcinoma if they will take time to examine the breasts carefully as part of every gynecological examination. By careful breast examination I mean simple inspection and palpation carried out in the systematic manner which I have described in Chapter 5 of *Diseases of the Breast*.* I do not believe that mammography or thermography are practical as screening techniques; thermography I have found to be valueless in differential diagnosis, and I use mammography only infrequently in patients in whom the physical findings are particularly puzzling.

Every time a gynecologist finds a small breast carcinoma in this kind of routine examination of the breast he adds considerably to his patient's chances of cure by radical mastectomy. My own data on this point are shown in Table 14–1.

In a short review such as this one I cannot, of course, deal with the whole

---

* Haagensen, C. D.: Diseases of the Breast. Philadelphia, W. B. Saunders Co., 1971.

TABLE 14–1.   *The Relation of the Size of Breast Carcinoma to 10 Year Survival Following Radical Mastectomy†*

NUMBER OF CASES	TUMOR SIZE	PER CENT 10 YEAR SURVIVAL
81	<2 cm.	75
252	2–3 cm.	67
183	4–5 cm.	46
110	>6 cm.	41
626		

† Personal series of cases of C. D. Haagensen, 1935–1957.

spectrum of benign lesions of the breast which have to be distinguished from carcinoma. Virchow long ago said that the breast is the wet nurse of the surgical pathologist because so many different lesions occur in it, and this is becoming increasingly true as we identify new types of breast disease. All that I can do here is to discuss the common breast conditions which have to be differentiated from carcinoma. These can be divided into physiological and pathological phenomena.

Physiological Changes in the Breast

Cyclical breast engorgement, manifested by increased sensitivity and a feeling of fullness in the breasts, as well as increased density and nodularity, normally begins three to five days before menstruation. The degree of engorgement varies greatly—some women scarcely notice these changes and, at the other extreme, there are women who are prostrated by them. The engorgement persists during menstruation, although it diminishes toward its end.

Engorgement adds so much to the difficulty of distinguishing between breast nodularity of physiological origin and actual breast disease that I long ago adopted the rule of not making appointments to examine the breasts during the week preceding or the week of menstruation. I recommend this rule to all gynecologists in examining the breasts.

Variations in the phenomenon of engorgement add to the difficulty of making this differentiation. Occasionally engorgement is not cyclical but persists for months and even years. It may be more marked in one breast, and even in one sector of one breast. Breast engorgement usually increases in degree during the last few years before the menopause. This is, of course, an age at which breast carcinoma is frequent and the clinician must be alert to detect it. I know of no valid evidence to indicate that women who have a marked degree of breast engorgement are predisposed to develop carcinoma.

Although the clinician's greatest worry is mistaking carcinoma for physiological engorgement, differentiation between these is not difficult. The nodularity that occurs with engorgement is usually a diffuse phenomenon most evident in the upper halves of both breasts. Carcinoma usually forms a single dominant tumor, which may develop anywhere in one breast. Moreover, engorgement has a labile and cyclical character, increasing and diminishing in relation to menstruation, while carcinoma is, of course, unchanged throughout the cycle. If the examiner is in doubt regarding the cyclical character of nodularity revealed by palpation he should reexamine his patient at different phases of her cycle.

The differentiation of nodularity of physiological origin and multiple cysts is much more difficult. Some women with cystic disease have a great many cysts of varying size in both breasts, resembling the nodularity of marked physiological engorgement. Moreover, cystic disease not infrequently is resurgent in the premenstrual phase of the menstrual cycle, old cysts enlarging and new ones forming at this time, again like the physiological nodularity of engorgement. In the patient who does not have a dominant tumor that makes some sort of diagnostic procedure imperative, the clinician may be hard put to distinguish between physiological nodularity and true cystic diseases and may decide to do nothing. He may attempt to placate his patient by telling her she has nothing more than "fibrocystic" disease. This is in fact the worst thing he can do if his patient has only harmless physiological engorgement, because she is left with the impression that she has real breast disease, and she may worry unnecessarily about it for the rest of her life. Clinicians should be extremely careful not to brand patients with any breast disease unless they are certain of their diagnosis. I will describe how the diagnosis of true cystic disease is established in my subsequent discussion of that disease.

Pathological Changes in the Breast

There are a great many benign pathological changes in the breasts, most of which do not predispose to carcinoma. In the present discussion I can only refer to the most frequent ones, and, of course, to those which are precancerous.

ADENOFIBROMA

The common tumor of the breast in women below the age of 25—although it occasionally develops later on in premenopausal years—is the benign adenofibroma. The age distribution of 619 patients with adenofibroma is shown in Figure 14-1. Adenofibromas are well delimited and slip around in the breast under the examiner's fingers. They are firm but not hard. Occasionally a young woman may have several, but not many, adenofibromas. Adenofibromas are not precancerous. The patient with a tumor of this kind should be reassured, not frightened. If she is below the age of 25 there is no rush having it removed, because carcinoma is exceedingly rare in patients below this age. The patient with a presumed adenofibroma should be referred to a surgeon who knows how to remove the tumor without leaving an unsightly scar.

GROSS CYSTIC DISEASE

There is more confusion regarding the diagnosis and treatment of gross cystic disease than any other disease of the breasts, a situation that can be attrib-

Figure 14-1. The age distribution of 619 patients with adenofibroma of the breast.

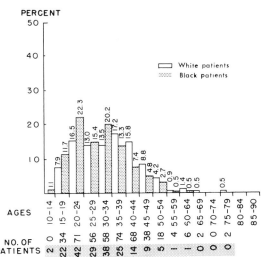

uted in large part to the pathologists, who have failed to distinguish this disease from a variety of other benign proliferative lesions of the breasts. Some of these, such as the dilatation of small ducts to form microcysts, and minor degrees of papillary intraductal proliferation which we label papillomatosis, do not constitute true disease in either a clinical or microscopical sense. Others, like adenosis and fibrous disease, are distinct diseases. But pathologists who are ignorant of the natural history of these different benign breast lesions usually throw all of them together in a pathological scrapbasket labeled fibrocystic disease or cystic mastitis, merely because they have in common some degree of proliferation of the epithelial or stromal elements of the breast. In so doing, pathologists make it nearly impossible for the clinicians to identify and sort out these different benign breast diseases. In the present discussion I will do so, and hope thereby to interest gynecologists in gaining a better understanding of benign breast disease.

Gross cystic disease of the breasts is a distinct disease *sui generis*. It is the most frequent disease of the breasts in Western women. It appears in the patient's late 20's and subsides with the completion of the menopause. The age distribution of my 2017 patients with the disease is shown in Figure 14-2. My youngest patient was 26. Gross cysts can be induced in postmenopausal women by the administration of estrogen; this was the actual etiology in the small group of postmenopausal women in my series.

A gross cyst is, as the name implies, a cyst large enough to be seen with the naked eye by the surgeon or pathologist. These cysts are almost always multiple and bilateral. The misguided surgeon who thinks that he can eliminate the disease by excising the cyst or group of cysts which he feels or sees does not understand the diffuse nature of the disease. Cystic disease has a very irregular course. Occasionally a patient will have only one clinically evident cyst and never develop another. Most patients will have one or two cysts from time to time. In a few patients both breasts are riddled with cysts.

A dominant tumor of the breast which has the clinical characteristics of a cyst—that is, it is rounded, somewhat moveable in the surrounding breast tissue, and perhaps fluctuant—first must be proved to be a cyst and then must be eliminated. The traditional method of achieving these objectives is by surgical biopsy

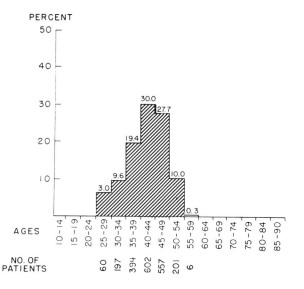

Figure 14-2. The age distribution of 2017 patients with gross cystic disease of the breast.

and excision in the operating room under general anesthesia. I have long since learned that operation for presumed cysts is unnecessary and indeed harmful. I aspirate such tumors in the office, using local anesthesia and inserting a 20 or 22 gauge needle. If I obtain the characteristic cyst fluid and the tumor disappears, I am content. Incidentally, I do not examine the cyst fluid microscopically—it is a waste of time. If my aspirating needle encounters a solid lesion, or if a palpable tumor still remains after I have aspirated some fluid, the patient is of course admitted to the hospital for a surgical biopsy. I have aspirated more than 10,000 cysts of the breast and have had no cause to regret having done so. It is true that, using this technique, I have failed in several cases to diagnose for a time a small carcinoma which happened to be situated in the vicinity of a cyst. However, I might also have missed the carcinoma in these patients if I had done a surgical biopsy and excised the cyst. Carcinomas do not evolve directly from individual cysts; the site of a carcinoma which develops in patients with cystic disease is not related to the site of previous cysts. But, as I will demonstrate, women with gross cystic disease are certainly predisposed to develop breast carcinoma.

The harm that may come from the policy of operating upon every cyst of the breast which presents as a dominant tumor is that women will not tolerate repeated breast operations for this benign disease. Most surgeons make disfiguring radial scars and remove so much breast tissue that after a number of these operations the patient rebels and refuses either to return for follow-up examination or to submit to further treatment when she develops a new tumor. If this is a carcinoma, she may well lose her chance of cure.

My conviction that gross cystic disease predisposes to breast carcinoma is based upon studies of 1693 women with documented gross cystic disease studied between 1930 and 1968, and followed for more than one year. Breast carcinoma developed in 72 patients. On the basis of the incidence of carcinoma in the general female population of the state of New York, only 17 breast carcinomas would have been expected in our 1693 women exposed to the risk of the disease (actual expected rate, 17.35 per 1693 women). Thus, carcinoma of the breast was found more than four times as frequently in our series of women with gross cystic disease as it is in women in the general population. The details of this calculation are presented in Table 14–2.

There are several interesting features of the carcinomas that developed in these women with gross cystic disease. Although a full documentation of my statements is beyond the scope of this discussion, I can point out here that the carcinoma was often situated in the opposite breast from the one in which there had been a previous cyst. Moreover, we found no significant relationship between the length of time in which the patient had had cystic disease of the breasts and the likelihood of her developing carcinoma. When carcinoma developed in these women with a history of cystic disease, it occurred at the normal age for breast carcinoma in our entire patient population. A final intriguing fact about gross cystic disease is that women with this disease have the same abnormally high family history of breast carcinoma that we have demonstrated in women with only breast carcinoma.

All these data suggest that, although gross cystic disease and carcinoma are separate diseases, and the latter does not evolve directly from the former, there are similar genetic or hormonal characteristics in the women in whom they occur.

TABLE 14–2.   *The Relationship of Gross Cystic Disease in 1693 Patients to the Subsequent Development of Carcinoma*

AGE	PERSON YEARS	OBSERVED BREAST CARCINOMAS	EXPECTED BREAST CARCINOMA
25–29	88.50		0.004
30–34	586.75		0.098
35–39	1552.50	2	0.594
40–44	2999.50	8	2.138
45–49	3946.50	12	4.185
50–54	3377.00	23	3.963
55–59	2125.00	14	2.977
60–64	1107.25	5	1.835
65–69	492.25	7	0.987
70+	207.00	1	0.569
TOTAL	16482.25	72	17.35

Observed incidence: 72
Expected incidence: 17.35
The observed incidence is four times the expected incidence.
Note: 23 carcinomas were found concomitantly with cysts, and these are excluded from the calculations.

The lesson from all of this is that although the predisposition to carcinoma in women with gross cystic disease is certainly not strong enough to justify prophylactic bilateral mastectomy, these patients must be followed with exceptional care, in hopes of detecting any carcinoma that may develop, at an early and curable stage. This means careful breast palpation every three months for the remainder of these patients' lives, since the likelihood of breast carcinoma increases with advancing age. To achieve this kind of lifetime follow-up is not easy. The responsible physician, be he internist, gynecologist, or surgeon, must win the trust and friendship of his patient, and he must be sure not to charge too much for this special service of breast examination.

I believe that if the gynecologist is to be responsible for these follow-up breast examinations in patients with gross cystic disease, he can learn how to do so just as efficiently as the internist or surgeon. But if or when the gynecologist discovers anything suspicious, or a dominant tumor, in the breast of one of these patients I do not believe that he should attempt to aspirate it or perform a biopsy. He should promptly refer the patient to a surgeon who is capable of dealing with all aspects of breast disease, including radical mastectomy for carcinoma, if it should be required.

ADENOSIS TUMOR

Adenosis is the pathologist's name for a special form of proliferation of the epithelium of the acini of the mammary lobules. The proliferating cells are quite regular and grow in a lobular pattern. The lesion is benign, but when it is distorted by fibrosis it appears to invade the surrounding breast stroma, and pathologists have occasionally been betrayed into diagnosing it as carcinoma. A typical area of adenosis is shown in Figures 14-3, 14-5, and 14-6.

Adenosis is ordinarily evident only to the pathologist, who sees it not infrequently as an incidental microscopical feature of breast tissue removed from

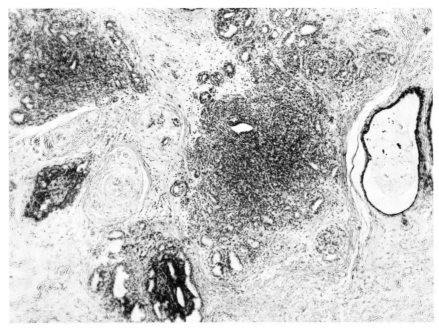

Figure 14-3.   Adenosis of the breast, showing its patchy character.

premenopausal women. Since there is no accompanying breast tumor, the presence of adenosis is not apparent to the clinician.

However, in occasional patients who are between puberty and menopause, adenosis progresses to the point of forming a dominant breast tumor. Figure 14-4 shows the age distribution of my series of 70 patients with adenosis tumor. These tumors are firm and not well delimited, and although they are not accompanied by skin retraction, they cannot be distinguished clinically from carcinoma. They must of course be biopsied. Grossly, this lesion is firm and slightly brownish in color. Frozen section will reveal its true nature. Since adenosis is always benign,

Figure 14-4.   The age distribution of 70 patients with adenosis tumor of the breast.

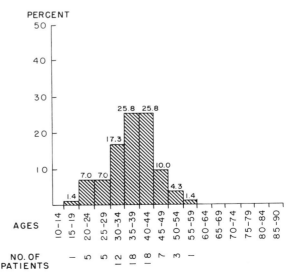

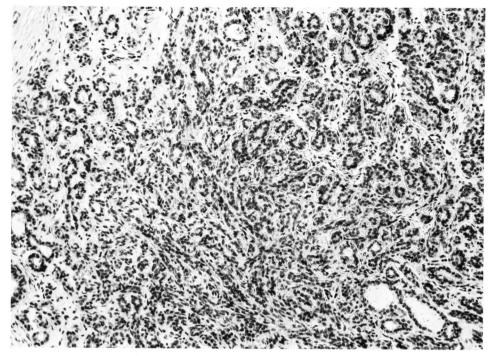

Figure 14-5.   Adenosis. Acinar epithelium proliferating in a lobular formation.

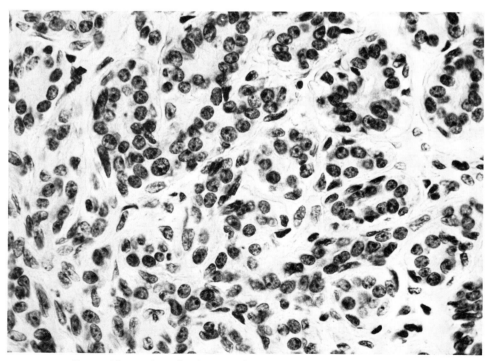

Figure 14-6.   The individual proliferating epithelial cells in adenosis.

local excision of the lesion is all that is required. Our follow-up studies have not revealed that the patients with adenosis are predisposed to subsequent carcinoma.

The diagnosis of adenosis tumor is best achieved by the collaboration of a surgeon and surgical pathologist who are accustomed to working together. The gynecologist who finds a tumor which may be one of these lesions had best refer the patient to a surgeon with such facilities.

FIBROUS DISEASE

The rather infrequent breast tumor which we call fibrous disease is usually relegated by pathologists to the scrapbasket of fibrocystic disease, and as a result it is usually not identified, although it is a separate disease with a natural history all its own. Like gross cystic disease and adenosis it occurs only during menstrual years; my youngest patient with fibrous disease was 23 and the oldest—who had been taking estrogen—was 56. The age distribution of my series of 119 patients is shown in Figure 14-7.

Fibrous disease makes itself evident as a poorly delimited tumor which seems to merge with the surrounding breast, in which it is somewhat fixed. It is firm but not hard. Skin retraction does not develop as it does with carcinoma. A special feature of this lesion is that in the majority of patients it is situated in the extreme upper outer portion of the breast. In 20 per cent of my patients with this lesion, fibrous disease occurred bilaterally in this portion of the breast.

Grossly, the lesion is dense and whitish, and poorly delimited. Microscopically, it consists of an area of proliferation of the fibrous stroma of the breast to form a dense fibrous matrix in which the gland fields are few and very small. Figure 14-8 shows the characteristic microscopical appearance of this lesion. It is easily recognized in frozen section by a surgical pathologist who is familiar with it. Local excision is all that is required. In our experience, fibrous disease has not predisposed to carcinoma.

Gynecologists who find a breast tumor with these characteristics had best refer the patient to a surgeon who collaborates with an experienced surgical pathologist.

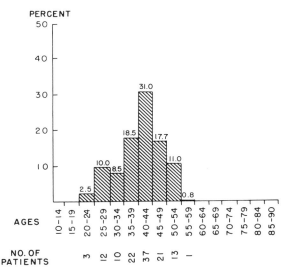

Figure 14-7. The age distribution of 119 patients with fibrous disease of the breast.

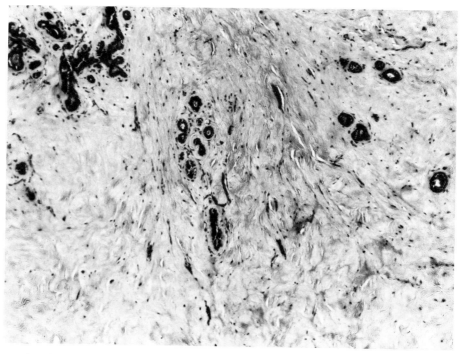

Figure 14-8.   The microscopic appearance of fibrous disease of the breast.

INTRADUCTAL PAPILLOMA

Intraductal papilloma is an only moderately frequent benign disease of the breast, but it has a considerable importance because of the difficulties which both clinicians and pathologists have in distinguishing it from carcinoma. There are four types of benign papillary proliferation of the mammary epithelium.

First, there is the minor degree of papillary heaping up of epithelium in dilated ducts, which is commonly seen in adult breast tissue. It is purely a microscopical phenomenon which produces no signs or symptoms and which is, as far as we know, of no prognostic significance. We call it papillomatosis and disregard it.

The three other forms of benign papillary proliferation are true diseases, each with its characteristic clinical features and natural history. The basic pathological phenomenon in all three is a stalked papilloma growing into a dilated duct and filling it up. The clinical feature common to all three is a nipple discharge, usually serous but sometimes bloody. Finally, when the papilloma grows large enough, it becomes palpable as a more or less well circumscribed dominant tumor. The tumor produced by an intraductal papilloma does not slip around in the breast as does an adenofibroma or a cyst, but it is not accompanied by skin retraction, as are so many carcinomas.

The most frequent of these three clinical forms of intraductal papilloma is the solitary type which grows in a terminal subareolar duct. Figure 14–9 shows the gross appearance of one of these lesions. This lesion may develop at any age, as indicated in the age distribution chart of my personal series of 179 patients

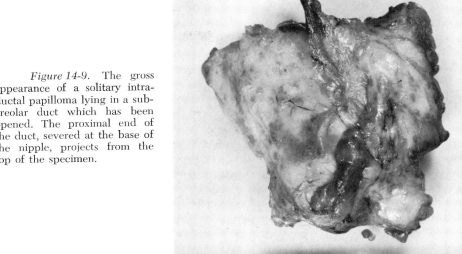

Figure 14-9. The gross appearance of a solitary intraductal papilloma lying in a subareolar duct which has been opened. The proximal end of the duct, severed at the base of the nipple, projects from the top of the specimen.

(Figure 14-10). In 81 per cent of my patients, the presenting symptom was a spontaneous nipple discharge, which was blood-tinged or bloody in approximately half of these. I should point out that the discharge must be spontaneous in order to have clinical significance; compression of the nipples will produce a very small amount of grayish thick material in many adult women. I do not compress the nipples as part of a routine breast examination. When a patient consults me because of a nipple discharge I carefully and gently palpate the subareolar region, seeking to find a small tumor. In 56 per cent of the patients who have consulted me because of a nipple discharge only, I have found such a tumor. Gentle pressure on it will produce a drop or two of serous or bloody discharge from the opening of a duct on the surface of the nipple which corresponds to the radial position of the subareolar tumor. In other patients with the characteristic nipple discharge, in whom a tumor cannot be identified, a subareolar pressure point will be found

Figure 14-10. The age distribution of 179 patients with solitary intraductal papilloma of the breast.

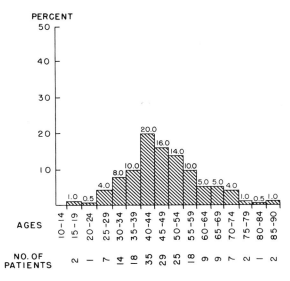

which produces the discharge. This information confirms the diagnosis and defines the position of the papilloma so that I can carry out a localized excision through a circumareolar incision. This does not deform the breast, and leaves a scar which is nearly invisible. I should add that I advise against examining the nipple discharge microscopically; pathologists sometimes mistake the degenerating epithelial cells in it for carcinoma cells, with the result that a tragic unnecessary mastectomy is done.

Occasionally a patient may have a solitary intraductal papilloma of long standing, which is larger and is situated in a much dilated duct that forms a cystic lesion located at some distance from the subareolar region.

A second type of intraductal papilloma is that which develops within the nipple itself and finally grows out onto the surface of the nipple through the opening of the duct in which it develops, and presents as a small, reddish, fungating mass on the nipple surface. Figure 14-11 shows one of these lesions. It has been called "florid papillomatosis," which is not a good name because it does not describe the pathological character of the lesion very well. We prefer the name "papillary adenoma of the nipple." Although the process begins in a single nipple duct as a papilloma, it soon involves a number of ducts and grows out into the nipple stroma and among them to form a poorly delimited, diffuse papillary neoplasm, as shown in Figure 14-12. When one of these lesions has been present for some time, fibrosis develops around and within it, compressing and distorting the papilloma and giving the impression of invasive carcinoma. Figure 14-13 shows one of these fibrosed benign papillary adenomas of the nipple simulating carcinoma. This mistake has been made by a good many pathologists, not only with papillary adenoma of the nipple but also with fibrosed solitary intraductal papilloma of the subareolar region, and as a result a wholly unnecessary mastectomy has been performed.

Papillary adenomas of the nipple are entirely benign and require only local excision. I have successfully dealt with a number of them by excising only the

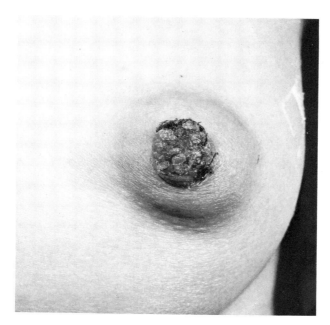

Figure 14-11. Papillary adenoma of the nipple fungating out onto the surface of the nipple.

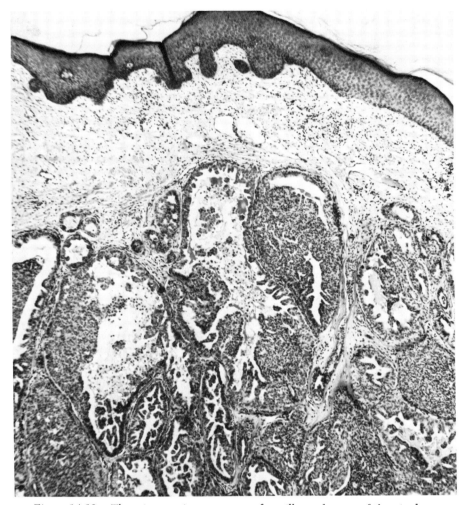

Figure 14-12.   The microscopic appearance of papillary adenoma of the nipple.

portion of the nipple that contains the lesion, although when the entire nipple is involved it has to be removed.

We have recently identified a third form of intraductal papilloma which we call "multiple intraductal papilloma." As the name indicates, it consists of a great many grossly visible papillomas, seemingly originating in many ducts in a sector of the breast. Figure 14-14 shows one of these lesions. It forms a palpable, fairly well delimited tumor which is usually situated in the breast at some distance from the subareolar region, where solitary intraductal papilloma is usually found. The clinical features which distinguish multiple from solitary intraductal papilloma are summed up in Table 14–3; these indicate clearly that two different diseases are involved.

The most important difference between solitary intraductal papilloma of the subareolar region, papillary adenoma of the nipple, and multiple intraductal papilloma is that the first two lesions do not predispose the patient to carcinoma, whereas multiple papilloma is, in our experience, clearly a precancerous process.

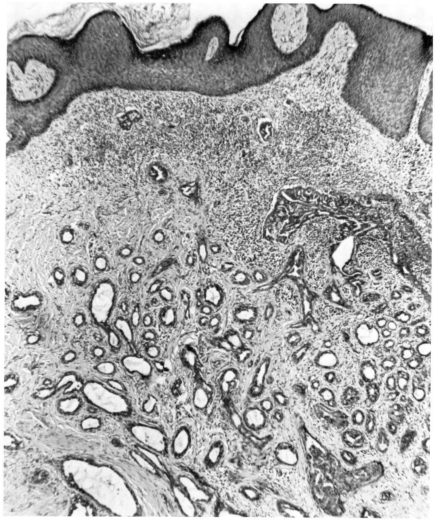

Figure 14-13.   Papillary adenoma of the nipple distorted by fibrosis so that it simulates carcinoma.

TABLE 14–3.   *Differentiation Between Solitary and Multiple Intraductal Papillomas*

CLINICAL FEATURES	SOLITARY INTRADUCTAL PAPILLOMA	MULTIPLE INTRADUCTAL PAPILLOMA
Mean age of patients	48 years	39.6 years
Nipple discharge	81%	36%
Situated in subareolar region	95%	26%
Bilateral occurrence	1.5%	26%

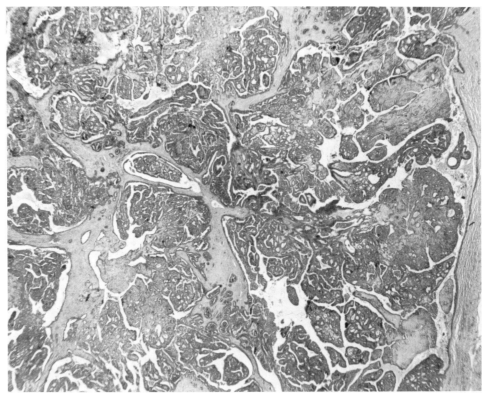

Figure 14-14.   Multiple papilloma of the breast.

In 38 per cent of our patients with multiple papilloma, carcinoma also developed, usually some years after the initial diagnosis of multiple papilloma had been made, and after it had been locally excised several times. The carcinoma was always of the special intraductal apocrine papillary and cribriform type that we have come to associate with multiple papilloma, and which presumably evolves from it. Our treatment of multiple papilloma continues to be local excision; we do not believe that mastectomy is justified. However, these patients must obviously be followed with great care and any recurrent tumor biopsied. The papillary apocrine carcinomas which develop in these patients are among the most favorable of all breast carcinomas, and radical mastectomy almost always cures them.

PAPILLARY CARCINOMA

Papillary carcinoma must be kept in mind in every patient with a nipple discharge. However, the likelihood of carcinoma is not as great as some authors have reported. Between 1956 and 1967, I was consulted by 157 patients with a nipple discharge; only 18, or 11.5 per cent, proved to have carcinoma. In seven the discharge was serous, in 10 it was bloody, and in one it was watery. Thus, a nipple discharge is only infrequently a sign of breast carcinoma.

When it is an indication of carcinoma, the carcinoma is usually of the papillary type, and it is almost always accompanied by a palpable tumor of the breast. In a series of 130 papillary carcinomas which I studied, a palpable tumor was present in all but three.

Although papillary carcinomas are a "favorable" type, they are fully malignant and occasionally metastasize. Radical mastectomy is the only reasonable treatment. Figure 14-15 shows one of these papillary carcinomas which metastasized to two axillary lymph nodes; the patient is well 25 years after radical mastectomy.

The role of the gynecologist in these papillary lesions of the breast should, I believe, be limited to their detection. When he is consulted by a patient with a nipple discharge, with or without an accompanying tumor, he should refer her to a surgeon who is properly qualified to undertake the complex diagnostic and therapeutic measures that are required for these neoplasms.

LOBULAR NEOPLASIA

This lesion, which, like adenosis, evolves from the epithelium of the mammary lobule, has been discovered comparatively recently and therefore is not very well known; its treatment also is not well understood, partly because the lesion has been given a deceptive name—"lobular carcinoma in situ." Names of diseases are important because in a descriptive sense they identify the lesion, and in a therapeutic sense they predicate its treatment. When Ewing first called attention to this lesion and published a photograph of it in 1919, he gave it no definitive name but stated that it was a "precancerous change." In 1941, Foote and Stewart labeled it "lobular carcinoma in situ," and their name has unfortunately been widely adopted, although English pathologists call it "epitheliosis." The lesion is certainly precancerous, as Ewing concluded, but it is not carcinoma. True

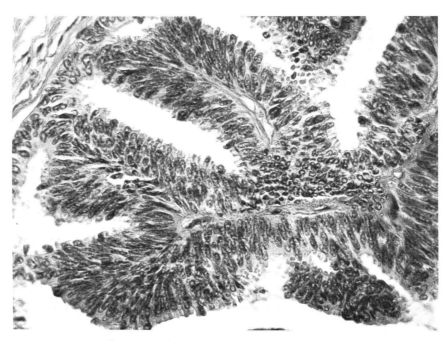

Figure 14-15.   Papillary carcinoma of the breast.

carcinoma, once established in the breast, grows progressively and often metastasizes. The lesion I am discussing does neither. Because of these and other features which are incompatible with a name that includes the term carcinoma, Dr. Lattes, the director of our department of Surgical Pathology, has suggested the name *lobular neoplasia*, and we urge its adoption.

Lobular neoplasia is a proliferation of epithelium lining the acini of the mammary lobules and the small ductules which emerge from them. The acini are lined with a single layer of small cuboidal cells and normally have lumens. In lobular neoplasia, these cells increase in number and also increase somewhat in size, although they usually maintain a comparatively uniform character, and they fill up the acini solid so that the lumens are no longer seen. Figure 14-16 shows, in low magnification, a group of lobules involved by this process. Figures 14-17 and 14-18 show, in higher magnification, these proliferating cells in what we call Type A lobular neoplasia, in which the cells are very regular, and in Type B, in which they vary more in size and shape. Figure 14-19 shows the same process evolving around a ductule emerging from a mammary lobule. These proliferating cells do not break out of the lobules and infiltrate the breast stroma in lobular neoplasia as I have described it.

These changes are too minute and too widely dispersed in the breast to form an aggregate visible with the naked eye. They do not form a palpable tumor, and are detected only by the pathologist who studies with sufficient care a speci-

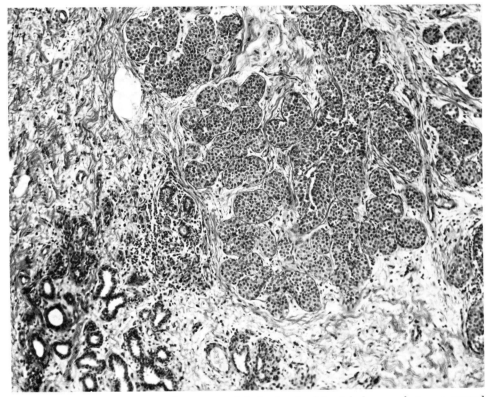

Figure 14-16. A group of mammary lobules involved by lobular neoplasia, contrasted with a normal lobule in the lower left portion of the photograph.

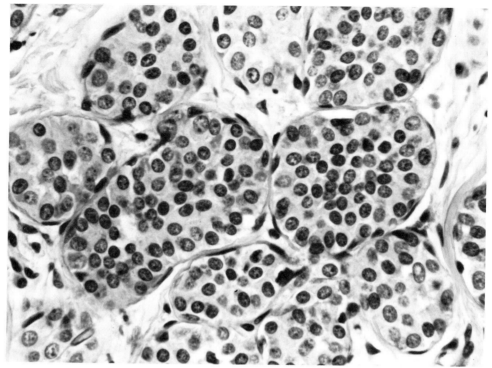

Figure 14-17. Lobular neoplasia, type A, in higher magnification, showing the individual proliferating cells.

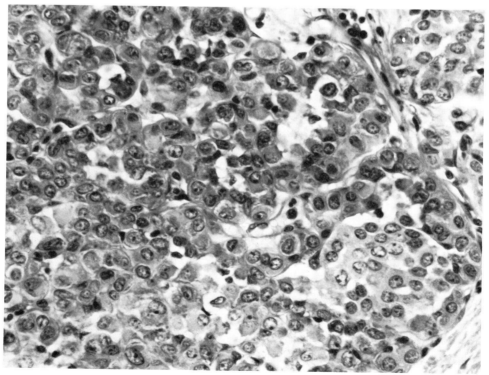

Figure 14-18. Lobular neoplasia, type B, in which the proliferating cells are more irregular.

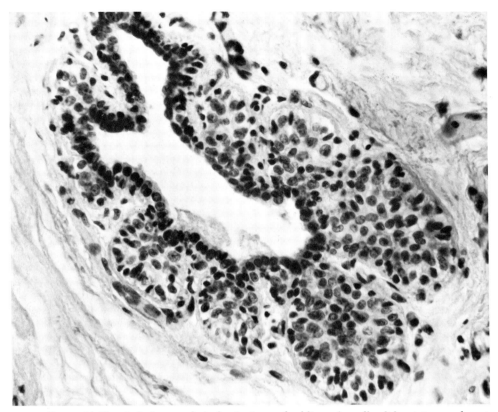

Figure 14-19. Lobular neoplasia beginning as budding of small solid acini around part of the circumference of a lobule.

men of breast tissue which has been removed because of some other lesion. Lobular neoplasia is therefore a pathological and not a clinical entity.

It is not a very frequent finding. When, in 1969, I last tabulated the cases that had been observed in our laboratory, there were only 55 over an 18 year period. There are several special features of the disease in addition to the fact that it does not infiltrate or metastasize. In our experience, it has occurred only in premenopausal women—the youngest was 33 and the oldest was 55. It apparently disappears after the menopause, like gross cystic disease. It often involves both breasts—just how often is difficult to ascertain, because lobular neoplasia can involve only a few lobules in an entire breast. We study such a small portion of each breast, even when we cut a number of blocks of tissue, that we may often miss it.

Nevertheless, lobular neoplasia, as we name it, certainly evolves into true carcinoma in a considerable proportion of patients. This is evident from the fact that we see it with ordinary fully developed carcinoma as often as we see it existing alone in the breasts of premenopausal women. We had 63 such patients when I made my 1969 tabulation. The 74 carcinomas that occurred together with lobular neoplasia in these patients were of a variety of types, but 50 per cent were a special type that we know evolves directly from lobular neoplasia. We see the small cells which crowd the acini breaking out of the lobules and invading the surrounding breast stroma, as shown in Figure 14-20.

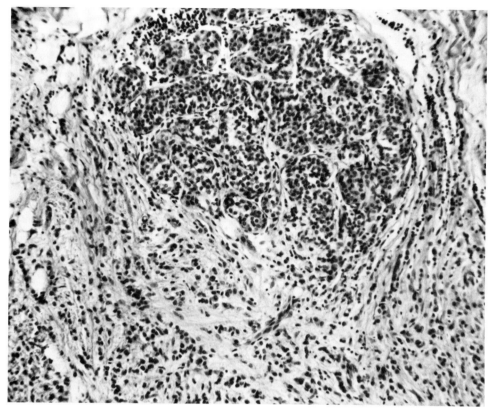

Figure 14-20.   Small cell carcinoma evolving from a mammary lobule affected by lobular neoplasia.

Another reason why we know that lobular neoplasia is precancerous is that the follow-up of patients with lobular neoplasia has shown that carcinoma develops in a considerable proportion of them. There are only two series of cases, that from Memorial Hospital (Hutter and Foote[8]) and our own from Columbia, which are large enough and have been followed long enough to give us some idea of how frequently this happens. These data are shown in Table 14-4.

The therapeutic dilemma which lobular neoplasia presents is a difficult one. The general practice has been to amputate the breast in which the lesion is found. This is not very logical because we know that this occult lesion is often bilateral, and that the carcinoma which follows may develop in the contralateral breast. If a woman with lobular neoplasia is to be entirely safe she must have both breasts amputated. This is a very severe penalty for younger premenopausal women, as these patients all are. The alternative is to do no surgery but to follow them with careful breast palpation every three months, and if a tumor develops to have it biopsied promptly. I have chosen to explain the facts concerning this disease as I know them to my patients and to offer them this latter alternative. Without exception they have all chosen it. To date, none of my patients has lost her life because of this choice. In those who have developed carcinoma, the disease has been of a favorable type and was detected at an early stage. I believe they have been cured by radical mastectomy.

Gynecologists, who in general are not as familiar with the complexities of

TABLE 14–4. *Follow-up of Lobular Neoplasia (Lobular Carcinoma In Situ) Occurring Alone, Not Accompanied by Simultaneous Carcinoma*

DATA	MEMORIAL HOSPITAL (HUTTER AND FOOTE)	COLUMBIA-PRESBYTERIAN MEDICAL CENTER (HAAGENSEN AND LATTES)
Number of patients exposed to risk of developing breast carcinoma	46	47
Length of follow-up	4–27 years	4–24 years
Mean length of follow-up	?	10 years
Subsequent carcinoma in breast with lobular neoplasia not amputated	10 of 40 patients (25%)	5 of 22 patients (23%)
Subsequent carcinoma in contralateral breast	4 of 46 patients (8.7%)	5 of 45 patients (10%)
Total number of breasts exposed to risk of developing carcinoma	86	69
Breasts in which carcinoma developed	14 (16.3%)	10 (14.5%)

breast carcinoma as are surgeons, will wisely avoid responsibility for the equally difficult problems of lobular neoplasia.

NONEPITHELIAL NEOPLASMS OF THE BREAST

There is a whole series of benign neoplasms of the breast which are of mesenchymal origin—lipoma, fibrous histiocytoma, leiomyoma, granular cell tumor, mesenchymoma, neurofibroma, and so forth. The lipomas and mesenchymomas are notably soft, well delimited, and movable within the surrounding breast tissue, but the other forms have no special clinical characteristics. None of them is precancerous, and local excision is all that is required.

Most of the mesenchymal tissues also give rise in the breast to truly malignant neoplasms, which behave here just as these soft part sarcomas behave in other tissues. Thus, there are liposarcomas, fibrosarcomas, and leiomyosarcomas of the breast. A particularly malignant form of malignant hemangioendothelioma occurs in the breasts of young women—fortunately very rarely. The lymphoblastomas sometimes also manifest themselves in the breasts.

A Family History of Breast Carcinoma

In his search for breast carcinoma the gynecologist must not overlook the significance of a family history of the disease. Our data have shown that patients whose mothers had breast carcinoma develop the disease twice as frequently as the general population, and that they develop it about 10 years earlier. A history of the disease in sisters or aunts also predisposes. Patients with this kind of family history should be followed more carefully. Ideally, they should be examined every three months for the remainder of their lives.

Summary

In this brief review I have emphasized the responsibility of gynecologists in the detection of breast disease. If they will only examine the breasts with care in all of their patients, they will surely find breast disease when it is present, and save lives when it is malignant.

I have recently been impressed by the unusual frequency of occurrence of certain benign lesions—adenosis and papillomatosis, for example—in the breasts of very young women who are taking contraceptives. I do not have enough experience to document it statistically, but I suspect that time will show that these estrogen-containing contraceptives alter the normal disease pattern in the breasts. Gynecologists have a special opportunity to study this question, and we hope that they will teach us something concerning it.

I hope that the gynecologists who read my discussion will understand why I believe that their role should be limited to detection, and that they should in general refer their patients to surgeons who have the help of experienced surgical pathologists for the necessary diagnostic procedures and treatment of the lesions they have discovered. My reason for this division of responsibility is not any lack of appreciation for the ability and surgical skill of gynecologists, but simply that they usually have not been as well equipped by training and experience for dealing with the complex diagnostic and therapeutic problems of breast disease as have properly trained surgeons. If my discussion has any value it has, I hope, demonstrated that some of these diagnostic and therapeutic problems of breast disease are very complex indeed.

I have not mentioned the present-day confusion among surgeons as to how best to treat carcinoma of the breast. There is considerable dissatisfaction with radical mastectomy among surgeons—mostly, I believe, among those who have not had enough special experience with breast carcinoma to know how to classify their patients as to the extent of their disease and to perform radical mastectomy only upon those whose disease is operable. Surgeons who do not have the patience to perform meticulous and thorough radical mastectomy also have inferior results. These dissident surgeons are turning to local excision supplemented by irradiation, to simple mastectomy, and to various curtailed modifications of radical mastectomy. These procedures are much less laborious for the surgeon and as such are a temptation to those who lack experience. I believe that there is today adequate evidence that the classical Halsted radical mastectomy gives better results than any of these more limited methods of surgical attack. Gynecologists will not, I hope, recommend or perform these limited operations. Carcinoma of the breast is a subtle and vicious disease and for the present our best hope of control over it is perseverance with painstaking and thorough radical mastectomy.

REFERENCES

1. Ewing, J.: Neoplastic Disease. Philadelphia, W. B. Saunders Co., 1919.
2. Foote, F. W., and Stewart, F. W.: Lobular carcinoma in situ. Am. J. Path. 17:91, 1941.
3. Haagensen, C. D.: Diseases of the Breast 2nd Ed. Philadelphia, W. B. Saunders Co., 1971.
4. Haagensen, C. D.: The physiology of the breast as it concerns the clinician. Am. J. Obstet. Gynec. 109:206, 1971.
5. Haagensen, C. D., et al.: Treatment of early mammary carcinoma: A cooperative international study. Ann. Surg. 170:875, 1969.
6. Haagensen, C. D., Lane, N., and Lattes, R.: Neoplastic proliferation of the epithelium of the mammary lobules. Surg. Clin. N. Amer. 52:497, 1972.
7. Hamperl, H.: Zur Kenntnis des sog. Carcinoma lobulare in situ der Mamma. Z. Krebsforsch. 77:231, 1972.
8. Hutter, R. V. P., and Foote, F. W.: Lobular carcinoma in situ. Long term follow-up. Cancer 24:1801, 1969.
9. Macgillivray, J. B.: The problem of 'chronic mastitis' with epitheliosis. J. Clin. Path. 22:340, 1969.

Management of Benign Lesions Related to the Diagnosis of Early Breast Cancer

A Biological Basis for Diagnosis and Management of Breast Disease

ERLE E. PEACOCK, JR.

University of Arizona College of Medicine and University of Arizona Medical Center

Benign disease of the breast is so common that the question of normal versus abnormal is probably more relevant to patients than is management of benign disease. This statement is not *entirely* true, however, because of the ubiquitous specter of cancer which hovers over all such considerations. The knowledge that over one-third of the female population carries microscopic cysts and harbors fibrous tissue proliferation without physical signs and symptoms, and that at least 20 per cent of women have grossly discernible abnormalities of breast tissue, argues strongly for the minimal significance of varying distributions of fibrous stroma and ductal configurations in the female breast.[6] There is strong suggestive evidence, however, that the incidence of carcinoma is two to four times more prevalent in breasts with abnormal proportions and amounts of fibrous and epithelial elements than in normal breasts, which keeps paramount the question of cause and effect relationship between noninvasive and invasive morphological changes.[4] Thus, for most women and their gynecologists, the major concern is not whether a symptom or sign such as nipple discharge or a breast mass can be classified pathologically or have a Latin name assigned to it, but, rather, if cancer is not present, how odds have been affected by what is found at any specific time during the development and regression of breast tissue. At present, the answer to this question cannot be found in the usual classification of breast disease or within the reach of any specialty group. The major thesis of this chapter, therefore, is that the greatest safeguard for women with identifiable changes in breast tissue probably lies in understanding the basic biology of breast tissue and the changes which occur, both normally and abnormally, during a life span.

Diagnosis and rational management of abnormal conditions of the breast can be worked out deductively on a biological basis. Classification and nomenclature, on the other hand, have added confusion and, in some instances, have actually resulted in tragedy for the individual patient.[13] This has been particularly true since frozen section techniques have improved to the extent that surgeons rarely look through a microscope themselves and ask only of a pathologist, "What is the diagnosis?" So long as both specialists understand and agree upon the terminology and nomenclature of breast disease, such a relationship works beneficially for most patients. Different understanding and inadequate communication because of individual variations in terminology, however, may leave a patient without the best medical care in spite of the superb specialty training her physicians may have. It seems worthwhile, therefore, to present a a scheme for diagnosis and management of breast disease based upon what is presently known about development and regression of breast tissue and the various biological phenomena which influence these processes, rather than upon the usual classifications of breast disease or the artificial limits of a specialty group. Such considerations are intended to imply that breast disease can be managed equally well by gynecologist or surgeon, provided that the fundamental biology of breast tissue is understood and a few technical maneuvers are mastered. A similar deduction is also implied: failure to understand or master biological principles and technical fundamentals is a positive indication to refer patients with breast disease to another physician, regardless of the other qualifications or credentials of the primary care physician.

No small consideration now is the increasing sophistication of women about medical knowledge and practice in the areas of breast disease.[14] Most women still want to believe that their physician knows best, but to what extent he does know best and the gaping holes in his knowledge are being revealed in medical articles in popular journals and in language nearly everyone can understand. The result is that a physician who attempts to cover deficits in understanding with dogmatic or empirical recommendations incites distrust and may even encourage "shopping." Thus, frank revelation of gaps in knowledge and willingness to concede that many women wish to participate in judgment decisions, particularly when they realize that no one has enough data to make some decisions on any better basis than intuition or empiricism, add to the stature of our profession in the eyes of many patients. It has been difficult for many surgeons to realize that some intelligent women actually prefer to live under a possible increased risk or even a known hazard of breast cancer rather than spend a portion of their lives entering hospitals for biopsies or losing an important segment of their body image. Thus, the best medical care for some women may involve frankness in discussing probable or known risk and having a physician assume the role of statistician or adviser on odds rather than an oracle of knowledge.

Diagnosis

Most important before considering management of breast disease is the need to make an accurate diagnosis. The major thesis of this article is that diagnosis must be based on explanation of physical signs and symptoms through sound biological reasoning, not on fitting a group of abnormal physical findings into a preset scheme or classification dominated by Latin names or eponyms. Such terminology may actually make physicians believe that classifying or identifying disease is synonymous with understanding.

Understanding the biology of breast disease involves at least six basic principles. They are: (1) breast tissue is composed essentially of three elements—epithelium, fibrous connective tissue, and fat; and most of the benign disorders of the breast are the result of disproportionate amounts of one or another. (2) Connective tissue can bind water as an inter- or intramolecular bond in varying amounts. Electrical charge on crystalline protein such as collagen in the fibrous tissue of the breast alters binding capacity, and therefore various amines such as histamine or serotonin can alter the water content of breast tissue significantly. (3) Normal growth and development, function, and cyclic changes in breast tissue are the result of the action of estrogen, progesterone, and prolactin. The ovary, with its corpus luteum, the adrenal, and the anterior hypophysis, therefore, influence breast tissue through the hormones they secrete. Thus, there is normally a significant variation in amount and type of breast tissue according to the cyclic changes in hormone levels. Considered in this light, the line between "normality" and "abnormality" is less distinct than conventional classifications may suggest, and some abnormalities may have less significance than their name implies. (4) Hemorrhage from a duct means epithelial ulceration has occurred, and continued ulceration of an epithelium-lined surface always must be considered neoplastic until positively proved otherwise. This incontestable biological principle is considerably more important than statistics which state the incidence of cancer in such lesions as intraductal papilloma, and so forth. (5) Epithelial growth is a continuous process in which a true understanding of what actually is happening and how fast it is happening often cannot be gleaned from a single "still frame" in the form of a hematoxylin-and-eosin stained slide. (6) Cancer is primarily the result of mutation of cells; and genetic influences are undeniable in mutatory changes. Other factors, such as viruses, radiation, and so forth, also are effective in inducing cell mutation, but genetic factors seem most important now in the history of patients with breast disease.

Of the six principles just listed, the effect of hormones is the most easily demonstrated and, in many instances, is the most dramatic. Tantalizingly, however, such changes are not completely understood. In both benign and malignant disease, until such time as cellular autonomy occurs, epithelial and connective tissue elements are affected dramatically by hormones. Much remains to be learned, however, about the varying sensitivity of substrates to hormones, and it may be that other hormones or precursor substances, yet to be accurately identified, are more important than estrogen, progesterone, and prolactin. Because the influence of prolactin seems to be primarily one of causing the mammary acini to start synthesizing milk, this hormone is thought to be relatively unimportant in the etiology of breast disease. Certain precursors of prolactin, however, may have a profound effect on breast tissue and could be the key to understanding some conditions not now explainable by known reactions of estrogen and progesterone.

The effect of estrogens on breast tissue in laboratory animals and human beings has been studied extensively.[2,8,12] Results show that estrogens have significant action on nipple development, pigmentation of the areola, capillary permeability, proliferation and ramification of ducts, and proliferation of fibrous tissue. Secondary effects include regulation of water content of breast tissue, leukocyte infiltration, and dilatation of terminal ducts and acini. Progesterone action seems limited primarily to maturation of acini, development of alveolar lobules, and regulation of estrogen effect. Interestingly, much of the effect of progesterone seems dependent on preparation ("priming") of the ductal system by estrogen.

So far, hormonal control of breast tissue seems to be a relatively simple process. The major complexity is introduced by realization that effects described above are not uniform in either qualitative or quantitative aspects. Levels of hormone vary within a single menstrual cycle, and substrate sensitivity seems to vary over the entire reproductive life span. Moreover, although estrogen and progesterone are essentially antagonists, as far as the ductal system is concerned the two hormones do not appear or disappear simultaneously. Because progesterone is dependent primarily on corpus luteum secretion, it is not surprising to learn that reduction in progesterone levels is among the most common hormone abnormality affecting breast tissue in women.[11] The failure to ovulate, therefore, can be predicted to have a profound effect upon breast tissue and undoubtedly explains a relatively frequent association of breast disease with infertility and menstrual irregularities.

Although gonadotropin, adrenal androgens, and other hormones produce secondary effects upon breast tissue which may or may not be important in the diagnosis and management of clinical abnormalities, estrogen and progesterone now seem the most important hormones and these will, therefore, be considered first in attempting to clarify the true nature and relation of benign and malignant conditions.

The earliest and most common breast condition, adolescent hypertrophy, is, of course, a natural phenomenon resulting from estrogen stimulation. The next condition which comes to our attention is usually a firm, movable nodule which occurs most often in the early 20's. Although such nodules may be single at first, they usually are multiple, occurring either in the same or both breasts, and later may actually coalesce to form nodular or shotty proliferations of fibrous tissue. These patients seldom have significant edema or evidence of inflammation. Microscopic examination reveals ductal proliferation, but periductal fibrous proliferation is so prominent that cystic dilatation of the ducts is encroached upon by fibrous tissue; the appearance may be one of intracannicular fibroma. Growth is rapid so that a capsule is formed early. Splitting the capsule reveals the contents to be under tension, although no evidence of secretory activity within the ducts of such a lesion has been noted. Clinically, the lesion is movable, nontender, hard, frequently in the area surrounding the areola, and seldom presents a problem in diagnosis or management. It is so typical grossly that microscopic examination is scarcely necessary for confirmation. The lesion usually is referred to as a fibroadenoma.

If a fibroadenoma is left undisturbed, it usually, after a period of years, begins to regress in size and may even show deposition of calcium salts while becoming harder and smaller. An exception, of course, is the occasional fibroadenoma which, for some reason, appears to become more susceptible to estrogen effect and grows to quite large dimensions. This occurs most often during pregnancy. Interestingly, although these lesions usually are removed during pregnancy in anticipation of accommodating a nursing infant, they regress more rapidly than normal breast tissue during postpartum involution. Although it is a relatively rare occurrence, some fibromas seem to become autonomous of hormonal control and begin to undergo sarcomatous change. The picture then becomes one of unrestrained growth, and the lesion may become enormous. In this situation, the ductal changes regress and the predominant findings are uncontrolled fibrous proliferation and multiplication of fibroblasts and fibrocytes. The prognosis is considerably more favorable for these tumors than for fibrosarcomas elsewhere in the body, but axillary metastases have been reported.[1] Thus, previous recommendations that treatment need consist only of local excision probably are not accurate. These lesions are termed cystosarcoma phylloides, and excision of the breast and adjacent lymph nodes in a manner generally referred to as modified radical mastectomy is required for cure. Although sarcomatous change in a fibroadenoma is rare, it is suggested that most fibroadenomas probably should be removed unless there is a good reason not to do so. In summary, smooth, movable, painless, hard nodules developing around the areola in young women are the result of localized sensitivity to estrogen or relative excess of estrogen stimulation. Diagnosis is not a problem. Excision for mechanical reasons before or during pregnancy and excision of the lesion at some convenient time, even when pregnancy is not involved, to protect the patient from rare but avoidable cystosarcoma transformation seems appropriate management at this time.

As patients go into their third and fourth decades, the lesions described above appear in a different way. Nodules appear to coalesce and involve entire quadrants of the breast; sometimes an entire breast or both breasts will be affected. The fibrous component is considerably less prominent than in fibroadenomas, and the terminal ducts become dilated so that they resemble cysts. Epithelium in the cysts is flat, and the histological picture often resembles sudoriferous sweat glands in the skin. Acini and lobules disappear as the ducts become prominent. Secretory activity is present and large cysts, several millimeters to a centimeter in diameter, may develop. Fluid within cysts is clear or brown in color. When dark fluid is found in a large cyst, the lesion has been termed a "blue dome cyst" or "blue dome cyst of Bloodgood." Assay of progesterone and progesterone-like substances in the breast tissue of these patients reveals relative deficiency of progesterone.[11] Lymphocyte infiltration is prominent, and the water content of the tissue varies, producing cyclic episodes of tenderness and pain, which can be quite severe just before menstruation. Palpation may reveal isolated cysts, but more typically a diffuse shotty thickening of an entire quadrant of the breast is found. Even though such lesions are fairly typical as a clinical entity, the question of cancer or progression to cancer makes the problem of cystic change a profound one. This is especially true because of the complex biology of the lesion and the advancing age of the patient. Because the lesion undoubtedly begins as the result of excess estrogen, or lack of progesterone, or some combination thereof, classification and nomenclature are unimportant, as are determinations of varying amounts of ductal or fibrous proliferations, secretion of cells, water content, or inflammatory components. It is not surprising that so many names, such as adenofibrosis, fibroadenosis, cystic mastitis, cystic disease, fibrocystic dysplasia, blue dome cyst, mastitis, and so forth, have arisen. These names are the result of understandable attempts to describe a particular variation of a basic biological process. The important and really the only major problem which progesterone deficiency produces, however, is the question of whether structural changes bear any relation to cancer of the breast. Strange as it may seem, the answer to this question is that we are not completely certain at this time.

Past epidemiological studies, based primarily upon raw data on incidence have suggested that carcinoma of the breast is as much as four times more prevalent in women with cystic disease than in the normal population.[7] More recent studies, however, in which data have been refined by modern statistical methods, suggest that if indeed there is an increased incidence of carcinoma in women with fibrocystic disease, the incidence is more nearly twice rather than four times that of normal women.[4] One recent study suggests that the incidence of carcinoma is actually less in women with cystic mastitis than in women without clinical evidence of fibrocystic disease.[5] Such data are difficult to interpret, which is why a cause and effect relationship between breast cancer and cystic mastitis definitely has not been established by epidemiological method. It is not inconceivable that the primary hormone imbalance can induce morphological changes which ultimately, as in the case of some fibroadenomas, become autonomous of hormonal control and thus proceed to frank neoplasia. One type of neoplastic change, intralobular carcinoma, which will be discussed in more detail in subsequent paragraphs, appears to be significantly affected by hormones for a relatively long time. Experience with this lesion suggests that some patients with hormonally induced morphological deviation may retain hormonal dependence even after frank neoplasia has appeared.

A third biological phenomenon occurs in breast tissue during the third and fourth decades and has a far graver potential than either connective tissue proliferation or ductal dilatation. This phenomenon is cellular hyperplasia. The epithelial cells in cystic disease previously described usually are flat and in monolayer configuration. There may or may not be water secretory activity, but serum or blood is not discharged into the ductal system. Hyperplastic change in epithelium, which appears as a piling up or palisading of cells in the lumen of ducts or cysts, is a distinct biological entity which changes the outlook for the patient and demands therapeutic considerations of a different order than previously considered. Like other conditions in the breast, this basic biological phenomenon exhibits varying degrees of morphological expression and occurs in different places in the duct-acini system. As before, the many names applied to such variations are not as important as the biological implications and the anatomic locations they signify. Epithelial hyperplasia in large ducts can be general or papillomatous, and the same is true for epithelium in large cysts and small ducts. In large ducts, the same condition is called adenosis or Schimmelbusch's (Cheatle's) disease; in large cysts epithelial hyperplasia is called intracystic papilloma. Although there may be some difference in prognosis which can be correlated with location of the lesion, all forms of epithelial hyperplasia present an order of seriousness greater than formation of cysts without epithelial hyperplasia. In all probability, epithelial hyperplasia is one of the late recognizable diseases before frank neoplasia occurs. Certainly the next step toward uncontrolled growth of hyperplastic epithelial cells is carcinoma in situ followed by invasion of periductal or periacinar tissue. This finding, of course, is the hallmark of invasive cancer.

The chances of epithelial hyperplasia becoming invasive cancer are not known exactly, but the data presently available strongly suggest that given enough time, the probability is high. It may take as long as 15 to 20 years for intraluminal cells which appear malignant (intralobular carcinoma) actually to invade surrounding tissue, but virtually 100 per cent of such lesions will become invasive cancer if unattended. Epithelial hyperplasia of cells in large ducts is not so kindly disposed from the standpoint of time. Invasive cancer will develop in these lesions in 30 to 50 per cent of patients and the time for invasion to occur may be measured in months rather than years. In addition, invasive cancer originating in large ducts shows little or no hormonal dependency and is a much more aggressive lesion than intralobular carcinoma. Thus it is important to know not only that epithelial hyperplasia is occurring but also where it originates. Unfortunately, epithelial hyperplasia usually is far more extensive than physical examination indicates. Many areas of epithelial hyperplasia form typical, easily palpable lumps, but epithelial hyperplasia progressing to invasive cancer can occur in breasts without palpable lumps because of the size and depth of the lesions. One of the most valuable biological principles in understanding and evaluating epithelial hyperplasia is significance of the type of nipple discharge.[3] Yellow lipid discharge or green or brown watery discharges are not characteristic of dangerous intraductal papilloma. Serum or blood is a positive sign of ulceration, however, and carries a much more serious prognosis. In a study performed by Donnelly at the University of Iowa Hospitals, 31 per cent of patients with serous or bloody discharge had intraductal papilloma and another 32 per cent had invasive carcinoma.[17] As pointed out by Womack in an analysis of these data, 50 per cent of women with hemorrhage from the nipple have cancer at the time they are examined, and the other 50 per cent have epithelial hyperplasia of a type which progresses to cancer in a high percentage of cases.[17] Such statistics introduce a far more serious consideration of the importance of nipple discharge than has been appreciated in the past. It is in this group of patients, therefore, that an opportunity exists to save some patients from breast cancer by aggressive precautionary therapy.

In summary, three basic pathophysiological changes can be recognized in breast tissue. They are fibrous tissue proliferation, ductal dilatation, and epithelial hyperplasia. The first two phenomena definitely are related to estrogen-progesterone balance, and progesterone deficiency appears paramount in most patients. The third phenomenon, epithelial hyperplasia, is, at best, only partially dependent on hormonal balance and is the most dangerous of the three. Identifiable changes, which probably are sequentially related in some patients, are hyperplasia, papilloma, carcinoma in situ, lobular carcinoma, and invasive cancer. Recognition and interruption of this sinister series of epithelial changes may offer a previously unrecognized opportunity to prevent carcinoma in some patients. With this idea as an introduction, a scheme for the diagnosis and management of breast disease, based upon biological principles of hormonal control, will be presented.

Physical Examination

Important items in the medical history of a woman with a breast mass are how the mass was discovered, duration of the mass, nipple discharge, whether or not pregnancy and lactation have occurred, cyclic changes in size or tenderness, extraneous hormone therapy, and history of breast cancer in close relatives. The method of discovery of the breast mass can reveal much about the extent of the patient's concern over breast disease and her probable attitude to future management. A history of breast cancer in mother, grandmother, aunts, or siblings is a significant factor in judging the risk of cancer for an individual patient.[10]

Examination of the breast usually confirms the diagnosis of fibroadenoma in a woman between 18 and 30 years of age without need for further diagnostic procedures. We do not recommend biopsy or removal of these lesions, particularly when they are multiple, for diagnostic purposes in young women. Patients often request excision of a fibroadenoma because of fear of cancer; this is certainly an adequate reason for doing so. Rapid growth, particularly in the areolar area in a patient anticipating pregnancy, is another reason for removing a fibroadenoma. In summary, in young women, a fibroadenoma can be treated pretty much according to the wishes of the patient. Most patients sooner or later desire removal of a fibroadenoma, and there is medical justification for doing so, even though relation to malignancy or fear of misdiagnosis is seldom a serious consideration.

A lump in the breast in a woman between 30 years of age and the menopause is a diagnostic problem; lumps in the breasts of postmenopausal women are therapeutic problems. Most lumps in middle-aged patients will turn out to be cancer, but the need to be certain is important. Most lumps appearing for the first time after menopause are carcinoma; fat necrosis is about the only other possibility. Physical examination and history may make diagnosis of a breast lump reasonably certain, but in the 30 to 50 year age group, additional insurance that cancer is not present is necessary. Thermography, mammography, aspiration biopsy, and open biopsy are adjuvants which can be utilized for this purpose. Thermography probably will become relegated primarily to mass screening use. Thermography is a little too expensive now to be used widely for this purpose, and it is slightly less accurate than mammography. Mammography is approximately 85 to 95 per cent accurate in locating and identifying breast carcinomas.[9] Mammography, of course, is not a substitute for histological examination, but it is useful in the examination of patients without a palpable mass, especially those who have an increased risk of cancer. Mammography also is helpful in following patients with a long history of multiple benign lesions, in whom repeated biopsy is not possible for practical reasons. Thus, in a patient with a palpable mass over the age of 30, an invasive technique, such as introduction of a needle or incisional biopsy, should be resorted to at the time of first appearance of a mass. Aspiration with a relatively large bore needle (No. 19) following the placing of a small amount of local anesthetic on the skin is an office procedure of great value. There is no reason why it should not be performed on all well defined masses.[16] A typical cyst will produce brownish fluid of low viscosity, and after aspiration is complete, the mass will disappear completely. We have not found cytological examination of aspirated fluid to be useful and, therefore, do not recommend that patients be subjected to additional expense which such studies require.

Failure to obtain fluid on aspiration or failure of a mass to disappear completely following aspiration is a positive indication for open biopsy of a new lesion. It is usually not necessary to admit patients to a hospital or prepare them for possible radical mastectomy and general anesthesia. Few surgeons have considered in all seriousness the severe emotional trauma which women experience during the period between discovery of breast mass and then being anesthetized without knowing whether a simple benign tumor will be excised or an operation about which she has many misgivings will be performed. Fear that this will happen and a natural uncertainty about the accuracy of decisions some other person will make in the operating room while the patient is narcotized have led to reluctance of some patients to seek medical advice and to shop for surgeons who fit the pattern hailed by authors of popular type medical articles. Unless there are highly suggestive physical signs of cancer, such as extension, skin or nipple retraction, and so forth, and the patient is past menopause, biopsy usually should be performed as an outpatient procedure under a local anesthetic. A circumareolar incision leaves no visible scar, provided the incision is placed just within the areola and not at the junction of nonpigmented skin and areolar tissue. Fine technique during closure consisting of the use of deep absorbable sutures in breast tissue to prevent hematoma, subcuticular sutures with fine white silk in the skin so that they will not show through transparent epithelium, and final skin closure with 6-0 silk sutures produces a scar which, for all practical purposes, is not visible. The technique of fine suture closure to eliminate suture marks and a wide scar is not difficult and should be mastered by anyone performing breast biopsies.[15] Assurance that a prominent scar will not follow open biopsy is reassuring and appreciated by most patients. Confirmation of a diagnosis of cystic disease is usually the result of biopsy; if carcinoma is found, there is no evidence that open biopsy with a one or two day delay compromises the effectiveness of present methods of treatment.

When carcinoma is suspected, a slightly larger bore needle can be utilized to obtain a core of solid tissue for examination. This procedure provides an immediate diagnosis, and allows the patient to discuss all aspects of treatment of carcinoma of the breast while fully clothed, and seated comfortably, sometimes with the support of her husband or other consultants, such as a family physician whose opinion she values. She is able to make plans and prepare herself for major surgery without the strain of uncertainty about the diagnosis. For the surgeon, there is reaffirmation of patient understanding and, of course, the saving of approximately 30 minutes of operating room time. Some patients prefer open biopsy under general anesthesia, followed by immediate radical treatment if cancer is found. In other words, they prefer to trust their surgeon alone and insist that diagnostic and therapeutic procedures be carried out while anesthetized. Such patients are becoming increasingly rare, and the failure of surgeons to appreciate the dread which most patients hold for conventional biopsy, frozen section, radical operation, and so forth, has resulted in tragic delays in diagnosis and treatment.

Diagnosis of a first lump or a recently appearing new mass is relatively straightforward. When cancer is found, aggressive treatment follows, but when cystic disease is confirmed, a number of problems arise. Again, the biological principles outlined for understanding reactions of breast tissue provide the most help in planning treatment and subsequently following the patient. Most patients require no therapy other than periodic reassurance that they have a relatively common disorder which does not hold life-threatening complications over them. Self-examination at regular intervals, reporting any new lumps to a physician, and yearly examination by a physician who may also wish to have mammograms or thermograms performed provide nearly maximum protection and allow most patients to place the responsibility for early recognition or prevention of cancer upon their physician's shoulders. New lumps should be aspirated and some new lumps should be biopsied. Certainly any new lump with different characteristics than others throughout the breast should be biopsied if a cyst is not found by aspiration. There are some patients in whom repeated biopsy becomes impractical as the appearance and disappearance of breast masses may be too rapid to make biopsy of each one practical. Clinical impression and roentgenological examination may have to suffice for these individuals; putting up with the possible threat of increased risk of cancer may be necessary in order to live any type of normal existence. Such considerations expose one of the seldom recognized hazards of chronic cystic mastitis—becoming so accustomed to the disease that normal precautions are not followed when new lumps appear. The possible increased incidence of carcinoma in patients with cystic disease is so small when raw data are refined by modern statistical techniques that any real differences between women with cystic disease and women without cystic disease may be significantly affected by such subtle factors. Although not enough data are available to support or disprove the effect of estrogens on prognosis of cystic disease, deductive reasoning strongly suggests that estrogen should not be administered and that progesterone might be helpful. Progesterone, administered in the form of 250 to 500 mg. of Delalutin intramuscularly on the twenty-first day of three or four successive menstrual periods, has helped a few patients but has been disappointingly ineffective in controlling symptoms or signs in most women. Testosterone actually has been the most effective hormone for treatment of fibrocystic disease. Unfortunately, androgenizing side effects have made this form of treatment unacceptable. We have found Phenergan in doses of 25 to 50 mg. taken by mouth 30 minutes before retiring to be effective in controlling premenstrual pain and tenderness. In addition, Phenergan provides a restful night's sleep, which may be no small factor in some patients. Recent investigation on the use of prolactin in chronic fibrocystic disease may add another dimension to hormone therapy.

Treatment

The problem of management when epithelial hyperplasia of any kind is encountered is much more serious than diagnosis and management of fibroadenomas and fibrocystic disease. Problems caused by hormonally induced abnormalities such as fibrocystic disease are less serious than danger of autonomous cell growth, which epithelial hyperplasia heralds. There is considerable disagreement among surgeons and pathologists about the outlook following discovery of epithelial hyperplasia; definitive answers to many important questions simply are not available at this time. On the basis of deductive reasoning on what we now know about the biology of breast tissue, however, we have become more aggressive than some others in treating our patients. Once epithelial hyperplasia has been identified, our judgment usually is that definite proof must be obtained either that the lesion is local and has been removed or that it is hormone responsive and has been relegated to inactive status by substitutional therapy. In practice, this means that multiple biopsies must be made repeatedly in some patients to produce this sort of information. Tissue is obtained by needle biopsies in at least four quadrants of each breast to obtain as complete a picture as possible of the overall histology.

Intracystic papilloma and epithelial hyperplasia of terminal ducts are more likely to be responsive to hormonal control than epithelial abnormalities in large collecting ducts. Terminal duct hyperplasia can often be caused to revert to a monolayer of thin cells by progesterone therapy. In some patients, an injection of Delalutin on the twenty-first day of four mentrual cycles will cause a reversion to normal, which persists until menopause, after which the condition usually disappears spontaneously. A course of progesterone therapy should always be followed, however, by multiple biopsies; if epithelial hyperplasia is still present after progesterone therapy, a strong case exists for performing subcutaneous mastectomy followed by insertion of silastic implants. If reversion of epithelium to normal resting state is accomplished and proved without doubt by biopsy, the patient should be followed carefully through the menopause without recommending further excisional therapy unless a new mass appears.

Intraductal papilloma involving large ducts is the most serious form of epithelial hyperplasia. Large duct epithelium seldom is responsive to hormonal control, and in our judgment the incidence of invasive carcinoma is too high in this area to treat lesions in the conventional manner of subareolar excision of a single lesion or quadrant excision of the breast. Subareolar excision of nodules seems especially dangerous, as it results in division of many, if not all, of the terminal collecting ducts, thus isolating large segments of the breast from a nipple outlet. When blood or serous material can be expressed from the nipple there is more likelihood of malignancy—both at the time it is discovered and for the future. This appears to us to be adequate reason for performing mastectomy. Not all surgeons agree with this relatively radical approach, but it is in this group of patients, perhaps, that we still have an opportunity to protect a few women from fatal breast cancer utilizing techniques presently available. The biology of breast tissue strongly suggests that, in the past, we may not have been aggressive enough with large duct epithelial hyperplasia. A plea is made, therefore, for placing treatment of a bleeding nipple in a high suspicion category. Only the results of numerous biopsies and correlation of the changing biological picture with morphological evidence of resting epithelium should deter the surgeon from an aggressive removal of breast tissue when large duct epithelial hyperplasia is found. Intraductal papilloma can be local and, of course, can be cured by a local excision, but the more than 50 per cent incidence of carcinoma in these patients and the wide distribution of the lesion throughout the breast in many patients argue strongly that, unless good evidence can be garnered to show that the disease is local, mastectomy should be performed.

Finally, what may be the last steps in the biological evolution of invasive breast cancer—carcinoma in situ and intralobular carcinoma—occasionally are found when biopsies are performed. Intralobular carcinoma arising from small ducts and acini may still be hormone dependent. In some investigations, approximately two-thirds of such lesions have responded to progesterone therapy.[18] Such therapy can be used as a sort of biological test for hormone dependency, much as thyroid tumors have been studied by administering desiccated thyroid. Because several years are required for intralobular breast carcinoma to become invasive carcinoma, such tests are justified and, in about two-thirds of women, can result in reversion of the lesion to normal while still retaining breast tissue. Failure to obtain complete transformation of epithelial hyperplasia (or any of its variants) to a nonproliferating state is a positive indication for simple mastectomy or possibly subcutaneous mastectomy followed by insertion of silastic implants. Thus, it is possible that improved survival *and* protection of body image may result from a more aggressive approach to intraductal papilloma in large ducts and biological testing and treatment of hormone dependent intralobular carcinoma rising in small ducts and acini.

Complex nomenclature, frozen section techniques, and ever-increasing awareness of the lay public to professional lack of understanding of breast disease have contributed to the confusion and sometimes less than optimal care for patients with breast problems. The major thesis of this presentation, therefore, has been that the biological basis for diagnosis and treatment of breast disease offers many advantages over memorizing a classification or series of eponyms and then trying to fit each patient into a preconceived slot. A thorough understanding of what presently is known about the influence of at least two major hormones on breast tissue and an appreciation of the significance of epithelial hyperplasia can do much to place diagnosis and treatment of breast disease on a more scientific basis than has been possible in the past. The results of such studies strongly suggest that two ways in which continued improvement may occur without major new discoveries are choosing a more aggressive approach to women with intraductal papilloma of large ducts and applying hormonal testing to determine whether epithelial hyperplasia in small ducts and acini is still responsive to hormone influences. Thus, the biological basis for diagnosis and management of breast disease adds an important dimension to our ability to understand and solve problems in this area.

REFERENCES

1. Amerson, J. R.: Cystosarcoma phyllodes in adolescent females. Ann. Surg. *171*:849, 1970.
2. Burnstein, N. A., Kjellberg, R. N., Raker, J. W., and Schmidek, H. H.: Human carcinoma of the breast, in vitro: the effect of hormones. Cancer *27*:1112, 1971.
3. Copeland, M. M., and Higgins, T. G.: Significance of discharge from the nipple. Ann. Surg. *151*:638, 1960.
4. Davis, H. H., Simons, M., and Davis, J. B.: Cystic disease of the breast: relation to carcinoma. Cancer *17*:957, 1964.
5. Devitt, J. E.: Fibrocystic disease of the breast is not premalignant. Surg. Gynec. Obstet. *134*:803, 1972.
6. Franz, V. K., Pickren, J. W., Melcher, G. W., and Auchincloss, H., Jr.: Incidence of chronic cystic disease in so called "normal breasts"; study based on 225 postmortem examinations. Cancer *4*:762, 1951.
7. Haagensen, C. D.: Diseases of the Breast. Philadelphia, W. B. Saunders Co., 1956.
8. Hollander, V. P., Smith, D. E., and Adamson, T. E.: Studies on estrogen sensitive trans-hydrogenase. The effects of estradiol-17β on α-keto-glutarate production in noncancerous and cancerous breast tissue. Cancer *12*:135, 1959.
9. Hutter, R. V. P., Snyder, R. E., Lucas, J. C., Foote, F. W., and Farrow, J. H.: Clinical and pathological correlation with mammographic findings in lobular carcinoma in situ. Cancer *23*:826, 1969.
10. Jacobsen, O.: Heredity in Breast Cancer: A Genetic and Clinical Study of Two Hundred Probands. London, H. K. Lewis, 1946.
11. Kier, L. C., Hickey, R. C., Keettel, W. C., and Womack, N. A.: Endocrine relationships in benign lesions of the breast. Ann. Surg. *135*:782, 1951.
12. Nelson, L. V., Carlton, W. W., and Weikel, J. H.: Canine mammary neoplasms and progestogens. J.A.M.A. *219*:1601, 1972.
13. Oberman, H. A.: Chronic fibrocystic disease of the breast. Surg. Gynec. Obstet. *112*:647, 1961.
14. Peacock, E. E., Jr.: Yet another form of Women's Liberation. Am. J. Surg. *124*:565, 1972.
15. Peacock, E. E., Jr., and Van Winkle, W.: Surgery and Biology of Wound Repair. Philadelphia, W. B. Saunders Co., 1971.
16. Wilson, N. D.: Aspiration of breast cysts. Am. Surgeon *38*:509, 1972.
17. Womack, N. A.: Benign lesions of the breast. J. Kansas Med. Soc. (Suppl.) *50*:64A, 1949.
18. Womack, N. A.: Personal communication (unpublished data).

Management of Benign Lesions Related to the Diagnosis of Early Breast Cancer

GEORGE V. SMITH AND ROBERT L. SHIRLEY

Harvard University and Boston Hospital for Women

Basically there is no controversy as regards medical care. The ideal is to provide the best care for all patients. How this can be accomplished, however, is indeed a controversial issue at present. Many of the so-called controversies concerning specific problems in medicine are referable to the still abysmal ignorance of human biology and of the means to prevent or correct pathological conditions. Benign lesions of the human female breast provide a striking example. The diagnosis of these and of cancer in the breasts of women is the challenge of this chapter. We take this opportunity to give strong support to the statement by Drs. Christian and Reid that the contributions of the obstetrician-gynecologist to the early diagnosis of female breast cancer could and should be substantial.

In recent years there has been an encouraging increase in the finding of *early* cancer of the breast. With the five-year survival rate exceeding 80 per cent in Stage I cases, mortality rates should eventually be reduced if this trend continues. Early self-detection made possible by educational programs, early detection through medical screening programs, and frequent resections result in the diagnosis of cancers much smaller than the classic ones. The actual management of cancer of the female breast continues to be fraught with controversy. At present the modified radical operation—viz., wide simple amputation with thorough resection of the axillary contents, and without removal of the pectoral muscles—is enjoying some popularity, though significant results are not available. Regardless of the type of surgery performed, however, any woman with a cancer in the medial half of the breast is referred for external irradiation, whatever the size of the tumor, at Boston Hospital for Women unless the lesion is microscopic—e.g., lobular carcinoma in situ. Lobular carcinoma has a propensity to develop in the contralateral breast.

At this hospital the policy of surgical investigation of mammary masses on the slightest suspicion of cancer seems to have been a factor in the increasing percentage of cases with negative axillary node findings: from 36 per cent (1905 to 1946) to 42 per cent (1947 to 1961) to 52 per cent (1964 to 1967) to 53 per cent (1967 to 1972). This trend is still low compared to the best reported value of 70 per cent negative axillary node findings.[7]

Benign Lesions

By far the most common and disturbing benign lesion is that which, from palpation, is suspected to be *mammary dysplasia* (also termed *chronic cystic mastitis* or *fibrocystic disease*). These terms cover diffuse or localized processes which on microscopic study have the following characteristics: sclerosing adenosis, apocrine metaplasia, cysts, fibrosis, and blunt duct adenosis—all lesions that are frequently reported and not alarming. Less frequent but more alarming are intraductal hyperplasia, intraductal papillomatosis, and lobular hyperplasia. These intermixed processes will be the subject of a later section of this chapter.

LESS COMMON BENIGN LESIONS

Galactoceles and sebaceous cysts require no comment. Fibrous histiocytoma, leiomyoma, lipoma, adenolipoma, granular cell tumor, neurofibroma, sarcoid, and tuberculosis are so rare as to need no discussion. In the past 16 years, only one case of tuberculosis has been seen at the Boston Hospital for Women, and even that one was questionable. Left for consideration are fibroadenoma, fat necrosis, squamous metaplasia with hyperkeratosis of the sinuses of lactiferous ducts, and lesions manifesting themselves by the exudation of fluid from the nipple.

Fibroadenomas occur most often in women under 30 years of age. They are firm, smooth, movable without distortion of skin, discrete, and usually less than 3 cm. in diameter. Although generally occurring singly, they may develop in both breasts, and as many as five or more may grow in one breast. Tenderness is variable and is more pronounced prior to the menses. There need be no rush to remove these masses; sometimes the diagnosis is proved wrong by the disappearance of a mass 1.5 cm. or less in diameter over the course of 3 or 4 months. Fibroadenomas, like other but less discrete fibrous areas, have a characteristic firm feel on insertion of a needle. When dealing with what seem to be fibroadenomas in both young and older women, however, the possibility of a deep, relatively circumscribed cancer must be entertained. If there is the slightest doubt, surgery must not be delayed. The insertion of a needle into a cancer gives a heart-sinking crunchy feel. The use of a needle in such instances will be discussed in more detail later in this chapter. Another consideration is that any mass which seems to be a fibroadenoma, especially if its size is over 2.0 cm., may be a cystosarcoma phylloides.

Fat Necrosis

The edema and firmness of a breast with many pinpoint holes owing to the swelling of the skin are characteristic of fat necrosis. The etiology of this local or diffuse inflammatory process is unknown. Occasionally the disease involves an area less than 25.0 sq. cm. and is less intense. To be sure, the breast should be examined repeatedly, and the necrotic area is expected to clear in less than eight weeks even without medication. However, if the disease is full-blown, regardless of the area involved, microscopic examination is imperative because of the fearful possibility of inflammatory carcinoma. A double elliptical incision 3.0 cm. long, with removal of a bit of skin and about 1.5 cm. of the underlying tissue, is sufficient surgery. Healing is accelerated by administering full doses of the broad-spectrum antibiotics.

Over the years, one of the authors (Dr. Smith) has drained an occasional subareolar breast abscess unrelated to the puerperium. He thought they had "just happened." In recent years he has made bold to question the few women who had nonpregnancy related midbreast abscesses; each admitted that suckling by her husband had preceded the infection. Therefore Dr. Smith has made it a point to undercut the nipple as part of the procedure. This technique was adopted after one of the women returned with another subareolar abscess. These women have not had recurrent infection.

Squamous Metaplasia with Hyperkeratosis of the Lactiferous Sinuses[4]

One must not be misled by the statements just made. Subareolar abscesses do occur without detectably introduced infection. These abscesses, which lie at the edge of the areola, may spontaneously drain, forming a sinus pointing at the edge of the areola. For proper treatment, one must keep in mind the possibility of squamous metaplasia with hyperkeratosis of the lactiferous sinuses. In reality the disease is similar to an infected wen, and—also similarly—occurs at any age. Cure depends on the removal of the ends of the ducts by making a flap of the areola and dissecting right under the skin of the nipple, removing about 2 cu. cm. of tissue, and inserting a small rubber drain. Delayed healing is usual.

Why so many women have chronically inverted or retracted nipples without any lesion to explain the situation is disturbing. In some instances the feature seems to be a matter of aging, with atrophy of the breast and shrinkage of the tissue behind the nipple dragging the nipple backward. The only requirement in managing this condition is continued periodic examination.

Quite a number of women have yellow-green debris on the nipples. This is easily scraped away and they should be told not to fear scrubbing their nipples. However, this finding always brings to mind the possibility of Paget's disease. If the debris cannot be easily removed and there is scaling and redness, biopsy is in order, even if no retroareolar mass can be felt.

Examination

It would be trite in a chapter of this sort to describe the technique of looking and feeling for mammary pathology. We are enthusiastic concerning the help which soapy water on breasts and fingers gives to palpation. This idea came from Dr. Paul A. Younge, who has used this method for over 20 years, with negative findings for axillary nodes in his mastectomies increasing from 33 to 54 per cent. With soapy wet skin, the ridges of previous sites of resection, the rosette of the lactiferous sinuses behind the areolar edge, and subtle differences in firmness and moveability are impressively clear. We are now advising our patients to do this themselves frequently when in shower or tub.

Too often women tell us that their breasts are not examined by other physicians. We feel that every patient should have her breasts carefully checked every time she is in the examining room for whatever reason.

To Act or to Wait

A daily problem is whether to wait and recheck or to investigate further at once. The length of delay before taking definitive action should be inversely proportional to the clinical concern index based on family history of breast cancer, past history of breast pathology, age, firmness, dominance, and change in relation to the ovarian cycle. It often is reassuring to reexamine breasts a few days after the menses and find soft homogeneity where confusing nodularity had previously been prominent. In any case, whenever the physician has any apprehension, immediate action is in order. We try not to aggravate mental turmoil. Cancer is not mentioned. We truthfully express ignorance of what the lesion actually is. Action may involve short temporization by needle aspiration and mammography or early admission for resection.

Twelve hour admission—"day surgery" excision of benign or probably benign lesions—has been very successful thus far in our hospital. In addition, it allows for early scheduling. The patient is reassured by the "low pressure" approach to minor surgery without the major threat of possible mastectomy, for which she must be admitted to the hospital for the more suspicious processes. Over a period of 24 months, only 12 of the 257 day surgery breast resections have had unsuspected cancers, all of them Stage I.

There is no evidence that mastectomy performed as long as two weeks after resection affects survival adversely. In fact, reports thus far have indicated longer survival in those undergoing delayed mastectomy.[11] In view of emerging immunologic concepts, this delay may receive some basic support from investigations in animals.

Mammography, Xeroradiography, Thermography

There is controversy over the value and possible harm in radiation examination of the breasts. Radiation studies can detect preclinical, especially deep, foci of cancer. Mammographic study can also serve as a baseline for comparison later on in patients whose breasts seem to have changed. However, the 15 per cent rate of errors, both positive and negative, makes these studies only an adjunct in evaluating lesions. Another problem is the lack of facilities for performing mammograms on really large numbers of women. Even more of a problem lies in the possible late effects of exposing breasts to significant doses of ionizing radiation. Studies have shown that women exposed to atomic bomb blasts, fluoroscopic monitoring of pulmonary tuberculosis, and radiation treatment of postpartum mastitis have developed cancer of the breast more often than could have otherwise been expected.[8,10,15]

The series of the late Dr. Gershon-Cohen included 1500 women who had each had 20 mammographic studies over one decade.[6] Various measurements lead us to believe that the dosage from one standard mammographic exposure lies between 3 and 18 rads. Therefore, a significant group of women has been exposed to between 60 and 360 rads of breast irradiation. Between 1975 and 1985 these women will help provide answers to a clear and worrisome human problem. Until these data are available we feel that repeated mammograms, and xeroradiography when it becomes easily available, involve a real risk. This situation calls to mind the greater than expected incidence of cancers of the thyroid that occurred in those exposed to irradiation of the thymus. At this hospital over the years we have been disturbed by the finding of cancers of bladder, ovary, and lower bowel among those who had received radiation for cancer of the uterine cervix. We would like to know whether the incidence of cancer of the ovary has been augmented among those exposed to radiation for infertility, myomas, and dysfunctional uterine bleeding. In this connection, the May 1973 Federal Drug Administration Drug Bulletin stated, "From 1300 to 6000 cancer deaths annually are caused by exposure of the American public to present levels of diagnostic x-rays. In addition, ill health results from genetic damage caused by the exposure."

Oral Contraceptives

A number of studies have concluded that there is no evidence which points to exogenous hormones as causative agents in cancer of the breast.[1,2,5,13,14] In keeping with this conclusion, Dr. Smith has had a series of breast cancers in women whose ovaries had been removed and who were ingesting no hormones. We would point out, however, that "the pill" is taken for the most part by younger women who, with exceptions, have not reached the age of increasing breast cancer incidence. We would also add that a goodly number of older women with cancer of the breast have been taking estrogens. Because of his concern that administered estrogen might enhance an already present propensity to breast neoplasia, Dr. Smith now admonishes his patients to consume the smallest amount of conjugated estrogens required to make the flushes bearable. This same concern applies as regards the enhancement by estrogen of a propensity to develop cancer of the endometrium.

These same authors[1,2,5,13,14] also noted a decrease in mammary dysplasia worrisome enough to require surgery among those taking oral contraceptives, as we have also. We have not been impressed with the effect of the sequential pills in this regard. Parenthetically, with present-day pills patients fare better with respect to mastalgia, tension, dysmenorrhea, and breakthrough bleeding if they resume their pills on the fifth day following the end of the previous "run."

Although the Federal Drug Administration has not interdicted the use of oral contraceptives because of the reported vascular complications apparently related to it, and some writers[1,5] have decided that the pill is not a vascular menace, one cannot deny the reliability of the careful studies performed by others who have found the pill statistically related to vascular tragedies.

Lesions Manifesting Themselves by the Exudation of Fluid from the Nipple

These lesions include cancer, fibrocystic disease (alias chronic cystic mastitis or mammary dysplasia), intraductal hyperplasia, intraductal papilloma, and simple dilatation of lactiferous sinuses, with some secretion. Bilateral milky discharge in relation to pregnancy or the ingestion of oral contraceptives is not considered to result from a lesion. In general, about 10 per cent of women with discharge from the nipple do have cancer. On the other hand, some women (aged 25 to 73) have episodes of exudation which are self-limited, requiring no surgery.

We believe that cytological examination of fluid from a nipple is worthwhile for what information it may give in addition to that gained from clinical examination. The first step prior to thorough palpation is to smear the secretion on a frosted glass slide, which is at once put into the ether-alcohol mixture like any Papanicolaou smear. Should a fair amount of fluid be obtained by suction, an equal volume of ether-alcohol solution or of 50 per cent ethanol is added and the specimen submitted for cell block pathology examination.

During a period of 20 years, Dr. Smith has submitted 137 nipple discharges from 46 women for cytological examination. Four of these patients had overt cancer, yet the Pap smears from the nipple in three patients were negative. One woman with a report of Class V carcinoma proved to have intraductal hyperplasia and papillomatosis in the resected portion of her breast and 5 years later underwent radical removal of the same breast. There was no nodal metastasis and she is well 5 years later. Three other women whose nipple smears were read as suspicious have remained free of cancer of the breast 3, 12, and 17 years later. Only one had a breast resection.

Resection of a breast was performed on 11 of this group of 46 patients. Nine had fibrocystic disease, of whom two also had intraductal hyperplasia, two had concomitant intraductal papilloma, and one had lobular hyperplasia. The remaining two had only intraductal papilloma.

The other 27 women in this series of 46 patients did not undergo surgery. We have no follow-up data on seven, however. Five were free of nipple secretion at 1 to 3 years, 13 at 6 to 10 years, and 2 at 15 and 18 years. Thus nipple discharge, even when occasionally bloody, appears to be self-limited in at least 33 per cent of cases. Therefore, if one is not impelled to perform surgery on the basis of examination or cytology or both, follow-up is in order, with a reasonable expectation of spontaneous remission of the leakage.

Cytology performed upon fluid sucked from the nipple by means of a double-barrelled device has not been reliable in following patients considered to be at risk for cancer. One of the authors (Dr. Shirley) has employed the device 129 times on 103 women, with some fluid return from 100 of the tries. Only 62 smears contained cells which could be interpreted. Two were reported to be Class III and both women proved to have only intraductal hyperplasia in the resected tissue. Two other patients developed cancer during the period of this study, the lesions being detected by the soap and water technique. The suction smears from each of these had been read as benign, although the cancers were active within the ductal systems. The discomfort, the time required, and the uncertainties of interpretation have reduced enthusiasm for suction in this hospital's breast clinic.

Chronic Cystic Mastitis, Fibrocystic Disease, Mammary Dysplasia

Over the years, chronic cystic mastitis has been the bugbear of physicians and women, and it still is. It may mask a developing cancer. Indeed, the full-blown disease carries a significantly greater risk of cancer. Its etiology is unknown. Why is it that so many women have it and so many others do not? No consistent endocrine abnormality has been detected. There are racial differences in incidence. It may even occur in women without ovaries who are not on estrogen therapy and in the elderly woman. The amount noted by palpation varies month by month and year by year. The breasts of many become soft before the menopause, but more often this does not occur until after menopause. Occasionally the disease flares up, rarely with actual lactation, during the months following complete hysterectomy with removal of tubes and ovaries. Usually the breasts become undisturbing by the second or third year following overiectomy or spontaneous menopause.

Bilateral simple amputation has solved the problem for some. This radical procedure has been refused by other patients, who have not required surgery during follow-ups from 10 to 25 years, despite having been at risk. Various endocrine therapies have been disappointing, with the exception of the nonsequential oral contraceptives, which one hesitates to prescribe because of the threat of vascular complications and the publicized controversy concerning their relationship to cancer.

Much fibrocystic disease is merely lumpiness, no dominant mass being present. There may be diffuse small lumpiness or, more often, large, irregular soft lumps felt most often in the upper, upper outer, and lateral portions. Any area which feels more firm or just "different" to one's fingers raises the red flag of suspicion and calls for action. A 20 gauge needle 1½ in. long might be first choice and mammography the second, temporizing choice. If the woman is still having menses, reexamination at the end of the following period may be the third choice. Suspicion may end or be confirmed, and surgery may be required. For the postmenopausal woman, surgery is safer; the incidence of carcinoma increases with aging.

Presumed Cysts of Sufficient Size for Puncture by Needle

Firm, rounded, discrete, movable, tender or nontender masses without attachment to overlying skin are likely to be cysts. (We wonder why the majority of women with cystic mastitis fail to have exudation from the nipple. Similarly, we wonder what is the significance of the universal inflammatory reaction seen under the microscope.) Some cysts are large and soft, and there may be more than one in either breast or in both breasts.

It is important not only to gain the patient's confidence but also to procure her consent to attempted aspiration, with the nurse present as witness. The patient may refuse, in which case a waiting period to "think it over" or surgery is suggested. Cancer, fibroadenoma, or localized fibrosis—not a cyst—are entertained in differential diagnosis, but the possibility of cancer is not conveyed to the patient. What a relief it is when fluid is obtained and the mass becomes a hollow space! However, the deep, discrete "cyst" may prove to be cancer.

The technique of aspiration is simple. The dominant area is trapped against the chest between the index and middle finger. Palpation then gives a bouncy, fluid-under-pressure sensation. The area is prepared with alcohol, and gentle introduction of the 20 gauge needle, attached to a disposable syringe of a size thought to be correct for the volume of the cyst, will give a feeling of firmness before puncture is accomplished. Strong suction is applied while the area is being kneaded, until the last drop of fluid is obtained. The fluid is mixed with an equal amount of 50 per cent ethanol and submitted for cytological examination. Although we cannot be certain, our experience suggests that emptied cysts usually do not fill up again.

During the last two years, six university centers have recorded their use of primary needle aspiration in the management of cysts.[3,9,12] Little had been written previously regarding this technique. Most of these authors have forgone cytological examination of the fluids. We opine, however, that such study is helpful even if it does on occasion result in false positive or false negative reports. Over the past 22 years, Dr. Smith has aspirated 607 cysts of 176 women and obtained cytological examination for 575 of the specimens. Fifteen of the 575 reports were "suspicious" or "positive," but none of these women has developed cancer during a follow-up period averaging 7½ years. Nine of the 176 women have had surgery for cancer of the breast, but none of them developed cancer on the side of aspiration within 10 years of the last emptying of a cyst. However, we have no follow-up data on 23 of the 176 patients. Twenty-seven others had resection after needle aspiration. From this experience, we can state that the use of needle aspiration in our office kept at least 126 women from surgery.

Return of Moisture Only from Inserting a Needle into a Mass in the Breast and Applying Suction

On 110 occasions, in 84 patients, the suction-puncture of a mass has yielded only a minuscule amount of moisture. This has been blown and spread on a frosted glass slide for cytological examination. We reiterate here that the introduction of a needle into a fibroadenoma or a localized area of fibrosis produces a bulldog type of bite on the needle, whereas a frightening grating sensation is produced by a cancer.

We have no follow-up data on 12 women for whom the moisture specimen was reported to be negative. Of 53 others whose findings were reported as negative, 28 have not come to surgery during intervals of one to over 10 years, 21 of the follow-ups being over two years, 15 of them over four years. Resection of the breast was performed on 25 patients, the diagnosis being most often fibrocystic disease and fibroadenoma. None of these patients had further breast trouble for one to 11 years later. The moisture from four was reported as disturbing; one had resection, the tissue still being diagnosed as of disturbing nature, but this patient's breasts were normal six years later. The breasts of the other three were normal four, six, and 16 years later. Two other patients with suspicious moisture had cancer surgery, one patient being terminal and the other free of recurrence at almost 6 years. Three with negative moisture findings had radical surgery and are apparently free of disease at five and six years (2 patients). Three others had moisture reported as negative but these patients underwent radical surgery 4½ years, 15 months, and 10 months later respectively. They are well at 6½, 5½ and 1½ years. The moisture specimens from seven patients were Class V. One patient, whose retroareolar mass was only 9 mm. and whose axillary nodes were negative, died of the disease four years later. The others are well at 4 to 7 years since surgery. It does not appear that use of a needle for cytology of mammary masses has been of special help in management. Resection of disturbing areas not only yields a definite diagnosis but also, in benign disease, removes tissue in which malignancy may develop. It is a constant satisfaction to observe how normal a breast can become after the resection of sizeable amounts of tissue followed by a plastic closure of the gap.

The impressive report of Zajicek and associates[16] on the cytological diagnosis of mammary tumors from aspiration smears makes the material reported here seem insignificant. But we wonder whether their elaborate studies, which now include cytophotometry, are really as important as conscientious clinical examination and surgery.

Summary

1. Cytological examination of nipple exudate in our series has not really helped in management. Neither has our management been aided by the cytology on the moisture removed by needle. The elimination of frank cysts, however, has been rewarding.

2. Repeated diagnostic radiation of breasts by mammography or xeroradiography raises the possibility of diagnostic carcinogenesis.

3. The nonsequential oral contraceptives seem to be not only safe but even helpful in women with fibrocystic disease.

4. Easily booked 12 hour admissions for resections have been a safe and practical procedure in preventive treatment of early cancer.

Conclusion

Constant awareness of possible serious disease in women's breasts, palpation with sensitive fingers, and surgery on the slightest apprehension are still of chief importance in the management of benign lesions.

REFERENCES

1. Andrews, W. C.: Oral contraceptives. A review of reported physiological and pathological effects. Obstet. Gynec. Surv. 26:477, 1971.
2. Arthes, F. G., Sertwell, P. E., and Lewison, E. F.: The pill, estrogen and the breast: epidemiologic aspects. Cancer 28:1391, 1971.
3. Bolton, J. P.: The breast cyst and the hospital bed. Arch. Surg. 101:382, 1970.
4. Crile, G., and Chatty, E. M.: Squamous metaplasia of lactiferous ducts (editorial). Arch. Surg. 102:533, 1971.
5. Drill, V. A.: Oral contraceptives and thromboembolic disease. I. Prospective and retrospective studies. II. Estrogen content of oral contraceptives. J.A.M.A. 219:583, 593, 1972.
6. Gershon-Cohen, J., Hermel, M. B., and Murdock, M. G.: Priorities in breast cancer detection. New Eng. J. Med. 283:82, 1970.
7. Gilbertsen, V. A.: Detection of breast cancer in a specialized cancer detection center. Cancer 24:1192, 1969.
8. MacKenzie, I.: Breast cancer following multiple fluoroscopies. Brit. J. Cancer 19:1, 1965.
9. Maier, W. P.: Needle aspiration of breast cysts. Consultant, April 1972, p. 106.
10. Mettler, F. A.: Breast neoplasms in women treated with x-rays for acute postpartum mastitis. J. Nat. Cancer Inst. 43:803, 1969.
11. Peters, M. V.: Delayed mastectomy. Breast cancer symposium. California Med. Assoc., May 1969.

12. Robbins, G. F., Rosemond, G. P., Copeland, M. M., Glassman, J. A., and Schnug, G. E.: Should breast cysts be aspirated? Mod. Med., March 20, 1972, p. 134.
13. Taylor, H. B.: Oral contraceptives and pathologic changes in the breast. Cancer 28:1388, 1971.
14. Vessey, M. P., Doll, R., and Sutton, P. M.: Investigation of the possible relationship between oral contraceptives and benign and malignant breast disease. Cancer 28:1395, 1971.
15. Wanebo, C. K., Johnson, K. G., Sato, K., and Thorslund, T. W.: Breast cancer after exposure to the atomic bombings of Hiroshima and Nagasaki. New Eng. J. Med. 279:667, 1968.
16. Zajicek, J., Casperson, T., Jakobsson, P., Kudynowski, J., Linsk, J., and Us-Krasovec, M.: Cytologic diagnosis of mammary tumors from aspiration biopsy smears, comparison of cytologic and histologic findings in 2111 lesions and diagnostic use of cytophotometry. Acta Cytol. 14:370, 1970.

Management of Benign Lesions Related to the Diagnosis of Early Breast Cancer

Editorial Comment

Although the interval from definitive treatment of breast cancer to recurrence of the disease may be extended, the cure rate has not been affected and the mortality rate remains unchanged. Curability hinges on the detection of cancer in its earliest stage, prior to lymph node involvement. One must conclude that the current system of medical care is not entirely conducive to diagnosis until the disease has passed this more favorable stage.

There is a parallelism here with detection—and to a degree, treatment—of cancer of the female reproductive tract, especially that of the cervix. It is recognized that some of the difficulties are patient-oriented, but others are due to medical limitations as currently practiced. We bemoan the fact that many women fail to have even one, to say nothing about a periodic, cytologic examination for cervical cancer. This may be due in part to the "lost decade"—namely, the ages of 30 to 40, a time when in situ lesions are becoming prevalent. This period is when many women are concerned with child rearing and hence fail to be examined. Furthermore, there has always been the question of who is to do the examination if all women are to be so screened. Apparently it must be the responsibility of the primary physician, whoever he may be.

In the evolution of medical care, it is evident that the obstetrician-gynecologist is becoming the primary physician for women. Hence, he must be carefully trained beyond the limits of his specialty; in this instance, he must examine the breast with particular thoroughness and provide advice for definitive treatment should the diagnosis of cancer of the breast emerge. Moreover, he must also represent the patient's interest in the management of her disease in this era of multidisciplinary approach. This is not to decry the latter, which in fact is a necessity for the treatment of this many-faceted disease. Indeed, if inroads are to be made in reducing the mortality from breast cancer, a system must be devised that will provide the ultimate in detection and treatment. It becomes increasingly clear that clinics must be designed for the care of patients with breast disease wherein the general surgeon, the specially trained gynecologic surgeon, the pathologist, the endocrinologist, and the patient's primary physician can work together harmoniously for the patient's welfare. The success of this arrangement is predicated on the medical dictum that "the diagnosis of breast malignancy, or any other, for that matter, must be the responsibility of all the physicians, while the treatment is the responsibility of the relatively few qualified by training interest and long-term motivation."

The basic issue for the primary physician is whether or not patients with various breast changes he can recognize are more prone to develop breast cancer. If so, the presence of these conditions and the possibility that they may develop or harbor a malignancy makes the diagnosis the more difficult and at times downright misleading.

Despite the differences in nomenclature and designation of the various breast lesions, there appears to be agreement on some of the lesions. Fibroadenoma or adenomafibroma is an acceptable term for somewhat firm, discrete, but often multiple lesions that occur before the age of 30 and which tend to enlarge during pregnancy. In fact, pathologically, breast tumors removed in pregnancy often fall into this category, but the lesions usually regress in the next decade of life. It is reassuring to be informed that these discrete masses are not precancerous.

The weight of the evidence—furnished in no small part by Dr. Haagensen —indicates that patients who have what he chooses to designate gross cystic disease rather than fibrocystic disease, who are frequently encountered throughout the childbearing period, have a greater incidence of breast cancer by some two to four times that encountered in the general population. The number of patients so afflicted with gross cystic disease are many; indeed, there are few patients with totally soft, pliable breasts. Hence, the problem of examination follow-up and overall management of these patients is a prodigious one. The third group of breast lesion is known by a variety of terms and its members are subject to differences in interpretation. Perhaps the term hyperplasia could be applied or be considered a common denominator. These lesions include a broad spectrum, from adenosis with proliferation of the acini epithelium to interductal cellular hyperactivity. Whether or not these various lesions can be recognized clinically is of some controversy, but within this maze of conditions and nomenclature resides what is in essence carcinoma in situ. In reality, the diagnosis may become a pathologic rather than a clinical one. Here the clinician is seriously in need of help by radiation examination of the breast. Furthermore, the recent demonstration of prolactin dependent human breast cancer strongly supports the biological approach to the etiology and classification of breast tumors.[1]

The diagnosis of breast lesions must be predicated on whatever is feasible for the primary physician. The incentive must be created for patients to carry out self-examination and immediately seek a physician's help when in doubt. In the event of the appearance of a lump in the breast, the diagnosis must begin with a careful history, followed by an equally careful physical examination. Differences exist in the interpretation of nipple discharge, but obviously it must not be ignored if indeed 10 per cent of women who have a nipple discharge prove to have cancer in the course of their lifetime. The generous use of needle aspiration where cystic disease is suspected is now generally accepted, adding immeasurably to patient management and diagnosis. It is anticipated that the cyst wall will collapse completely with aspiration, and whenever this fails to occur, further diagnostic investigations are indicated.

Also, the utilization of 24 hour biopsy, usually on an outpatient basis, is now being accepted. Several series are now in progress in which early cancer lesions have been uncovered—a most regarding experience. This, together with a careful physical examination of the breast, may well bypass mammography and thermography. These latter examinations have their enthusiastic supporters and undoubtedly should be used in special clinics for screening purposes.[2,3] This is stated more for the possibility that the techniques will improve over those that are current. Certainly the primary physician need not feel thwarted in his efforts if these methods are unavailable.

While there may be some division of opinion in the approach to patient management, influenced perhaps by the particular training of the individual and the hospital environment within which he works, all of the writers have made substantial contributions to the understanding of breast disease. Their contributions reflect enormous personal experience and wisdom, and it is reassuring that they all agree that the greatest assets in detecting early cancer of the breast are to be found in complete history and careful physical examination.

It is strongly urged that the women's unit of any hospital set up a cancer screening program to detect early lesions in both the breasts and the other organs of the female reproductive system. Not only will this contribute immeasurably to patient care, but it will also serve as an educational device. The presence of such a clinic should be a prerequisite for resident accreditation; otherwise residents in whatever field will graduate with the blasé attitude that a breast examination consists of superficial palpation and observation.

REFERENCES

1. Salih, H., Flax, H., Brander, W., and Hobbs, J. R.: Prolactin dependence in human breast cancers. Lancet 1:1103, 1972.
2. Thermography (editorial). New Eng. J. Med. 286:880, 1972.
3. Nathan, B. E., Burn, J. Ian, and Macerlean, D. P.: Value of mammary thermography in differential diagnosis. Brit. Med. J. 2:316, 1972.

15

Management of Endometrial Adenomatous Hyperplasia and Carcinoma In Situ of the Endometrium

Alternative Points of View:

    By John R. Davis
    By S. B. Gusberg and S. Y. Chen
    By Alfred I. Sherman

Editorial Comment

Management of
Endometrial Adenomatous Hyperplasia
and Carcinoma In Situ of the Endometrium

Precursors of Endometrial Adenocarcinoma

JOHN R. DAVIS

University of Arizona College of Medicine and Arizona Medical Center

In assessing our level of sophistication concerning endometrial carcinoma and its precursors, it is helpful to refer to the model afforded by abnormal epithelial proliferations of the uterine cervix. The declining incidence of cervical cancer is attributed in part to recognition of its potentially cancerous (i.e., precancerous) alterations. Comparing abnormal endometrial glandular proliferations with similar conditions in the cervix might indicate the quality of our experience and depth of insight concerning endometrial lesions.

As a model, three aspects of cervical epithelial abnormalities that are pertinent are: (1) histopathological definitions (dysplasia, carcinoma in situ, and invasive cancer), (2) cytopathological applications in screening and monitoring, and (3) biopsy procedures (random punch, conization, and guided biopsy by staining or culposcopy).

HISTOPATHOLOGICAL DEFINITIONS. In the cervical model, precise, well accepted definitions prevail for dysplasia, carcinoma in situ, and invasive cancer. In contrast, definitions of endometrial gland hyperplasias, carcinoma in situ and early cancer are neither as sharp nor generally accepted. Cystic and adenomatous hyperplasias pose no problem in histopathologic definition. In cystic hyperplasia the glands are enlarged and epithelium is actively proliferating in the form of tall columnar cells with mitotic activity. In the adenomatous type, the gland units are increased in number, and the epithelium is actively hyperplastic. Up to this point, the analogy with cervical dysplasia serves well, but exact equivalents of atypical adenomatous hyperplasia and carcinoma in situ of the endometrium are lacking in the cervix in terms of precise, accepted definitions. These two pathologic entities appear to bridge the gap of severe dysplasia and carcinoma in situ of the cervix.

Atypical adenomatous hyperplasia is frequently defined as piled-up columnar epithelium exhibiting altered polarity and cellular pleomorphism in tightly packed, crowded glands showing internal papillations as well as external budding.

Carcinoma in situ, a term coined by Hertig, is a histopathologic entity consisting of atypical adenomatous glands composed of large eosinophilic cells with pale nuclei—a sort of apocrine metaplasia of the columnar epithelium.

It is difficult to sort out the precancerous significance of endometrial lesions, since definitions are not universally accepted. Hertig's cystic hyperplasia, adenomatous hyperplasia, anaplasia (atypical adenomatous hyperplasia), and carcinoma in situ classification[1] is frequently condensed to a scheme including the first two plus atypical adenomatous proliferations (variously termed atypical adenomatous hyperplasia, carcinoma in situ or AAH-CIS).[2] This condensed scheme appears to be workable, but we should not lose sight of the variety of histopathologic patterns encompassed by atypical adenomatous hyperplasia or carcinoma in situ. Until more is known about pathogenetic mechanisms, life history, and response to therapy, it is best to keep an open mind with regard to the AAH-CIS milieu.

The precancerous potential of cystic hyperplasia is shrouded in confusion if care is not directed to the setting in which it occurs. A frequent finding at menopause, it is not considered ominous, but in postmenopausal women it appears to carry a substantial precancerous potential.

Evidence for a continuum of abnormal epithelial alterations in the cervix is well accepted and is based on (1) incidence and prevalence data, (2) retrospective, prospective, and concurrence studies, and (3) cytopathologic correlations. That a continuum of abnormal gland changes occurs in the endometrium is suggested by similar evidence—by incidence-prevalence data and by circumstantial associations. Dallenbach-Hellweg[3] compiled the world literature relating to the circumstantial associations between cystic hyperplasia, adenomatous hyperplasia, and AAH-CIS. Of these, adenomatous hyperplasia was most frequently found to be associated with carcinoma in the retrospective and concurrent studies (70 to 80 per cent); cystic hyperplasia and AAH-CIS were less frequent (15 to 28 per cent). In the prospective study cystic hyperplasia (including perimenopausal occurrences) was associated with cancer in less than 5 per cent of cases; adenomatous hyperplasia and AAH-CIS were associated with carcinoma in approximately 20 per cent of cases. The stage of the continuum at which irreversibility occurs in the endometrium is not known exactly, although Hertig and others suggest that carcinoma in situ is the point of no return.

Early invasion is difficult to document in curettage material. Breach of basement membranes and stromal invasion in the case of early squamous carcinoma of the cervix is a valuable and workable criterion; but basement membranes and endometrial stromal invasion in the endometrium serve us poorly as indicators of malignancy.

CYTOPATHOLOGIC CORRELATES. The correlations between cytopathologic preparations and biopsies as found in cervical lesions are poorly developed for the endometrial epithelial abnormalities. Of interest is the classification metamorphosis relating to cervical lesions. The numbers scheme (0 to 5) of Papanicolaou has generally been abandoned in terms of the positive-inconclusive-negative reporting system. The "yes" and "no" aspects of the latter system were satisfactory, but the "maybe's" caused more problems than they solved. In recent years the reporting system has been further refined in many laboratories. So long as there are proper cytologic preparations and sources, diagnostic terms are reported with a high degree of reliability and correlation. A cervical cytologic report of "consistent with moderate dysplasia" is more useful to the clinician than one termed "inconclusive." Thus, the "state of the art" in cervical cytopathology is an appropriate model on which to design reporting systems for other sites. In addition, the sophistication of diagnostic methods for cervical cytopathology, which allows screening, correlation with biopsy, and monitoring of post-therapy effects, is an appropriate goal to try for as regards endometrial cytopathology.

Is the endometrium an unsatisfactory site for comparable cytopathologic studies? The positive yield in diagnosing endometrial carcinoma is 60 per cent using cervicovaginal preparations (vaginal pool and cervical scraping). The yield is increased to upwards of 80 per cent by cervical scraping and endocervical aspiration.[4] However, with regard to abnormal endometrial proliferations short of carcinoma, little is known because endocervical aspirations are usually not performed routinely. If endometrial cytopathologic methods are to be developed to the level of excellence of those for cervical cytopathology, greater utilization of aspiration is necessary.

In order to gain further knowledge of the cytopathology of endometrium, we must first become experienced with the character of normal endometrial cells. Then, building on this base, the cytopathologist will be able to contribute to recognition of the cancer precursors. Further appreciation of the continuum and life history of endometrial lesions will follow the development of a perceptive cytopathologic method of study as it has in the case of the cervical continuum.

The relative merits of endocervical aspiration for sampling exfoliated endometrial cells versus the Gravlee jet aspiration of the fundal cavity have received little attention. The advantage of the Gravlee aspiration lies in the return of tissue fragments; from a purely cytologic standpoint, however, the cells obtained by this technique are difficult to evaluate. Thus, the Gravlee aspiration method is more comparable to a suction curettage.

BIOPSY PROCEDURES. In a sense, the random punch biopsy of the cervix is comparable to suction curettage of the endometrium, and both suffer from sampling limitations. If the punch biopsy of the cervix is positive for carcinoma, or if the suction curettage is positive for carcinoma of the endometrium, random biopsy has proved helpful diagnostically. However, if the random biopsy shows an epithelial abnormality short of carcinoma, it cannot be considered that cancer is not present. Limitations of sampling or distortion by the sampling technique may require exclusion of carcinoma by more elaborate biopsy.

Cervical conization may be considered comparable to sharp, complete endometrial curettage, and the limitations of the two procedures are similar. When adenocarcinoma of the endometrium is present, its stage (whether limited to the endometrium or deeply invasive into the myometrium) cannot usually be determined by curettage alone. Depth of invasion is frequently made retrospectively following hysterectomy.

Many of the interpretative problems that pathologists have are imposed by the size and condition of the sample. Although most endometrial diagnostic problems involve type of hyperplasia rather than presence or absence of cancer,[5] it is common knowledge that on occasion distinction between AAH-CIS and carcinoma cannot be made with assurance. In this instance, a sharp curettage may be productive of more satisfactory study material than a suction technique. Our inability to judge the biological potential on the basis of histopathologic examinations of bulky curettage material will remain in a small percentage of cases. These borderline lesions are regarded with caution in patients over 40 years.

Unfortunately, no analogous diagnostic techniques comparable to guided biopsy (staining and culposcopy of the cervix) are presently available for the endometrium. In the absence of directed biopsy procedures, the lack of well developed cytopathologic correlates looms as a greater deficiency. Some peace of mind is afforded when cervical biopsy showing squamous dysplasia and cervical cytologic findings suggests nothing worse; if an endometrial biopsy shows adenomatous hyperplasia, the endocervical or endometrial aspirate is usually not used to advantage, either to establish the correlation or to deny it.

In summary, the model of cervical epithelial abnormalities is suggested as a means of assessing our capabilities and deficiencies in early diagnosis of endometrial abnormalities. There is much to support the concept that both cervical and endometrial precancerous lesions fall into comparable patterns, and little evidence to suggest otherwise. By striving for sharp, precise histopathological definitions for endometrial glandular abnormalities, and by applying cytopathologic study to the endometrium as intensely as we do to the uterine cervix, hopefully insight into endometrial epithelial abnormalities will be attained with as much sophistication. Factors in pathogenesis, life history, and response to treatment of endometrial precancerous conditions may be better appreciated once diagnostic procedures for the endometrium are fully fashioned after the cervical model.

REFERENCES

1. Hertig, A. T., Sommers, S. C., and Bengloff, H.: Genesis of endometrial carcinoma. III. Carcinoma in situ. Cancer 2:964, 1949.
2. Sommers, S. C.: The significance of endometrial hyperplasias. In Lewis, G. C., et al. (eds).: New Concepts in Gynecological Oncology. Philadelphia, F. A. Davis, 1966.
3. Dallenbach-Hellweg, G.: Histopathology of the Endometrium. New York, Springer-Verlag, 1971.
4. Reagan, J. W., and Ng, A. B. P.: "The Cells of Uterine Adenocarcinoma," Monograph. Basel, Switzerland, S. Karger, 1965.
5. Hark, B., and Sommers, S. C.: Endometrial curettage in diagnosis and therapy. Obstet. Gynec. 21:636, 1963.

Management of Endometrial Adenomatous Hyperplasia and Carcinoma In Situ of the Endometrium

S. B. GUSBERG AND S. Y. CHEN

Mount Sinai School of Medicine and The City University of New York

There seems little doubt that the definition and acceptance of adenomatous hyperplasia as an endometrial cancer precursor can bring this malignant disease under increasing control, in the same manner that the recognition of dysplasia and carcinoma in situ of the cervix has already changed the formerly bleak outlook for cervix cancer. However, the technology of screening must differ at least for the present time.

As a diagnostic tool for cervix cancer precursors, the Papanicolaou cytologic smear has a high degree of sensitivity and accuracy even for focal lesions of limited extent. While endometrial cancer can be diagnosed by the cytologist with considerable accuracy if the cytologic sample is obtained directly from the endometrial cavity, there are very few cytologists who can accurately diagnose endometrial cancer precursors. It would seem appropriate, therefore, to screen all women at the perimenopausal age for adenomatous hyperplasia by obtaining a histologic sample, with special reference to those at high risk. Such routine surveillance may be possible without anesthesia if the newer suction methods prove technically sound and free of significant discomfort for the patient.

With respect to those groups who are at high risk for adenomatous hyperplasia, and who presumably are possible candidates for endometrial cancer in later life, one must make note of the presence of any of these factors: (1) infertility; (2) obesity; (3) failure of ovulation; (4) dysfunctional uterine bleeding; and (5) long-term estrogen administration.

Definitions

Understanding of the morphology and biologic significance of adenomatous hyperplasia has been delayed by semantic differences and even histologic considerations. It may be of help, therefore, to define the terminology we use for these precursors.

521

In the mild (Type I) form, one may see only areas of an intense micro-cystic pattern as the glands proliferate actively. In the moderate (Type II) form, epithelial infolding, protrusion into the lumen, and occasional budding reflect a more intense metaplastic change, whereas the severe (Type III) form is charac-terized by the full blown picture of epithelial protrusion and budding, glands back-to-back, and a pallor of the glandular epithelium or eosinophilic staining in the conventional hematoxylin-eosin preparations, indicating its anaplastic quality.

It seems clear that adenomatous hyperplasia is a cancer precursor, but we have refrained from calling it carcinoma in situ because of the impure criteria for invasion, which defy precise designation in the endometrium, and because adeno-matous hyperplasia is frequently reversible, especially in younger women, by the administration of progestins or by induction of ovulation. In short, it would appear to have preserved some measure of physiological control, whether it is a dysfunctional or neoplastic lesion, or—more likely—a transitional one.

We have reserved the diagnosis of *carcinoma in situ* in our laboratory for those lesions in which a cluster of glands exhibits anaplasia and free replication without apparent local control, yet appears confined to a focus of well differenti-ated malignant change in the manner described in the past as adenoma malignum. This lesion is not reversible, though it may be removed at times by local excision —i.e., curettage. This therapeutic observation should be considered in evaluating the result of treatment of this lesion by hormonal means.

Treatment

PREMENOPAUSAL AGE.   In those patients of reproductive age with failure of ovulation, oligomenorrhea, or dysfunctional bleeding associated with adenoma-tous hyperplasia, it is possible to revert the endometrium to normal by inducing a progestational response. Clearly, in those for whom fertility is an issue, the use of a gonadotropin is indicated, whereas the remainder are best served by instituting a cycle of progestin therapy. A minority of patients initially will prove refractory to this treatment, but persistence will usually effect the desired reversion to nor-mal endometrium.

PERIMENOPAUSAL AGE.   In those patients with Type II and Type III ade-nomatous hyperplasia, we have found it prudent to perform hysterectomy to stop the bleeding, which is frequently recurrent, and to prevent endometrial cancer in later life, for it is clear that these patients are at high risk. For minor (Type I) change, we may only observe the patients, with repeat histologic sampling at six months and one year intervals. We have not adopted a plan of progestational treatment for patients with adenomatous hyperplasia at the menopause because of frequent refractoriness, recurrent bleeding, recurrent adenomatous hyperplasia, and the clear advisability of removing an organ at high risk for malignant change in later life, at which time surgical risk is increased.

POSTMENOPAUSAL AGE.   Some cases occur with ovarian pathology, such as theca-granulosa cell tumors, and the endometrial adenomatous hyperplasia will be removed with the uterus at operation.

In the case of adenomatous hyperplasia produced by estrogen, one may stop the medication and await reversion to normal.

If adenomatous hyperplasia is found on diagnostic curettage of a postmenopausal woman who has suffered postmenopausal bleeding without other event, one must assay the patient's operability against the advantage of prophylaxis. Of course, her age, general medical condition, opportunity and willingness for repeat observation, and psychoemotional state must be considered, for in such a patient the balance of advantage and disadvantage of any treatment, surgical or otherwise, becomes increasingly sensitive and requires seasoned clinical judgment. We prefer to perform hysterectomy if the patient is otherwise well and understands the indications, but we have managed many patients with observation only when our criteria for operation were not plainly in evidence.

Discussion

It would appear that semantic problems for these lesions, which clearly lie in the transitional zone of endometrial neoplasia, might be resolved by calling them Stage 0 cancer of the endometrium. It is unfortunate that each school of study of this disorder, and the pupils associated with each, have fragmented this field taxonomically. This has caused delay in acceptance and wide recognition of the importance of these disorders and has retarded the opportunities for labeling the menopausal patient at high risk, for earlier diagnosis of the invasive stage, and for improvement in the cure rate of this malignant disease.

Evidence that adenomatous hyperplasia, as defined in this report, is a clear cancer precursor may be derived in several ways:

1. Prospective studies of these patients reveal an average progression of 18.5 per cent of cases to frank endometrial carcinoma, with a cumulative risk of 30 per cent at 10 years.

2. Accumulation of individual case reports that show histologic progression from cystic glandular hyperplasia to adenomatous hyperplasia to adenocarcinoma with interval observation and study.

3. Coexisting lesions in the same endometrium with adenomatous hyperplasia and adenocarcinoma side by side.

4. Retrospective studies of patients with carcinoma of the endometrium, who have been under observation in the past, have frequently reported the finding of dysfunctional bleeding at the menopause and adenomatous hyperplasia in a proportion exceeding that anticipated.

Therefore, sequential observation to identify the high risk patient by histologic sampling of the endometrium at the menopause could lead to control of malignant diseases of the endometrium.

REFERENCES

1. Gusberg, S. B.: Precursors of corpus carcinoma, estrogens and adenomatous hyperplasia. Am. J. Obstet. Gynec. 54:905, 1947.
2. Gusberg, S. B., and Kaplan, A. L.: Precursors of corpus cancer. IV. Adenomatous hyperplasia as Stage 0 carcinoma of the endometrium. Am. J. Obstet. Gynec. 87:662, 1963.
3. Vellios, F.: Endometrial hyperplasias, precursors of endometral carcinoma. Path. Annu. 7:201, 1972.

Management of
Endometrial Adenomatous Hyperplasia
and Carcinoma In Situ of the Endometrium

Alfred I. Sherman

Wayne State University and Sinai Hospital of Detroit

The management of the patient with adenomatous hyperplasia or with carcinoma in situ of the endometrium is dependent on a variety of factors, the most significant of which is the question of whether or not adenomatous hyperplasia is accepted as a neoplastic premalignant condition. It is our opinion that adenomatous hyperplasia and carcinoma in situ of the endometrium represent two successive phases of the preinvasive stage of endometrial cancer. The situation, we believe, is analogous to carcinoma of the cervix, in which dysplasia is the forerunner to carcinoma in situ, which in turn leads to invasive cancer of the cervix. Because our management of these endometrial lesions entirely reflects and depends on a particular interpretation of this concept, a detailed explanation is in order.

Although the true relationship of hyperplasia of the endometrium to carcinoma remains controversial, the recognition of some relationship, at least to a relative degree, is inescapable. To some extent, the difficulties involved in linking the two entities is attributable to semantics, but primarily it results from the absence of specific criteria by which to designate clear-cut, distinctive histological patterns. The term "endometrial hyperplasia" as commonly used encompasses a wide variety of histological patterns. Many attempts have been made to clarify and simplify this nomenclature so as to conform to specific histological types, but these have resulted only in the adoption of a variety of new and often conflicting terms. However, although a number of these analogous terms continue to persist, some agreement in their use by pathologists is beginning to occur.

The histological appearance of premenopausal or postmenopausal endometrium, which results from continued exposure to estrogen from either endogenous or exogenous sources, presently is recognized and accepted as a well-defined and distinctive entity. This typical response of the endometrium to estrogen, characterized by abundant proliferation of both glands and stroma and the associated cystic changes of the glands within this copious stroma, most frequently is recognized and aptly described as "cystic hyperplasia of the endometrium." Nevertheless, terms such as "benign hypertrophy or hyperplasia" and "Swiss cheese hyperplasia" continue to be used. Regardless of the name, any relationship of this type of endometrium to the type which we call adenomatous hyperplasia or to carcinoma of the endometrium itself is to be strongly denied. It is of utmost importance that these two forms of hyperplasia be completely distinguished and separated.

The type of endometrium in which hyperplasia of the glands far exceeds the stromal growth portrays a completely different picture from that of cystic hyperplasia. Here the glands are seen back-to-back, with very little stroma, which may be extremely fibrous. The terms usually applied to this type of endometrium include "adenomatous hyperplasia," "glandular hyperplasia," "atypical hyperplasia," "anaplasia," and "carcinoma in situ." Furthermore, prefixed to each of these may be found the term "premenopausal" or "postmenopausal." These terms as used by individual authors, generally are meant to carry with them certain connotations of the degree of severity of the condition as the authors have interpreted them. Fortunately there is generally more acceptance of the fact that a correlation does exist between a number of morphological and cytological characteristics and the severity of the lesion. The gradation of the severity is measured by the extent of the abnormal changes in a variety of histological characteristics, which are as follows:

1. The ratio of glands to stroma. The degree to which the glands are packed together, which is of course dependent upon the amount of intervening stroma, determines to some degree the severity of the condition.

2. The degree of irregularity of the glands. This is dependent on the amount of infolding, budding, or papillary projections that occur within the glands.

3. Mitoses. The mitotic rate and the number of abnormal mitotic figures markedly influence the assigned severity.

4. The cytoplasmic nuclear ratios. The ratio of nuclear to cytoplasmic material, the relative hyperchromicity of the nuclei, the amount of clumping of the nuclear material, and the abnormal staining characteristics of the cytoplasm all contribute in determining the degree of abnormality.

5. The loss of polarity and stratification of the cells and the lack of uniformity of shape and size of the cells further indicate the gravity of the lesion.

The severity of each of these histological characteristics may vary considerably in any one specimen, with grades ranging from mild to severe. However, the degree of anaplasticity which their total effect elicits, together with the diagnostic term selected to label any particular specimen, depends mostly on personal and subjective impressions rather than on any objective changes. Therefore, the diagnosis might vary considerably from one examiner to the next. Nevertheless, in any classification of these lesions, and notwithstanding any specific subjective diagnostic criteria, there will of necessity be a range of abnormalities, from that of a lesion totally benign in appearance to one which is highly suspect of malignancy. Furthermore, it is our contention that the degree of histological aberration of these lesions parallels their biological aggressiveness.

It is within this latter group of lesions that the greatest controversy exists, and for understandably good reasons. Foremost of these is the fact that seldom is there a clear-cut, definitive degree of change noted within any one specimen. No specimen ever falls completely into an entirely black or white category, but rather there are variable degrees of grey. The arbitrary designation of these conditions, therefore, into either a benign or a potentially malignant category is extremely hazardous. Instead, all phases of this lesion should be considered on a par, without regard to the fact that at any one stage there will be within this continuum relative degrees of abnormality. Furthermore, since the entire gamut of this disease exists, with all its phases in continuity, we believe that the lesion in its entirety should be incorporated as a single lesion and referred to as intra-epithelial carcinoma of the endometrium, with the implication of course that it is a forerunner or precursor of frank carcinoma.

In this concept, endometrial carcinogenesis is viewed as if some inductive stimulus initiated the neoplastic process, in which the glandular response in its earliest phase is represented by minor hyperplastic changes, usually designated as "atypical," "mild," or "adenomatous," and it is believed that with persistent stimulation, the endometrium changes progressively to eventuate in its endpoint, which is an endometrial cancer. Therefore, endometrial hyperplasia of the adenomatous variety and carcinoma in situ of the endometrium are regarded as important and antecedent lesions in this sequence.

The endometrial lesions in which the histological patterns are most severely affected are at times difficult to distinguish from frank invasive cancer. Illustrative of this difficulty is the occasionally encountered diagnosis of "Nicht Karzinoma aber besser heraus."* Here the pathologist admits his inability to distinguish the two. In some medical centers, these lesions are labeled as carcinoma in situ of the endometrium. In others, this final step between a frank carcinoma and its noninvasive counterpart is recognized and referred to as "adenoma malignum." Therefore, from a practical and realistic viewpoint, there is all the more reason that this entire carcinogenic process should be envisioned as a single transitional state, during which all phases within this continuum and their histological counterparts should be considered as intra-epithelial carcinoma of the endometrium. For convenience, the connotations of "early or mild," and "late or severe" should be acceptable. The analogy with cervical dysplasia through its progressive stages to invasive cancer of the cervix is inescapable, despite the fact that this supposed correlation remains an unsettled and still disputed question. Similar to the suggestion that the entire range of cervical disease be referred to as cervical intra-epithelial neoplasia (C.I.N.), we are urged to call the endometrial counterparts intra-epithelial carcinoma of the endometrium (I.C.E.).

Speculation as to the cause of this lesion or the identification of its inductive agent or stimulus is probably not in the province of this article. Suffice it to say here that estrogens have been most notoriously implicated, for a variety of reasons. Pros and cons on which to argue the point are amply found in the literature, but the basic evidence on which the carcinogenic action of estrogens is based lies with its known relationship to endometrial growth, regardless of the morphologic form which that growth may take. It is our considered opinion that the morphological appearance of the glandular stromal hyperplasia that consistently results from pure estrogens usually is a completely different entity from that of neoplastic glandular dysplasia and from the lesion we have here identified

---

* Not carcinoma but better removed.

as adenomatous hyperplasia. This we consider to be the earliest phase of intra-epithelial carcinoma of the endometrium.

In counterdistinction to the above, it is our theory that androgens and not estrogens play the major role, either alone or in combination with estrogens, in the carcinogenesis of endometrial cancer. A number of factors lead us to this conclusion, a discussion of which, however, is beyond the scope of this paper. But, regardless of whether a dominant role can be assigned to either estrogens or androgens, the implication of a disturbed hormonal milieu is highly suspect.

In accepting the concept of an ongoing carcinogenic process, it becomes necessary to speculate on whether a spontaneous reversal of this process is possible. Though indisputable evidence is lacking for the mechanisms of carcinogenesis, the fact that histological reversals do take place is unquestionable, but the factors which play a part in this reversal are not known. It is entirely possible that in the earliest stages of its origin, the original stimulus, regardless of its nature, may be interrupted and the lesion may be held at abeyance or may regress. Furthermore, those factors which influence the progression of this disease to invasion similarly are not known at this time, though two possibilities exist. Either the host tissues maintain a barrier-type resistance, perhaps of an immune type, for a period of time and then for some unknown reason lose this resistant capacity, or the cells themselves through possible enzyme or mutant changes gradually gain the ability of invasiveness.

Our approach in managing patients with these lesions obviously reflects and stems directly from our viewpoint, which in essence may be stated as "adenomatous hyperplasia or carcinoma in situ of the endometrium is a malignancy in a state of benignity but with the inherent capability to eventually develop into frank invasive cancer." In this phase of the disease it is only potentially malignant, and the time interval in which it remains in this state is variable and not determinable. Therefore, with this in mind, a variety of factors may play a role in the ultimate management of the patient. However, the diagnosis alone should neither dictate the type of treatment nor suggest an emergency situation. Several different approaches are possible.

At this stage of the disease, its total excision by a complete hysterectomy should offer a 100 per cent chance for cure. Likewise, entire removal of the lesion by a curettage is certainly technically possible. A curettage would be easier on the patient, and would entail less risk. However, execution of this procedure would be less controllable and complete extirpation less assessable. Therefore, dilatation and curettage might offer somewhat less than a 100 per cent chance for cure.

Chemotherapy with progestins also has been proposed as a curative procedure. Such pharmacological use of progestins for the treatment of these premalignant lesions has been shown to interfere with the further progression of the disease, and to evoke a presumable cure in a certain percentage of these patients when given in exceedingly large doses. However, approximately 25 per cent of all cases are found to be unresponsive to such therapy. The mechanism by which progestins accomplish this reversal of the ongoing process is as yet not known; nor are those factors known which relate to its success or failure. Unfortunately there is no consistent association of features to demonstrate correlation with either success or failure. Furthermore, there is at present insufficient knowledge regarding optimal dosage, optimal duration of treatments, or the long-range results to be expected.

Accordingly, the selection of the most appropriate therapeutic approach for any patient should be determined by the specific clinical factors pertinent to that particular patient. If future childbearing is no longer a factor, menses are not psychologically important to the patient, and her medical condition is such that an operative procedure does not carry undue risk, we would recommend a total hysterectomy. The choice between a vaginal or an abdominal approach may be immaterial. This would depend on other factors, such as the size of the uterus, previous surgical procedures, or the need for additional procedures, such as the correction of a cystourethrocele or rectocele. Also, since the majority of patients with these lesions will be perimenopausal or postmenopausal, we would recommend a hysterectomy combined with salpingo-oophorectomy. However, recommending salpingo-oophorectomy, or deciding to include it, is not because it is pertinent to this particular lesion; rather, other factors play a role in this decision.

Considering that we have never seen intra-epithelial carcinoma of the endometrium in a woman under the age of 40, unless concomitantly associated with some endocrinopathy, most commonly the Stein-Leventhal syndrome, our recommendations here would be to correct the endocrinopathy. A variety of different methods are applicable. These include:

1. Cyclic administration of progestins or progesterone.

2. The use of ovarian resection, either by medullary excision or by wedge resection.

3. The administration of clomiphene, which would probably require intermittent courses in a long-range program.

Other endocrinopathies may require other methods of correction.

The danger of accepting a thorough curettage as a definitive therapeutic measure lies in the difficulty of determining its thoroughness and the completeness of removal of the lesion. The possibility of persistence would of course exist, and the progression of the disease to cancer might proceed either from residual elements or from continuation of the stimulus on the residual endometrium. However, it may be justifiable in situations in which definitive therapy is either undesirable or dangerous. As long as one understands the possibility of such persistence, ample precautions may be taken to alert one of this possibility. Furthermore, under these circumstances, progestin therapy would certainly be of additional value, and we definitely would recommend its use in combination with dilatation and curettage.

In summary, therefore, we feel that adenomatous hyperplasia and carcinoma in situ of the endometrium are preinvasive forms of adenocarcinoma of the endometrium, and that adenomatous hyperplasia represents the earliest phase of this premalignant stage of the disease. Hysterectomy is the treatment of choice, but under certain specific conditions, patients with these lesions may be treated by the combination of a thorough curettage and progestin therapy, or by progestin alone, bearing in mind, however, that this is not definitive therapy.

Management of
Endometrial Adenomatous Hyperplasia
and Carcinoma In Situ of the Endometrium

Editorial Comment

Adenomatous hyperplasia has been proposed to be a counterpart of cervical dysplasia in the sense that both may regress to a normal histologic anatomy but at the same time they may harbor a malignant potential. Being able to identify a potential malignancy in a given specimen would indeed be an invaluable advance in understanding the biology and etiology of cancer and certainly in improving patient management. As the contributors indicate, it is common to classify the degree of histologic change, but it remains a somewhat open question whether these categories are infallible in determining whether the tissue will regress or advance to cancer in situ. Except for those with extensive experience in the management and study of patients with these lesions, most clinicians in most hospitals will have to make their decisions on patient management largely on the basis of a diagnosis of adenomatous hyperplasia, without recourse to grading of the lesion by the pathologist or the clinician himself. Indeed, when arguments arise by pathologists and others as to whether the lesion represents an extreme degree of adenomatous hyperplasia or carcinoma in situ, unquestionably the time to act has arrived. The clinician is well advised to perform an immediate hysterectomy without wasting time on preoperative irradiation. An exception to this approach might be a patient who is an extremely poor surgical risk and those in whom irradiation or hormone therapy might be the only recourse to therapy.

If hormone therapy—i.e., progestational agents—has a place in the treatment of adenomatous hyperplasia, it appears to be in the young woman who may desire children. However, those who are identified as being at risk and menopausal patients are not suitable candidates for hormone therapy. Rather, in those patients in whom the uterus is freely movable and usually of normal size, the risk of hysterectomy is slight to negligible. Undoubtedly, this is the treatment preferred by most women over the constant uncertainty of long-term management implied by endocrine therapy. The risk of developing endometrial cancer remains and some patients will come to hysterectomy even when they choose endocrine therapy, so students, physicians, and patients must not be misled on this point of supposed controversy.

The overzealous use of estrogen therapy in the management of the menopause all too commonly precipitates uterine bleeding and creates a degree of anxiety in the minds of the patient and her physician. As recommended, the cessation of such therapy is indicated, and the patient should be followed closely with repeated endometrial biopsies.

Whether patients with adenomatous hyperplasia should undergo curettage in the hope that this will encourage the endometrium to assume a normal pattern is sometimes discussed, and also whether the procedure should be repeated. Any degree of success this approach may have had is open to question. Certainly after the second curettage in the patient with excessive bleeding and an endometrial biopsy consistent with adenomatous hyperplasia, a hysterectomy is indicated, provided that the patient has finished childbearing. Otherwise, progestational agents might be employed on a relatively short-term basis.

16

Diagnosis and Management of (a) In Situ (Stage O), (b)Microinvasive, and (c) Stage I of Cancer of the Cervix

Alternative Points of View:

By Douglas E. Cannell

By John L. Lewis, Jr., and James H. Freel

By George D. Wilbanks

Editorial Comment

Diagnosis and Management of (a) In Situ (Stage O), (b) Microinvasive, and (c) Stage I of Cancer of the Cervix

DOUGLAS E. CANNELL

University of Toronto Medical School and
Ontario Cancer Treatment and Research Foundation

Controversy is defined in the Oxford dictionary as "disputation, dispute, contention, discussion (especially conducted in writing) in which opposite views are advanced and maintained by opponents."

The diagnosis and management of carcinoma in situ, microinvasive, and stage I cancer of the cervix provide excellent examples of controversy. The differences of opinion stem from a variety of factors—geographic, economic, and disciplinary—accentuated by lack of communication. Thus, it is exceedingly difficult for the unbiased observer to arrive at soundly based conclusions. It may well require another 10 to 20 years' follow-up of well documented cases to establish with assurance the course and significance of carcinoma in situ in relationship to invasive cancer. Such long-term studies are warranted by present uncertainties in the efficacy of screening programs in general and their role in early detection and management, and in the reduction in mortality from carcinoma of the cervix in particular.

Differences of opinion exist between cytopathologists in respect to definition and diagnosis and how these relate to the natural history of the disease. In the instance of diagnosis of microinvasion pathologists offer varied views and conclusions.

Gynecologists support many different methods of detection and diagnosis; disagreement in the techniques of management and the results obtained is profound. In the management of Stage I carcinoma of the cervix, gynecologists and therapeutic radiologists have put forward conflicting claims for the superiority of their own methods of treatment.[1]

Carcinoma in Situ

THE PATHOLOGIST'S VIEW

The definition of epidermoid carcinoma in situ established in 1961 by the International Committee for Histological Definitions is as follows: "Only those cases should be classified as carcinoma in situ which, in the absence of invasion, show a surface epithelium in which throughout its whole thickness no differentiation takes place. The process may involve the cervical glands without creating a new group." Alternatively, it is suggested that "a carcinoma in situ is a lesion confined to the epithelium of the uterine cervix, morphologically resembling invasive cancer."[2]

Koss, in a further comment, suggests that "In the final analysis, carcinoma in situ and, therefore . . . dysplasia, is a highly subjective diagnostic entity. If dysplasia is graded into minimal, slight and marked then reasonable agreement can only be reached in the first two categories. The moderate and marked dysplasia will be considered by many as a carcinoma in situ."[2]

Hulme and Eisenberg[3] state that "when one understands and appreciates 'the facts of life' concerning the diagnosis of carcinoma in situ of the cervix and related lesions, it becomes apparent that the actual diagnosis of severe dysplasia, carcinoma in situ, or carcinoma in situ with questionable invasion is less important than the understanding of the natural history of premalignant cervical neoplasia and its place in the spectrum leading to invasive cancer."

The divergence of opinion in the interpretation of textbook views or those of the International Committee for Histological Definitions is illustrated in Hulme and Eisenberg's report. They submitted for review by two pathologists 22 slides sent to them as carcinoma in situ (CIS) by various pathologists in Connecticut. In nine instances they both agreed with the diagnosis; both pathologists agreed that the diagnosis was not CIS in three. In one case, both agreed that the diagnosis of CIS was questionable; in nine cases, one felt that the diagnosis *was* CIS and the other felt it was not. Cox[4] reported differences in opinion of British pathologists in 54 of 200 specimens submitted between 1955 and 1967. Similar studies elsewhere demonstrate corresponding lack of agreement in the diagnosis of microscopic invasive carcinoma of the cervix.

There are differences of opinion also in respect to the number or percentage of patients in whom CIS proceeds to invasive carcinoma of the cervix.[5]

THE GYNECOLOGIST'S VIEWPOINT

Owing to different interpretations of results, a variety of treatment regimens, ranging from observation (after having excluded invasive cancer)[6] to an extended radical hysterectomy or irradiation,[7,8] have developed. More recently, a more conservative approach to management has been advocated by several authors, using the colposcope for selective biopsy, followed by cryosurgery, conization, or hysterectomy as indicated.[9,10,11,12]

The more conservative approach applies in particular to pregnant patients with abnormal cytological findings. In many instances, conization, which is more hazardous during pregnancy, may be avoided completely or performed postpartum.

The diversity of management is summed up succinctly by Knapp and Feldman,[13] who state, "We have come to a conclusion: currently, the treatment of carcinoma in situ of the cervix commences in doubt, persists in uncertainty and ends in confusion."

Knox[5] suggests that "to summarize the available evidence on the natural history, it is fairly clear that carcinoma in situ may progress to invasive cancer, but it is not known how often this happens, nor after what interval it is likely to happen, nor how often the in situ lesion regresses. The significance of the epithelial dysplasia is even less certain." It may be that some gynecologists, supported by insufficient clinical or pathological evidence, embarked on active treatment programs which were unwarranted.

In the light of present knowledge, reconsideration of the significance and management of carcinoma in situ may be indicated.

Knapp and Feldman feel that a controlled clinical trial is warranted and ethical because "we do potential harm by over treating or under treating." Knox shares their view. Others, on the contrary, submit that it is now too late and would be unethical to embark on such a trial.[14,15]

A survey of the Departments of Obstetrics and Gynaecology at the five medical schools in Ontario[16] reveals a reasonably consistent attitude in the management of CIS. In the younger patient desiring future pregnancies, *if* previous colposcopic investigation or conization (where it was required) *has ruled out* an invasive lesion, the patients are followed with cytology/colposcopy and no further surgery is performed. In older patients, or those whose families are complete, *conization to rule out invasion* is followed either immediately or six weeks later by total hysterectomy with a wide cuff of vagina. The type of hysterectomy, vaginal or abdominal, depends upon the preference of the operating gynecologist. In other institutions—and in some patients for a variety of reasons—simple total hysterectomy is carried out as a primary procedure; the wisdom of this latter course is open to question. A recent survey of over 1000 patients with invasive cancer of the cervix, admitted for treatment to clinics of The Ontario Cancer Treatment and Research Foundation and The Princess Margaret Hospital, reveals justifiable cause for concern.[17] In a significant proportion of patients so treated, our information suggests that the survival results are considerably less satisfactory than if the initial treatment were extended hysterectomy or radiotherapy.

The minimal differences in the approaches to management of CIS at university centers in Ontario are not accepted by some gynecologists elsewhere in Ontario. In too many instances, immediate simple total hysterectomy is performed without further investigation, with the unsatisfactory results noted above. In other instances, patients with varied but lesser degrees of dysplasia than CIS are treated with unnecessarily radical procedures.

COMMENT

In the light of the present rather widespread uncertainties in the diagnosis of carcinoma in situ, the varied approaches to treatment, and the wide differences of opinion as to the eventual progression of the lesion to invasion, it would seem justifiable to adopt more conservative approaches to treatment. Indeed, when one considers that we may expose from 30 to 70 per cent of women with a diagnosis of CIS to needlessly extensive surgery, with possible morbidity and mortality, the adoption of the course suggested by Knapp and Feldman would appear to be justified. Unfortunately, there seems little prospect of such a sensible course being accepted; only those who feel that the verdict of CIS is still unproved would adopt such a proposal. The convinced will continue, as they now do, to practice more extensive surgical treatment.

Microinvasive Carcinoma of the Cervix

Carcinoma in situ with microinvasive foci is defined by Boyes and associates[18] as being "confined to those lesions in which one or more small invasive tongues of cells have broken through the basement membrane. They are usually multiple, but in no place do they produce a confluent lesion."

Morton[19] considers that the depth of involvement must not exceed 5 mm. in the stroma. Others[20,21] quoted by Boyes as using the terms "microinvasive" or "early invasive cancer" have used the criteria suggested by Morton. In Ontario the definition of Boyes is accepted by both pathologist and clinician.[22,23] It may be said that there is agreement that such lesions may be treated as carcinoma in situ unless the microscopic foci occur in close proximity to or involve lymphatics or blood vessels. In these circumstances, they are considered as truly invasive carcinoma and treated as such either by irradiation, by surgery, or by a combination of both.

According to TNM (tumor, nodes, metastasis) classification of carcinoma of the cervix of the Union Internationale Contre le Cancer, microinvasive and other *invasive lesions which cannot be recognized* except by histological examination fall into group TIa (Stage 1a).* Another synonymous term is occult carcinoma of the cervix. It is or seems to be important to differentiate between this group and those classified as TIb lesions, which are clinically recognizable invasive tumors confined to the cervix. This division of TI (Stage 1) lesions has some bearing upon the methods of treatment and the results of therapy. This classification has not been used long enough in our clinics to supply any firm conclusions at the present time.

EXPERIENCE IN ONTARIO

In the years 1968 to 1970, 194 patients classified as TIa (Stage 1a) (microinvasive, and occult) were reported from our clinics, The Princess Margaret Hospital, and clinic and teaching hospital registries. The bulk of these (150, or 77.3 per cent of the total) were treated at or reported from our clinics or The Princess Margaret Hospital. The treatment varied, depending upon the institution providing the information, and was complete in 191 of 194 patients.

Surgical treatment was elected in 67 or 35.1 per cent of patients with information recorded; the largest proportion of these were from the clinic or teaching hospital registries. Radiotherapy was the method of choice in 110 patients, or 57.6 per cent, all of whom were from our clinics or The Princess Margaret Hospital. Combined surgery and radiotherapy was employed in 14 patients or 7.3 per cent. In the greater percentage of the latter, the invasive character of the lesions was discovered postoperatively on histological examination of the surgical speci-

---

* Classification of American Joint Committee for Cancer Staging and End Results (1963).

men. Presumably adjunctive treatment with radiotherapy was employed to provide more adequate treatment for surgery, which was less than extended hysterectomy.

MORTALITY.   Six patients died, of whom five had received treatment; one of these died of cerebrovascular accident at 89 years of age. Two deaths occurred owing to recurrent or metastatic disease in patients treated by radiotherapy, and two deaths occurred in the group treated by surgery or a combination of surgery and radiotherapy. The information obtainable in respect to this group of patients is necessarily incomplete at the present time. Further follow-up will be necessary to evaluate the management of these patients, as well as those who have been treated subsequently. In the patients treated surgically, the age of the patient seemed to be the major consideration for the selection of this mode of treatment. The younger patients were treated surgically. The older or postmenopausal patients were treated by radiotherapy.

COMMENT

From this small series with admittedly inadequate follow-up, the crude mortality rate to date has been six patients or 3.1 per cent. There is no obvious difference between the results of surgery or radiotherapy. It is at the present time difficult to assess fairly the achievement or failure of the different methods of therapy. Further study and follow-up may demonstrate significant differences in results, which may justify changes in treatment regimens.

There is, as noted above, a tendency to apply surgery in the treatment of younger patients. In the greater number of the Foundation's Treatment Centers, treatment is decided after consultation between radiologists and gynecologists. In some instances, for a variety of reasons, the decision is made unilaterally, without prior consultation, a course which is undesirable. The best treatment, irrespective of the personal feelings or prejudices of gynecologist or radiologist, is achieved when both have mutual respect and have confidence in each other's judgment and competence.

TI (Stage 1) Carcinoma of the Cervix

Results of radiotherapeutic treatment have been reported annually for some years from all our clinics, except The Princess Margaret Hospital, to the Cancer Committee of the International Federation of Gynaecology and Obstetrics. Five year survival rates are now available from patients seen in the period between 1960 and 1966 at both our clinics and The Princess Margaret Hospital.

In that period of time in some (but not in all) clinics, division between lesions classified as TIa and TIb was recorded. As a consequence, this report will present only the results of treatment of *all* TI cervical lesions.

It is worth recording that in his introduction to the symposium on invasive carcinoma of the cervix, Peckham[24] stated: "It is sad but true that the number of cobalt teletherapy units in the United States far exceeds the number of competent radiotherapists, just as the total number of radical hysterectomies performed for invasive carcinoma of the cervix each year exceeds the number performed in a satisfactory manner. Once initiated, unsatisfactory therapy can neither be supplemented nor altered successfully." Peckham's comments in this respect, at least where Ontario and Canada as a whole are concerned, do not apply.

In the 10 provinces of Canada adequate, competent radiotherapeutic services are now available and these have been available in nine for many years. In the majority of university centers and elsewhere, a limited number of gynecologists with adequate training and clinical competence perform major operations for sound treatment of gynecological cancer. It speaks well for the conscience of the medical profession that the vast majority of surgical procedures for these malignant conditions are performed by individuals competent to render good service to patients and public. This may be *one* of the *relatively few* benefits of the gross intrusion of government into the field of medical care in this country.

In assessing the relative advantages of radiotherapy vs. surgery in the treatment of carcinoma of the cervix, we must appreciate that radiotherapy is—or should be—employed at present in the majority of patients with carcinoma of the cervix. In reality, surgery is used primarily in the treatment of early lesions—those with limited extension or, more rarely, in T4 lesions with central disease. Both methods have advantages in competent hands. In Ontario it may be said that there is reasonable agreement between the therapeutic radiologist and oncological gynecologist with regard to the utilization of their respective methods of management.

The TI (Stage 1) patients seen at the Foundation's clinics and The Princess Margaret Hospital from 1960 through 1966 numbered 1209. Of these, 931 or 77 per cent survived for five years.

Ten year survival rates are available from some but not all of the treatment centers at the present time.

There are few reports of surgical treatment of TI (Stage 1) cervical lesions reported from Canada. In 1969 Bean and associates reported the results of the treatment of 148 patients of all stages from the Toronto General Hospital.[25] Of these, 110 were patients classified as having TI (Stage 1) lesions. Of those 61 at risk for five years, 40 were alive and well, 14 were lost to follow-up and seven were known to be dead—a five year salvage rate of 65.6 per cent.

Unfortunately, there were no statistics quoted for patients treated primarily by surgery. The indications for surgical treatment were pregnancy, adenocarcinoma, and failed radiotherapy. The period covered by their report and that of the treatment centers are different. In the intervening time, improvement in both methods of management has occurred. It would be of interest to compare the results for the same periods of time. The low rate of loss of patients to follow-up in the study of Bean and colleagues is some indication of the excellence of follow-up at the Foundation's centers. This may again indicate another benefit of a government service and its facilities, as opposed to that of solo practitioners, albeit in a university center.

COMMENT

The study of available information does not permit fair comparison of results in these two series. It does demonstrate a very satisfactory five year survival rate in patients treated by radiotherapy. There are circumstances in which age, pregnancy, and early or late complications may influence the treatment modality to be employed. In a well organized treatment center with adequate pretreatment consultation, the patient does and should benefit from this consideration. Disagreement and controversy between gynecologists and therapeutic radiologists have decreased in recent years, and greater appreciation of the potentialities and indications for treatment in both disciplines should result in enhanced benefit to our patients.

Conclusions

Further prospective studies should determine the natural history of carcinoma in situ. In the meantime, a trend toward more conservative management of this condition has become apparent. It should be increased and encouraged. Until more definitive knowledge is obtained, many women will undergo unwarranted radical treatment.

In TI (Stage 1) lesions, either approach should produce satisfactory results if properly employed. The method used should depend upon the adequacy of the professional services available to the individual patient. Hopefully, controversy in this area will disappear in the near future.

REFERENCES

1. Savage, E. W.: Microinvasive carcinoma of the cervix. Amer. J. Obstet. Gynec. *113*:708, 1972.
2. Koss, L. G.: Significance of dysplasia. Clin. Obstet. Gynec. *13*:874, 1970.
3. Hulme, G. W., and Eisenberg, H. S.: Carcinoma in situ of the cervix in Connecticut. A review. 1949–1962. Amer. J. Obstet. Gynec. *102*:415, 1968.
4. Cox, B. S.: Carcinoma in situ of the cervix uteri. J. Obstet. Gynec. Brit. Comm. *74*:723, 1967.
5. Knox, E. G.: Screening in medical care. Oxford, Nuffield Provincial Hospital Trust, 1968.
6. Green, G. H.: Invasive potentiality of cervical carcinoma in situ. Int. J. Gynec. Obstet. 7:157, 1969.
7. Way, S., Hennigan, M., and Wright, V. C.: Some experiences with preinvasive and microinvasive carcinoma of the cervix. J. Obstet. Gynec. Brit. Comm. 75:593, 1968.
8. MacKay, E. A.: Personal communication.
9. Hollyock, V. E., and Chanen, W.: The use of the colposcope in the selection of patients for cervical cone biopsy. Amer. J. Obstet. Gynec. *114*:185, 1972.
10. Townsend, D. E., Ostergard, D. R., Mishell, D. R., and Hirose, F. M.: Abnormal Papanicolaou smears. Evaluation by colposcopy biopsies and endocervical curettage. Amer. J. Obstet. Gynec. *108*:429, 1970.
11. Lickrish, G.: Personal communication.
12. Kramer, W. M., and Kay, S.: Anaplasia clinic—aid in the diagnosis and treatment of preinvasive cervical lesions. Cancer 20:202, 1967.
13. Knapp, R. C., and Feldman, G. B.: The problem of optimal management of carcinoma in situ. Clin. Obstet. Gynec. *13*:889, 1970.
14. Miller, A. B.: Personal communications.
15. Sackett, D. L.: Personal communications.
16. Personal reports from Professors of Obstetrics and Gynecology in Ontario medical faculties.
17. Cannell, D. E.: Unpublished reports.
18. Boyes, D. A., Worth, A. J., and Fidler, H. K.: The results of treatment of 4389 cases of preclinical and cervical squamous carcinoma. J. Obstet. Gynec. Brit. Comm. 77:769, 1970.
19. Morton, D. G.: Incipient carcinoma of the cervix. Amer. J. Obstet. Gynec. 90:60, 1964.
20. Mussey, et al.: Microinvasive carcinoma of the cervix. Late results of operative treatment of 91 cases. Amer. J. Obstet. Gynec. *104*:738, 1969.
21. Levitt, S. H., and Rubin, P.: Early invasive carcinoma of the cervix. Radiology 85:711, 1965.
22. Thompson, D.: Personal communication.
23. Allan, H.: Personal communication.
24. Peckham, B. M.: Invasive carcinoma of the cervix. Clin. Obstet. Gynec. 10:881, 1967.
25. Bean, J., et al.: Results of surgical treatment of carcinoma of the cervix. Amer. J. Obstet. Gynec. *103*:465, 1969.

Diagnosis and Management of
(a) In Situ (Stage O), (b) Microinvasive,
and (c) Stage I of Cancer of the Cervix

John L. Lewis, Jr., and James H. Freel

Memorial Sloan-Kettering Cancer Center

There is now general agreement that carcinoma in situ, microinvasive carcinoma, and Stage I carcinoma of the cervix represent a continuum of diseases that occur both sequentially and at times simultaneously in relatively young women.[1] Much of the controversy with regard to treatment of these conditions arises from difficulty in establishing clear borderlines between the diagnostic categories. It is axiomatic that the natural history, likelihood of spread, and consequently the proper therapy of a cervical cancer in an individual patient will be based on the most advanced lesion found in the biopsy specimen. For this reason, logical combination of cytologic smears, colposcopic exam, punch biopsies of nonstaining areas of the cervix, endocervical curettage, and cold knife conization of the cervix are necessary if the true diagnosis is to be established and appropriate therapy given. Although there is little disagreement as to the diagnosis of carcinoma in situ and Stage Ib invasive carcinoma of the cervix (in which there is a visible lesion and frankly invasive tumor limited to the cervix), the disease intermediate between these two categories raise many questions, not only of definition but also concerning the proper methods for diagnosis and treatment. We will try to outline these differences and then discuss our current management.

Although it is not our purpose to propose any new classifications for cervical cancer, another way of looking at these diseases is to divide them into (1) those which have a grossly visible lesion, that is, Stage Ib carcinoma of the cervix, and (2) those with an invisible lesion, which would include every condition that precedes frankly invasive carcinoma with a visible lesion. The anatomy of the cervix is such that it can be seen and palpated, and its exfoliated cells can be examined cytologically by the Papanicolaou technique. This enables one to diagnose a nonvisible, invasive lesion of the cervix or a precursor such as carcinoma in situ or dysplasia. It is the cytologic exam, which has had great success in detecting asymptomatic invisible cervical cancer or its precursor states, which has resulted in the decreased death rates from cervical cancer in women who have regular examinations.[2] There is now evidence that dysplasia of the cervix is an even earlier stage of cervical neoplasia than carcinoma in situ, and presumably its eradication by local treatment such as cryosurgery or cauterization will prevent the ultimate development of carcinoma in situ and invasive cancer of the cervix.[3,4]

The usefulness of the cytologic examination of exfoliated cells in detecting early lesions has led to a false sense of security in some physicians. Although its false positive rate is negligible, a single cytologic exam has an up to 5 per cent false negative rate even in the face of invasive cancer. Because of this, any visible lesion of the cervix should be biopsied at the time of first examination rather than relying on a cytologic exam to establish its true nature. Similarly, a negative result on a cytologic exam has often been considered to be evidence that a woman does not have a pelvic malignancy. Since a cervical scraping will be positive in less than 40 per cent of women with endometrial carcinoma and less than 1 per cent of those with ovarian carcinoma, it follows that proper screening for pelvic malignancy must include not only a thorough history and complete physical examination but also other diagnostic procedures in addition to a Papanicolaou smear. This same reasoning can be used to discourage self-administered cytologic exams. Finally, the growing body of evidence that most cervical neoplasms progress very slowly from the stage of dysplasia to carcinoma in situ to early invasive cancer of the cervix should not lull one into feeling that it is always possible to treat these early lesions at one's leisure. There are now several studies from the Scandinavian countries in which closed populations of women had annual screening exams and invasive lesions of the cervix were found to have developed within a year of obtaining a negative cytologic exam.

The technique of colposcpy has added precision to the evaluation of patients with nonvisible lesions of the cervix. Following others' leadership, we have now established a colposcopy clinic for evaluation of patients with abnormal Papanicolaou smears. Since early cervical neoplasms develop in the transition zone found at the squamocolumnar junction, this instrument is most useful when the squamocolumnar junction and the entire transition zone are visible, that is, when the lesions are located on the ectocervix and possibly extend onto the vaginal fornices. It is of limited use when the lesion is located entirely in the endocervical canal or when a margin extends into the canal. This limitation can be overcome with an endocervical curettage utilizing a small, sharp curette which does not require dilatation of the cervix. In our experience, the benefits of colposcopy have included the identification of the source of abnormal Papanicolaou smears, selection of appropriate sites for punch biopsies, and the mapping out of the distribution of abnormal epithelium, which should be removed at the time of either cold knife conization of hysterectomy. Its use has decreased the necessity for conizations in the evaluation of mild and moderate dysplasias. We have continued to utilize cold knife conization when the diagnosis of severe dysplasia or carcinoma in situ has been made on the basis of colposcopically directed punch biopsies or when the epithelial lesion extends into the endocervical canal.

Carcinoma In Situ

Carcinoma in situ of the cervix is a neoplastic lesion of squamous epithelium in which undifferentiated cells extend from the basal layer through the entire thickness of the squamous epithelium. Although there may be rare situations in which some pathologists will use this term to refer to lesions in which there is minimal differentiation on the surface, general agreement relegates the term to severe forms of dysplasia. The important therapeutic observation in this disease is that it is curable by removing all of the abnormal epithelium, whether by conization or by hysterectomy. Experimental studies are now being performed in which the abnormal epithelium is destroyed with either cauterization or cryosurgery, but longer follow-up periods will be necessary before this method of treatment can be relied upon.[3,4] It should be emphasized that these studies are appropriate in centers which have specialists involved who not only utilize reliable cytologic evaluation but also are experienced in the use of colposcopy, endocervical curettage. and thermal destruction of the lesions.

Although cytologic evaluation is reliable in determining whether there is an abnormality of squamous epithelium of the cervix, in most hands this technique is not reliable in determining the exact nature of the lesion. For this reason, histologic diagnosis is utilized for determining the exact nature of the disease. We now see the patient who has an abnormal Papanicolaou smear in the colposcopy clinic and take punch biopsies from the areas showing the greatest abnormality, and we also perform an endocervical curettage. Practitioners who do not have colposcopy available should rely on staining the cervix and upper vagina with Lugol's stain and then taking biopsies of the nonstaining areas. Again, endocervical curettage is recommended, for it can establish the dagnosis of a more advanced lesion in the endocervix. Taking a biopsy of the junction of the staining and nonstaining areas assures one of getting at least some tissue from the transformation zone. If the punch biopsy shows carcinoma in situ, our current policy is to carry out a cold knife conization as well as a fractional dilatation and curettage to rule out any foci of invasion.

Treatment of carcinoma in situ depends upon several factors. Not the least important of these factors is the desire of the woman to preserve the uterus, whether for reproductive function or for emotional or psychological reasons. Although a total hysterectomy with removal of the entire lesion of the cervix and any extension onto the vaginal fornices has been the usual practice in the United States, it should be recognized that this practice is considered too radical by gynecologists in most other countries. We feel that conization alone can be utilized if the following criteria are met:

1. The entire lesion is encompassed in the conization specimen and there is no evidence of disease at the surgical margins;

2. The endocervical curettage is negative; and

3. The patient is reliable and is motivated to return for the necessary follow-up, including cytologic examinations.

Since cervical neoplasms tend to develop in women who have been very active sexually and often in women of early parity, many patients request simple hysterectomy, by either the abdominal or the vaginal route, not only because they wish to end the possibility of further childbearing but also to avoid the 15 to 30 per cent rate of persistence of disease found in hysterectomy specimens after conization.[5] It is not clear whether these same rates occur when the margins are carefully inspected histologically and endocervical curettage has been carried out. Regardless of the type of therapy utilized, these patients should be examined at three monthly intervals for the first year and every six months thereafter because of the frequency of subsequent development of the same lesions in the vagina.

Although carcinoma in situ has been shown to progress to invasive cancer in a leisurely fashion in most patients, it is our clinical impression that carcinoma in situ arising in previously irradiated tissue does not follow this same chronology. This is particularly pertinent following successful irradiations of an invasive cancer of the cervix.

Microinvasive Carcinoma of the Cervix

There is probably no area in the field of gynecologic oncology in which there is as much confusion in definition and uncertainty as to proper therapy as in patients who have a nonvisible lesion of the cervix with extension of neoplastic cells into the superficial stroma of the cervix. Even the term "microinvasive" means different things to different reliable investigators.[6] To some gynecologists, microinvasion implies all those lesions in which there is invasion but in which no visible lesion is present. Thus, to these, "microinvasive" means the stage of invasive cancer in which the diagnosis is made only by microscopic examination. Others call "microinvasive" only those lesions in which the neoplastic cells have extended no further than a certain distance into the stroma. Even here, different investigators set different limits. Differences arise according to the significance of involvement of lymphatic channels, vascular channels, or the presence of growth patterns termed "confluence." Similarly, there is no agreement as to whether the measurement should be made from the surface of the epithelium, the basement membrane, or the nearest endocervical gland involved with carcinoma in situ. There is agreement that involvement of endocervical glands alone does not constitute invasion.

The Cancer Committee of the International Federation of Gynecologists and Obstetricians has proposed a subdivision of Stage I carcinoma of the cervix, in which those patients who do not have a visible lesion and in whom no cancer is found on endocervical curettage are grouped in Stage Ia, and all other patients with invasive cancer of the cervix are grouped in Stage Ib. Stage Ia is further divided into Stage Ia$_1$, in which there is only early stromal invasion, and Stage Ia$_2$, in which there is occult cancer. One interpretation of Stage Ia$_1$, illustrated in Figure 16-1, shows a breakthrough of a tongue of invasive neoplastic cells through the basement membrane, but in which there is continuity with the overlying carcinoma in situ. This is our own interpretation of early stromal invasion, but it should be recognized that not everyone agrees with this. Stage Ia$_2$ similarly is interpreted in Figure 16-1, as an area of invasion at various depths below the basement membrane without any apparent connection to the overlying layer of carcinoma in situ. It should be obvious that these early lesions of the cervix can only be made properly by careful study of a conization specimen. This must include free margins. In addition, there is the obvious problem of tangential cuts, which make neoplastic cells which are still in contact with overlying epithelium appear to be invasive.

The apparent interest in subdividing the early lesions of invasive carcinoma of the cervix is to determine if there are degrees of invasion in which the likelihood of undiagnosed local extension or metastases to lymph nodes is so low that

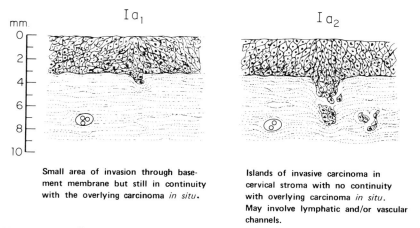

Small area of invasion through basement membrane but still in continuity with the overlying carcinoma *in situ*.

Islands of invasive carcinoma in cervical stroma with no continuity with overlying carcinoma *in situ*. May involve lymphatic and/or vascular channels.

Figure 16-1.   Illustration of an interpretation of the two substages of the classification of Stage Ia carcinoma of the cervix: Stage Ia$_1$, early stromal invasion; and Stage Ia$_2$, "occult" cancer.

the disease can be treated successfully with a simple hysterectomy—that is, as if it were no more significant than carcinoma in situ. It is our opinion that the final answer is not available at this time. Our own policy is to treat with simple hysterectomy those patients with Stage Ia carcinoma of the cervix who meet the following criteria: invasion limited to tongues of tissue extending through the basement membrane, but with continuity to the overlying carcinoma in situ; or presence of islands of invasion which extend no deeper than 1 mm. from the basement membrane and do not show evidence of lymphatic or vascular permeation. Whether less rigid criteria for conservative management will be acceptable is a matter which is being widely investigated. This is clearly a gray area, in which one often must make a decision on the basis of incomplete information, even to deciding which of two possible errors is more acceptable: to overtreat some lesions with the possible risks of complications or to undertreat some lesions and lose the opportunity for cure.

Stage I Carcinoma of the Cervix

Stage I carcinoma of the cervix includes those cases with a gross lesion which can be diagnosed by biopsy or endocervical curettage and also the non-visible lesions included in Stage Ia. If a visible lesion is biopsied and the diagnosis is invasive carcinoma, there is no indication for conization, a procedure that not only requires an extra anesthesia but also increases the risk for morbidity in subsequent therapy, whether this is carried out by means of radical surgery or radiation therapy. When conization is carried out as a diagnostic procedure prior to either a simple or a radical hysterectomy, the definitive procedure is performed within 48 hours of the conization. If this is not feasible, we delay surgery 6 weeks to allow complete healing not only of the cervix but also of the inflammatory changes in the parametrium and pelvic side walls.

All clinical staging of patients with invasive carcinoma of the cervix is carried out under anesthesia, and all procedures are done in conjunction with members of the Department of Radiation Therapy. If a previous punch biopsy of a visible lesion has shown invasive carcinoma, the procedure consists of careful inspection and palpation, a dilatation and curettage to rule out pyometrium or an unlikely second primary lesion, cystoscopy, and proctoscopy. Particular attention is paid to palpation of the urethra and bladder base while the cystoscope is still in place in order to detect early anterior spread.

The choice of appropriate therapy for patients with Stage Ib carcinoma of the cervix is a matter for careful consideration and honest evaluation of the facilities and skills available. Whether therapy is carried out by means of radical hysterectomy and pelvic lymphadenectomy or by a combination of intracavitary and external radiation therapy, there can be no question but that the results will be better if treatment is given on a service specializing in cancer care. This need not be a hospital devoted solely to cancer, but there should be gynecologists and radiation therapists with special training, skills, and equipment available in order to attain maximal cure rate.

In the past, there have been strong advocates of either a purely surgical or a purely radiotherapeutic approach to invasive carcinoma of the cervix. Many of these debates or arguments generated more hostility than information. It is obvious that cancer care for all malignancies will be best when radiation therapists and gynecologic oncologists cooperate in an effort to determine the best form of treatment for each individual patient, as well as for each stage of cancer of the cervix. Randomized studies utilizing either radiation therapy or surgery for Stage I carcinoma of the cervix have been shown to give equal results in terms of survival rates.[7] Unfortunately, efforts to predict responsiveness to one treatment modality or the other either have not proved consistent or have been extremely difficult to reproduce.

One of the major problems in determining the likelihood of cure of a patient with cervical cancer is the uncertainty of determining the presence of metastatic disease in lymph nodes prior to therapy. In Stage Ia lesions with minimal invasion, the likelihood is very small, but as one progresses to Stage Ib lesions, the incidence of lymph node metastases increases to as high as 20 per cent. Although there is evidence that these nodes will be cleared of cancer in some patients with radiation therapy, the persistence of positive nodes after full radiation therapy remains a source of worry. Lymphangiograms have not been consistently reliable in our hands for predicting the presence of lymph node metastases. This is owing to their inability to demonstrate small metastatic deposits as well as their failure to stain nodes which are completely replaced by tumor.

Although we utilize radiation therapy as our primary treatment in patients with advanced cancer of the cervix, it is our current policy to carry out a radical hysterectomy and bilateral pelvic lymphadenectomy in most patients with Stage I and Stage IIa carcinoma of the cervix. As a general guideline, we utilize this in women under the age of 60 who have no health problem which would increase the risks from anesthesia or the surgical procedure. Without going into the technical details, we feel that this operation requires the removal of the uterus, cervix, and upper third of the vagina with an *en bloc* dissection of the paravaginal and paracervical tissues as far lateral as the hypogastric vessels. It also requires the removal of the posterior extension of the parametrium from the presacral region and also the complete excision of lymph nodes in the common iliac, external iliac, obturator, hypogastric, and parametrial chains. Although the complication rate after this surgery is higher than that after good radiation therapy, the fact is that surgical complications are decreasing in incidence and are more amenable to correction than the infrequent but serious complications of radiation therapy. It might be noted that in the last 60 consecutive radical hysterectomies and pelvic lymph node dissections carried out as primary therapy for invasive carcinoma of the cervix on the Gynecology Service at Memorial Hospital, there has not been a single urinary tract or gastrointestinal tract fistula created.

Summary

Early neoplasms of the cervix are viewed as a continuum beginning with dysplasia and carcinoma in situ and extending to frankly invasive carcinoma of the cervix with a visible lesion. There is a spectrum of disease between carcinoma in situ and Stage Ib carcinoma of the cervix; in these it may be possible to identify lesions in which the likelihood of local spread or lymph node metastases is so small that the lesions can be successfully treated as if they were only carcinoma in situ. An outline of appropriate diagnostic measures is given and our current treatment protocol is discussed.

REFERENCES

1. Richart, R.: Natural history of cervical intraepithelial neoplasia. Modern Treatment 5:748, 1968.
2. Boyes, D. A., Worth, A. J., and Fidler, H. K.: The results of treatment of 4389 cases of pre-clinical cervical squamous carcinomas. J. Obstet. Gynec. Brit. Comm. 77:769, 1970.
3. Richart, R. M., and Sciarra, J. J.: Treatment of cervical dysplasia by outpatient electro-cauterization. Am. J. Obstet. Gynec. 101:200, 1968.
4. Ortiz, R., Newton, M., and Tsai, A.: Electro-cautery treatment of cervical intraepithelial neoplasia. Obstet. Gynec. 41:113, 1973.
5. Singleton, W. P., and Rutledge, F.: To cone or not to cone—the cervix. Obstet. Gynec. 31:430, 1968.
6. Savage, E. W.: Microinvasive carcinoma of the cervix. Am. J. Obstet. Gynec. 113:708, 1972.
7. Newton, M., Hickman, B. T., and Bolten, K. A.: Radical hysterectomy versus radiotherapy in Stage I cervical cancer: preliminary results. Obstet. Gynec. 24:503, 1964.

Diagnosis and Management of
(a) In Situ (Stage O), (b) Microinvasive,
and (c) Stage I of Cancer of the Cervix

GEORGE D. WILBANKS
Rush Medical College

Introduction

Early cervical neoplasia continues to be an important and often perplexing clinical entity. Deaths from cervical cancer have decreased 10 to 15 years after institution of intensive Papanicolaou smear screening programs. However, the rate of occurrence of cervical cancer in all patients has decreased only slightly, but this has been accompanied by an increase in the percentage of patients who are found to have early lesions, i.e., carcinoma in situ, microinvasive cancer, and Stage I cancer.[2,6,11,15] Dysplasia, which is the earliest recognizable stage of this continuum of cervical neoplasia, continues to occur at approximately the same rate.[13] Although it is not feasible to go into the details of the biology and epidemiology of the lesions discussed in this chapter, their backgrounds should be familiar to all who manage patients with this disease. The most recent assessment was that of the Conference on Early Cervical Neoplasia.[15]

The suspicion of these early lesions originates mainly from an abnormal Papanicolaou smear, which should lead to definitive diagnostic studies and treatment. However, it is of utmost importance in the diagnosis and management of these lesions that the clinician know the methods of reporting and the accuracy of the pathology laboratory with which he deals. Many experts have stressed this matter of accuracy of diagnosis, but it bears repeating in any discussion of this disease. The cytology report should indicate some diagnosis of the lesion suspected. Biopsy specimens must be properly labeled and oriented to give perpendicular sections. Ideally, step serial sections should be made from cone biopsies, and as a minimum, the whole specimen must be blocked and sections made every 2 to 3 mm. The clinician should review personally all borderline lesions with the pathologist.

As a basis for this discussion, carcinoma in situ is defined classically as those lesions in which the undifferentiated neoplastic cells extend throughout the entire thickness of the epithelium. However, theoretically and practically, we prefer to consider the disease as comprising a spectrum beginning with mild dysplasia and ending with invasive carcinoma. Patients with severe dysplasia are managed in a manner similar to those with carcinoma in situ.

The abnormal Papanicolaou smear indicates the need for further evaluation of the cervix; even the most accurate cytologic evaluation needs tissue study before definitive management is begun. Ideally, the specimen should be only the minimal amount of tissue, obtained by the simplest technique, required to give an accurate diagnosis. The technique for obtaining the specimen should be generally applicable to the practice of the majority of physicians who treat patients with carcinoma in situ. Younge has been able to do this successfully with the unaided eye, Schiller's stain, and multiple punch biopsies.[14] Colposcopically directed biopsies, with or without endocervical curettage, are other successful methods of diagnosis.[15] Each requires special training or special equipment. Cold knife conization has become the accepted diagnostic method, but it is by no means perfect. The "planned" cold knife conization must be designed for the specific cervix and include a liberal margin around affected epithelium, on both the exocervix and the endocervix. The cone must be oriented and blocked properly and sufficient sections taken.

Carcinoma In Situ

Treatment of carcinoma in situ ideally would consist of local removal of the lesion. However, in practice, most series indicate that residual neoplasms are found in the hysterectomy specimen removed following cold knife conization in from 10 to 50 per cent of the patients. Therefore the definitive treatment should be hysterectomy with a liberal vaginal cuff. Ovarian function may be preserved. Treatment may be individualized to the patient if the management is planned from the outset. A young woman who desires further childbearing may have a therapeutic conization. If the cone specimen shows ample margins of normal epithelium, the patient may be followed carefully by repeat Papanicolaou smears and allowed to have her family. However, no matter what the treatment, recurrences or new primary lesions in the lower genital tract (vagina and vulva) are more frequent than in the population at large, so these patients must be followed indefinitely. Boyes and associates[1] found further disease (carcinoma in situ to invasive cancer) in 1.9 per cent of 1192 patients who had been followed for five years after treatment for carcinoma in situ and in 8.2 per cent of 233 patients followed for 10 years.

Irradiation has been used successfully in patients who are not surgical candidates. Del Regato and Cox[4] treated 27 patients with carcinoma in situ using transvaginal roentgen therapy. Within the range of follow-up from 2 to 16 years, no patients developed invasive cancer, although one had persistent carcinoma in situ with microinvasion. Two patients became pregnant and delivered normal babies. Although it is not the ideal treatment, this method should be known to those who treat patients with carcinoma in situ.

Electrocautery has also been used successfully as treatment. Younge[14] has followed 22 patients from 9 to 19 years after treatment of carcinoma in situ with extensive, complete electrocauterization and has had no recurrences. Richart and

Sciarra[9] treated 170 patients with cervical dysplasia using similar electrocauterization techniques. In 151 patients (89 per cent), the lesion was eradicated with the first treatment, 19 (11 per cent) required a second treatment, and two had persistent disease requiring conization or hysterectomy. Electrocautery may serve as therapy for special situations when it is desirable to postpone definitive surgery.

Cryosurgery of the cervix is the most recent nonoperative method of treatment of early cervical neoplasia. The technique has been reported primarily for treatment of dysplasia, but it has been used successfully for a few patients with carcinoma in situ. A recently symposium[12] indicates that cryosurgery is a simple, painless technique which appears successful in preliminary studies. It requires precise preoperative evaluation, utilizing colposcopically directed biopsies, with or without endocervical curettage. Final analysis of the immediate and long term results of this therapy requires further critical evaluation and longer follow-up. If proved successful, cryosurgery would be economical in saving time as well as money and in addition offer low risk for the patient.

Microinvasion

The diagnosis of "microinvasion" can only be made on an adequate cone specimen which is studied by step serial sections. The exact definition of "microinvasion" has varied in the past, but concepts as outlined by Boyes and colleagues[1] are generally accepted. They define "carcinoma in situ with microinvasive foci" as those lesions in which "one or more discrete small invasive tongues of cells have broken through the basement membrane." A confluent lesion or permeation of lymphatic vessels is regarded and treated as Stage Ia. The key issue in the definition of microinvasion relates to the correlation of the disease so defined with the occurrence of metastases in the regional nodes and ultimately recurrence, or persistence, after simple therapy. In a review of the literature, Savage[10] selected 580 patients with variously defined "microinvasions" who had pelvic nodes available for study. Only 7 (1.2 per cent) had positive nodes. There were no positive nodes in 71 of these patients whose lesion penetrated 4 mm. or less. Because of the rare metastases from microinvasion, simply hysterectomy with liberal vaginal cuff is adequate treatment for microinvasion when the lesions are so defined. Boyes and associates[1] had three recurrences in 205 patients, 88 of whom were followed more than five years. Parker had no recurrences in 34 patients so treated, with 11 being followed more than five years.[15] The hysterectomy specimen should be examined similarly to the cone biopsy for evidence of possible residual neoplasia. The patient must be followed carefully, for epithelial neoplasias in the genital tract occur more frequently in these patients than in a control population.

Stage I

Stage I carcinoma of the cervix is now divided into Stages Ia and Ib. Stage Ia is occult carcinoma in which there is no visible lesion, the diagnosis being made by pathologic study, usually cold knife conization. Stage Ib is the clinically visible lesion which is confined to the cervix. Once Stage Ia is reached in the progression of cervical neoplasia, the occurrence of metastases to the lymph nodes and recurrences or persistence after conservative therapy necessitate radical treatment of the paracervical tissue and pelvic lymph nodes.[1]

The debate continues as to the efficacy of irradiation therapy versus radical surgery in these lesions. Proponents of both modalities have good results with low complication rates. Until a randomized, double blind study is performed, the final answer cannot be given. Newton and co-workers[7] do report a small randomized series of patient with Stage I disease treated by either radiation or radical hysterectomy. In the 70 patients followed for more than two years, the results are comparable in each group.

Radical surgery has the disadvantage of being a major operative procedure with possible genitourinary complications. It cannot be utilized in all patients. Surgery has the advantages of preserving ovarian function and allowing evaluation of the extent of the disease. Radiation carcinogenesis on residual pelvic organs and radiation destruction of pelvic marrow do not occur.

Radiation therapy has the advantages of being almost universally applicable to all patients, of requiring minimal anesthesia, and of lacking immediate complications. However, late bowel complications and pelvic fibrosis may occur. The current studies on the merits of the new high intensity sources of irradiation and the various techniques of application have not extended over long enough periods for conclusive evaluation, but use of these high intensities may increase late complications as well as increase survival rates.

Late recurrences after irradiation therapy, the possibility of irradiation induced carcinomas of other pelvic structures, the destruction of pelvic bone marrow, and the destruction of ovarian function suggest that young patients (35 and under) with Stage Ia and early Ib lesions should be treated surgically. The Duke University series[8] showed a slightly better salvage rate in patients treated surgically in the group followed 10 to 22 years. These young patients also have the potential for sufficient longevity that carcinomas may be a threat 15 to 20 years after radiation therapy. Although statistically difficult to substantiate, the findings of several studies indicate that patients may have recurrent cervical lesions or other pelvic tumors[3,5] as a result of radiation therapy undergone many years previously. Also, the patients treated 15 to 20 years ago received lower doses of radiation than currently used. Radiation carcinogenesis varies with the amount of irradiation given, so this problem may increase in the future.

Therefore, patients with Stage I cervical carcinomas should be carefully staged and discussed individually in conference with a competent gynecologic oncologist and radiation therapist. The above factors, plus any other relevant problems, such as fibroids or other pelvic masses or disease, must be considered in treatment plans.

Summary

The diagnosis of all forms of early cervical neoplasia (dysplasia, carcinoma in situ, microinvasion, and Stage Ia) requires evaluation by careful pathologic study of a well designed cold knife conization, or, perhaps, colposcopically directed biopsies. Treatment of carcinoma in situ and severe dysplasia is hysterectomy with a vaginal cuff. In special situations, therapeutic cold knife conization may be employed. Other methods of local destruction of the diseased epithelium, such as irradiation, electrocautery, or, most recently, cryosurgery, may be used in individual problem patients. However, universal acceptance of any of these techniques requires further evaluation and time in follow-up. Microinvasion seems safely treated as carcinoma in situ when defined as one or more discrete small invasive tongues of cells that have broken through the basement membrane, without confluence or vascular space involvement. Once the disease is classified as Stage I, the treatment must involve radical therapy and inclusion of regional lymph nodes. Radiation therapy is universally applicable to invasive cancers, but there are indications for radical surgery in selected young patients with early Stage I lesions. All patients with these forms of early cervical neoplasia should have careful evaluation of the extent of the lesion and individualized therapy by teams of physicians who have expertise in all modalities of therapy. Long-term, careful follow-up of these patients is mandatory.

REFERENCES

1. Boyes, D. A., Worth, A. J., and Fidler, H. K.: The results of treatment of 4389 cases of pre-clinical cervical squamous carcinoma. J. Obstet. Gynec. Brit. Comm. 7:769, 1970.
2. Christopherson, W. M., Mendex, W. M., and Ahuja, E. M.: Cervix cancer control in Louisville, Kentucky. Cancer 26:29, 1970.
3. Covington, E. E.: Recurrences of carcinoma of the cervix after 15 years. Amer. J. Obstet. Gynec. 87:471, 1963.
4. del Regato, J. A., and Cox, J. D.: Transvaginal roentgen therapy in the conservative management of carcinoma in situ of the uterine cervix. In Ackerman, L., and del Regato, J. A., eds.: Cancer: Diagnosis, Treatment and Prognosis. 4th Ed. St. Louis, C. V. Mosby Co., 1970.
5. Holan, J.: Late tumours after radiological treatment of gynecologic malignomas. A clinical study of postactinic changes with special reference to the development of so-called radiogenic tumour. Neoplasma 14:399, 1967.
6. Kolstad, P.: Cytological mass screening of a defined population. Acta Obstet. Gynec. 43(Suppl. 3):50, 1969.
7. Newton, M., Hickman, B. T., and Bolten, K. A.: Radical hysterectomy versus radiotherapy in Stage I cervical cancer; preliminary results. Obstet. Gynec. 24:563, 1964.
8. Parker, R. T., Wilbanks, G. D., Carter, B., and Yowell, R. K.: Radical hysterectomy with and without preoperative radiotherapy in the treatment of cervical cancer. A report of 265 patients followed 10–12 years. Amer. J. Obstet. Gynec. 99:933, 1967.
9. Richart, R. M., and Sciarra, J. J.: Treatment of cervical dysplasia by outpatient eletcrocauterization. Amer. J. Obstet. Gynec. 101:200, 1968.
10. Savage, E. W.: Microinvasive carcinoma of the cervix. Amer. J. Obstet. Gynec. 113:708, 1972.
11. Silverberg, E., and Holleb, A. I.: Cancer Statistics 1972. Cancer 22:2, 1972.
12. Sonek, M. G.: Cryosurgery in the treatment of abnormal cervical lesions. An invitational symposium. J. Reprod. Med. 7:147, 1971.
13. Stern, E., and Neely, P. M.: Carcinoma and dysplasia of the cervix. Acta Cytol. 6:357, 1963.
14. Younge, P. A.: The conservative treatment of carcinoma in situ of the cervix. Nat. Cancer Conf. Proc., 682, 1956.
15. Conference on Early Cervical Neoplasia, American Cancer Society, 1968. Obstet. Gynec. Surv. 24(Part 2):617, 1969.

Diagnosis and Management of
(a) In Situ (Stage O), (b) Microinvasive,
and (c) Stage I of Cancer of the Cervix

Editorial Comment

The question of how frequently women should have a cytological examination for cervical cancer detection has yet to be fully answered. The "do it yourself" method of securing material from the vagina for examination is a bow to the fact that many women, especially those in the lower economic brackets, would otherwise not be screened. While the yield of positive smears justifies use of this method, it is hardly the answer to the early identification of cancer of the female reproductive tract. In this era, marked by a trend to relinquish physician responsibility to paramedical personnel—or perhaps in an effort to fill a clinical void—individuals concerned with the care of women must be trained to obtain a working history and to do a creditable pelvic examination, including inspection and assessment of the appearance of the cervix in addition to obtaining a smear for cytologic examination.

The contributors have reinforced and extended the ideas expressed in Chapter 17 with respect to the identification of early cervical lesions. The various nonvisible early neoplastic lesions have been precisely defined, which removes much of the controversy on what is being treated.

Although it is accepted that conization and cryosurgery are therapeutically capable of eradicating cervical dysplasia and carcinoma in situ, it would appear that both procedures carry about the same 10 per cent or more failure rate. It must also be remembered that these results come from cancer centers, so that the therapeutic failure rate for the country as a whole may indeed be substantially higher. Certainly the question of recurrence following such therapy must also be considered in overall patient management. Also, these procedures unfortunately have been performed on occasion in the presence of an early invasive lesion.

Whatever the differences of opinion are regarding the above-mentioned procedures, there appears to be general agreement that the patient must be motivated to submit to long-term follow up. Not unlike the patient with adenomatous endometrial hyperplasia, these individuals are confronted with a degree of emotional uncertainty, and they continue to wonder about the curative effect of hysterectomy. Patient motivation basically hinges on physician confidence, and that means confidence in one physician. From the patient's viewpoint, cancer is not a disease that lends itself to management by committee of physicians. Rather, the patient desires her own physician, but is totally willing and even expects him to utilize consultants and those with special skill in order to provide her with the highest type of quality care.

When considering the question of follow-up, the interval from the initial recognition of carcinoma in situ to invasive cancer is predicated on averages derived from large numbers of patients. These are less meaningful when the individual patient is being considered, for it cannot be established when the pre-invasive lesion or carcinoma in situ began or the number of months that will supervene before invasion is undeterminable.

Both cryosurgery and conization are often presented as a procedure with few if any complications. Actually, cryosurgery has produced its fair share of pelvic infection, as indeed has conization. Moreover, many patients who have undergone cryosurgery complain bitterly of prolonged and copious irritating vaginal discharge. Certainly the physician should postpone speculum examination until 4 to 6 weeks after the procedure, or he may be discouraged by the appearance of the unhealed cervix.

Assuming that the cytopathologist and the gynecologist can agree on the diagnosis of the lesion in question, the treatment of carcinoma in situ and micro-invasion is similar—either the local methods as mentioned above or hysterectomy with ovarian conservation. As indicated by the contributors, opinions vary where the management of Stage I lesions is concerned. There appears to be a definite trend, described briefly by Dr. Lewis, toward surgical management in younger women who are physically suitable. However, whether ovarian conservation should be practiced may be open to question and controversy. Radiation is the primary modality employed in the treatment of Stage I lesions in older women (50 to 60 years of age or beyond).

17

The Cone Versus Multiple Punch Biopsy in the Diagnosis of Cervical Neoplasia

Alternative Points of View:

    By Ernest W. Franklin, III

    By George C. Lewis, Jr.

    By J. W. Roddick, Jr.

Editorial Comment

The Cone Versus Multiple Punch Biopsy in the Diagnosis of Cervical Neoplasia

ERNEST W. FRANKLIN, III

Emory University School of Medicine

MANAGEMENT OF THE PATIENT WITH ABNORMAL CERVICAL CYTOLOGY

Management of the patient with abnormal cervical cytology remains a controversial issue because of uncertainty concerning the precise nature of intra-epithelial neoplasia in terms of definition and natural history, as well as the effects thereon of various diagnostic and therapeutic modalities. The initial objective in management of the patient with an abnormal cervical cytology is to accurately predict the site and nature of the lesion present, with particular care to detect or exclude the presence of invasive carcinoma. One cannot dictate a single mode of management for this problem because of variations in applicability and economic feasibility. Techniques which are utilized by a small number of highly trained individuals to screen a large series of high risk patients are not applicable in the case of the individual practitioner seeing only an occasional patient with abnormal cervical cytology. For a variety of reasons, the necessary equipment may be lacking, particularly such specialized instruments as the colposcope, for undertaking precise and refined studies.

Equally important is the question of the type of training appropriate for resident physicians in order to qualify them in the management of the patient with an abnormal cervical cytology. Too often their training reflects the policies and practices of a large center involved in an investigational protocol or has been obtained with exceptional facilities available within that institution, which are not generally available. Thus, programs which encourage the resident to proceed directly from cervical cytology to conization of the cervix because of a high rate of correlation between the cervical cytology and the histologic findings fail to recognize that the physician may face this problem under an entirely different set of circumstances on completion of his training. Similarly, a training program in which management is dependent upon the availability of cryostat evaluation of conization specimens can provide excellent results, but diagnosis of invasive cancer short of conization will be infrequent, since biopsy will be neglected. Conversely, not every practitioner will be using a colposcope, as effective and easy to master as that instrument may be.

Speaking from personal experience, in my faculty the patients with abnormal cytology were managed by highly specialized teams protecting the "purity" of their study of cervical neoplasia. I had little opportunity to manage the patient with abnormal cervical cytology and completed my residency without ever performing a cervical conization. Subsequent to the conclusion of this study, the investigators have pointed out the efficacy with which patients can be managed without cervical conization, and yet it is questionable whether the conclusions of a specialized team can be extended to involve the general obstetrician and gynecologist, not to speak of the physician less well equipped by training. It is therefore not the purpose of this discourse to dictate what is appropriate or inappropriate in the management of the patient with abnormal cervical cytology. Rather, I will attempt to summarize data pertinent to the natural history of intraepithelial and early invasive cervical neoplasia, at the same time reviewing the efficacy and feasibility of several diagnostic and therapeutic modalities utilized in management. While the cervical and vaginal cytology may detect endometrial, tubal, or ovarian carcinoma, the adenomatous histologic origin of such atypical cells is usually discernible. For this reason, as well as because of its greater frequency, primary consideration will be given to detection of epidermoid malignancy within the genital tract.

INTRAEPITHELIAL NEOPLASIA: THE NATURAL HISTORY OF THE DISEASE AND ITS SUSCEPTIBILITY TO A NUMBER OF MODIFYING FACTORS

Initial observations by Meyer[1] and Schiller[2] resulted in the thesis that carcinoma in situ arose in squamous epithelium, with subsequent evolution into invasive carcinoma. Prospective studies of preinvasive lesions of the cervix, as well as retrospective studies of invasive lesions, have defined a spectrum of epithelial abnormalities ranging from dysplasia through carcinoma in situ to invasive cancer of the cervix. Just as the association of intraepithelial carcinoma with invasive carcinoma made the former lesion suspect, the association of the dysplastic lesions with carcinoma in situ provided a significant impetus to incrimination of dysplasia as a pathway to carcinoma of the cervix. The transition of cervical dysplasia into carcinoma in situ and invasive cancer has been demonstrated both morphologically and by epidemiologic data that have demonstrated such facts as an incidence of carcinoma in situ 22 times greater in populations with dysplasia than in populations with previous negative cytology.[3]

Of considerable therapeutic significance is the question of the probability of progression of a lesion through the spectrum of intraepithelial neoplasia to invasive cancer and, conversely, the probability of regression to normalcy of such a lesion, as well as the nature of those factors initiating, accelerating, and reversing carcinogenesis. Estimates of the probability of progression to invasive cancer by carcinoma in situ have ranged from 100 per cent[4] to "less than 10 per cent"[5] with a latency of 5 to 20 years.[4,6] The variability in these conclusions is attributable not only to differences in diagnostic criteria and observation interval but also to the criteria for coming under observation in the first place (i.e., how the population of normal or abnormal patients was defined), as well as to the effects of the diagnostic studies themselves upon the natural history of the disease. A cervical biopsy may completely remove some lesions in a single specimen, thus complicating observations of the spontaneous behavior of the lesion, as well as having potential therapeutic significance.

In order to define the natural history of the disease, Richart and Barron[7] observed by cytology and colposcopy alone 557 women whose findings in three consecutive cytologies were considered to indicate cervical dysplasia. They reported a consistent transition from lesser to greater degrees of atypicality and dysplasia in observing progression of these lesions to carcinoma in situ and, indeed, a number of early invasive cervical carcinomas. Regression to lower stages of atypicality or normalcy was rare, especially among the more dysplastic lesions. The conclusions of this study were consistent with those of Fidler and associates[8] and of Dunn.[9] The latter observed that the average duration of carcinoma in situ prior to invasion was five years, while preclinical invasive cervical carcinoma had an average duration of two years.

Observation of the patient with dysplasia utilizing both cervical cytology and biopsy rather than the former alone may, indeed, present a somewhat different picture. Following cervical biopsy, regression to normal has been observed in from 30 to 50 per cent of patients with dysplasia, and yet some 20 to 33 per cent of cases recurred.[3,7,10] While such observations might result in part from false negative examinations, they also suggest that simple removal of the focus of intraepithelial neoplasia is far from definitive therapy. While Barron and Richart noted a median transit time to carcinoma in situ for all dysplasias unmodified by excisional biopsy of 44 months, introduction of periods of regression by extraneous influences may well extend the transition time among those uncured. Progression of dysplasia to carcinoma in situ with subsequent invasion has been noted to take place during such periods of recurrence[10] and may occur despite apparent regression following limited therapy, such as cervical conization, cryosurgery, or cautery.

These observations on the transition probability and latency for the spectrum of the intraepithelial neoplasia prior to invasion thus refute conclusions minimizing the potential hazard of dysplasia and carcinoma in situ based upon brief observations of limited numbers of patients which failed to demonstrate progression to invasion.[5] The evidence is persistent that the lesion is real; the problem in the management of the patient with the abnormal cervical cytology is to rule out the presence of invasive cervical carcinoma and then plan appropriate treatment.

DIAGNOSTIC TECHNIQUES IN THE EVALUATION OF THE PATIENT WITH ABNORMAL CERVICAL CYTOLOGY

Several considerations are paramount in deciding on techniques for evaluation of the patient with an abnormal cervical cytology. First, the methods must be generally applicable, meaning that they must be techniques which can be widely taught and practiced. Second, such techniques must have the lowest possible morbidity and mortality rates and be economically feasible. Finally, and most important, such techniques must accurately establish the nature of the problem at hand while reducing to the lowest possible probability the presence of occult invasive cancer. Additional consideration must be given to the effect of the diagnostic techniques both on the natural history of the disease and on subsequent treatment of the disease in order that the latter may not be compromised.

Perhaps the most conservative approach to the management of the patient with abnormal cervical cytology—if conservative is meant to denote that plan of treatment which has long been recognized as having the least margin of error in the hands of all physicians, regardless of training—has involved conization of the cervix. Included among the advocates of cold cone biopsy of the cervix in the management of abnormal cervical cytology have been those who recommended proceeding directly to cold conization in the presence of suspicious cytologic findings suggesting dysplasia or greater disease within the cervix. The validity of this approach has been justified by the reporting of a high frequency of correlation between histologic and cytologic findings in such studies, with the conclusion being made that the finding of any degree of cervical neoplasia from dysplasia to invasive cancer justified conization of the cervix.

Such an approach to the management of the patient with the abnormal cervical cytology, which is indeed perhaps more aggressive than "conservative," can best be justified if the appropriate treatment of cervical dysplasia is to be conization of the cervix,[11] a premise as yet unsubstantiated. Such an approach can be rejected as uneconomical, with too great a risk of morbidity and mortality if more selective methods of detection of invasive cancer and treatment of dysplasia are available. Indeed, studies of the natural history of dysplasia show that it may well revert to normal following incidental trauma, such as cervical biopsy and cauterization, while cryosurgery[12] or cauterization[13,14] for the management of this spectrum of the disease shows some promise in early evaluation, with over 90 per cent success in eradication of the lesion reported on early follow-up. Several points should be emphasized in regard to the latter management, however. The first is that such treatment can only be undertaken if the presence of invasive carcinoma has been excluded, and this in itself may require conization. Second, the role of such management will only be determined after follow-up of carefully selected populations of patients for five to ten years at a minimum. Finally, the technique of adequate cryosurgery and cauterization requires freezing the stroma to a depth of at least 0.5 cm. to encompass disease within the glands,[5] and this may not be achieved in a satisfactory percentage of patients by utilizing the cryosurgical units now widely distributed. It is not too early to sound a warning about potential abuse of this technique of management, and particularly the patient who is seen with an abnormal cervical cytology but does not have adequate evaluation prior to superficial cryosurgery. Examples of such mismanagement are already beginning to be seen with increased distribution of cryosurgical units.

In addition to the increased morbidity and mortality rates and greater expense incurred in proceeding directly from abnormal cytology to conization of the cervix, such an approach also affects the planning of subsequent therapy if invasive cancer is discovered, for both radical surgery and radium therapy must be delayed four to six weeks following conization. Should the patient be pregnant prior to conization, she may have begun labor either at term or prematurely, leaving the clinician with the dilemma of incipient delivery through a recently coned cervix, possibly containing invasive cancer.

The calculation of prevalence rates among pregnant patients demonstrates some five cases of dysplasia and three cases of carcinoma in situ per 1000 patients, with approximately one case of invasive cervical cancer per 2500 to 5000 pregnancies.[15] The importance of screening for cervical cancer in pregnancy and appropriate diagnostic evaluation cannot be overemphasized.

The management of the pregnant patient with an abnormal cytology offers additional challenges because the changes of pregnancy alter the gross and microscopic anatomy. Careful clinical evaluation for a gross lesion, a firm area within a softened cervix, and careful review and repetition of the cytology are only a beginning, though a negative cytology following a positive one as always must not obscure the significance of the former. Endocervical evaluation by either curettage or conization is of necessity limited. In this age group, and when there is eversion of the patulous cervix, the anatomic and histologic exocervix can optimally be evaluated by selective biopsy of the transitional zone using Schiller's stain, while colposcopy is of particular value.

Conization has little to add, as it must be a short and superficial specimen, sampling the same area that lies within reach of the punch biopsy. Jones and associates[15] demonstrated that the accuracy of a single set of cervical biopsies during pregnancy was 80 per cent, with a 90 per cent accuracy achieved with two sets of biopsies. There were no known abortions, nor was there a need for transfusion among 998 patients evaluated. Eighteen patients in that series had invasive cancer, in 17 of whom the diagnosis was established by multiple punch biopsies. In the one remaining patient, the possibility of microinvasion was considered after biopsy, and more extensive invasion was proved on conization. Conization should be reserved for such cases in which the possibility of invasion or the degree of invasion has not been satisfactorily elucidated by punch biopsies. The finding of carcinoma in situ in the cervix of a pregnant patient should not prevent vaginal delivery, and the same can probably be said of microinvasive carcinoma once the existence of further invasion is excluded by conization of the cervix. The presence of more extensive invasion within the cervix necessitates early treatment of the patient, even if the pregnancy must be terminated. Given carcinoma of the cervix in a pregnant patient, the most significant factor contributing to an adverse prognosis is a delay in treatment. Other than that, the pregnant patient should have no poorer prognosis after appropriate treatment than her nonpregnant counterpart with a comparable stage of disease.

The decision to carry out conization in the pregnant patient must be made with some care, for even when excluded from the first trimester this procedure carries an increased maternal morbidity rate, including hemorrhage requiring transfusion and cicatrix of the cervix with cervical dystocia or laceration. The additional risk of spontaneous abortion and premature labor makes it clear that when the potential benefit of this procedure is weighed against the potential risk, conization is justified only in those in whom the presence of invasive cancer cannot be excluded by careful clinical evaluation, including punch biopsy.

It has been the experience of the author that physicians trained to manage the patient with abnormal cervical cytology proceeding directly to conization in the absence of a gross lesion soon become unable to recognize the gross lesion within the cervix. The fundamentals of close observation and palpation of the cervix and adjacent structures are neglected; such clinical evaluation becomes of little significance, as "the patient is going to have a conization of the cervix anyway." Advanced cervical lesions of Stages I, IIa, and IIb have thus remained undetected until conization. To avoid the latter dilemma, the conization of the cervix should be preceded by careful clinical evaluation of the uterus on an outpatient basis, including at least careful observation and palpation of the cervix, vulva, vagina, and urethra, with application of Schiller's stain. Subsequent punch biopsies of the cervix at the squamocolumnar junction, as directed by observation or staining techniques, should be carried out, as should endocervical curettage. The efficacy of these procedures can be improved by utilizing the colposcope, although this is not essential. The potential benefit of these techniques in adequately assessing the extent of cervical neoplasia must be evaluated in the context of their applicability to all specialists in gynecology and obstetrics. If an approach is feasible only in the hands of a specialized team, it has little to recommend itself for general use.

Such a clinical trial has recently been the subject of review in the Department of Gynecology and Obstetrics at the Emory University School of Medicine. At the Grady Memorial Hospital in Atlanta, Georgia, all patients with abnormal cervical cytology are evaluated in the biweekly Dysplasia Clinic by resident physicians. In the two-year period from July, 1969, through June, 1971, 5802 patients were evaluated according to the afore-mentioned guidelines. Cold conization biopsy was performed when severe dysplasia or carcinoma in situ was found on punch biopsy or when cytology suggested carcinoma in situ or undetected invasive cancer. During this observation period, an attempt was made to evaluate the efficacy of these studies in detecting occult subclinical cervical carcinoma.

Utilizing the guidelines described previously, we found 405 patients who were admitted for cold conization biopsy. Of these, 5 per cent had no neoplasia, 24 per cent had mild-moderate dysplasia, and 68 per cent had severe dysplasia–carcinoma in situ. Eleven patients (2.7 per cent) were found to have invasive carcinoma, though in nine the extent of invasion was less than 5 mm. Among the 11 patients, the presence of invasive carcinoma had been specifically suggested in seven by either the cytology and/or cervical and endocervical biopsies. Of the 2 patients who had carcinoma invading to a depth greater than 5 mm., one had a diagnosis of carcinoma in situ with superficial invasion on conization and was found at hysterectomy to have invasion extending approximately 8 mm. into the cervical stroma. Thus, the cervical conization is not infallible. The other patient was found to have epidermoid carcinoma in situ and a second lesion, adenoid basal carcinoma, extending deep into the cervical stroma on conization biopsy. With subsequent observations of at least one year, there have been cases of undetected invasive cervical carcinoma among the 5802 patients originally evaluated.

These results are felt to justify utilization of outpatient diagnostic procedures, including punch biopsy of the cervix, in association with cytology in selecting those patients who should appropriately be subjected to conization biopsy of the cervix. Resident physicians in training were able to screen a large population of patients with no evidence at present that they let subclinical invasive carcinoma go undetected. Equally significant is the fact that during the four year period from January, 1968, through December, 1971, the resident staff accurately diagnosed 99 patients with Stages Ib, IIa, and IIb epidermoid carcinoma of the cervix without resorting to conization of the cervix. In addition, they were able to select with considerable specificity a population at greatest risk of having significant intraepithelial neoplasia with an approximately 3 per cent incidence of occult invasive carcinoma. Only one of 405 patients had a cancer invading greater than 5 mm. into the cervical stroma which was detectable by conization but undetected by punch biopsy and endocervical curettage. Utilization of these techniques, if properly performed, does contribute to the optimal management of the patient with abnormal cervical cytology.

Feeling that it was indeed possible to improve our selection of patients and decrease the necessity for conization by utilizing the colposcope, we initiated a prospective study to evaluate the impact of colposcopy on outpatient evaluation of the patient with abnormal cervical cytology. In addition to review of the previous abnormal cervical cytology, a cytologic specimen was obtained prior to punch biopsies of the cervix directed by colposcopy and Schiller's stain, with subsequent endocervical curettage. Any conclusions regarding the validity of such studies should also point out the importance of proper technique, including reliable cytopathologic tests. Incomplete or inadequate studies require repetition or increased use of conization. The colposcope is of particular value when the squamocolumnar junction can be visualized, as in the premenopausal patient, including the pregnant woman. If the lesion extends up the endocervical canal beyond visualization with the colposcope, or if the endocervical curettings contain neoplastic epithelium, invasive cancer cannot be excluded without conization. Optimal biopsies can be obtained with an instrument which is sharp enough to avoid crushing and distortion of the tissue while obtaining a specimen of adequate size and depth and appropriately oriented for histologic study. The Kevorkian biopsy forceps and endocervical curette are particularly satisfactory for these studies.

In reviewing the final histologic diagnosis based on conization or hysterectomy following colposcopically directed punch biopsy and endocervical curettings, it was found that these preoperative studies had been able to detect the most advanced lesion in 93 per cent of the cases. In 74 per cent of the patients, the lesion had been removed by the punch biopsy and endocervical curettage. Among the 7 per cent of 125 patients who had a more advanced degree of neoplasia, only one had invasion, and that was limited to a depth of 2 mm. It was also significant to note that in 12 per cent of the patients the endocervical curettings contained the most advanced degree of cervical neoplasia, thus reinforcing the value of this technique.

On the basis of these results, it has been concluded that the appropriate diagnostic procedures for evaluation of the patient with an abnormal cytology include a repetition of the cervical cytology, careful inspection and palpation of the cervix, preferably including use of the colposcope, the application of Schiller's stain and selective punch biopsies with endocervical curettage. While expert use of the colposcope may markedly curtail the necessity of undertaking conization of the cervix, this instrument has not yet received the widespread acceptance and utilization which it deserves. These techniques are extremely accurate in detecting invasive carcinoma of the cervix, especially that extending beyond 5 mm. into the cervical stroma and requiring radical therapy. They are also extremely accurate in detecting the extent of preinvasive cervical neoplasia. Most important, these techniques can readily be taught to and utilized by the majority of those training within the specialty of obstetrics and gynecology.

Cold conization of the cervix must be reserved within the armamentarium for use when the above studies suggest but fail to confirm or exclude the possibility of invasive carcinoma, when adequate studies cannot be obtained on an outpatient basis, and as a possible diagnostic and therapeutic modality for the patient with carcinoma in situ for whom hysterectomy is not appropriate. Under the latter circumstances, conization may reduce the risk of undetected invasive cancer to a minimum with a potential for temporary or permanent eradication of cervical intraepithelial neoplasia. Pertinent to the use of conization for this purpose is the realization that persistent intraepithelial neoplasia has been reported in from 15 to 40 per cent of hysterectomy specimens following cold conization.

The validity of cytopathologic findings in evaluating the status of the cervix following conization, cautery, or cryosurgery is also of concern. Confusion may exist during the early healing phase owing to an abundance of giant repair cells or foreign body reaction giving atypical cells difficult to differentiate from true invasive cancer. Such reaction may be a partial explanation for the high reported incidence of intraepithelial neoplasia in some series of hysterectomies following conization. Of equal concern is the false negative cytology report, particularly that which may fail to detect a lesion owing to inflammation or extension of normal epithelium over an underlying malignancy. This concern prompted a recent review of 176 patients at the Grady Memorial Hospital who had had cytologic examination after conization and preceding hysterectomy. The hysterectomy was performed at an interval of less than three months in 126 patients, and of greater than three months in 50 patients. The cytology accurately predicted the presence or absence of residual neoplasia in 88 per cent of cases. This was comparable to the accuracy achieved with cytology prior to conization; the accuracy did not seem to be affected by whether the specimen was obtained before or after the three month interval. Of interest was the fact that cytology did consistently demonstrate the presence of an invasive carcinoma within a uterus which had remained undetected by biopsy or conization.

It is the view of the author that the optimal treatment of carcinoma in situ of the cervix that carries the least risk of recurrence is total hysterectomy, preferably via the vaginal route, with a wide vaginal cuff, to include all Schiller positive areas or a minimum of 2 cm. of the vaginal membrane in the presence of a negative Schiller strain.[18] Among 273 patients with carcinoma in situ of the cervix treated in this fashion at the Grady Memorial Hospital and followed for three to 10 years there have been no recurrences of epidermoid carcinoma of the vagina. This finding is in agreement with that of Boyes and colleagues,[16] who reported a series of 4389 patients with preclinical epidermoid carcinoma of the cervix. Treatment of carcinoma in situ by hysterectomy plus partial vaginectomy resulted in a recurrence rate of only 0.84 per cent. A recent report of 483 patients treated by simple hysterectomy but without partial vaginectomy[17] and followed for a shorter period of time noted a recurrence rate of 2.27 per cent, an index of probability of <0.001. The conclusion suggested is that total hysterectomy with partial vaginectomy offers a significantly better degree of long-term control of epidermoid carcinoma in situ than hysterectomy alone, with no increase in operative morbidity or mortality rates. When 144 cases of total vaginal hysterectomy and partial vaginectomy were compared with 99 cases of vaginal hysterectomy without colporrhaphy or vaginectomy carried out for benign disease by the resident staff at the Grady Memorial Hospital between January, 1970, and December, 1971, no difference in morbidity or mortality rates was revealed. The optimal degree of control of the disease reported by this technique should rule out the need for any more radical surgical procedure for intraepithelial carcinoma.

Conization of the cervix as treatment for carcinoma in situ should be reserved for the patient who is amenable to close follow-up and who desires to retain her reproductive capacity if occult invasive carcinoma is excluded. It represents a risk of recurrence of up to 10 per cent.[19] While the short-term efficacy of the cold conization with or without subsequent cauterization for control of intra-epithelial neoplasia has been discussed in initial reports, the validity of cryosurgery for dysplasia or carcinoma in situ remains a completely untested thesis and must be subjected to carefully controlled scrutiny prior to general clinical application. In any event, it would be applicable only after the presence of invasive carcinoma of the cervix has been excluded by appropriate diagnostic techniques.

Microinvasive carcinoma invading to a depth of less than 5 mm. into the stroma may be adequately treated with simple total hysterectomy, preferably with partial vaginectomy. The delineation of this selected group of patients must be made with conization prior to electing conservative therapy. A recent review of 60 such cases treated at the Grady Memorial Hospital revealed equal success in treatment among patients receiving limited versus radical therapy, with a greater frequency of complications among the latter.

As the treatment for carcinoma in situ and early microinvasion is the same, diagnostic techniques which fail to detect the earliest stage of invasion do not place the patient in jeopardy. Essentially all cases with invasion extending to a depth of greater than 0.5 cm. into the cervical stroma should be detected prior to hysterectomy by diagnostic techniques such as those described above. Occasionally, however—as was the case among our series of patients—a patient will be seen in whom the lesion is undetected even by conization. Such patients can very adequately be treated with radiation therapy[20] with an excellent chance of cure. While these considerations may provide considerable reassurance, they should never become an excuse for neglecting a complete evaluation of the patient with abnormal cervical cytologic findings, an evaluation which must attempt to effectively exclude the presence of invasive cancer and must be accomplished with the greatest economy of resources and with the lowest morbidity and mortality rates. As always, the reliability of the conclusions must reflect the adequacy of the studies undertaken, while the final plan of treatment may be individualized to the patient's needs.

Use of the cervical punch biopsy and endocervical curettage following abnormal cervical cytology suggesting dysplasia or worse can effectively detect and rule out the presence of carcinoma of the cervix extending beyond 5 mm. into the cervical stroma. As noted previously, in the evaluation of 5802 patients with abnormal cervical cytology at the Grady Memorial Hospital, it was possible for the resident staff to detect all Stages Ib, IIa, and IIb carcinomas of the cervix with these techniques. Of the 405 patients thought to have less than a Stage Ib carcinoma of the cervix who had carcinoma in situ or suspected invasion on cytologic examination or severe dysplasia or carcinoma in situ on biopsy, significant stromal invasion had effectively been excluded by these techniques of evaluation in all but two cases. Conization failed to detect one of these two lesions. In addition, one death owing to pulmonary embolus occurred following conization.

While such techniques may be considered a cornerstone of evaluation of the patient with an abnormal cervical cytology, it is evident that colposcopy can play a significant role in improving the precision of these diagnostic studies. Conization of the cervix will continue to be important whenever the presence of invasion is suggested by the cervical cytology or the cervical or endocervical biopsies, including the presence of neoplastic cells in the endocervix. By necessity, conization must play a larger role in the hands of physicians who evaluate patients with abnormal cervical cytology less frequently, and it provides assurance against the presence of invasive cancer. It should not supplant the role of initial cervical and endocervical biopsies, since a significant percentage of the early invasive carcinomas and the majority of more advanced lesions can be detected with these diagnostic techniques.

REFERENCES

1. Meyer, R.: Histological diagnosis of early cervical carcinoma (Charles Sumner Bacon Lecture). Surg. Gynec. Obstet. 73:129, 1941.
2. Schiller, W.: Early diagnosis of carcinoma of cervix. Surg. Gynec. Obstet. 56:210, 1933.
3. Stern, E.: Epidemiology of dysplasia. Obstet. Gynec. Surv. 24:711, 1969.
4. MacGregor, J. E.: A study of clinically and cytologically detected cancers in the city of Aberdeen. Acta Cytol. 10:246, 1966.
5. Green, G. H.: The significance of cervical carcinoma in situ. Amer. J. Obstet. Gynec. 94: 1009, 1966.
6. Boyes, D. A., Fidler, H. K., Lock, D. R.: Significance of in situ carcinoma of the uterine cervix. Brit. Med. J. 1:203, 1962.
7. Richart, R. M., and Barron, B. A.: A follow-up study of patients with cervical dysplasia. Amer. J. Obstet. Gynec. 105:386, 1969.
8. Fidler, H. K., Boyes, D. A., and Worth, A. J.: Cervical cancer detection in British Columbia. J. Obstet. Gynaec. Brit. Comm. 75:392, 1968.
9. Dunn, J. E., Jr.: The relationship between carcinoma in situ and invasive cervical carcinoma. Cancer 6:873, 1953.
10. Johnson, L. D., Nickerson, R. J., Easterday, C. L., Stuart, R. S., and Hertig, A. T.: Epidemiologic evidence for the spectrum of change from dysplasia through carcinoma in situ to invasive cancer. Cancer 22:901, 1968.
11. Villasanta, U.: Malignant potential of cervical dysplasia: Diagnosis and treatment. South. Med. J. 61:1018, 1968.
12. Kaufman, R. H., and Conner, J. J.: Cryosurgical treatment of cervical dysplasia. Amer. J. Obstet. Gynec. 109:1167, 1971.
13. Richart, R. M., and Sciarra, J. J.: Treatment of cervical dysplasia by outpatient electrocauterization. Amer. J. Obstet. Gynec. 101:200, 1968.
14. Channen, W., and Hollyock, V. E.: Colposcopy and electrocoagulation-diathermy for cervical dysplasia and carcinoma in situ. Obstet. Gynec. 37:623, 1971.
15. Jones, E. G., Schwinn, C. P., Bullock, W. K., Varga, A., Dunn, J. E., Friedman, H., and Weir, J.: Cancer detection during pregnancy. Am. J. Obstet. Gynec. 101:298, 1968.
16. Boyes, D. A., Worth, A. J., and Fidler, H. K.: The results of treatment of 4389 cases of preclinical squamous carcinoma. J. Obstet. Gynec. Brit. Comm. 77:769, 1970.
17. Creasman, W. T., and Rutledge, F.: Carcinoma in situ of the cervix: An analysis of 861 patients. Obstet. Gynec. 39:373, 1972.
18. Lyon, J. B., Hajjar, S., and Thompson, J. D.: Vaginal hysterectomy and partial vaginectomy for carcinoma in situ of the uterine cervix. South. Med. J. 58:937–944, 1965.
19. Kullander, S. N., Nils-Otto, S.: Treatment of carcinoma in situ of the cervix uteri by conization: A five-year follow-up. Acta Obstet. Gynec. Scand. 50:153, 1971.
20. Durrance, F. Y.: Radiotherapy following simple hysterectomy in patients with Stage I and II carcinoma of the cervix. Radiology 102:165, 1968.

The Cone Versus Multiple Punch Biopsy in the Diagnosis of Cervical Neoplasia

Detection, Diagnosis, and Therapeutic Decision in Cervical Malignant Disease

GEORGE C. LEWIS, JR.
Thomas Jefferson University Medical College

The gynecologist must at times play a role akin to that of the challenged duelist. He can be said to have a choice of weapons—the methods for coming to grips with a spectrum of cervical lesions from dysplasia to frankly invasive cancer. The multiple phases of cellular alteration require a variety of study techniques and treatment programs to detect and eradicate abnormalities. Actually, the very array of diagnostic and therapeutic techniques has taught the physician more about the pathogenesis of cervical malignancy than is known for cancer arising in other sites.

In the past, admonitions that urged both patient and physician to do their utmost to discover and treat cervical cancer were directed at action on a relatively gross level. In effect, the disease too often had spread beyond the primary site, to regional lymphatics or remote locations. The results of treatment paralleled that of relatively late disease patterns. Currently, diagnostic decisions relative to cervical malignancy are coming to be based less on macroscopic considerations and more upon microscopic findings.

Just over two decades ago the patient's watchword was abnormal bleeding; the physician's role was to take a careful history in search of such events, to perform a pelvic examination, and to biopsy the suspect lesion. These basic steps —history, physical examination, and biopsy—are still important, but they are the starting point for a series of other procedures. Difficulty in defining limits of abnormality led to development of a technique in which stains are applied to the cervical mucosa. This allowed more specific localization of the biopsy sites, a principle still important today. The addition of cervical staining techniques provided the gynecologist with a method that would include testing of all suspicious malignant areas as determined by direct visual observations. Despite the aid of stains, the areas selected for biopsy could be incorrect ones or malignancies could be missed. Removal of relatively innocuous material next to a malignancy can be as much of a defeat for the patient as failure to biopsy. If nothing else, the false reassurance of the benign report may intensify both the patient's and the physician's feelings that all has been done that is required.

Subsequently, two procedures—colposcopy coupled with microscopy and cytopathologic techniques—became available. These were in limited use at the time when the main attention was still being devoted to the patient's symptoms. Both shared the same fate in that they were only slowly accepted as a means for microscopic discovery and localization of a tumor. These methods, however, permitted the clinician to appreciate details of cancer and premalignant lesions at the cellular level, including repeated or serial observations. Colposcopy and colpomicroscopy have become of particular value in tracing the ebb and flow of normal and dysplastic tissues.

Cytology of course has been associated with mass screening, particularly for the asymptomatic patient. This technique has been visualized as a means of eliminating cervical cancer totally, but many practical aspects hinder this concept.[4,5]

The two screening techniques, when added to the basic attack upon cancer, began to change the clinical and laboratory picture. As experience was gained, the procedures helped define such entities as carcinoma in situ and dysplasia. A solitary focus could be contrasted with origin from multiple foci. Further investigations revealed a spectrum of change, namely, in the extent of invasion and in degrees of dysplasia. Gray zones of decision could be identified. When was a lesion malignant? Was it possible for some phase of abnormal tissue to change to normal? Would an identifiable type of lesion progress to cancer? These methods of identification began to provide ample material through biopsy for study of the pathogenesis of cervical cancer.

While the popularity of colpomicroscopy and cytopathology increased and they found wider acceptance and use, the discoveries they produced led to an expansion of the tissue biopsy techniques. With colpomicroscopy the site for punch biopsy can be definitely selected.[7] Very restricted areas of tissue can be sampled with little disturbance of the remaining surface structure.

Four-quadrant biopsy was introduced to sample and study the squamocolumnar junction adequately. This approach was also based on the assumption that it would be so rare for a small focus of early invasive cancer to be found adjacent to an in situ lesion and dysplastic tissues that the cancer would be missed altogether. With small cervices and generous removal of tissue, the effect for all practical purposes may be equivalent to a four piece "cone."

The so-called "cold" knife cone technique was probably introduced initially as a study procedure by physicians who had made extensive use of the high-frequency cutting current to cone the cervix. Their colleagues in pathology, complaining of "cooked" tissues, brought about a natural shift to the cold technique. In theory, this provided an unbroken ring of tissue that would indicate any neoplasm present. If the tissue was removed and sent to the pathologist as one perfect specimen, there existed the possible associated hazard that he would follow the "one piece–one tissue section" rule. The gynecologist must be certain to work in close collaboration with the pathologist and see that the patient's tissues are sectioned adequately for thorough study. When inexperienced or when worried about pregnancy, some gynecologists tended to remove inadequate amounts of tissue. A few severe postconization hemorrhages damped the ardor of some gynecologists for this procedure. If the tissue removed for diagnosis of in situ carcinoma and dysplasia was adequate, conization could serve as therapy in selected situations.[11] This same asset made it difficult to investigate cellular progression or regression, for if the lesion was totally removed, there was nothing left for study. Certainly at present "punch" biopsy of the obvious lesion is the procedure of choice. However, conization for most patients is still unnecessary and relatively hazardous. Nevertheless, despite absence of a visible lesion, the cytology may suggest invasive disease; the physician so alerted should find cone biopsy necessary, especially when the cytopathologist has suggested the possibility of a more advanced lesion than in situ disease.[2,8,10]

In summary, a historical path has been traced in a very condensed form, and the present procedures have been considered from a very general point of view—and possibly not adequately in terms of everyday value. The contacts of members of the medical profession with our female patients are so variable and so numerous that we cannot define a universally acceptable, rigid standard for detection and diagnosis of cervical cancer. Time and economic factors play different but important and interacting roles. A directed biopsy under colpomicroscopy may prove to be effective, practical, and less expensive than the most extensive cone biopsy performed in an operating room. Mass cytologic screening surveys by trained technicians may uncover more premalignant lesions than any physician, office, or hospital oriented program. Indeed, there are indications that automation and refinements in laboratory processing may soon streamline cytologic examinations by technicians, which will no doubt prove of value in reducing costs of survey programs. Finally, diagnostic procedures that are highly effective in the hands of one physician may be less so in the hands of others. For example, the quality and quantity of cone biopsy will depend upon the surgeon's experience and attitude.

Physicians tend to espouse and adhere to one method of screening and biopsy evaluation. They do this, of course, feeling that the approach they have chosen is highly accurate. However, anyone arguing the merits of a cancer diagnostic procedure must realize that various systems are open to factors that may bias the results. Bilbo and associates[1] reported, in a survey of 148,735 patients, that there was no evidence of dysplasia, carcinoma in situ, or invasive cancer in 97 per cent of patients screened by cytology. Accordingly, if every smear had been read as negative, there would have been only a 3 per cent error in terms of these pathologic changes. Even when cytopathologic changes alone are considered, it is possible, because of a high incidence of relatively benign lesions, to be generally more accurate by issuing a more conservative pathologic evaluation than might fit the true situation. In Bilbo and co-workers' material, if the 3602 patients with dysplasia, the 849 patients with carcinoma in situ, and the 228 patients with invasive cancer had been reported as having dysplasia and carcinoma in situ, the overall accuracy would still have been 95 per cent. Essentially, these analyses mean that the results of screening, biopsy, or conservative observation of populations may be more impressive as to accuracy than is really the case because the odds favoring a relatively benign condition are high. As a result, one should not depend upon one procedure or evaluation alone. Combinations of cytologic studies and colpomicroscopy biopsy offer greater opportunity to uncover the pre-malignant, nonvisible lesion that might otherwise be missed.

Detailed comparative analyses of all the pros and cons of various biopsy techniques may soon be outmoded. There are indications that using surveillance techniques for lesions that are at the starting point of carcinogenesis may avoid the potential hazards of cancer.[3] There are at present suggestive findings that significant proportions of mild to moderate dysplasia regress or at least stabilize.[6,9]

The possibility of eliminating cervical cancer has already been heralded by proponents of mass screening. The obvious drawback has been the failure to obtain, up to now, 100 per cent physician and patient participation in survey programs. Although supplemented by biopsies for study purposes as indicated above, surveillance and conservative "medical" procedures may be the only requirements for avoiding cervical cancer in the future. Should this happen, today's battlefield, with the gynecologic oncology team arrayed against cancer in women, should deservedly become a thing of the past.

REFERENCES

1. Bilbo, M., Keebler, C. M., and Wied, G. L.: Prevalence and incidence rates of cervical atypia: computerized file analysis on 148,735 patients. J. Reprod. Med. 6:184, 1971.
2. Chao, S., McCaffrey, R., Todd, W. D., and Moore, J. G.: Conization in evaluation and management of cervical neoplasia. Am. J. Obstet. Gynec. 103:574, 1969.
3. Fox, C. H.: Biologic behavior of dysplasia and carcinoma in situ. Am. J. Obstet. Gynec. 99:960, 1967.
4. Green, G. H.: Invasive potentiality of cervical carcinoma in situ. Internat. J. Gynaec. Obstet. 7:157, 1969.
5. Green, G. H., and Donovan, J. W.: Natural history of cervical carcinoma in situ. J. Obstet. Gynaec. Brit. Comm. 77:1, 1970.
6. Hall, J. E., and Walton, L.: Dysplasia of the cervix: a prospective study of 206 cases. Am. J. Obstet. Gynec. 100:662, 1968.
7. Hillemanns, H. G.: Biopsy methods and their selective application in diagnosis and therapy of cervical carcinoma: contribution to actual significance of colposcopy. Geburtsh. u. Frauenheilkd. 28:1104, 1968.
8. Hulka, B. S.: Punch biopsy and conization as diagnostic procedures after abnormal cervical smears. Obstet. Gynec. 36:54, 1970.
9. Johnson, L. D., Nickerson, R. J., Easterday, C. L., Stuart, R. S., and Hertig, A. T.: Epidemiologic evidence for the spectrum of change from dysplasia through carcinoma in situ to invasive cancer. Cancer 22:901, 1968.
10. Neubert, C.: Findings following diagnostic cervical conization. Geburtsh. u. Frauenheilkd. 28:428, 1968.
11. Villasanta, U.: Malignant potential of cervical dysplasia: diagnosis and treatment. South. Med. J. 61:1018, 1968.

The Cone Versus Multiple Punch Biopsy in the Diagnosis of Cervical Neoplasia

J. W. RODDICK, JR.

Southern Illinois University School of Medicine

Since Papanicolaou demonstrated that the normal appearing cervix may harbor intraepithelial lesions which can progress to invasive cancer, conization of the cervix has been the sine qua non for the diagnosis of these lesions. The concept that conization is necessary to make an exact diagnosis of such lesions is based on the fear that less inclusive tissue study may sample areas not involved by a more serious lesion—namely, invasive carcinoma. There can be little doubt that a properly performed cervical cone biopsy will almost always reveal the presence of an invasive cancer high in the cervical canal, remembering that the worth of a conization specimen in evaluating a given lesion is directly related to the manner in which it is done and the amount of tissue that is removed and studied. With the development of increased accuracy in the interpretation of cytologic specimens, the availability of colposcopic and colpomicroscopic directed biopsies, as well as other techniques, a real question can be raised as to the necessity of performing conization on every patient with an atypical smear or an abnormal biopsy. Periodic reviews of what are thought to be unbreakable rules or axioms, made in the light of more recent knowledge, are necessary to prevent the perpetuation of dogma unsupported by good evidence.

The question to be asked is: "Does every patient with suspected intraepithelial neoplasia of the cervix require conization for definitive diagnosis before a satisfactory treatment plan can be developed?" There is little doubt that most cases of invasive cervical cancer progress through stages of dysplasia and carcinoma in situ before developing into more serious and significant lesions. There is also little doubt that significantly invasive cervical cancer may occur in the endocervical canal beyond the vision of the examiner. It is because of the fear of missing the latter that most authors recommend the routine performance of cervical conization in all patients suspected of having less serious degrees of intraepithelial neoplasia.

In most instances, lesions that fall short of invasive cancer not only are asymptomatic but also produce no visible lesion. For the most part, the suspicion that an epithelial lesion exists begins with the finding of abnormal cytology. The management of such a situation is the real subject of this discussion. The changing roles of cytology, biopsy, conization, and ancillary techniques will be discussed in turn.

The Role of the Cytologic Examination

Papanicolaou originally designed a reporting method for cytology which utilized classes ranging from I to V, with variable increases in abnormality as one ascended the scale. While this scheme was satisfactory in the early years, increased sophistication in the interpretation of smears has made it less than ideal with the passage of time. In Papanicolaou's classification, an ambiguous Class III report with no further description leaves the responsible clinician with little solid evidence one way or the other as to the presence or absence of significant epithelial lesion or abnormality. A large number of "diagnostic conizations" are the direct result of a Class III report. The yield of histologic abnormalities in these cases depends largely upon the ability and willingness to make a decision of the cytologist who made the original interpretation. All too often Class III is used as a mechanism to avoid such decision making, and a large number of patients therefore undergo unnecessary conization.

Greater proficiency in the interpretation of cytologic specimens has led many to abandon the method described above in favor of reporting methods that use nomenclature paralleling that used in tissue examination. It is possible to indicate, with a high degree of accuracy, cytologic patterns which are consistent with dysplasia, carcinoma in situ, or invasive cancer.[11] Combined with a description and explanation of the findings, a report such as this is far more meaningful than is one utilizing the older nomenclature. Armed with a cytologic report predictive of a tissue diagnosis, the question of whether to perform a biopsy or a cone, or do nothing, becomes easier to answer.

The Role of Cervical Biopsies

As early as 1964 Dilts and associates[4] reevaluated the use of four-quadrant punch biopsies of the cervix to replace conization for the definitive diagnosis of preinvasive squamous cell carcinoma of the cervix in some instances. Since that time, others have indicated that under certain circumstances biopsies are adequate to make this diagnosis. Dilts and his co-workers studied 244 cases of punch biopsy of the cervix with a diagnosis of preinvasive, questionably invasive, or minimally invasive squamous cell carcinoma. One of 163 patients diagnosed as having preinvasive cancer (0.6 per cent) was found to have serious invasion in the hysterectomy specimen; one of 25 questionably invasive (4.0 per cent), and one of 11 minimally invasive (9.1 per cent) turned out to be seriously invasive. Thus, a total of three in 199 cases originally thought to contain insignificant invasion were found to have serious invasion in the hysterectomy specimen. These findings were based on what the authors considered adequate amounts of tissue with adequate tissue orientation. As a result of their studies, the authors concluded that four-quadrant punch biopsies of the uterine cervix, when properly obtained and studied, are adequate in the diagnosis of preinvasive squamous cell carcinoma of the cervix. They stress the fact that in the event that there is any question, or when minimal invasion is present in the biopsy, further study by means of conization is mandatory. Similar findings were subsequently reported by Griffith and colleagues,[6] who found a serious error in only one of 144 patients. These findings correspond to error rates in cone specimens reported to be as high as from 0.7 per cent to 1.7 per cent in several series.[1,5,7] Others have corroborated these findings and strongly suggest that adequate punch biopsies, in combination with cytologic studies, frequently are sufficient for the definitive diagnosis of carcinoma in situ.

The Role of Conization

One would have little difficulty in finding dozens of articles in the literature over the past years which state unequivocally that conization is vital for the proper diagnosis of carcinoma in situ and in order to eliminate the possibility that invasive cancer might be present. These articles cite varying instances in which unsuspected invasive cancer was found in conization specimens. It can also be argued that a large number of patients are adequately treated by means of a combined diagnostic and therapeutic conization, eliminating the need for subsequent hysterectomy or more radical method of treatment. As previously noted, there can be little argument that an adequate cone specimen will rarely fail to reveal the occult invasive cancer originating high in the endocervix. Those cases in which invasive cancer is found in the hysterectomy specimen of a patient whose cervix was previously coned most likely represent technical inadequacy in the performance of the diagnostic procedure. In reviewing large numbers of surgical specimens, it has not been uncommon in the author's experience to find specimens labeled as "conization" which consist only of small fragments of unoriented and unorientable squamous epithelium with little or no endocervical epithelium or cervical stroma present. These specimens unfortunately represent an attempt to follow the letter of the law rather than its spirit. An improperly performed and studied conization not only is not superior to adequate biopsies but also is truly an inferior procedure, since it gives the physician a false sense of security. To be adequate, a cone specimen must contain a significant portion of the squamous epithelium of the portio vaginalis cervicis, as well as the entire endocervical epithelium up to the internal os, along with the fibrous connective tissue stroma underlying all these areas. The properly obtained specimen must then be adequately blocked so that multiple specimens are obtained, sampling the entire cervix, and preserving proper orientation in order to facilitate interpretation of the tissue. Unless all of these conditions are met, conization must be considered inadequate.

The Role of Combined Techniques

Adding to the increased value of cytologic interpretation are several additional techniques which make definition of the extent of a given cervical lesion more precise. Some of these, such as the Schiller test, are not new, whereas others, such as colposcopy and colpomicroscopy, have developed over the past few years to a point where they are becoming increasingly useful clinically.

The performance of biopsies of material characterized by failure to take up iodine has increased the yield of abnormal findings on biopsy. In a number of instances, the correlation of the biopsy findings with the abnormal cytology will be sufficient to settle the question of the degree of atypia present and make conization unnecessary. Other stains, such as toluidine blue, may also be used in a similar manner.

Colposcopic or colpomicroscopic selection of biopsy sites also can aid in the elimination of errors. In a recent study, Krumholz and Knapp[9] performed colposcopically directed biopsies in 74 patients with abnormal smears and performed random biopsies in 51. Ninety per cent of those with directed biopsies showed no significant difference between the diagnosis on biopsy and that on conization, while 17.5 per cent of those with random biopsies had significantly more advanced disease on conization. In no instance in the directed biopsy group was invasive cancer found, whereas three of the random biopsy group demonstrated microinvasive disease on conization. In a study of 317 patients, Hollyock and Chanen[8] were able to eliminate the need for conization in 65 per cent of patients with noninvasive lesions by the use of colposcopy and directed biopsy. It is important to emphasize, however, that patients who exhibit these characteristics require conization for proper evaluation:[9] (1) no colposcopic lesion in the presence of an abnormal smear, (2) disease extending into the endocervix with its limits not visualized, (3) lesions too extensive for meaningful biopsy, and (4) lesions in which the cytologic smear suggests invasive disease but biopsy reveals a lesser grade.

The combination of endocervical curettage with four-quadrant biopsy of the cervix has recently been recommended by a number of authors. By means of this technique, the diagnosis of invasive disease high in the endocervix, away from the biopsy site, can be suggested or excluded. In a study of 89 patients with carcinoma in situ evaluated only by this technique, Thompson[10] demonstrated that in no instance was invasive cancer found on hysterectomy. It was interesting to note—though it was to be expected—that in those patients, 69 per cent showed residual disease in the hysterectomy specimen, whereas of 50 patients in whom hysterectomy was preceded by conization, only 44 per cent had residual disease. It must be stressed that in situations in which abnormal epithelium is found on endocervical curettage specimens, conization must be performed. However, the majority of patients will not have such findings and will thus be spared the added risk of conization. Thompson's conclusion, which has been shared by a number of other authors, is that occult invasive cancer can be adequately ruled out by means of adequate four-quadrant biopsies combined with vigorous endocervical curettage. The use of the Schiller staining technique to delineate biopsy sites is an additional aid that may be employed. This technique, when properly carried out, can be utilized by those who do not have the equipment available or the expertise for performing colposcopy.

Comment

The final diagnosis of an intraepithelial lesion of the cervix cannot be made until the presence of an invasive lesion has been ruled out. Thus, it is necessary to perform any diagnostic test or procedure required to accomplish this goal. Much of the preceding discussion has laid stress on the word "adequate." What is an adequate conization? The answers to these questions must be left to the individual physician, and depend upon his past experience and upon his ability to correlate cytologic abnormalities with tissue findings.

Adequate biopsies, as defined by many of those who depend upon biopsies for definitive diagnosis of intraepithelial neoplasia, are those which contain enough tissue for proper identification of squamous epithelium, endocervical epithelium, and the squamocolumnar junction in at least four quadrants and preferably upon multiple sectioning as well. Adequate conization is more difficult to define, since what may be considered a conization by one physician is often less adequate than a four-quadrant biopsy in the opinion of another. Conversely, one individual's idea of conization may be equivalent to a total cervical amputation performed by another. Thus, definition is essential when one is considering the validity of an argument that conization is mandatory for the proper diagnosis of intraepithelial neoplasia of the cervix. It is interesting to note that in many studies of carcinoma in situ, an incidence of residual disease varying from 16 per cent to 44 per cent[4] is reported in hysterectomy specimens following conization. It would not seem unreasonable to ask, "Why could not the intraepithelial lesion that is left be an occult invasive lesion which was missed?" If the conizations done in those series were adequate, would not the cervix essentially be free of any epithelial abnormality? The fact that this is the case in some situations is pointed out by the consistent reporting, in various series, of a few instances of invasive cancer found following diagnostic conization. Of course, one should not criticize a technique just because it is often performed improperly. One may, however, criticize a dictum demanding the performance of that procedure regardless of its effectiveness or need in some situations.

The relatively recent recognition and acceptance of the lesion diagnosed as microinvasive carcinoma of the cervix has added another dimension to the problem of the ultimate diagnosis and treatment of early cervical neoplasia. This lesion, which is no longer truly intraepithelial but which is not considered significant insofar as spread or metastasis is concerned, makes the proper diagnosis and management of the patient with an invisible cervical lesion even more difficult. It is very likely that lesions such as this have led to considerable confusion in the past where the adequacy or inadequacy of biopsies compared to conization specimens is concerned. It is not the purpose of this discussion to enter into the controversy surrounding the definition or treatment of microinvasive cancer, but I mention it here to point out the added confusion it has brought into the picture.

In no disease or condition should one allow a single method of diagnosis or treatment to become so entrenched as to obscure or preclude any further thought concerning its validity. Improvement in existing technology, the development of new techniques, the combination of existing techniques for more efficiency, and a better understanding of the biology and the pathophysiology of a disease necessarily create the demand for reevaluation in terms of its clinical management. It is unfortunate that all too often certain tests or procedures become so fixed in our thinking that we fail to reevaluate their applicability from time to time. The answer to the question posed earlier in this discussion—regarding whether conization is required in every patient suspected of having intraepithelial neoplasia of the cervix—is no. This is not to say that many, if not most, patients do not require conization. If invasion can be effectively ruled out by other methods, conization need not be done. However, in the event that there is any question regarding the presence of invasive cancer, *adequate* conization with *adequate* study of the tissue is vital to the best interests of the patient. Those who do not have available the advantages of advanced cytopathologic techniques, colposcopy, or detailed tissue examination of biopsy specimens are best advised to continue conization in every case of suspected cervical epithelial abnormality. When these techniques are available, however, properly studied and selected patients can be treated definitively for intraepithelial cervical neoplasia without the necessity of conization.

Summary and Conclusion

1. Methods of diagnosing intraepithelial neoplasia of the cervix and differentiating it from invasive cancer have been enumerated and discussed.
2. The values and pitfalls of diagnostic conization have been emphasized.
3. When certain definite criteria are met, selected patients with cervical epithelial abnormalities need not be subjected to conization in order to properly evaluate the extent of their lesion.
4. It is stressed that in the event of any question of invasion, or question of inadequacy of specimens, conization must be done before definitive therapy is undertaken.

REFERENCES

1. Baker, W. S., and Hawks, B. L.: The prognostic significance of glandular involvement in cold knife conization biopsies in carcinoma in situ of the uterine cervix. Am. J. Obstet. Gynec. 73:1266, 1957.
2. Christopherson, W. M., Gray, L. A., and Parker, J. E.: Role of punch biopsy in subclinical lesions of the uterine cervix. Obstet. Gynec. 30:806, 1967.
3. Devereux, W. P., and Creighton, L. E.: Carcinoma in situ of the cervix. Am. J. Obstet. Gynec. 98:497, 1967.
4. Dilts, P. V., Jr., Elesh, R. H., and Greene, R. R.: Re-evaluation of four-quadrant punch biopsies of the cervix. Am. J. Obstet. Gynec. 90:961, 1964.
5. Ferguson, J. H., and Demick, P. E.: Diagnostic conization of the cervix. New Eng. J. Med. 262:13, 1960.
6. Griffiths, C. T., Austin, J. H., and Younge, P. A.: Punch biopsy of the cervix. Am. J. Obstet. Gynec. 88:695, 1964.
7. Hester, L. L., and Read, R. A.: An evaluation of cervical conization. Am. J. Obstet. Gynec. 80:715, 1960.
8. Hollyock, V. E. and Chanen, W.: The use of the colposcope in the selection of patients for cervical cone biopsy. Am. J. Obstet. Gynec. 114:185, 1972.
9. Krumholz, B. A., and Knapp, R. C.: Colposcopic selection of biopsy sites. Obstet. Gynec. 39:22, 1972.
10. Thompson, N. J.: Personal communication.
11. Tweeddale, D. N., and Dubilier, L. D.: Cytopathology of Female Genital Tract Neoplasms. Chicago, Year Book Medical Publishers, 1972.

The Cone Versus Multiple Punch Biopsy
in the Diagnosis of Cervical Neoplasia

Editorial Comment

The salvage of patients from cancer of the cervix has largely been dependent on identification of the disease in its early stages. The view has been expressed that this cancer could be eliminated if every woman had periodic examinations, including a cytologic smear. However, this presupposes high patient motivation and the availability and proper application of current diagnostic methods.

The primary physician in most instances must resolve the question of whether he is prepared to refer his patients who have a verified positive or suspicious cytological cervical smear to a cancer center or service especially equipped to apply the various modalities of diagnosis and treatment. This includes the obstetrician who, even if he has a large practice, will uncover in the course of his career perhaps no more than a dozen patients with uterine cancer, of both the cervix and the corpus. The question is posed whether he should harbor the attitude that he can serve the patient's welfare just as well as those who by training and research interest can devote their total efforts and energies to the study and treatment of women so afflicted.

Again we are confronted with the proposition that all primary physicians must be involved in the early detection of malignant disease, but the treatment must reside in the hands of the specialists listed above, working in centers equipped with all of the modalities of cancer diagnosis and treatment. In fact, the treatment may be dictated in large measure by the laboratory and pathologic findings observed in the course of establishing the precise diagnosis.

The instrumentation that has evolved in recent years has permitted a greater utilization of the methods for diagnosis, replacing the dogmatic principles of previous years, especially regarding punch biopsy versus conization of the cervix. For some years, the proponents of each of these methods were so rigid in their attitudes that it became evident that the patient had to be the ultimate loser. It was not surprising, therefore, that many physicians adopted the policy that when a suspicious smear (class 3?), often unverified or repeated, is seen, one should proceed forthwith to perform a conization. The other extreme is reflected by the remarks of one contributor that he did not perform a single conization in the course of his residency training. Perhaps the barriers of bias have crumbled somewhat, although not without skeptical resistance, through the introduction of the colposcope and colpomicroscopy. Admittedly—though grudgingly—these methods perhaps permit a clear delineation of the suspicious lesion, after which a punch biopsy can usually provide a diagnostic answer. At the same time, this more sophisticated approach favors the concept that a patient with a suspicious smear and a nonvisible lesion should be referred to a cancer service for further diagnosis and appropriate treatment.

18

The Place of Culdoscopy and Laparoscopy in Diagnosis and Patient Management

Alternative Points of View:

    By S. J. Behrman

    By Wayne H. Decker

    By John M. Leventhal

Editorial Comment

The Place of Culdoscopy and Laparoscopy in Diagnosis and Patient Management

S. J. Behrman

The University of Michigan Medical Center

Both laparoscopy and culdoscopy in its various forms have been available for many decades; yet it was not until the introduction of the fiberoptic cold light, which removed the hazard of dissipated heat and increased the intensity of light, that both procedures suddenly leapt into prominence, expanded their usefulness, and have become the sine qua non in diagnostic aids for the gynecologist. Each of these procedures, for various good reasons, has won its rabid protagonists, who have added new and varied modifications, at the same time inundating the literature with claims for the superiority of their own specific techniques over the others. Understandably, then, from this continued interest, research and advancement of technology a new and third endoscopic technique has emerged—i.e., hysteroscopy. Since all three techniques have made an enormous impact on modern medicine as diagnostic and therapeutic modalities, it is to be expected that considerable controversies exist over their relative values. It is precisely this aspect of endoscopy—rather than instrumentation or specific techniques—which will be the main purpose of this discussion.

Laparoscopy or Laparotomy? It is quite obvious that the impact of these procedures over surgery either for diagnosis or therapy is that it reduces the number of hospitalization days, with the subsequent advantages not only to the patient's pocketbook but also to hospital bed utilization. The fact that now most of these endoscopic procedures can also be done under local anesthesia and as an outpatient procedure further underscores their economic advantages. Even these benefits, however, are far overshadowed by the fact that endoscopy reduces the need for surgical exploration, so that the rapid subsequent mobility reduces the patient's chance of postoperative complications due to thromboembolism, ileus, and so forth. Above all, it enhances the diagnostic acumen of the gynecologist.

Endoscopy is used as a diagnostic procedure for:

1. Acute and chronic pelvic pain.
2. Suspected pelvic endometriosis.

581

3. Suspected tubal obstruction, to test tubal patency preoperatively.
4. Infertility of unknown etiology.
5. Second looks at carcinoma of the pelvis and ovary.
6. Peritoneal irrigations for cytology in suspect carcinoma of the ovary.
7. Biopsy of gonads in genetic disorders.
8. Liver biopsies.

Many of these conditions would not have been diagnosed without the use of an endoscope, while some can be treated through the laparoscope. The endoscopic procedure has been advocated over surgery for (1) major cases of pelvic endometriosis which can be fulgurated simply through the laparoscope, (2) the severing of mild adhesions in cases of tubal obstruction, (3) removal of intrauterine devices which might have perforated the uterus, (4) uterine suspension, (5) division of uterosacral ligaments, (6) removal of ova for in vitro fertilization followed by intratubal implantation, and (7) open wedge resection of the ovary.

As with all new procedures, the ever-present danger of overenthusiasm is evident, and it is essential that we assume a sense of responsibility in judging what procedures to do as well as when and how to do them. This admonition is intended to be cautionary rather than to be taken as final judgment, and due and deliberate thought should be given prior to undertaking any of the listed procedures. However, it can be safely said that the wide acceptance of the endoscopic procedures gives testimony to their practicability as a substitutional procedure or a preparatory procedure prior to undertaking a laparotomy.

LAPAROSCOPY OR CULDOSCOPY? Obviously any discussions of this question will be heavily weighted by the individual's experience, depending largely on whether he had first learned culdoscopy and then laparoscopy, had been trained in culdoscopy and never tried laparoscopy, or belongs to the new school, which recommends laparoscopy exclusively, without ever attempting culdoscopy. Ignoring this heavy bias, there are certain very definite points of reference which can settle this issue—viz., the purpose for which the procedure is done, such as diagnosis or therapy; the circumstances under which the procedure is to be done and the facilities available; the skills of the operator; whether anesthesia is available; and finally the social factors involved and demands of the patients served. Clearly, then, where minimal hospital facilities prevail, culdoscopy has the advantage as a diagnostic procedure because of the relative ease in performing the procedure under local anesthesia. When visible scars are a source of concern to the patient, clearly culdoscopy is preferable. Semantically, it should be clearly understood that when one speaks of a therapeutic procedure, i.e., tubal ligation or wedge resection of the ovary through the culdoscope, one is in fact talking of a culdotomy. With this in mind, the vaginal approach cannot be faulted, and after all is the métier of the gynecologist. Again it should be emphasized that when local anesthesia is the only type available, even though the abdominal approach is possible, the vaginal approach is indeed simpler and certainly easier on the patient.

Less favorable to the culdoscopist is the fact that when there is less mobility it is more difficult to manipulate the internal genital structures through a culdoscope or a culdotomy than through a laparoscope. In chronic pelvic disease with fixed lesions and nodulation in the cul-de-sac, the culdoscope cannot be introduced with safety. Furthermore, lesions in the cul-de-sac (i.e., endometriosis implants, which often are the reason for doing the diagnostic procedure in the first place) are indeed very difficult to see through the culdoscope, and certainly it is virtually impossible to see the anterior surface of the uterus and the bladder—common implantation sites for endometriosis—through the culdoscope. Less important, but still worthy of mention, is the fact that on occasion the scar following culdotomy results in dyspareunia and may start a new train of symptoms in the patient.

Definitely working in favor of the laparoscope, admitting the fact that general anesthesia must be used more frequently than local, is its superb visual field, sometimes even better than that of laparotomy, for the lens and therefore the eye can be trained virtually upon each organ or lesion being studied. In addition, the mobility of instruments when the patient is in the dorsal position is of course far greater than when working through a somewhat narrow cavity, and the visibility of lesions in the cul-de-sac is outstanding. But where laparoscopy really stands out is in diagnostic procedures in children, in whom, of course, the culdoscope is not feasible. Admittedly, laparoscopy is a more difficult procedure, but with training it becomes a facile instrument in the hands of any gynecologist.

Whether one or another procedure may be considered "best" is really of no real concern, for ideally the gynecologist should know how to use each procedure at the appropriate time, i.e., he should be able to provide individual management, which after all is the core of good medical practice.

WHEN TO PERFORM THE PROCEDURE

When interval sterilization is decided on, because of inability to schedule patients at a specific time of the menstrual cycle, many have performed dilatation and uterine curettage prior to laparoscopy or culdoscopy in the firm belief that this would take care of any unexpected pregnancy. However, experience clearly indicates that even following dilatation and curettage a pregnancy may be missed. Therefore, the time to do any of the procedures of sterilization is during the proliferative phase of the menstrual cycle, in which case the only question is which technique to use—laparoscopy, culdoscopy, or hysteroscopy?

Postpartum sterilization definitely should be done by laparoscopy rather than culdoscopy because of the size of the uterus and its increased vascularity. Many would state, and rightly so, that a "mini-laparotomy" is even better than a laparoscopy, a view with which I agree. Performing a mini-laparotomy with tubal sterilization immediately after delivery, under spinal anesthesia or even local anesthesia, is the simplest procedure. Direct vision adds greater safety, with no further expense or hospitalization time for the patient. In my opinion this is the safest method for the postpartum period. However, if laparoscopy or culdoscopy is to be used, the question to be asked is what is the most appropriate time to do this procedure—i.e., at day 1 or 5, or at 6 weeks? Reports in the literature suggest that postpartum abdominal surgery is associated with higher incidence of thromboembolic phenomena than is laparoscopy. As stated, the ideal time to perform the procedure is within the first 12 to 24 hours after delivery, but if this cannot be effected, and especially if there has been a difficult delivery with ruptured membranes and potential infection, it might be well to delay the procedure until day 5 or until 6 weeks for fear of creating a pelvic abscess with consequent attendant morbidity.

When sterilization is performed post partum, attempting to reach the fallopian tube through the cul-de-sac can be extremely difficult and bloody. Even performing the ligation through the laparoscope is fraught with approximately three times the complication rate, owing to the presence of the enlarged uterus. For this reason it might be far simpler to insert a Hegar dilator into the postpartum uterus and tent the anterior abdominal wall by bringing the uterus forward; make a half-inch incision in the midline and under direct vision, using local anesthesia, perform a mini-laparotomy, deliberately tying and cutting the tube. Although, logically, hysteroscopy will be easiest in the immediate postpartum period, it is also the least desirable because the postpartum uterus is in fact an open wound and the precipitation of infection or of intravascular emboli is certainly a hazard. Above all, of course, is the fact that at present very little experience is available with such procedures post partum. Thus, postpartum sterilization definitely favors mini-laparotomy as a first choice and then laparoscopy over culdoscopy, mainly because of the size of the uterus and its vascularity. However, when one considers interval sterilization, the choice of laparoscopy versus culdoscopy becomes a much more emotional one, governed by experience and circumstances. Because hysteroscopy is still only in its infancy, very few people have experience with this procedure, but if results hold up it is safe to state that this may well supplant both laparoscopy and culdoscopy in the very near future. Whichever method is chosen, certain major controversies of detail exist for each procedure, which will now be discussed.

Laparoscopy

SITE OF INCISION

It is not surprising that, as more physicians become familiar with the technique, the preferred site of incision will vary. Ignoring these personal propensities, one might discuss some of the basic factors that determine incision. Principally for cosmetic reasons, the prime incision is made in the lower fold of the umbilicus, but whether it is made transversely or vertically is of little consequence. This type of incision is ideally suited for the 6 mm. probe used for diagnostic viewing. When one uses the 10 mm. instrument, either as a "one-hole" technique or for purposes of photography, the cosmetic value of making the incision there is somewhat lost. Consequently, a vertical incision 2 or 3 mm. beneath the umbilicus or parallel and lateral to it is quite acceptable. The lateral incision might be preferred primarily because the trocar would go through the rectus muscle and the chance of herniation is much less than when a hole is placed through the linea alba.

PNEUMOPERITONEUM

Certainly it has been said that without pneumoperitoneum an adequate exposure cannot be attained. Perhaps one of the most difficult steps of the entire procedure is getting an adequate pneumoperitoneum. While actual techniques will not be considered here, there is room for discussion of the medium to be used. Certainly carbon dioxide is the most universally used because of its rapid absorption, known safety factor, lack of flash point, and the traditional experience with CO_2 insufflation and gynecography. However, many have tried nitrous oxide because by itself it is also an analgesic agent and less irritating to the diaphragm. While research data are still meager it appears that the main hazard of nitrous oxide for laparoscopic sterilization is its low flash point, and as such it might be well not to use this medium. In countries where ancillary instrumentation might be difficult to obtain, gynecologists have been known to use plain air, either pumping it in by a small hand pump, or letting air enter after making a small incision first down to the fascia. The fascia is then elevated with Allis clamps and the incision is extended through it into the peritoneal cavity, allowing air to enter while inserting the trocar under direct vision. Although these latter methods do work, there is little question that they are to be avoided because of their potentially lethal risk of air embolism.

INSTRUMENTATION

The selection of instruments, whether the Cohen-Eder drill, the Palmer drill, or the Semm coagulation and separate scissors, is purely one of personal preference. However, it is imperative that the shaft of either the coagulator or the trocar, or preferably both, be covered with fiber glass to prevent burns. The preferred telescope is the 180° scope of either Wolf or Storz, and it may vary in size from 5 to 10 mm. in diameter. The CO_2 insufflator is the automatic one designed by Semm, with its major advantage indicating the amount of CO_2 insufflated. A new type devised by Steptoe will be released shortly, which in addition will determine the pressure inside the abdominal cavity. I also strongly urge the use of solid state coagulating equipment in preference to the at present commonly used Bovie equipment, in which the voltage is too high and leakage can occur, with the hazard of severe shock.

INSTRUMENTS APPLIED TO THE CERVIX. It is necessary to have some instrumentation of the uterine cavity to permit manipulation of the uterus while observing through the laparoscope. Many use a small conventional curette or a uterine sound, despite the ever-present danger of perforation of the uterus. Far safer would be a cannula which permits not only manipulation of the uterus but also instillation of indigo carmine to determine tubal patency. However, in a new clamping instrument designed by Hulka, one arm is a uterine sound and one arm a tenaculum, allowing a simple one-step application of cannula and tenaculum without danger of uterine perforation. The use of a suction vacuum cap is an elegant way of attaching a cannula to the uterine cervix by negative suction, but practically it is a little more difficult because of variations in the size of the cervix.

ANESTHESIA

This is still the most important area of controversy. For culdoscopy, use of local anesthesia is ideal and indeed it is seldom necessary to use general anesthesia in these cases. While local anesthesia can be used for laparoscopy, as evidenced by the extensive experience of Wheeless, it is my firm conviction that it is safer to use general anesthesia for laparoscopy despite its attendant hazards and despite the fact that it requires hospitalization. One of the dangers of instilling CO_2 into the uterine cavity is that absorption from the peritoneal cavity leads to hypercarbia, especially if there is rapid distension of the abdomen. This may cause vagal stimulation, with resultant decreased ventilation of the lungs, leading in turn to hypoxia. As a consequence, cardiac arrhythmias are not uncommon. If general anesthesia is used for laparoscopy by the beginner and too much CO_2 is instilled over too long a period, this may lead to increased levels of circulating catecholamines, producing clinical effects of hypertension and increased suscepti- bility to cardiac irregularities (Schwimmer). Thus, the basic measures that should be taken to prevent hypercarbia are (1) adequate premedication, (2) controlled ventilation, using an endotracheal tube and so avoiding hypoxia, and (3) where feasible, continuous EKG monitoring and precordial auscultation for prompt diag- nosis and attention to irregularities.

TECHNIQUE OF TUBAL STERILIZATION

Whether tubal sterilization is done through a culdotomy or through a cul- doscope or through the laparoscope, there is still considerable controversy as to which method is the most appropriate. It is remarkable that despite surgical pro- cedures, e.g., Pomeroy and Madlener techniques, there is still a failure rate of about 1 to 2 per cent. Since the advent of the laparoscope and the increased demands for tubal sterilization, electrocoagulation has become the method most often used. At first an attempt was made to coagulate only the tube, along its entire length, and good results were reported with this technique. Subsequently with the use of the Palmer drill, the tube was coagulated and also a half centimeter of it was removed, with both the proximal and distal ends being coagulated simultane- ously. Certainly the results from this technique have been as good as or even better than the surgical approach. I prefer coagulation along with incising the tube at two areas with a scissors, which simultaneously cuts and coagulates it as it incises into the tube. This again is merely a matter of preference, but in 1500 cases performed to date, only one failure has been reported.

Because interest has been expressed in using tubal ligation as an interim technique, the possibility of a reversible tubal ligation has been seriously enter- tained, and as a consequence many approaches have been developed that employ a tantalum or self-loading silastic clip. The results of reversible reconstructive surgery following the removal of these clips are not yet at hand. However, it is of interest to note that the failure rate of clips is somewhat greater than that of coagulation and cutting, and there have even been reports of ectopic pregnancy when clips have been used. Tubal ligation with clips is, however, a much simpler procedure and avoids any danger of burning of bowel or other tissue. There is little question that the ingenuity of man will sooner or later develop a clip tech- nique that will be foolproof and reversible, though this has not yet been done.

ONE OR TWO HOLES? There has been considerable debate over whether a single trocar perforation should be used, or, alternatively, a trocar perforation plus one additional perforation suprapubically. For the patient who must submit to this procedure under local anesthesia, a single hole certainly is preferable, since the least amount of disturbance is desired. In experienced hands, the use of the "single hole technique" works, without question, but for the beginner it is far easier to use the "two-hole technique." The problem basically lies in the fact that if there is movement of bowel or difficulty in exposing the tubes, manipulation of the second instrument (i.e., the coagulator or scissors) is limited through a single hole. With the two-hole technique, it is possible not only to manipulate the tube out of harm's way but also to use the second puncture to move bowel or omentum out of the field of view and away from potential danger.

CLOSURE OF THE WOUND.   When using the vaginal approach, there is little question that one or two sutures at the apex of the vagina is all that is required, and this is easily effected with absorbable suture.

If a 5 mm. scope is used, frequently no form of closure is required following laparoscopy other than a Band-Aid to approximate the cut edge for 24 hours. When a 10 mm. incision has been made, frequently it is necessary to put in one or two subcuticular absorbable sutures. Use of Dexon slow absorbable sutures has been favored by some. If these are to be used it is strongly recommended that they do not perforate the skin because of the danger of infection. Many operators use three tantalum clips, removing them in 24 hours. However, regardless of the choice of method, one thing should be remembered, viz., the thinner the patient and the larger the trocar used, the greater the chances, remote though they may be, for herniation of a piece of omentum or loop of bowel through the wound. It is also important to remember that a suture can be put into the bowel accidentally with the greatest of ease if subcuticular sutures are being used. Attention should be paid to this possibility.

Culdoscopy

Much of what has been said regarding anesthesia, suture, coagulation, clips, and so forth, for laparoscopy applies to culdoscopy as well. Other than the prime decision of whether to use culdoscopy or laparoscopy there still remains one main area of controversy. Which is the method of choice, section of the tube, coagulation, or clips?

As the fimbriated ends of the tubes are frequently the easiest to deliver into the vagina through the culdotomy incision, it is common practice to do a fimbriectomy. Although this is quite acceptable, it should be emphasized that the fallopian tube is a dynamic structure and secretes fluid, and ligating only the fimbriated end is an ideal way of creating a hydrosalpinx. In time this may cause such pain as to demand a total hysterectomy. It is recommended, therefore, that all procedures be done in the midportion or proximal end of the tube.

Hysteroscopy

This technique is definitely an outpatient procedure, to be done under local anesthesia. Much needs to be learned about details and variations of methodology, but already one aspect is at issue. What medium is to be used to distend the uterine cavity?

The original study used 30 per cent Dextran, which has the same optical density and light transference as the lens of a telescope. However, it is expensive and is not available to all countries. Five per cent glucose in distilled water (not saline) has been found to be as good, as in addition it is inexpensive and always available. More recently, CO_2 under 100 mm. Hg pressure has been found to be equally effective in distending the uterus. However, special and expensive equipment is needed, and once more one is faced with potential risks of hypercarbia and CO_2 embolism.

As long as endoscopy remains popular and is used by more gynecologists, there will be controversy and as a result more improvements. While no claim is made for the ultimate, experience modified by indications, economic considerations, and other variables has led to these diverse views. We should fully appreciate that when one starts with certainties one ends with doubts; it is only by starting with doubts that one can hope to achieve certainties.

The Place of Culdoscopy and Laparoscopy in Diagnosis and Patient Management

WAYNE H. DECKER

New York University Medical College and University Hospital

Historical Background

Culdoscopy and laparoscopy have evolved as a result of a constant endeavor to develop better methods for inspecting the female pelvis. Gynecologists have long relied on palpation for the diagnosis of gynecological pathology. While the tactile senses have become highly developed in the experienced clinician, many conditions remained obscure and indefinite when there was sole reliance on the sense of touch.

During the past 70 years there have been reports from numerous investigators who have attempted direct or indirect visualization of the pelvis by means of puncture through the abdominal wall or through the vagina. About 1910 Jacobaeus[1] was able to introduce a telescope through an abdominal puncture used for paracentesis in patients with ascites, by means of which the abdominal viscera could be visualized. He reported on 17 patients examined by this method. This was the beginning of laparoscopy. Kelling[2] was able to develop a technique using air introduced into the abdominal cavity which replaced the ascitic fluid necessary in the technique described by Jacobaeus. Other investigators, including Bernheim,[3] Orndoff,[4] Alvarez,[5] and Petersen,[6] also reported rather extensive use of a procedure variously termed celioscopy, peritoneoscopy, and splanchnoscopy, utilizing pneumoperitoneum to permit inspection of the abdominal and pelvic viscera. This method gained some popularity until the early 1920's, when Case[7] drew attention to four deaths which had resulted from air embolism. Even though investigators had begun to utilize carbon dioxide with complete safety, the procedure fell into disfavor and its use continued only on a limited basis.

Those who continued to use peritoneoscopy found it to be a procedure of some value, particularly in the inspection of the upper abdomen and the liver.

The largest series of cases appeared to be that of Ruddock,[8] published in 1934, in which he described the results of 500 examinations using a technique similar to that of Kelling.

The vaginal approach to examination of the pelvic viscera had long been established as a safe, convenient procedure, and posterior colpotomy had been utilized by gynecologists for the evacuation of hematomas and the drainage of pelvic abscesses. Von Ott[9] in 1903 referred to the successful employment of the transvaginal approach for the visualization of the pelvic organs. He used reflected light from a head mirror to visualize the organs through an opening in the vaginal vault. The patient in this instance was placed in a steep dorsal Trendelenberg position. During his work Von Ott had described a negative pressure phenomenon which occurred with the extreme vertical position. Few other investigators, however, tried Von Ott's technique, and his method of diagnosis gained little acceptance.

In 1935, Decker,[10] through the use of cadavers, was able to demonstrate to his satisfaction that the knee-chest position caused the abdominal viscera to be displaced cephalad and created a significant negative intra-abdominal pressure. When a puncture was made in the vaginal septum, an inrush of air could be detected, and the pelvic viscera could readily be visualized by means of a simple right angle telescope fitted with a small incandescent light bulb. After some experimentation, Decker found that the knee-chest position could be maintained with relative ease and did not require any unusual tables or supports.[11] Furthermore, and of extreme importance, the procedure was reasonably painless and could be performed readily under local anesthesia. As a matter of fact, some early experiences with culdoscopy indicated that the knee-chest position contraindicated the use of general anesthesia, particularly inhalation anesthesia, because the position made it difficult to maintain an adequate airway.

During the 20 years or so following Decker's original report of the successful use of culdoscopy, the technique gained increasing popularity in gynecological centers throughout the world. An experienced culdoscopist found satisfaction in the ability to make accurate diagnoses by a relatively simple means and with little danger or discomfort for their patients.

During this same time, however, many persons less experienced and knowledgeable in the use of the techniques attempted to perform culdoscopy by their own self-taught methods. In many instances, these were very crude, and examples have been seen where culdoscopy was attempted on a patient in the dorsal lithotomy position and with the patient suspended by various unusual trapeze-like apparatuses. Indeed, one instance is reported in which an individual made two successful culdoscopic examinations while passing the trocar through the anterior cul-de-sac between the cervix and the bladder, miraculously avoiding injury to the bladder.

Because of the inexperience of many individuals who failed to obtain adequate training in the use of these procedures, there remained areas of resistance among a significant segment of physicians, who felt that culdoscopy was of little value as a diagnostic method and that the results could not be relied upon. The numerous reports, however, by those well trained and versed in the procedure and aware of the principles involved gave ample evidence of culdoscopy as a diagnostic procedure of unusual value.

Technique of Culdoscopy

A number of factors have been responsible for the failure of the novice to appreciate the value of culdoscopy. Principal among these have been the lack of proper training and understanding of the principles involved prior to applying culdoscopy as a diagnostic tool. Frequently the inexperienced culdoscopist fails to gain access to the pelvis because of his lack of concern about a number of seemingly minor details. First among these is failure to pay proper attention to the instruments used. It is extremely important that the trocar employed for the cul-de-sac puncture have a keen edge. When the instrument is allowed to become dull, the vaginal mucosa may be punctured with ease, but the delicate peritoneum, which offers less resistance and tends to ride ahead of the instrument, is pushed forward rather than allowing the dull instrument to pass through.

The culdoscopist must also be concerned with the proper positioning of the patient. Carelessness in this matter results in the lack of proper distention of the vagina and as a result a thicker, less well-defined site for puncture.

The third important consideration for successful cul-de-sac puncture is the proper selection of the site for puncture. Inexperienced operators tend to make the puncture too close to the cervix for fear of injury to the rectum. This results in penetration at the point where the peritoneum becomes fixed to the posterior cervix, and intraperitoneal penetration does not occur. The puncture must be made at the point of greatest concavity of the distended mucosa of the posterior cul-de-sac. This site must be utilized even though it may appear to be too close to the rectum or cervix.

Even if successful puncture is made, the culdoscopist may be dissatisfied with many aspects of the visual diagnosis. Some experience is required in order to estimate and judge the size of the various structures because of the magnification factors in the lens system. Structures viewed very close up may appear larger than they actually are; conversely, when viewed from a distance, they tend to appear somewhat smaller. Only after repeated observation and experience will the physician eventually be able to judge these factors with considerable accuracy.

The beginning culdoscopist also has considerable difficulty in orientation because he must realize that structures located on the patient's right side appear on the operator's right side or on the right side of the field of vision. This is a matter which can readily be overcome after a short period of experience.

The physician may be somewhat alarmed by a patient's complaints of postoperative pain if considerable care is not taken to relieve the pneumoperitoneum at the conclusion of the procedure. This is often omitted by those unfamiliar with the technique. When the culdoscopic examination is completed, the patient is placed on her abdomen, with her head slightly lower than the buttocks. Using a pillow or pressure to the abdomen, with the cannula still in place in the puncture site, the patient is told to cough or strain. The air which had created the pneumoperitoneum can be readily expressed, and the patient will usually be quite comfortable or experience only minor upper abdominal and shoulder pain when she assumes the upright position. When proper care of the pneumoperitoneum is omitted, the patient may experience excessive discomfort, which may last for several days. This can be quite discouraging and annoying for the patient and physician alike. Emphasis must be placed on relieving the pneumoperitoneum at the conclusion of the examination. The patient should be advised that post-examination pain can be readily relieved by lying perfectly flat. Not even a pillow to raise the head should be used. Well meaning attendants often encourage the patient to walk about in order to relieve this discomfort, but this should be cautioned against, as it will only aggravate the symptoms.

All through the early years of development and utilization of culdoscopy, the telescope was equipped with a small incandescent lamp as a means of illumination. Although this was usually adequate, it sometimes proved cumbersome and gave a limited illumination because any increase in amount of light created heat, which in turn caused considerable patient discomfort. The frequent failures of this delicate lamp were also a source of inconvenience. About 10 years ago, after the fiberoptics had been developed for the transmission of light as well as of an image, there was a marked improvement in the instruments used for culdoscopy. Fiberoptics permitted a greater degree of illumination, without the heat created by the incandescent lamps. The light transmitted through fiberoptics is "cold light." The light source was also considerably more dependable, and light failures became a matter of little concern. An incidental benefit of the development of fiberoptics was the increased utilization of photographic equipment through culdoscopy. This made possible pictorial records heretofore extremely difficult to obtain.

Laparoscopy

During the years when culdoscopy was becoming a standard diagnostic method in many clinics, laparoscopy was seldom employed. Curiously, with the use of fiberoptics, which made culdoscopy a more convenient and dependable procedure, laparoscopy enjoyed a renaissance. This too resulted principally from the use of fiberoptics.

Together with improved instrumentation, laparoscopy provided a means of diagnosis which was a little easier for the gynecologist who is either unable or unwilling to master the techniques involved in culdoscopy. In laparoscopy the problem of orientation is more or less overcome because the pelvic organs are viewed in the more conventional way, as they would be during a laparotomy. Chief among the disadvantages of laparoscopy is the need for general anesthesia. Although some operators have utilized local anesthesia, it is generally conceded that this is insufficient for the patient's comfort and for the successful completion of the examination. In order to displace the intestine from the pelvis, a gas must be introduced into the abdomen by the use of nitrous oxide or carbon dioxide under positive pressure. In addition, the procedure of laparoscopy does require an abdominal incision, though a small one, usually through the umbilicus. Frequently a secondary incision is made to utilize various probes and operative instruments as well.

In summary, it might be said that whereas culdoscopy is easier on the patient, laparoscopy is easier for the physician. Those physicians who find culdoscopy too difficult to master will often be able to utilize laparoscopy more effectively.

Use of Culdoscopy for Diagnosis

In the beginning, culdoscopy found its chief value in the diagnosis of ectopic pregnancies. It became a useful procedure to place the patient in the knee-chest position and perform a culdoscopy when ectopic pregnancy was suspected.[12] The visual interpretation of an ectopic pregnancy was relatively easy. Although tubal gestation may have occurred, frequently it was not actually visualized, but the presence of clots and blood was sufficient to make a diagnosis on a strongly presumptive basis. For this reason culdoscopy has become a fairly standard procedure in most clinics in order to make an exact diagnosis of ectopic pregnancy. In these situations, the use of general anesthesia required for laparoscopy would hardly seem warranted in most instances.

In our clinic, when a patient presents herself with the classic history and physical findings of a tubal gestation and there is physical and laboratory evidence of rupture and hemorrhage, appropriate surgical treatment is instituted. However, when the evidence is not so clear-cut, other measures are employed. Culdocentesis that reveals gross blood which fails to clot is usually sufficient indication for laparotomy. Occasionally the surgical findings do not confirm the clinical diagnosis of tubal pregnancy, but regardless of the exact etiology, the hemoperitoneum is usually sufficient to warrant surgical intervention.

Probably more than half of all tubal pregnancies do not create a typical symptom complex or cause characteristic physical signs. It is in these circumstances that culdoscopy can be most rewarding. A definitive diagnosis based on culdoscopic findings can avoid considerable waiting and delay, and often eliminates unnecessary laparotomy. It is doubtful that laparoscopy is employed as readily when there is limited provocation.

As the original culdoscopists gained experience, the use of culdoscopy extended into other areas. It is frequently used for the diagnosis of obscure pelvic complaints. Chronic pelvic pain for which there was little or no palpable evidence of pathology offered a diagnostic challenge for culdoscopy.

Every gynecologist is confronted with repeated instances of women who complain of pelvic pain for which there is no symptom pattern or physical findings to offer clear evidence of an exact diagnosis. Such conditions as endometriosis and chronic salpingitis often present themselves in this fashion. "Chronic pelvic congestion" is a diagnosis applied when more definite findings are absent. Not infrequently, pelvic symptoms of a bizarre nature result from various psychogenic factors. The gynecologist will usually assign such a diagnosis with reluctance, however, as most patients will resist this conclusion unless it is based on very substantial evidence. Culdoscopy frequently provides such evidence, and the gynecologist will be more secure in his approach to the management of the true nature of his patient's problem.

On the other hand, more obscure conditions are often uncovered when their presence is unsuspected. We have encountered numerous instances of endometriosis, chronic pelvic inflammatory disease, and pelvic tuberculosis, and even the marked venous distention of "chronic pelvic congestion" is sometimes detected by culdoscopy.

It soon became apparent also that the field of infertility offered rich rewards for the competent culdoscopist. In our clinic today, culdoscopy has become a routine part of almost all infertility evaluations. Unless there is some overriding contraindication or an obvious defect in the male partner, culdoscopy is almost always employed in the evaluation of the infertile female. It has been through the use of culdoscopy in large numbers of infertile patients that previously unsuspected causes of infertility have been recognized.

At best, most infertility workups require weeks or even months before thorough evaluation is completed. However, a carefully planned routine can accomplish a great deal in a few days and can afford a substantial saving of time for the anxious patient. It has been found to be of particular value for patients who come from some distance and have limited time to spend away from home.

The following is a routine adopted from that recommended by Decker[10]: The patient reports for her first appointment at about the time of her expected ovulation, as determined from her usual menstrual pattern. That is, she will report on day 11 or 12 if she has a 25 or 26 day cycle or day 13 to 15 if she has a 28 day cycle, and so forth. She is instructed to have intercourse 4 to 5 hours before her first appointment. At the first interview a complete history is taken and a thorough physical examination is performed. Vaginal smears are made for a study of hormonal effect and cervical smears are made for cytology review. The cervical mucus is examined for viscosity and for the presence and condition of spermatozoa. A point is made to examine the patient in the knee-chest position to acquaint her with the position to be maintained during culdoscopy and to establish the presence of a freely distensible vaginal vault (ballooning sign). Prior arrangements will have been made for the patient to enter the hospital. Specimens are obtained for complete blood count, urinalysis, and protein bound iodine.

The following morning, culdoscopy is performed under local anesthesia. Culdoscopic lysis of adhesions and biopsy may be performed at this time. Also, if indicated, a dilatation and curettage, cervical biopsy, and cauterization may be done with the use of additional local paracervical block anesthesia. Infusion with indigo carmine under direct vision is always performed, even though the tubes appear grossly normal. At this time, starch may also be introduced into the pelvic cavity for examination the following day to test tubal function.[13] The patient is discharged from the hospital on the first post-operative day.

Later in the cycle an endometrial biopsy may be obtained.

With this routine, seminal, cervical, uterine, tubal, and ovarian factors can be substantially evaluated in a short time and during a single cycle. Depending on the findings, further studies may be required.

Diagnosing Causes of Infertility

The value of culdoscopy in the fertility workup is apparent in a review of a recent series of 221 infertile women who underwent culdoscopy as a part of their infertility workup. The husbands of these patients were found to have reasonably normal fertility. The culdoscopic findings are summarized in Table 18-1.

Those patients with ovarian dysfunction, not including Stein-Leventhal syndrome, showed 15 instances of ovarian hypoplasia, two cases of ovarian agenesis, five of microcystic ovaries, and three reported as ovaries with "thickened tunica."

Stein-Leventhal ovaries are perhaps best and most conclusively diagnosed

TABLE 18-1. *Culdoscopic Findings in 221 Infertile Women*

Ovarian dysfunction	24
Stein-Leventhal ovaries	20
Perisalpingeal disease	42
Fimbrial disease	31
Endosalpingeal disease	30
Endometriosis	31
Uterine fibroids	9
No abnormal findings	27
Failed culdoscopy	7
TOTAL	221

by visual inspection. The appearance of large, smooth, white ovaries without evidence of follicular activity is characteristic of this condition. These patients are usually amenorrheal and show some degree of obesity, hirsutism, and acne. However, lesser degrees of the condition appear to occur when these features are absent or are present to a minimal degree, but the characteristic ovaries are present and infertility results. In these instances, culdoscopy offers an ideal means of diagnosis.

Peritubal disease usually presents as adhesions involving the tubal serosa and the ovaries. This results in kinking and immobilization of the tubes and interference with ovum transport. These patients usually show evidence of tubal patency on insufflation or hysterosalpingography. Although the minimal changes seen on hysterosalpingography are sometimes suggestive of peritubal disease, these may be indicated by marked stretching and fixation of the tube or sometimes by displacement of the tube into an unusual location. Unfortunately these findings are seldom diagnostic. These minimal derangements in tubal function are usually completely overlooked when the patient is subjected to only the conventional diagnostic procedures, yet they may represent the only factor to account for infertility.

Fimbrial disease of the tubes accounted for 31 of the significant findings in this group. Fimbrial disease is defined as a condition which involves primarily the tubal ampulla and fimbriae. This may result in tubal occlusion or only in fimbrial agglutination and phimosis, conditions which are difficult to detect by other means. Culdoscopy offers a valuable aid for detecting the presence of these conditions, and also provides an excellent opportunity to assess the extent of involvement and indicate the best method of treatment.

In 30 instances of endosalpingeal disease there was complete tubal occlusion. Although this can usually be detected by hysterosalpingograms, the extent of involvement and the type and feasibility of surgical repair can best be evaluated by culdoscopy, not only because there is direct visualization, but also because the perfusion of indigo carmine indicates the site and extent of occlusion.

Endometriosis was detected in 31 instances. All degrees of this condition are encountered. When extensive disease is noted, appropriate medical and surgical treatment may be planned. Although minimal disease does not often seem to require treatment, it occurs with such frequency that its relationship to infertility is suspect. Perhaps the same mechanisms that result in endometrial implants in the ovaries and tubes may also be responsible for interference with ovum transport or other fertility factors.

It is surprising that even extensive endometriosis with its resulting adhesions and uterine displacement usually does not prevent culdoscopic visualization.

Uterine fibroids of the size seen on culdoscopy usually represent an incidental finding and are seldom of significance.

Of perhaps more importance are the seven instances of failed culdoscopy (Table 18-1). Our experience now indicates that when the cul-de-sac puncture fails or the pelvic organs cannot be visualized, significant pathology is usually present. In five of the seven instances cited subsequent laparotomy proved this to be true.

In only 27 patients in this group was there no significant pathology detected by culdoscopy.

Other pelvic disease not related to infertility may be detected and evaluated by culdoscopy. These include functional and functioning ovarian tumors, acute salpingitis, the evaluation of dysmenorrhea, and other instances in which visualization of the pelvic organs may be of value.

Culdoscopy as a method of pelvic diagnosis has been established as valuable, effective, and reliable when properly performed. The average gynecologist may find that laparoscopy requires less skill, but the patients will experience less stress and less manipulation, and there will be less need for anesthesia when culdoscopy is used if the necessary skills have been mastered by the operating gynecologist.

REFERENCES

1. Jacobaeus, H. C.: Uber die Möglichkeit die Zystoskopie bei Untersuchung Seröser Höhlungen Anzuwenden. München. Med. Wchnschr. 57:2090, 1910.
2. Kelling, G.: Uber die Möglichkeit die Zystoskopie bei Untersuchungen Seröser Höhlungen Anzuwenden. München. Med. Wchnschr. 57:238, 1910.
3. Bernheim, B. M.: Organoscopy-cystoscopy of the abdominal cavity. Ann. Surg. 53:764, 1911.
4. Orndoff, B. H.: Pneuomoperitoneum in xray diagnosis. J. Roentgenol. 2:265, 1919.
5. Alvarez, W. C.: The use of CO_2 in pneumoperitoneum. Amer. J. Roentgen. 8:71, 1921.
6. Petersen, R.: Advantage of gas inflation in obstetric and gynecologic diagnosis. Canad. Med. Ass. J. 2:893, 1922.
7. Case, J. T.: A review of three years' work and articles on pneumoperitoneum. Amer. J. Roentgen. 8:714, 1921.
8. Ruddock, J. C.: Peritoneoscopy. West. J. Surg. 42:392, 1934.
9. Von Ott, D.: Die unmittelbare Beleuchtung der Bauchhohle der Harnblase, des Dickdarms und der Gebarmutter zu diagnostichen under operativen Zwecken. Monatschr. f. Geburtsch. u. Gynek. 18:645, 1903.
10. Decker, A.: Culdoscopy. Philadelphia, F. A. Davis Co., 1967.
11. Decker, A., and Cherry, T.: Culdoscopy—a new method in the diagnosis of pelvic disease. Preliminary report. Amer. J. Surg. 64:40, 1944.
12. Riva, H. L., Kammeraad, L. A., and Anderson, P. S.: Ectopic pregnancy: report of 132 cases and comments on the role of the culdoscopic diagnosis. Obstet. Gynec. 20:189, 1962.
13. Decker, A., and Decker, W. H.: A tubal function test. Obstet. Gynec. 4:3538, 1954.

The Place of Culdoscopy and Laparoscopy in Diagnosis and Patient Management

JOHN M. LEVENTHAL

Harvard Medical School and Boston Hospital for Women

It was six men of Indostan
    to learning much inclined,
Who went to see the elephant
    (though all of them were blind)
That each by observation
    might satisfy his mind.

John Godfrey Saxe
"The Blind Men and the Elephant"

The problem encountered by the learned men of Indostan was in some respects similar to the problem faced by every obstetrician and gynecologist at manual pelvic examination. No matter how experienced he may be, the examiner is forced to identify the objects of his examination without use of his sense of vision. What he feels must of necessity be identified only through his "mind's eye" by an incredibly long and deceptive chain of sensory obstacles. Interpretation of pelvic bimanual findings is a complicated central process for the observer—one which, by its very nature, can never be perfect. Translation of what the observer feels is accomplished, in part, by comparison with what he "sees" in his mind and what he has actually seen or felt in previous experience. Correct interpretation is often encumbered by obesity, pain, inability of the patient to relax, or even by the disease process itself. The adherent knuckle of small bowel, fixed to the lateral aspect of the uterus, feels as much like a solid tumor of the ovary, a hydrosalpinx, or a subserous leiomyoma, as what it actually is. The tender vague mass in the right adnexal area in the patient with fever, leukocytosis, and spotting could as well be an early acute salpingitis or a bulging tubal pregnancy as it could be acute distal appendicitis. An adherent endometrioma can be interpreted as postoperative adhesions or even a stool-filled sigmoid. More significantly, perhaps, the easily palpated "normal pelvis" in the woman unable to conceive could harbor a myriad of endometriotic implants clustered on the anterior bladder peritoneum or in the cul-de-sac. No matter how skillful the observer, there is usually nothing specific found at bimanual examination to reveal the presence of total fimbrial occlusion. Not only are the hands deceptive, but in certain cases even our visual acuity may lead us to false conclusions. The tube which is clearly patent on the uterotubogram might indeed be thwarted by adhesions which prevent it from reaching the ovary.

It is true that the practitioner's bimanual findings become only a part of the diagnostic whole, and the process of deductive logic utilizes historical data, symptoms, and experience to arrive at a diagnostic possibility. It is also true, however, that pathologically dissimilar pelvic diseases often elude the diagnostician by presenting striking similarities in symptoms, signs, and bimanual findings. The analogy of the partially "diagnosed" elephant of Indostan is even more relevant when consideration is given to the possibility or even probability that bimanual findings will suggest different disease processes. The importance of knowing the whole picture in order to arrive at correct diagnoses, and to plan proper treatment, obviously cannot be overemphasized. The age-old necessity of having to base treatment on bimanual findings of unseen disease in the pelvis has yielded at last, though only in part, to the pelvic endoscope. The ability to combine experience, touch, and imagination with true visual observation has, in many cases, brought the dark unseen reaches of the pelvis out into the light of objective evaluation.

Long the instrument of other disciplines, the endoscope has only relatively recently been applied to diagnosis of disorders of the female pelvis. The culdoscope and laparoscope have allowed the gynecologist to replace his "mind's eye" with an "eye" capable of far greater acuity. Although endoscopic observation of the bladder had been described in the nineteenth century, credit for the introduction of intra-abdominal endoscopy belongs to the German surgeon Kelling. In 1902, Kelling described the use of a Nitze cystoscope in viewing the abdominal cavity of the living dog.[1] He called the procedure "celioscopy," and interestingly enough described the use of a pneumoperitoneum of filtered air. In the succeeding decade he applied his technique to the intra-abdominal observation of human subjects, and reported his work in 1910.[2] The term "laparoscopy" was introduced that same year by Jacobaeus, who, apparently working without knowledge of Kelling's experiments, described intra-abdominal endoscopy on patients with ascites.[3] Neither Jacobaeus nor Bernheim, who was the first American to describe the use of laparoscopy,[4] utilized a preliminary pneumoperitoneum, and it is ironic to note that even Kelling, in his subsequent work in the early 1920's, abandoned this most important of preliminary procedures. Cohen, in his outstanding monograph,[5] and Horwitz,[6] in his review of the subject of gynecologic laparoscopy, have eloquently detailed the rich history of the development of this procedure.

The current widespread popularity of the procedure began in the mid-1960's, and in this country can be attributed primarily to the enthusiasm of Cohen at the Michael Reese Hospital in Chicago. His monograph, his tireless teaching efforts, and his enthusiasm for laparoscopic cinematography will remain as true contributions to operative gynecology. It is interesting to note that Cohen, whose interest has been primarily in the field of infertility, was an accomplished and enthusiastic culdoscopist prior to his introduction to laparoscopy by Palmer in France, in 1966. Like many others since who have become familiar with the numerous advantages of laparoscopy, he has found the two procedures to complement each other, and feels that the indications for their use are similar.

We now tend to view pelvic laparoscopy as a newer technique than that of culdoscopy, and it is hard to believe that the reverse is true. Decker, who can rightfully be called the father of modern culdoscopic technique, became interested in the vaginal route because of his apparent dissatisfaction with the results of laparoscopy. Utilizing the knee-chest position to empty the pelvis of bowel and create a spontaneous pneumoperitoneum, Decker and Cherry in 1944 were the first modern physicians to place an endoscope through the posterior vaginal fornix into the cul-de-sac and view directly the panoply of pelvic disease previously revealed only to the surgeon who performed a laparotomy.[7] Limited by its point of entry, and incapable in most cases of bringing into view the entire pelvis, culdoscopy nonetheless has proved immensely useful in the diagnosis and planning of treatment in the infertile woman. The diagnoses of endometriosis, ovarian neoplasia, and tubal pregnancy were all greatly enhanced by the use of culdoscopy. Following Decker's perfection of the technique, the use of culdoscopy as a diagnostic procedure became widespread and highly developed. Many clinicians working in the field of infertility incorporated culdoscopic investigation of the pelvis into the routine workup of the female patient unable to conceive. The procedure, when it could be performed, offered the first practical and simple method for overcoming the limitations of bimanual examination. Both Decker and Clyman are to be credited with the introduction of various operative techniques at culdoscopy, and for the first time it became practical to perform ovarian biopsy, cauterization, and other minor pelvic procedures without resorting to open surgery.

The ancient but well known Chinese proverb which states "One picture is worth more than ten thousand words" has had no better application in clinical medicine than in the field of pelvic endoscopy. Cohen applied his expertise in photography to documentation of pelvic findings, and in 1953, with Guterman, he described a technique for obtaining excellent photographs of culdoscopic findings.[8] They utilized initially a rather large culdoscope of some 14.5 mm. in diameter which required an incandescent distal lightbulb. Photographic techniques steadily improved with advancing optical system technology, and reached their present advanced state with the introduction of fiberoptic illumination. Clyman's introduction in 1963 of his pan-culdoscope greatly facilitated culdoscopic photography and allowed the use of a movie camera to demonstrate both the technique and certain diagnostic findings.[9] Indeed, just as in the case of laparoscopy a few years later, many clinicians were introduced to the technique of culdoscopy by way of films made by leaders in the field and widely distributed at meetings and postgraduate courses.

Instrumentation

There is now a wide variety of endoscopes available which are designed specifically for either culdoscopy or laparoscopy. Almost without exception each incorporates a fiberoptic bundle and a distal light source, thus eliminating the danger of an intraperitoneal burn, and providing much greater reliability than the previously used incandescent bulbs.

CULDOSCOPES. Most culdoscopes have a 90 degree field of vision, allowing viewing to be done laterally about the axis of insertion. Depending upon the specific optics of the endoscope employed, some backward vision along this axis is possible, thus allowing theoretically for visualization of areas already passed with the scope. Such visualization, which would usually include areas deep in the cul-de-sac, is in practice quite limited.

LAPAROSCOPES. Most laparoscopes utilize a direct viewing field (180 degrees) or have a slightly offset field of vision (usually 135 degrees). Since the pelvic viscera are approached from above, this affords the surgeon a panoramic view of the entire pelvis, much as would be seen at laparotomy. In the past two years, there have been significant technological improvements in optical systems, allowing for the use of quite small caliber endoscopes. Indeed, one company now offers a collated fiber bundle, surrounded by a fiberoptic light collar, which is encased in a 15-gauge needle. The cannula which holds this needle permits the continuous introduction of gas, making the entire assembly ideal for diagnostic laparoscopy under minimal local anesthesia. The field of vision through this instrument, although not as well illuminated as with larger laparoscopes, is virtually the same, and it is anticipated that the smaller amount of pneumoperitoneum which would be necessary would be easily tolerated by the patient without premedication.

INSUFFLATORS. The gas-regulating insufflator designed by Semm is generally used by laparoscopists. This device, which can be used with either carbon dioxide or nitrous oxide, regulates the gas flow rate, indicates the back-flow pressure, and displays the amount of gas delivered. Because of its design, it eliminates the danger of sudden, uncontrolled pneumoperitoneum.

LIGHT SOURCES. Many light sources are available to provide the endoscopist with a complete spectrum of lighting possibilities, including high-intensity lights for photography. Most of these units provide for the distally generated light to be transmitted to the endoscope by way of a fiberoptic bundle. Rechargeable, stroboscopic flash units for photography are available for strobe lights located either proximally or distally.

INSTRUMENTS FOR SURGICAL MANIPULATION. Numerous instruments are available for use through a second puncture site, enabling the surgeon to perform a variety of diagnostic and operative procedures, such as biopsy, resection, cauterization, exploration, and removal of foreign bodies within the abdominal cavity. Clark, in Buffalo, has recently described instrumentation for placing sutures, under direct vision, at laparoscopy. The technique, which requires two additional puncture sites, is not difficult to master, and adds still another dimension to operative laparoscopy.[10]

Culdoscopy

Culdoscopy may be defined as endoscopic visualization of the pelvis using a telescope placed through the posterior vaginal fornix into the cul-de-sac of Douglas. The procedure is indicated primarily for diagnostic purposes, but it can be utilized for minor operative manipulation, such as biopsy, electrofulguration, and tubal coagulation. Unfortunately, there has been some confusion in the recent literature with regard to operative culdoscopy. Some culdoscopists, notably

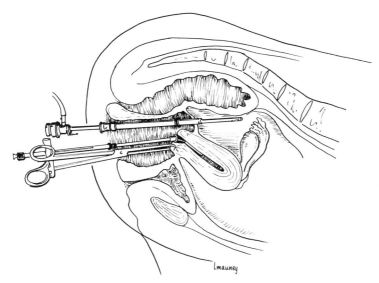

Figure 18-1.   Diagrammatic representation of culdoscopy. Patient in knee-chest position.

Clyman, have described various surgical procedures performed concomitantly with culdoscopy which involve surgical incision of the cul-de-sac, amounting to colpotomy. In these instances, culdoscopy has been employed to view the pelvis prior to and during the performance of open culpotomy. More complex procedures, such as incisional biopsy, tubal ligation, and fulguration or excision of endometriosis, are possible with this combination. For the purposes of this discussion, however, the more strict definition of culdoscopy, which excludes open incicision, will be used.

At this time, culdoscopy is probably more widely employed than laparoscopy in the United States, although the latter procedure is enjoying an enormous growth in popularity. When no surgical manipulation is planned culdoscopy may be performed with local anesthesia, on an outpatient basis, in either a clinic or a minor surgical unit. Although exact data are difficult to obtain, it is probably true that culdoscopy is most often performed under local anesthesia, and it may well be that this simple anesthetic requirement has provided the main impetus for the continued use of the procedure.

INDICATIONS AND CONTRAINDICATIONS

Indications for any surgical procedure must presuppose that the method represents the best possible means for establishing a diagnosis or providing treatment. For this reason, indications for culdoscopy must then take into consideration whether or not the patient would be better served by the only slightly more complex procedure of laparoscopy. This decision will, of course, also be based upon the training of the individual and the facilities available. Certainly, should there be any other contraindication to the abdominal approach, culdoscopy should be considered. It should be remembered that there are definite anatomic limitations to the field of vision at culdoscopy. If the suspected pathology lies within these limitations, and the patient's physical and emotional status allows for assumption of the knee-chest position and local anesthesia, then culdoscopy may be the procedure of choice. Obviously, for a gynecologist working in an institution in which laparoscopy is not available, all the previous indications for culdoscopy, which include suspected ectopic pregnancy, infertility, and suspected pelvic endometriosis, remain valid. However, we are now in an era in which most hospitals that perform culdoscopy are equipped and staffed to perform laparoscopy as well. Because the indications for both procedures overlap so completely, decision as to the procedure of choice will often be based on other factors than the disease itself.

As with any procedure, there are specific contraindications to culdoscopy. The most important of these is the presence of a mass or fixation of the uterine fundus in the cul-de-sac. Because of the likelihood of introducing infection into the peritoneal cavity, and the impossibility of preparing a sterile vagina, the presence of a florid vaginitis or cervicitis contraindicates the procedure. Culdoscopy should not be performed in any other than the knee-chest position, and therefore must be avoided in patients who are unable, for any reason, to assume this posture.

ANESTHESIA

The popularity of culdoscopy in the past two decades has been in part a result of the convenience and low morbidity attendant to the use of local anesthesia. Local infiltration of the vagina, cervix, and cul-de-sac is therefore the method of choice. Pelvic field block, administered as hypobaric spinal or caudal anesthesia, has found some popularity in a few centers where the necessary expertise is available, but this is an uncommon method today. Because of the necessity of placing the patient in the knee-chest position, the use of general anesthesia is both undesirable and contraindicated.

Appropriate premedication, prior to the use of either local or hypobaric spinal anesthesia, is extremely important for the patient undergoing culdoscopy. At the Boston Hospital for Women, meperidine, diazepam, and scopolamine are most commonly used preoperatively. The latter agent is used for its amnesic effect as well as an anticholinergic.

Anesthetics of choice for local infiltration are usually either mepivacaine or lidocaine in 1 per cent solution. For hypobaric spinal anesthesia, a 0.1 per cent pontocaine in dextrose solution is used to achieve sensory anesthesia only. For augmentation of either method of anesthesia, intravenous diazepam is often used —5 mgm. given on arrival in the operating room, and 5 mgm. administered slowly during the procedure.

TECHNIQUE

The procedure of culdoscopy, in its present form, is traced to the description of Decker and Cherry in 1944.[7] Little modification, except for improved instrumentation, has occurred since that time. The following technique is the one currently in use at the Boston Hospital for Women:

1. PREOPERATIVE PREPARATION. Neither preoperative enema nor genital shave is performed. Premedication is administered approximately one hour preoperatively, as indicated previously.

2. OPERATING POSITION. On arrival in the operating room, an intravenous infusion of 5 per cent dextrose in water or Ringer's lactate is started, and the patient is placed on the table in the knee-chest position. Shoulder braces are used to prevent forward motion of the patient, and upright leg holders are positioned in such a way as to prevent lateral movement of the patient while on the table. Appropriate padding for the shoulders, chest, and legs is provided and adjustable straps are positioned from the leg holders to the thighs for steadiness. The foot of the table is depressed, enabling the surgeon to operate from a standing position between the patient's legs.

3. ANTISEPTIC PREPARATION OF THE FIELD. The vagina and the skin of the buttocks and vulva are prepared with a povidone–iodine solution.

4. LOCAL ANESTHESIA.
    a. The vagina and cervix are well visualized with either a Sims or side opening bivalve speculum.
    b. Downward traction of the posterior lip of the cervix with a tenaculum is done in such a way as to stretch the uterosacral ligaments and expose the entire posterior fornix of the vagina.
    c. Both uterosacral ligaments are then infiltrated with a 1 per cent solution of either mepivacaine or lidocaine, and the area of the culdoscopic puncture site is injected through to the peritoneal surface of the cul-de-sac. The paracervical area at the 4 and 8 o'clock positions is then infiltrated with approximately 5 cc. on each side for cervical anesthesia.

5. INSTRUMENTATION.
    a. If the examination is intended to include an evaluation of tubal patency, either a Jarco or Cohen-Eder patency cannula or a No. 10 Foley catheter is placed through the endocervical canal into the uterus. Alternatively, this may be done after pelvic inspection.
    b. With the cervix on traction, the posterior vaginal fornix should balloon inwardly toward the peritoneal cavity. If the surgeon then inserts a finger into the rectum and draws the bowel posteriorly, the danger of rectal perforation is virtually eliminated.
    c. A pneumoperitoneum is now created by inserting an 18 gauge spinal needle through the midportion of the vaginal fornix into the peritoneal cavity. The point of puncture, which is the center of the trocar site, should be midway between the uterosacral ligaments. When the peritoneal cavity is entered, air insufflated by way of the needle will displace the concavity of the vaginal fornix.
    d. Continuing to displace the rectum posteriorly with one finger, the surgeon plunges the trocar and cannula through the mucosa with a sharp movement. Air will continue to enter the peritoneal cavity when the trocar is removed.
    e. The culdoscope is introduced through the cannula, and the vaginal speculum is removed.
    f. It should be remembered that most culdoscopes have a 90 degree viewing angle. The surgeon should orient the direction of view, prior to introducing the culdoscope, so that the posterior aspect of the uterus is viewed first. Simple rotation of the culdoscope from side to side should bring the adnexal structures into view.

g. Once the fimbriated ends of the tubes have been identified bilaterally, indigo carmine or methylene blue dye, diluted in saline, can be introduced under gentle pressure through the previously placed cannula or catheter.

h. When the examination has been completed, the culdoscope is removed and the pneumoperitoneum is expressed by compressing the patient's abdomen. The cannula is then withdrawn, and the puncture site closed with a single figure-eight suture of chromic catgut.

i. When paracervical anesthesia has been given, it is possible to perform endometrial biopsy or uterine curettage. We do this with the patient in the knee-chest position.

6. POSTOPERATIVE ORDERS.   The intravenous infusion apparatus should be removed before the patient leaves the recovery room, and she should be encouraged to ambulate as early as possible. Douches and intercourse are prohibited for two weeks, after which the patient should be examined by the physician for any late complications.

COMPLICATIONS

In our experience there have been very few complications following culdoscopy. In our own small series of somewhat more than 125 culdoscopies, performed both at the Boston Hospital for Women and the Michael Reese Hospital, there have been four complications. Three of these involved postoperative bleeding from the vaginal puncture site, one of which resulted in a hematoma of the cul-de-sac. The remaining complication, or technical error, was that of rectal perforation with the trocar. This was closed under direct vision following a small colpotomy at the puncture site.

In planning endoscopic evaluation of the pelvis, it should be remembered that culdoscopy offers a limited view of the viscera. It is rarely possible to identify more than the fimbriated end of the fallopian tube or any of the structures in the cul-de-sac. The view of the uterus is that of the posterior and lateral portions of the fundus, including occasionally, the round ligaments. The uterosacral ligaments may be visualized by carefully withdrawing the cannula 1 or 2 cm. Decker has stated that it is possible to view the anterior wall of the uterus, but this has never been the case in our experience. It usually is possible to view both ovaries quite clearly, and with practice the culdoscopist can maneuver the scope in such a way as to manipulate the ovary for viewing most of its surface. The sacral promontory and portions of the large and small bowel can be observed, and occasionally, when it is in a pelvic position, the vermiform appendix can be seen.

Gynecologic Laparoscopy

Gynecologic laparoscopy, which is also known in the literature as celioscopy and peritoneoscopy, may be defined as endoscopic visualization of the pelvic viscera using a telescope placed through the lower abdominal wall into the peritoneal cavity. As indicated previously, its widespread use in the United States is relatively new, but it is probably true that it has now or soon will replace culdoscopy as the primary gynecologic endoscopic procedure. Although the indications for the procedure were initially diagnostic, hardly a month passes without the appearance in the literature of another report on laparoscopic surgical technique. Within the past few years, and with the ever-increasing list of indications for laparoscopy, there has been a parallel expansion in instrumentation and technology. Vastly improved optical and illumination systems, smaller caliber telescopes, and a staggering array of ancillary instrumentation attest to the current intense interest in the subject.

Typical of the increasing interest in laparoscopy is the experience at the Boston Hospital for Women. In the two years since the reintroduction of laparoscopy (1970), more than 1055 cases have been performed, and the technique has become a part of the regular resident training program.

Almost universally, once the procedure has been mastered by gynecologists already familiar with the technique of culdoscopy, there has been agreement that the better view and wider application of laparoscopy make it the technique of choice in most situations. That it has not replaced culdoscopy entirely has probably been due to the fact that the potential complications are more serious, and the anesthesia requirements more rigorous. However, within the past two years there has been an increasing use of local anesthesia for laparoscopy, and a tendency to use the procedure on an outpatient or day-admission basis. We feel it would be unfortunate, however, if this enthusiasm resulted in the abandonment of culdoscopy. In our hospital, where it has been an important, frequently used procedure for many years, culdoscopy continues to be taught and used. Although it is less widely employed since the introduction of laparoscopy, we feel that culdoscopy should not fall into disuse.

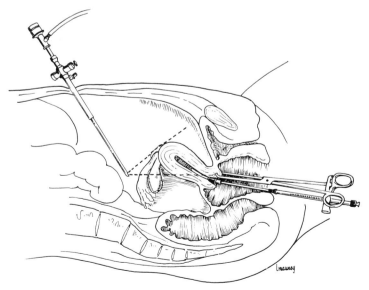

Figure 18-2. Diagrammatic representation of laparoscopy. Patient in modified dorsal lithotomy position.

INDICATIONS AND CONTRAINDICATIONS

Because of the ever-increasing interest in the use of laparoscopy, it seems prudent to sound a note of caution when outlining the indications for the procedure. There has been a disturbing tendency on the part of enthusiastic gynecologists to ignore the limitations of this essentially closed surgical procedure. While it is true that many procedures are technically possible at laparoscopy, it is also true that some of them may not always be in the best interest of the patient. Certainly from the standpoint of diagnostic exploration of the pelvic cavity, laparoscopy usually affords the most complete view. In the evaluation of the infertile patient, laparoscopy is often preferred to either culdoscopy or laparotomy, and it has become an invaluable and definitive diagnostic procedure in cases of suspected ectopic pregnancy. It is in the area of operative manipulation that the most caution needs to be exercised. Although some procedures formerly performed only at laparotomy can be done with equal safety at laparoscopy, careful consideration must always be exercised before abandoning the open approach. Although the view at laparoscopy is similar to that afforded by laparotomy, it is in fact not the same. Manipulation of instruments through secondary puncture sites, no matter how great the dexterity of the laparoscopist, will seldom be as safe or as informative as through an incision. There will therefore always be conditions which, although they do not specifically contraindicate the procedure, are more safely handled in other ways.

Specific contraindications to laparoscopy have changed somewhat with advancing technology and experience. For instance, we would no longer list prior abdominal surgery as a contraindication. In our experience roughly 85 per cent of abdominal operations leave no residual adhesions involving the anterior abdominal wall. Of the remainder, most abdominal scars are adherent to only a thin veil of omentum, and extremely few are involved with adhesions of the bowel or other abdominal viscera. With respect to infection, after encountering numerous cases of acute salpingitis or appendicitis during the investigation of acute abdominal pain, we no longer regard peritonitis *per se* as a contraindication to laparoscopy. In this latter situation, it should be mentioned, however, that if inflammation is encountered, care should be exercised not to disturb the inflammatory response or manipulate the inflamed viscera except for obtaining cultures.

In view of these statements, the following conditions remain contraindications to laparoscopy:
1. Hiatus hernia.
2. Intestinal obstruction.
3. Inability to establish pneumoperitoneum.
4. Inability of the patient to tolerate anesthesia.

ANESTHESIA

To provide safe, adequate anesthesia for laparoscopy, we prefer endotracheal anesthesia utilizing controlled ventilation in a "balanced" technique with Pentothal or Surital for induction; succinylcholine to facilitate intubation; and nitrous oxide, oxygen, and a narcotic such as meperidine for maintenance. A 0.1 per cent succinylcholine intravenous drip is administered for muscular relaxation to permit controlled ventilation. This technique has been used with no complications except for one patient, who developed persistent apnea, and who was subsequently found to have a congenital atypical cholinesterase.

It has been demonstrated[11] that the carbon dioxide introduced into the peritoneal cavity is readily absorbed. Controlled hyperventilation has been found to be an essential part of the anesthetic technique to minimize the hypercarbia, respiratory acidosis, cardiac arrhythmias, and even cardiovascular collapse that may be seen in patients allowed to ventilate spontaneously with halothane, nitrous oxide and oxygen.[11] It has been shown in a study by Baratz and Karis[12] that with adequate controlled respiration the arterial pCO_2 does not rise significantly even in the presence of carbon dioxide in the peritoneal cavity at a pressure of 50 cm. water. Alexander and associates[13] reported a consistent rise in arterial pCO_2 accompanied by a fall in arterial pH. These investigators could not, however, rule out hypoventilation. This could have occurred as a result of the marked diaphragmatic elevation they demonstrated while studying respiratory impedance.

There has been increasing use of both regional and local anesthesia techniques for laparoscopy during the past three years. Wheeless reported satisfactory use of local anesthesia for a sizeable group of patients undergoing tubal sterilization with the one incision technique.[14] His patients received meperidine and diazepam premedication with local periumbilical infiltration of lidocaine. Wheeless makes the point, with which we agree, that the use of local anesthesia offers the advantage of allowing laparoscopy to be performed in the clinic situation, where facilities for general anesthesia are not available. We have had a smaller and equally successful experience with local infiltration and similar premedication, but have insisted on the timely availability of facilities for performing more extensive surgery should this be necessitated by a complication of laparoscopy.

Regional block, administered as lumbar spinal anesthesia, has been successfully used in our institution on a few occasions. This technique, requiring full anesthesia facilities, probably has less application to laparoscopy than either local or general endotracheal anesthesia, but it is available for the patient in whom the latter method is contraindicated.

With either spinal or local techniques, less pneumoperitoneum must be used, both because of the discomfort it causes the patient and because of the diminished ability to clear accumulating levels of arterial pCO_2 with spontaneous respirations. This restriction, however, does not materially reduce the effectiveness of the procedure. In addition, with local or regional anesthesia, less manipulation of the pelvic viscera is tolerated by the patient. Although, for this reason, Wheeless feels there is a great advantage in the one incision technique, we have not found this to be the case, and consider the safety advantages that accompany the second puncture technique to outweigh the disadvantage of more extensive abdominal wall infiltration.

TECHNIQUE

The specific details of laparoscopic technique vary from institution to institution. Our interest in laparoscopy began in 1967, and the basic technique used is that learned under the tutelage of Dr. Melvin Cohen in Chicago. Since that time we have used a wide variety of instruments produced by many manufacturers. During the following discussion of our basic technique, it should be borne in mind that, for every individual, the procedure must be learned at the operating table from an experienced laparoscopist. There is no substitute for this. Regardless of what technique is developed, for any specific purpose, the paramount consideration must always be to maintain the widest possible margin of patient safety.

1. PATIENT PREPARATION. Patients undergoing elective laparoscopy are asked to maintain a low residue diet for the 24 hours prior to entering the hospital. Because we have found a high incidence of distended large bowel at laparoscopy within 24 hours of a cleansing enema, no enema is given before surgery. If necessary, an abdominal shave down to the pubic crease is performed but no perineal preparation is necessary. We have found that in the majority of cases, if the patient can void just prior to leaving for the operating room, catheterization is unnecessary. Preoperative medication depends on the choice of anesthesia, as discussed previously.

2. OPERATING ROOM PREPARATION AND PATIENT POSITIONING. The instruments are placed in the sterilizing solution when the patient arrives in the operating room, and are left for 10 minutes. The patient is placed initially in the supine position on the operating table for induction of anesthesia, and then is moved to a modified dorsal lithotomy position with the legs flexed slightly at the hips in moderate abduction. The legs are supported by padded braces in the popliteal space. It is important that the buttocks be moved slightly over the break in the operating table in order to allow subsequent depression of the tenaculum and cannula handles for movement of the uterus. The ground plate for the electrocautery is placed under the patient, and the unit checked for proper performance before the procedure. The foot switch for this device is placed only on the surgeon's side of the table. The fiberoptic light source and the gas supply are checked and the insufflator charged to full capacity with the flow valve off. Skin preparation of the abdomen, perineum, and vagina is done with povidone–iodine solution, and the patient is appropriately draped.

3. INSTRUMENTATION.
   a. The vagina and the cervix are visualized, and the anterior lip of the cervix grasped transversely with a single tooth tenaculum. After sounding the uterus for depth and direction, a patency cannula of either the Cohen-Eder or Jarco variety, fitted with an appropriate acorn tip, is placed in the endocervical canal and locked to the tenaculum (Figure 18–3). An alternative to the tenaculum-cannula method is the vacuum cup device designed by Semm. Either method is satisfactory and allows for the manipulation of the uterus during the procedure.
   b. A Verres cannula, with the sharp point locked out, is inserted subcutaneously for a distance of about 1 cm. in the midline at the lower margin of the umbilicus (Figure 18–4). The blunt end of this instrument is then unlocked, and the abdominal skin grasped just above the pubic symphysis and lifted by the surgeon. The needle is then aimed toward the pelvic concavity and should pierce the abdominal wall at approximately a right angle, with the lower abdominal skin elevated. Once the needle has been inserted to almost its entire length, the tip is moved from side to side within the peritoneal cavity to ensure that it is free.

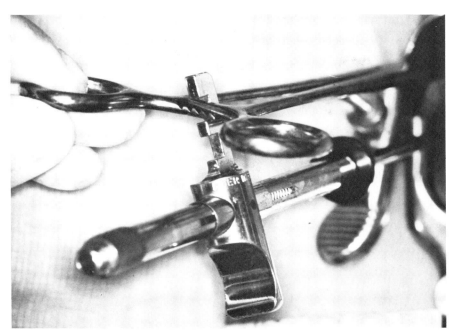

Figure 18-3.   Cohen-Eder cannula and tenaculum locked together for manipulation of uterus and for tubal insufflation.

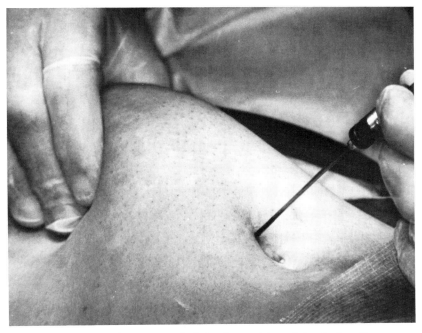

Figure 18-4.   Verres cannula being inserted into abdominal cavity.

c. The insufflator tubing, connected through a two-way stopcock, is connected to the cannula and the gas flow begun. The cannula and abdominal skin are released by the surgeon so that the needle lies of its own weight in a position parallel to, and just underneath, the abdominal wall. Immediate attention should be directed to the insufflator, where gas back-flow pressure should not be more than 20 mm. Hg. Pressures in excess of this value indicate retroperitoneal or intravisceral positioning of the cannula tip, and repositioning should be accomplished at once.

d. Symmetric expansion of the abdomen should be observed, and, when there is about a liter of gas in the peritoneal cavity, percussion should demonstrate the loss of liver dullness. The abdominal wall is checked for crepitus as the gas continues to flow. Unless the patient is extremely small, at least 3 liters of pneumoperitoneum should be established.

e. The Verres cannula is removed and, using a No. 15 blade, a curvilinear incision is made in the lower umbilical margin, with the cannula puncture site at its midportion. The length of this incision will depend upon the caliber of the laparoscope employed. A trumpet-valve cannula and trocar are inserted subcutaneously for a distance of approximately 1 cm. through the incision, and, with the abdominal wall lifted as before, the trocar and cannula are pushed through the abdominal wall in the direction of the pelvic concavity (Figure 18–5). The gas flow tubing is connected to the cannula, and observation of back-flow pressure made immediately.

f. With the fiberoptic bundle connected and the light on, the trocar is removed and the laparoscope inserted through the cannula (Figure 18–6). Immediate visualization is made of the bladder and the underside of the anterior abdominal wall. If the bladder is full or is obstructing the view of the anterior pelvis, it should be emptied with the use of a straight catheter.

g. If desired, a second puncture site may then be established under direct vision in either lower quadrant. This is preceded by transillumination of the abdominal wall to locate and avoid the inferior epigastric vessels.

h. Using a blunt manipulating probe through the second puncture site, and with the patient in 5 to 10 degree Trendelenberg position, the bowel is swept out of the cul-de-sac and upward over the pelvic brim into the general abdominal cavity, thereby creating a clear view of the posterior pelvis.

i. With an assistant depressing the handles of the tenaculum and cannula, the fundus of the uterus can be placed in the extreme anterior position, thus affording the operator with a complete panoramic view of the cul-de-sac and supporting ligaments of the uterus. Elevation of the handles will depress the fundus and expose the entire bladder flap and anterior cul-de-sac.

j. Using the manipulating probe, all surfaces of the ovaries can be viewed. Directing the laparoscope into the right lower peritoneal gutter, the vermiform appendix can be seen, and the right and left lobes of the liver and dome of the gallbladder can be visualized.

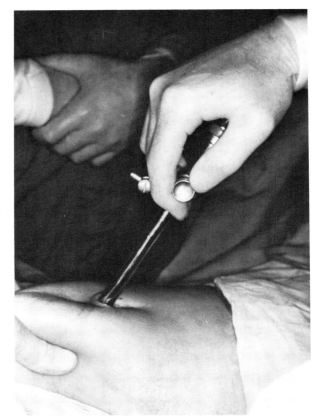

Figure 18-5. Trumpet-valve cannula and trocar being inserted into abdominal cavity.

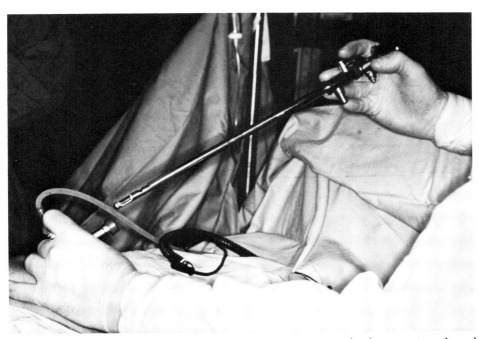

Figure 18-6. A 135 degree photographic laparoscope ready for insertion through trumpet-valve cannula.

k. When the procedure has been completed, the laparoscope is withdrawn, and while holding the trumpet-valve cannula in the open
   position, the surgeon compresses the abdomen to expel as much of
   the gas as possible. The cannulas are then removed and the wounds
   are closed with interrupted sutures of fine silk, subcutaneous catgut,
   or clips.

4. POSTOPERATIVE ORDERS. The key to lowered morbidity following laparoscopy is early ambulation. Removing the intravenous infusion apparatus in the
recovery room, avoiding heavy analgesia, having the patient void only in the bath-
room, and getting her up and walking as soon as she returns to her room are all
measures which keep postoperative complications minimal, and ensure her early
release from the hospital. Approximately 95 per cent of our patients are discharged home on the day of surgery.

COMPLICATIONS OF LAPAROSCOPY

A review of the literature seems to suggest that perhaps the most important basic cause of complications of laparoscopy is inexperience with the procedure. However, complications can and do occur even with the most experienced
laparoscopist. Unfortunately, unlike open surgical techniques, teaching at the
operating table is complicated by the fact that usually only one person at a time
can observe procedures within the peritoneal cavity. Attempts to remedy this
situation have resulted in the development of both rigid and flexible (fiberoptic)
teaching devices which split the viewed image so that two individuals may
observe at the same time. Better than this, but prohibitively expensive, is the use
of closed circuit television connected to the laparoscope through a flexible fiberoptic bundle. At the Boston Hospital for Women, we have found that the use of
color slides and movies, depicting the entire sequence of events from patient
preparation through intra-abdominal observation, is a useful adjunct for the introduction of the procedure to inexperienced personnel.

Prevention of laparoscopic complications rests on thorough understanding
of the indications for, the limitations of, and contraindications to the procedure.
Once these are understood, there is no substitute for actual experience gained
under the direct guidance of an experienced laparoscopist.

Complications of laparoscopy may be considered under four general categories: (1) complications of pneumoperitoneum, (2) complications of abdominal
wall puncture, (3) complications of intra-abdominal manipulation, (4) minor
complications.

COMPLICATIONS OF PNEUMOPERITONEUM

Induced pneumoperitoneum is not a procedure limited to abdominal
endoscopy. Prior to the introduction of antibiotics, pneumoperitoneum was an
important ancillary method for the treatment of pulmonary tuberculosis, and as
such has been widely described in the literature. With respect to laparoscopy,
however, the most common complication arising from the induction of pneumoperitoneum is failure to reach the peritoneal cavity. Inasmuch as both carbon
dioxide and nitrous oxide are rapidly absorbed from body tissues, introduction of
gas into the abdominal wall is usually of minor consequence. In the obese patient,
in whom this is most likely to occur, rather large quantities of gas can collect

undetected in the subcutaneous tissues. On occasion, this subcutaneous emphysema can dissect into the vulva or upward onto the chest wall. In the very thin patient, there is a danger of introducing the needle through the peritoneal cavity into the retroperitoneal tissues. This is a more serious complication and can result in a pneumomediastinum or dissection of gas around the great vessels. If the pneumoperitoneum needle is introduced or directed away from the midline, the danger of perforating the iliac vessels is great. Should this occur, failure to recognize the complication immediately can result in the introduction of enough gas to result in fatal air embolism. The possibility of perforation of the bowel or other pelvic viscera by the pneumoperitoneum needle is increased if previous abdominal surgery had been performed or when inattention to the direction of placement of the needle had occurred. At one time or another, in the long history of pneumoperitoneum, virtually every intra-abdominal structure has been inadvertently perforated. In the majority of cases the major complication has been that of intraperitoneal hemorrhage. Hiatus hernia is a contraindication to pneumoperitoneum because of the danger of diaphragmatic rupture with resultant pneumothorax.

In most instances, complications of penumoperitoneum can be avoided by paying close attention to the resistance to gas flow. Using the Semm insufflator and the Verres cannula, unobstructed flow into the peritoneal cavity results in a back pressure of no more than 20 mm. of Hg. Higher pressures encountered at the commencement of gas flow should be immediately suspect, and the cannula should be carefully replaced.

COMPLICATIONS OF ABDOMINAL WALL PUNCTURE

Perforations of abdominal viscera with a small pneumoperitoneum needle are of less consequence than perforations made with the use of larger instrumentation cannulae. Although they occur less frequently, because of the protection afforded by adequate pneumoperitoneum, lacerations made by a sharply pointed trocar can result in massive intraperitoneal hemorrhage or intestinal contamination of the peritoneal cavity. For this reason we agree with Cohen that laparoscopy should not be performed unless the surgeon and operating room personnel are prepared for immediate laparotomy.[5] We have encountered one instance of omental perforation, and five injuries to the fundus of the uterus, resulting in bleeding, which was controlled by electrocoagulation at laparoscopy. We have had one case of perforation of redundant transverse colon and one case of perforation of the stomach by the main puncture site trocar. These were repaired at laparotomy.

Even after transillumination of the abdominal wall to avoid laceration of the inferior epigastric vessels, perforation for a second puncture site may result in abdominal wall bleeding of sufficient magnitude to require incision and vessel ligation. In two instances we have seen brisk bleeding from an abdominal wall vessel occur along the puncture site cannula into the peritoneal cavity, and an arterial vessel encountered once in the subumbilical incision required separate ligation.

It should be emphasized again that laparoscopy is, except under exceptional circumstances, a *midline* procedure. Ancillary puncture sites, outside the midline, should be established only under direct vision of the inner side of the abdominal wall.

COMPLICATIONS OF INTRA-ABDOMINAL MANIPULATION

Assuming that usual care in handling tisues is employed by the surgeon at laparoscopy, most complications arising within the peritoneal cavity occur because he attempts to do more than the technique permits. Hemorrhage and hematomas resulting from lysis of adhesions or tubal resection are not uncommon. Attempts to obtain biopsies from areas too vascular to be controlled by cautery, or from sites at which coagulation in proximity to the bowel may eventuate in necrosis and subsequent intestinal perforation, are further examples of imprudent judgment. It is our practice to treat bowel burns by laparotomy, resection of the burned area, and direct closure of the bowel. Inadvertent intraperitoneal burns are of course best avoided by very strict adherence to the principle that only the surgeon who is actually visualizing the tissue should initiate the electric current. *Avoidance of complications arising from laparoscopic surgery is best accomplished by becoming thoroughly familiar with visualization techniques before attempting surgical procedures.*

MINOR COMPLICATIONS

The most frequent minor complication encountered by most laparoscopists is that of postoperative shoulder pain owing to diaphragmatic irritation. Some authors report this as being virtually universal, while others, including ourselves, find that this occurs in 10 to 40 per cent of cases.

Perforation of the uterus with the patency cannula is an occurrence which we have observed on as many as a dozen occasions. It is easily detected during the establishment of the pneumoperitoneum by the sound of gas escaping through the cannula, or by visualizing the tip of the cannula with the laparoscope (Figure 18–7). Inadvertent perforation of the nonpregnant uterus at laparoscopy raises the suspicion that perhaps this event occurs in gynecologic practice more frequently than we might believe. When uterine perforation occurs at laparoscopy we have withdrawn the cannula under direct vision from above, noting a small amount of bleeding on only one occasion.

Postoperative ecchymosis along the tract of the laparoscope cannula is virtually universal, but hematoma formation is rare. Skin burns resulting from electrical shorting from the coagulation instrument to the metal sleeve of the cannula also occur, but these are rare and are averted by employing a nonconductive cannula or taking care that at least an inch of insulating material on the coagulation instrument is exposed before applying current.

All of the general complications of any surgical procedure apply as well to laparoscopy. Anesthetic complications are no different than for any other procedure, and, although they are rare, they underline the necessity for the presence of an experienced anesthesiologist.

Laparoscopic Procedures in Gynecology

INFERTILITY

Perhaps the most important use for laparoscopy has been in the field of infertility. In as many as 25 to 35 per cent of women in whom no cause for sterility has been discovered, endoscopic evaluation of the pelvis has revealed some previ-

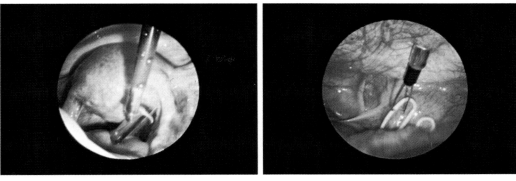

Fig. 18-7.   Fig. 18-8.

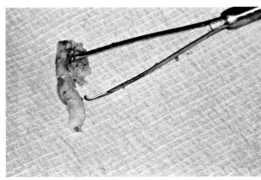

Fig. 18-9.   Fig. 18-10.

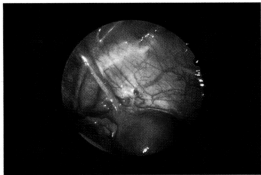

Fig. 18-11.   Fig. 18-12.

Figure 18-7. Perforation of uterus with Cohen-Eder cannula at laparoscopy.

Figure 18-8. Endometriosis involving left round ligament and anterior cul-de-sac in otherwise normal pelvis.

Figure 18-9. Electrosurgical resection of right fallopian tube using Eder biopsy tongs.

Figure 18-10. Resected segment of fallopian tube with attached mesosalpinx. Lumen clearly visible.

Figure 18-11. Removal of perforated IUCD from right upper pelvis, using Eder biopsy tongs through right lower quadrant second puncture cannula.

Figure 18-12. Lysis of cul-de-sac adhesions using Semm scissors through second puncture cannula.

ously unsuspected abnormality. For this reason, laparoscopy has virtually become a standard part of most infertility investigations. In 28 of 84 such cases (33 per cent), we have been rewarded by finding pelvic endometriosis, postoperative adhesions, unsuspected tubal occlusion, uterine abnormalities, or evidence of ovarian dysfunction.

Laparoscopy has proved to be especially helpful in evaluating tubal function and patency in the infertile patient. The office tubal insufflation test (Rubin test) and uterosalpingography both have serious drawbacks in defining tubal disease. Auscultation of gas escaping from the tube will reveal nothing of unilateral closure, fimbrial phimosis, or tubal position. The uterotubogram, which is an unpleasant experience for the patient, and, according to Shirley,[15] can be a source of considerable radiation if done by the fluoroscopic method, does not define the anatomic relationship between the tube and ovary, and is often misleading. Since the use of oil-based radiopaque dyes, which allow for delayed films, should be condemned because of the danger of tubal damage, most radiologists now use a water-soluble viscous medium. The transcervical instillation of this material is painful, and its viscosity, which necessitates the use of high pressures, is often responsible for tubal spasm and apparent nonspillage. Even when the x-ray reveals normal patency bilaterally, the anatomic relationships of the tube and ovary are not clearly delineated. Certainly a tube which is patent but adherent to the bowel or lateral pelvic side wall cannot be expected to participate normally in ovum transfer, and may well be responsible for the patient's inability to conceive. The gynecogram, which was popularized by Stein,[16] and which combines a radiopaque medium with pneumoperitoneum, thus silhouetting the pelvic viscera, does permit a rough evaluation of the tubo-ovarian relationship, and is to be preferred to the ordinary uterotubogram. Unfortunately this technique is not widely used, and is seldom available. Neither of these x-ray techniques, however, can substitute for the direct visualization and close-up inspection of the adnexal structures afforded by laparoscopy. Fimbrial phimosis and salpingitis isthmica nodosa are diagnoses which can be made only under direct vision. For tubal lavage and patency testing, we use a dilute solution of either indigo carmine or methylene blue dye, which has the viscosity of body fluids and is highly visible. The solution is instilled transcervically, under gentle pressure, while viewing both tubes simultaneously. In most cases, the dye can be seen through the tubal serosa, and some evaluation of patency can be made by noting the ease with which it spills from the fimbriated end of the tube. Close-up inspection, while injecting dye, will often reveal the presence or absence of tubal spasm. Shirodkar[17] has stated that blanching of the cornual area of the uterus, without fimbrial spillage, is strongly suggestive of isthmic nodular salpingitis. The normal open tube, when lavaged just after menstruation has ceased, will be seen to transmit the dye promptly, and to allow for free and rapid spillage from its fimbriated end.

In our own series, the most commonly observed pelvic disease has been endometriosis. In many cases, the only evidence of the process has been observed on the anterior aspect of the uterus, or in other places in the pelvis in which culdoscopic examination would have been inadequate (Figure 18–8). Although it does not seem likely that a single discrete area of endometriosis on the anterior bladder peritoneum could have any influence on infertility, we make it a practice to biopsy any implants observed, so that histologic confirmation of active endometriosis can be made the basis for appropriate treatment. Once biopsy of a typical area has been made, fulguration of all other implants can be done under direct vision. When performing electrocoagulation of endometriosis, extreme caution must be exercised in treating areas on the serosa of the bowel. As a rule only very small discrete implants of the bowel should be approached in this fashion, and in such cases the coagulation current should be reduced so that only the area of the implant itself is coagulated. Deep coagulation of the muscularis will likely result in late necrotic perforation.

When the infertility problem involves suspicion of oligo-ovulation or anovulation, visual inspection of the ovary for evidence of ovulatory activity is often informative. Each ovary should be manipulated, with the second puncture site probe, in such a way as to observe its entire surface. An ovary which is functioning normally will contain obvious evidence of ovulation, and often, if the procedure is timed appropriately, a corpus luteum or corpus hemorrhagicum will be seen. On two occasions, when laparoscopy was performed at the calculated time of ovulation, we have observed graafian follicles apparently ready to rupture. Conversely, an ovary which is not functioning is also apparent on visual inspection. Often such ovaries will be small and have a convoluted brain-like surface, without showing evidence of previous ovulation. Androgenized ovaries such as are found with polycystic ovary syndrome or adrenal hyperplasia are usually enlarged bilaterally, and have smooth white surfaces on which are seen areas of telangiectasia. Biopsy of the ovary, under direct vision, with a variety of biopsy-coagulation instruments, is easily accomplished at laparoscopy. Care must be taken, when performing biopsy of the ovary, to avoid vascular areas, such as the hilum, from which uncontrollable bleeding might ensue. Ovarian biopsies, taken at laparoscopy, have been entirely satisfactory from the histologic standpoint, and often have been diagnostic of such conditions as neoplasia, Stein-Leventhal syndrome, and early ovarian failure.

CHRONIC PELVIC PAIN

Patients with chronic lower abdominal pain present a challenge to the gynecologist. In this group of women are those who complain of dull, or intermittently sharp, nagging pain over extended periods of time. Usually the pain is unilateral and unassociated with the phases of the menstrual cycle. However, it may be bilateral, dull, and nagging throughout the cycle, and then exacerbated with menstruation. The value of laparoscopic evaluation of this symptom complex is somewhat in dispute. Liston and associates in their series of 134 patients with chronic abdominal pain, found no apparent cause in 76 per cent.[18] Pent observed normal findings in approximately 50 per cent of his cases.[19] In 19 cases we have seen of long-standing pain, we have found normal pelves in 11 instances (58 per cent). We have had, however, an unusual experience with some of the patients with presumably normal findings. In six of the 11 patients, all young women with chronic persistent pelvic pain, we found surprisingly large quantities of serous or serosanguinous fluid in the cul-de-sac (30 to 75 cc.). In each case, in order to better visualize the cul-de-sac, the fluid was aspirated, but no other positive findings were noted. Five of the six patients experienced complete and lasting relief of their pain following laparoscopy. It is of course not easy to relate the disappearance of pain with the removal of what appeared to be innocuous peritoneal fluid. In none of these cases was there any evidence of recent rupture of an ovarian cyst, and it is perhaps interesting to speculate upon the psychotherapeutic effect of laparoscopy alone in such patients.

The most frequent cause of chronic pain found at laparoscopy is unsuspected pelvic inflammatory disease. Endometriosis is the second most common finding, confirming the possibility that this disease may produce pain throughout the menstrual cycle rather than only during the period. Pelvic adhesions, either postinflammatory or postoperative, are usually cited as an additional cause of chronic pain. As always, one is hard put to ascribe a cause and effect relationship between adhesions and pain. However, it is true, in a few cases, that simple lysis of these adhesions results in alleviation of the symptoms. The question of whether or not it is prudent to employ laparoscopy in the investigation of chronic abdominal pain is really a moot one. When such a symptom exists, and its cause remains obscure, the temptation to take a look is not only irresistible but justifiable.

It should be emphasized that whenever the gynecologist deems it appropriate to perform laparoscopy on the patient with chronic pelvic pain, he should be prepared to perform electrocoagulation, biopsy, and sharp lysis of minimal adhesions. He should utilize the laparoscope to visualize in detail all the pelvic organs, the appendix, and the large bowel. To this end, we have found it necessary to establish a second puncture site, through which various accessory instruments can be placed.

ACUTE PELVIC PAIN

Perhaps one of the best, but unaccountably neglected, uses for laparoscopy is in the patient with an early acute abdomen. The sudden onset of lower quadrant pain, with or without nausea and vomiting, fever, and leukocytosis, most often results in a bewildering overlapping of diagnoses of many intrapelvic conditions. Often the differential diagnosis includes unruptured tubal pregnancy, early appendicitis, a leaking physiologic cyst of the ovary and acute salpingitis. Laparoscopy is not definitive treatment for any of these conditions, but laparotomy is indicated only for the first three, which are the least common. In cases in which the developing complex dictates an open abdominal approach, laparoscopic observation is superfluous and should be condemned. However, as is often the case, when the diagnosis is in doubt and delay is dangerous, diagnostic laparoscopy can often afford immediate resolution of the problem. If laparoscopy reveals the necessity for surgery, the instruments are withdrawn, and laparotomy is performed with no significant delay. On the other hand, if acute pelvic inflammation is encountered, the patient is not jeopardized by the laparoscopy, cultures can be obtained, and, more importantly, the patient is spared the morbidity and expense of unnecessary laparotomy.

It cannot be overemphasized that the laparoscope is not a substitute for prudent clinical judgment. It is, however, an extremely valuable adjunct, which, when used in conjunction with other findings, can result in rapid, certain diagnoses.

PELVIC MASS

The proper evaluation of a pelvic mass, should, in most cases, involve exploratory laparotomy. Since the resurgence of interest in laparoscopy in this country, there has been a disturbing tendency to evaluate such masses endoscopically. Generally speaking, this practice should be condemned. Most gynecologists would agree that the finding through bimanual examination of an adnexal mass larger than 5 cm. is deserving of open exploration and probably the mass should be resected. Masses smaller than this are usually physiologic extensions of normal ovarian activity, and will regress spontaneously with time or after ovarian suppression. While it is possible to aspirate ovarian cysts at laparoscopy, only rarely can such practice be condoned, and then only if small and in a young woman. In an older patient, a harmless appearing cyst could well be an early cystadenocarcinoma. On the rare occasions when we have aspirated persistent ovarian cysts, we have made it a practice to submit the fluid for cytology, and to biopsy the wall of the cyst, so that histopathologic confirmation of benignancy could be made. We have made it a rule to avoid laparoscopy in all cases of solid-appearing masses, and to reserve the procedure for those instances in which there has been persistence of a definitely cystic mass, less than 5 cm., in a young woman. It is our strong feeling that, even in these cases, when any doubt persists at laparoscopy exploration should be performed.

PREOPERATIVE EVALUATION FOR RECONSTRUCTIVE SURGERY

Because of the complete view afforded at laparoscopy, evaluation of the tubes in patients considered for fimbrioplasty or cornual transplantation can aid the gynecologist in planning his surgical approach. On a number of occasions, we have encountered tubes so badly damaged by previous inflammation that fimbrioplasty would have been an exercise in futility. These patients have been spared the complications of surgery and the disappointment of failed reconstruction. On two occasions, in patients referred for unification operations, in whom the diagnosis of bicornuate uterus had been made by uterotubogram, laparoscopy revealed a normal uncleaved fundus, and thus indicated only the presence of a uterine septum. In one of these cases, the basis for the infertility was subsequently found to be severe oligospermia, and the patient later conceived and carried a normal pregnancy following homologous insemination. Because of this sort of experience, we feel that no reconstructive surgery for infertility should be undertaken without prior laparoscopic evaluation and, if desired, photographic documentation of the problem.

TUBAL STERILIZATION

The most frequently performed, and increasingly popular, laparoscopic surgical procedure at present is interim tubal sterilization. In part, the enthusiasm for the procedure has been a result of the coincidental changes in social acceptance of permanent sterilization, and in part by the low morbidity and shortened hospitalization possible with the laparoscopic approach. In general, two types of laparoscopic tubal sterilizations have been described. One procedure, as originally described by Semm[20] and others, involves only electrocoagulation of a portion of the tube, without division or resection. The other, which we employ, entails the resection of a segment of proximal tube and allows positive histologic identification of the tissue—a point which could have medicolegal significance. With respect to recanalization and pregnancy, partial tubal resection is to be vastly preferred to coagulation alone.

There have been many descriptions of interim laparoscopic tubal sterilization in the recent literature.[5,20,21] Although minor differences in technique exist,
and different instruments are used, all accomplish essentially the same objectives.
Briefly, our technique, which involves the use of a second puncture site and tubal
resection, is as follows:

1. Following initial visualization of the pelvis for interfering adhesions or
unsuspected pathology, a second puncture site is established in the right lower
quadrant. Using a manipulating probe, a complete inspection of the pelvic viscera
is carried out. Special care is taken to specifically identify the fallopian tube over
its entire length. Visual inspection of the upper abdominal viscera may be accomplished at this time.

2. Using a coagulating grasping forceps, inserted through the second puncture site cannula, the tube is picked up at a point approximately 1 cm. from the
cornu of the uterus. In order to avoid inadvertent resection of the round ligament,
we make it a point to identify the fimbriated end of the structure we have grasped.
Electrocoagulation of approximately 2 to 3 cm. of tube, and its associated mesosalpinx, is performed by placing the coagulation instrument at two or three places
along this length of tube (Figure 18–9).

3. Resection of a portion of the coagulated segment of tube is then accomplished using one of the many types of biopsy instruments. We use the Eder
biopsy tongs, which allows the resection of a sizeable segment of tube, or the
Storz biopsy forceps for this purpose.

4. Careful, close-up inspection of the resected area for complete hemostasis should be done, and any bleeding points are electrocoagulated.

5. The entire procedure is then repeated on the opposite side, and the
tissue submitted as before in a separate container (Figure 18–10).

It cannot be overemphasized that careful checking for complete hemostasis at the end of the procedure is absolutely essential. Late bleeding can be a
serious complication of the procedure. Preoperatively the patient should be prepared for the possibility of laparotomy if necessary to control bleeding. In our
own series of 356 cases, this has been needed on only two occasions.

Most of our patients undergoing this procedure are admitted on the day of
surgery and are discharged from 3 to 6 hours after their operation. In those rare
instances in which histologic examination of the tissue has failed to reveal luminal
epithelium, the patient is informed, and uterosalpingography is carried out three
months postoperatively. Should x-ray evidence of patency be demonstrated, reex-
ploration by laparoscopy should be performed, and, if necessary, the open tube
resected.

The laparoscopic approach to tubal sterilization has also been described in
the early puerperium.[23,24] At the Boston Hospital for Women, postpartum sterilization by laparotomy has traditionally been performed during the same anesthesia used for delivery. To date, laparoscopic tubal sterilization in the immediate
puerperium has not been used. Keith and co-workers, at the Cook County Hospital, have reported a series of patients who underwent partial tubal resection by
laparoscopy from one to seven days following delivery.[25] In 167 patients, they
reported only three cases in which bleeding at the operative site required laparotomy, and one case of late bleeding which resulted in hematoma. They concluded that the procedure was safe and preferable to laparotomy, particularly
in reducing the postoperative stay.

Laparoscopic tubal sterilization combined with early therapeutic abortion was first reported by Steptoe and Imran,[26] and more recently by others.[25] Our own experience includes 27 such cases. The procedure is essentially the same as that used for interim sterilization, with some precautionary modifications. The uterus is evacuated vaginally before laparoscopy is begun. *Under no circumstances* can pneumoperitoneum be established transcervically because of the near certainty of fatal air embolism. Uterotonic agents, in the form of an oxytocin infusion and methylergonovine intramuscularly, are used to gain the maximum uterine involution prior to starting the laparoscopic procedure. Visualization of the proximal portions of the tubes is more difficult because of the weight of the enlarged uterus, but this can be partly overcome by exerting downward and outward traction on the anterior lip of the cervix during the procedure. Particular caution must be taken to produce a large area of coagulation before resection of the tube, because of the increased vascularity. We feel that the psychologic aspects of postabortal sterilization are extremely important, and the procedure is probably best reserved for the married multipara with a contraceptive-failure pregnancy.

REMOVAL OF ECTOPIC INTRAUTERINE CONTRACEPTIVE DEVICES

In 1967 Smith described the removal of an ectopic intrauterine contraceptive device (IUCD) at laparoscopy,[27] and in 1971 we described a similar series of cases.[28] To date we have removed 18 Lippes loops and four Dalkon shields from the peritoneal cavity, including one Dalkon device which was imbedded in the posterior wall of the uterus.

Uterine perforation of an intrauterine contraceptive device occurs in approximately 1 in 1000 insertions. Complications arising from this event have been extremely rare, but when present, have generally been those of bowel obstruction. In 192 perforations, following 6449 insertions, Scott reported 15 cases of bowel obstruction,[28] and others have cited similar cases. Despite the low complication rate, most gynecologists would agree that, when perforation occurs, the device should be removed. Previously this has been accomplished only by laparotomy.

The possibility of uterine perforation must be considered when, in the absence of a history of expulsion, the loop strings of an IUCD are not found to be protruding from the cervical canal. If there is no evidence of pregnancy, localization of the device by x-ray should be accomplished prior to attempting removal, either at laparoscopy or laparotomy. We have found that the simplest way to exclude malpositioning of the device within the uterine cavity is to obtain anterior-posterior and lateral views of the pelvis with a uterine sound in place or by hysterography. Direct visual localization of the device can then be accomplished at laparoscopy.

Once located, the device is teased free of any filmy adhesions, and then is removed by grasping it at one end with the biopsy tongs, pulling it up against the second puncture site cannula, and removing cannula, tongs, and device at the same time (Figure 18–11). Although we have not yet encountered the problem, it is possible that the device may be so entrapped in omental adhesions that removal at laparoscopy would be impossible or dangerous because of bleeding. Should this be the case laparotomy would then be appropriate.

LYSIS OF PELVIC ADHESIONS

Fine, avascular pelvic adhesions, such as are seen following previous surgery, can be quite easily divided at laparoscopy using small coagulating scissors (Figure 18–12) manipulated through a second puncture site. Cautious judgment, however, must be exercised in the selection of adhesions to be treated in this manner. Thin, fibrous, peritubal bands, which appear to impair tubal motility, and translucent omental adhesions, usually can be lysed safely at laparoscopy. On the other hand, thickly adherent areas, especially if they involve the bowel, are quite vascular and make the closed approach dangerous. Since inadvertent perforation of the bowel may occur in pelvic surgery of any type, adhesions between loops of bowel or other viscera should not be divided at laparoscopy. Multiple adhesions of the tubal fimbria, which are most often postinflammatory in origin, should be lysed only at laparotomy, where sharp dissection with fine instruments, and complete hemostasis can be accomplished.

SECOND-LOOK PROCEDURES

Because of the routinely excellent view of the pelvic and abdominal viscera afforded by the laparoscope, successive reexamination of patients who have undergone previous surgery for intra-abdominal cancer is possible by laparoscopy. Photographic documentation and biopsy of areas suggestive of recurrence can be performed on repeated occasions, with minimal risk in terms of morbidity. It should be remembered that, if palpation of residual or regressing tumor tissue is important, laparoscopy is of no value, and exploration should be carried out. We have had the opportunity to follow two patients with resected ovarian carcinoma by repeated laparoscopic biopsy, aspiration of peritoneal fluid, and photography.

UTERINE SUSPENSION

Ventrosuspension of the uterus, at laparoscopy, has been described by Steptoe[29] and others.[17] The technique involves drawing a loop of round ligament through abdominal wall puncture sites established 3 cm. above the midpoints of the inguinal ligaments on each side. The round ligament is then sutured, under direct vision, to the anterior rectus sheath with nonabsorbable sutures. The procedure is simple and, if indicated, presents definite advantages over older open techniques.

REMOVAL OF SILASTIC HOODS

Bagley has recently described the use of laparoscopy for removal of Mulligan hoods following fimbrioplasty.[30] He reported one case in which this was accomplished using the Eder biopsy tongs to hold the silastic hood while dividing and removing the anchoring sutures with biopsy forceps. The hood was then removed from the peritoneal cavity by pushing it through the 1 cm. laparoscope cannula.

SUTURING AND LIGATION

In an attempt to devise better methods for securing hemostasis, and to expand the scope of possible surgical procedures at laparoscopy, Clark has recently described three instruments which can be used to perform suture ligation of tissue within the abdominal cavity.[10] The procedure described has been demonstrated to me, and is ingeniously simple. With the achievement of appropriate skill, it can be applied to the lysis of adhesions, excision of small pedunculated tumors and cysts, segmental biopsies of the ovary, and tubal ligation, perhaps opening a whole new era of laparoscopic surgery.

CYTOLOGIC SMEARS OF THE OVARY

Wagman and Brown, in England, in an attempt to augment the early detection of ovarian cancer, have described a method of obtaining cytologic smears of the surface of the ovary at laparotomy.[31] Although the smears were of readable quality, in 457 cases in which the ovaries appeared normal, no abnormal smears were found. Despite this, we feel the idea has merit, and perhaps should become a routine adjunct to gynecologic laparoscopy. To date we have obtained only enough smears to prove the concept feasible.

Culdoscopy or Laparoscopy?

In recent years, as gynecologic laparoscopy has gained in popularity, often at the expense of culdoscopy within a particular hospital, a mild controversy among gynecologists has arisen over the relative merits of the two procedures. In some centers, where culdoscopy has been widely employed, there has been some reluctance to acknowledge any advantage to the abdominal approach. Some gynecologists, usually those not familiar with laparoscopy, have held that there is little difference in the diagnostic potential of the two techniques, and that the risks involved with laparoscopy outweigh its usefulness. Although such pronouncements seem to spawn the elements of a controversy, they are emotional ones, and fail to carry the weight of experience. In the view of gynecologists familiar with both procedures, there are specific advantages and disadvantages to each. Although both find primary application in visualization of the pelvic viscera, the selection of one or the other depends upon the training of the operator, the limitations imposed by the general health of the patient, and the specific problems posed by the disease process under study. There is no disputing the fact that laparoscopy offers a more complete view of the pelvis and enables the surgeon to perform a wider variety of manipulative and surgical procedures. However, in certain cases this advantage may not be important, and culdoscopy may be entirely adequate. Unfortunately, the arguments favoring one procedure over the other have often been less than objective. All too often they are advanced by those who have never performed, or in some cases, never even observed, laparoscopy. This is prejudice, and like all prejudice, is based upon a paucity of information and understanding. The widely proclaimed argument that culdoscopy offers the advantage of requiring only local anesthesia, and therefore short hospitalization, fails to acknowledge the fact that many laparoscopies are being performed today under local anesthesia on an outpatient surgery basis.

The time has come to lay these arguments aside and acknowledge that there are indeed many advantages to laparoscopy, which speak in their own behalf. The procedure is being taught and practiced in virtually every center

TABLE 18-2.   *Comparison of Various Factors Involved in Culdoscopy and Laparoscopy*

	CULDOSCOPY	LAPAROSCOPY
Anesthesia	1. Local (usually used) 2. Hypobaric spinal (rare)	1. General endotracheal (usual) 2. Spinal 3. Local
Patient position	Knee-chest	Modified dorsal lithotomy
Patient comfort	Uncomfortable, awake	Comfortable, even when awake
General risk to the patient	Small	Greater or the same as for culdoscopy, depending on the anesthesia used and the ancillary procedures performed
View of pelvic viscera	Limited to distal adnexae and upper posterior pelvis; no view of cul-de-sac	Usually unlimited
View of abdominal viscera	Minimal	Excellent, including some of the upper abdominal organs
Operating time for diagnostic procedure in experienced hands	15 to 30 minutes	15 to 30 minutes
Recovery time	2 to 6 hours (local anesthesia)	4 to 8 hours (general endotracheal anesthesia)
Surgical possibilities	Limited to biopsy of the ovary and upper posterior pelvis	Numerous procedures in both pelvis and abdomen
Applicability to outpatient surgery	Excellent	Good
Cost of equipment	$1000 to $2000	$2500 to $5000
Photographic potential	Fair	Excellent
Complications	Minimal from the culdoscopy itself	More numerous than culdoscopy
Indications	Limited (see section in text on indications)	Numerous (see section in text on indications)
Contraindications	1. Inability of patient to assume knee-chest position 2. Obstructed cul-de-sac 3. Florid vaginitis or cervicitis	1. Hiatus hernia 2. Intestinal obstruction 3. Inability to establish pneumoperitoneum 4. Inability of the patient to tolerate anesthesia
Usefulness in ectopic pregnancy	Limited somewhat by inability to see the entire tube	Diagnostic
Usefulness in endometriosis	Contraindicated when there is involvement in the cul-de-sac. Of no value for anterior pelvis involvement	Diagnostic. Allows ability to biopsy and easily fulgurate implants. Indicated with cul-de-sac involvement
Usefulness for tubal lavage	Good. Occasionally cannot see fimbria	Excellent. Can see dye through serosa in isthmal portion of tube
For partial tubal resection	Poor (rarely used)	Excellent. Rapidly becoming method of choice for interim sterilization
Usefulness for location of ectopic IUCDs	Fair	Excellent

of gynecology in the world. Constant improvements in technique, application, and anesthesia are being made and reported almost daily. There is certainly a rightful place in the gynecologic armamentarium for culdoscopy, but it is folly not to accept the fact that much of its former usefulness has been replaced by the even greater advantages of laparoscopy.

Table 18–2 compares the two procedures with respect to several of the factors which must be taken into consideration when selecting the route of pelvic endoscopy.

Summary

Pelvic endoscopy has come of age, and should rest securely in the armamentarium of gynecologic surgery. Clear visualization of the pelvic viscera not only is a technical reality, and easily accomplished, but also can now be considered an integral part of the diagnostic investigation of many pelvic conditions.

It is important to remember, however, that no matter how finely developed they may become, culdoscopy and laparoscopy can never replace good clinical judgment and diagnostic expertise. They are only extensions of the senses which provide for objective observation and remote manipulation. They can never provide interpretation. They must be used or withheld with intelligence, and performed with skill. The analogy of the blind men and the elephant, however applicable it may have been to the gynecologist relying solely on bimanual pelvic examination, no longer has relevance to the specialist trained in pelvic endoscopy.

REFERENCES

1. Kelling, G.: Uber Oesophagoskopie, Gastroskopie, und Kolioskopie. Münch. Med. Wschr. 49:21, 1902.
2. Kelling, G.: Uber die Möglichkeit, die Zystoskopie bei Untersuchung Seröser Höhlung Anzuwenden. Bemerkung zu dem Artikel von Jacobaeus. Münch. Med. Wschr. 57: 2358, 1910.
3. Jacobaeus, H. C.: Uber die Möglichkeit die Zystoskopie bei Untersuchung Seröser Höhlung Anzuwenden. Münch. Med. Wschr. 57:2090, 1910.
4. Berheim, B. M.: Organoscopy: cystoscopy of the abdominal cavity. Ann. Surg. 53:764, 1911.
5. Cohen, M. R.: Laparoscopy, Culdoscopy, and Gynecography. Philadelphia, W. B. Saunders Co., 1970.
6. Horwitz, S. T.: Laparoscopy in gynecology. Obstet. Gynec. Surv. 27:1, 1972.
7. Decker, A., and Cherry, T.: Culdoscopy: a new method in diagnosis of pelvic disease. Amer. J. Surg. 64:40, 1944.
8. Cohen, M. R., and Guterman, H. S.: A pelvic photoscope. Obstet. Gynec. 1:544, 1953.
9. Clyman, M. J.: A new panculdoscope: diagnostic, photographic, and operative aspects. Obstet. Gynec. 21:343, 1963.
10. Clark, H. C.: Laparoscopy—new instruments for suturing and ligation. Fertil. Steril. 23:274, 1972.
11. Hodgson, C., McClelland, R. M. A., and Newton, J. R.: Some effects of the peritoneal insufflation of carbon dioxide at laparoscopy. Anaesthesia 25:382, 1970.
12. Baratz, R. A., and Karis, J. H.: Blood gas studies during laparoscopy under general anesthesia. Anesthesiology 30:463, 1969.
13. Alexander, G. D., Noe, F. E., and Brown, E. N.: Anesthesia for pelvic laparoscopy. Anesth. Analg. 48:14, 1969.
14. Wheeless, C. R.: Outpatient laparoscope sterilization under local anesthesia. Obstet. Gynec. 39:767, 1972.

The section on anesthesia for laparoscopy was written in collaboration with Jess B. Weiss, M.D.

15. Shirley, R. L.: Ovarian radiation dosage during hysterosalpingography. Fertil. Steril. 22:83, 1971.
16. Stein, I. F.: Gynecography: x-ray diagnosis in gynecology. Surg. Clin. N. Amer. 23:165, 1943.
17. Shirodkar, V. N.: Plastic surgery of fallopian tubes. West. J. Surg. 69:253, 1961.
18. Liston, W. A., Bradford, W. P., Downie, J., and Kerr, M. G.: Laparoscopy in a general gynecologic unit. Amer. J. Obstet. Gynec. 113:672, 1972.
19. Pent, D.: Laparoscopy: its role in private practice. Amer. J. Obstet. Gynec. 113:459, 1972.
20. Semm, K.: Die laporoskopie in der Gynäkologie. Geburtsh. Frauenheilkd. 27:1029, 1967.
21. Steptoe, P. C.: A new method of tubal sterilization. Proceedings of the Fifth World Congress on Fertility and Sterility (Stockholm) 133:1183, 1967.
22. Wheeless, C. R.: Elimination of second incision in laparoscopic sterilization. Obstet. Gynec. 39:134, 1972.
23. Keith, L., et al.: Postpartum laparoscopy for sterilization. J. Int. Fed. Obstet. Gynec. 8:145, 1970.
24. Keith, L., et al.: Puerperal tubal sterilization using laparoscopic technique: a preliminary report. J. Reprod. Med. 6:133, 1971.
25. Keith, L., et al.: Laparoscopy for puerperal sterilization. Obstet. Gynec. 39:616, 1972.
26. Steptoe, P. C., and Imran, M.: Combined procedure of aspiration termination and laparoscopic sterilization. Brit. Med. J. 3:751, 1969.
27. Smith, D. C.: Removal of an ectopic IUD through the laparoscope. Am. J. Obstet. Gynec. 105:285, 1969.
28. Leventhal, J. M., Simon, L. R., and Shapiro, S. S.: Laparoscopic removal of intrauterine contraceptive devices following uterine perforation. Am. J. Obstet. Gynec. 111:102, 1971.
29. Scott, R. B.: Critical illnesses and death associated with intrauterine devices. Obstet. Gynec. 31:322, 1968.
30. Steptoe, P. C.: Laparoscopy in Gynaecology. Edinburgh, E. & S. Livingstone, Ltd., 1967.
31. Bagley, G. P.: Mulligan hood removed through the laparoscope. Obstet. Gynec. 39:950, 1972.
32. Wagman, H., and Brown, C. L.: Ovary cytology. Brit. J. Cancer. 25:81, 1971.

The Place of Culdoscopy and Laparoscopy in Diagnosis and Patient Management

Editorial Comment

The rapid developments in optical technology have placed new and successively better instruments in the hands of today's gynecologists. Combining use of these tools with increasing competence and dexterity, the endoscopist can now enter the alimentary tract at both ends, as well as the lung, the bladder, and now the peritoneal cavity with singular ease and safety. Observation, manipulation, biopsy, lysis of adhesions, culture, cytologic study, and tissue coagulation are routine procedures carried out through the point of entry which is most efficacious for the organ system to be explored or condition involved. With this understanding, there ceases to be a controversy regarding one approach over another (for example, laparoscopy versus culdoscopy), but rather an individualization of the procedures.

When obesity prevents pneumoperitoneum through the subumbilical Verres needle, CO_2 may be easily instilled through the cul-de-sac, with laparoscopy to follow. Multiple dense anterior wall adhesions simply indicate a culdoscopy approach, whereas the adherent posterior uterus would mediate the laparoscopic abdominal procedure. Common sense and good judgment are necessary for the most efficient and safest patient management.

While all three authors have pointed out that local anesthesia may be used with either procedure, the editors would agree with those who prefer intratracheal general anesthesia for laparoscopy. The presence during the procedure of a skilled anesthesiologist leaves a wide margin of safety for the patient with cardiac arrhythmias or hypoventilation, and allows more adequate volumes of pneumoperitoneum, making possible not only better visualization but also more adequate displacement of the bowel from the pelvis. Also, controlled respiration prevents unexpected sudden pushing of the bowel against the cautery tip at the moment of coagulation. Organ manipulation is facilitated as well. Moreover, the anesthesiologist skilled in improved techniques is able to maintain adequate relaxation with minimal depression of the patient. By forced ventilation at time of abdominal compression at the end of the procedure he also aids in more complete evacuation (with the cannula open) of the CO_2 from the peritoneal cavity and thus facilitates rapid safe recovery to ambulatory status. At the same time, his presence makes possible an immediate laparotomy, if one is necessary, providing a margin of safety and one which makes hiatus hernia a theoretical contraindication only.

The complications of laparoscopy have been enumerated and, though they are rare, they are potentially lethal. Major hemorrhage, air embolism, and emphysema are prevented by care in placing both the Verres needle and the trochar as well as by aspirating with a syringe before injecting CO_2. As Pent points out, the majority of reported fatalities were in conjunction with liver biopsy, but still a significant number of deaths follow unrecognized bowel burns with delayed necrosis and fulminating peritonitis. Sloughing of the abdominal wall along the coagulating cannula site has been reported (Munsick) from unrecognized shorting of the coagulation tip to the metal cannula. The new plastic cannula still affords only partial protection against this entity. Prompt surgical excision of the entire tract is necessary to prevent prolonged disability. The small size of the coagulation tongs of the right angle laparoscope used in the single puncture of Wheeless makes complete coagulation of the tube more difficult, and has produced an increased number of failures. Also, there is greater danger of bowel burns owing to the limited field of vision immediately below the cautery tip.

The contributors to this chapter have presented the historical progression of the art of celioscopy, at one time divergent in approach, but now being combined, with better instrumentation and technical expertise, into one overall procedure tailored to the individual patient, incorporating the various aspects of laparoscopy and culdoscopy in such a way as to give the most information in the safest possible manner. This complementary usage of the two techniques should lay to rest the controversy and will effect better patient management.

19

Medical Versus Surgical Management of Endometriosis

Alternative Points of View:

    By George W. Mitchell and Martin Farber

    By Brooks Ranney

    By E. J. Wilkinson and R. F. Mattingly

Editorial Comment

Medical Versus Surgical Management of Endometriosis

George W. Mitchell, Jr., and Martin Farber

Tufts University School of Medicine

The term "endometriosis" presumably refers to a single disease entity, but the wide range in the distribution of the implants and the great variation in symptoms hinder a discussion of management in general terms. The specific problem to be treated must be delineated. The histology is unpredictable because of varying proportions of glands and stroma and because of the differences in responsiveness of individual implants to the steroid hormones,[1] both of which make it nearly impossible to collect large numbers of similar cases and which affect the therapeutic results. Because the medical literature contains no well controlled studies of either the medical or the surgical management of endometriosis, the clinician must individualize his cases and use common sense, with the help of the few clues that can be gleaned from the literature, recognizing that many of these reports exhibit a personal bias. Since adenomyosis is considered by most pathologists and interested gynecologists to be a separate disease entity from endometriosis, although often coexisting with it, this discussion will deal only with the subject of external endometriosis.

Almost all endometriosis is histologically benign, but it is convenient to prepare a staging taxonomy similar to that used for malignant disease to clarify the anatomical entity to be considered for treatment. This system can be outlined as follows:

Stage I. One or more small superficial implants (less than 5 mm.) on the pelvic peritoneum.

Stage II. Larger superficial implants involving uterosacral ligaments, rectovaginal septum, and/or ovaries.

Stage III. Endometriomas of the ovary greater than 5 cm. in diameter with or without superficial involvement of broad ligament and adjacent organs.

Stage IV. Penetration of vagina, bowel, or urinary tract and distant metastases (lymph nodes, umbilicus, surgical wounds, and so forth).

Stage V. Endometriomas giving rise to adenocarcinoma.

It is impossible to obtain statistics on the incidence of symptoms associated with the various stages of endometriosis, since most reported series comprise patients who consulted the clinician because of specific complaints. The assumption that symptoms tend to increase through succeeding stages is not necessarily true. Patients with minimal disease may have severe symptoms and patients with no symptoms may have advanced disease discovered incidentally at the time of a routine pelvic examination. All claims for cure, by whatever method, must be considered in this context, since the permanent alleviation of symptoms is more important in the treatment of benign disease than the eradication of the disease process.

Symptoms attributed to endometriosis include dysmenorrhea, pelvic pain, dyspareunia, and infertility. In the rare Stage IV cases, the symptoms are commensurate with the degree of dysfunction of the organ involved. The mechanism by which Stage I and Stage II lesions produce dysmenorrhea or pelvic pain is unclear, since under the microscope many of them appear relatively inert and show no tendency to bleed or propagate. The occurrence of dysmenorrhea, which is related to the force of uterine contractions independent of the external pelvic environment, is difficult to comprehend as an effect of endometriosis unless one supports the unproved hypothesis that these pockets are an additional source of prostaglandins. Dyspareunia and infertility can be more rationally related to the presence of endometriosis because of the tendency of this tissue to obliterate the cul-de-sac and significantly shorten the vagina, and because of the possibility of dislocation or entrapment of organs necessary for reproduction. The relationship between endometriosis and symptoms is further obscured by the reported frequency of coexisting pelvic abnormalities such as leiomyomas, pelvic inflammatory disease, adenomyosis, hyperplasia of the endometrium, and endometrial polyps.[2]

A presumptive diagnosis of endometriosis frequently is made after a pelvic examination in women who are absolutely asymptomatic, and it seems likely that there are at least as many undetected cases among the female population that has not been examined as there are cases identified. The allegation that socioeconomic status plays a part in the development of endometriosis ignores the fact that individuals at the lower end of the scale do not have routine physical examinations and are, therefore, much less likely to undergo surgery for this condition. This provides a clue for the proper management of asymptomatic patients who incidentally are found to have Stage I or II disease—which is, in general, to do nothing.

The armamentarium available to the gynecologist may be divided into four descriptive categories: nihilistic, prophylactic, medical, or surgical, plus various combinations of these modalities. No long-term studies are available to determine the rate of progression or the incidence of spontaneous remission in Stages I and II, which certainly contain the vast majority of cases. Significant data are difficult to collect because of the inaccuracy of pelvic examinations. Even in the hands of a self-acknowledged expert the histologic confirmation of presumptive diagnoses does not exceed 75 per cent, and the diagnostic accuracy is not more than 20 per cent if left to relatively inexperienced or to successive different examiners.[3] The strong likelihood is that the majority of cases in early stages will progress at a slow rate and will require no treatment.

The question of the need to treat asymptomatic Stages I and II in order to prevent the eventual development of minor symptoms in some cases or more serious complications such as acute rupture of cysts or carcinoma arising in endo-metrial implants can be considered under the general heading of prophylaxis. The risks attendant upon either medical or surgical intervention are greater than the chances that an asymptomatic Stage I or II individual might develop life-threatening complications. The use of drugs or surgery to prevent the possible onset of pain at a later date also seems unwarranted. The beneficial effect of early childbearing in preventing endometriosis has been generally accepted for at least 20 years,[4] but the evidence for this is certainly not conclusive. Many individuals with known endometriosis become pregnant without difficulty, and endometriosis is encountered quite commonly in multigravid women. To counsel marriage and early childbearing to a woman with asymptomatic Stage I or II endometriosis seems, therefore, rather radical, but since it is accepted that increasing age and infertility go hand in hand, such advice might be said to contain at least some logic.

Microscopic examination of implants of endometriosis removed inciden-tally at the time of cesarean section first suggested the possibility that the hor-mones of pregnancy might have a profound effect upon the disease.[5] The decidual changes associated with areas of necrosis indicated the possibility that marked stimulation might be followed by complete necrosis and absorption. The availability in the 1950's of powerful progestational agents capable of suppressing ovulation indefinitely and inducing a so-called pseudopregnant state prompted the experimental application of these agents to the cure of endometriosis in the hope of producing changes in implants similar to those observed during true preg-nancy. A number of early reports on the use of progestogens to treat endometri-osis were enthusiastic in their claims of alleviating pelvic pain and increasing fertility.[6,7] Complete regression of the lesions was noted in as many as 75 per cent of the patients treated. These claims were based on diagnoses made by culdos-copy prior to the beginning of treatment and after the completion of a treatment course lasting approximately six months, during which time ovulation was sup-pressed by the continuous use of progestogens in increasing doses. Since there is a discrepancy of approximately 8 per cent between the diagnosis of endometri-osis made at laparotomy and the histologic diagnosis,[3] it may be safely assumed that culdoscopy without biopsy was associated with at least as large a percentage of error. Observations over a longer period of time indicated that when treated patients were followed for an additional six months or more, the signs and symp-toms of endometriosis recurred in a significant number of cases.[8,9]

Laboratory data indicated that when endometriosis was produced experi-mentally in the Rhesus monkey by permitting retrograde flow of the menstruum into the peritoneal cavity, treatment with intramuscular Norethindrone for 5½ to 7 months produced partially necrotic decidua. Six or seven months after Norethin-drone therapy was discontinued the presumably absorbed necrotic decidua was replaced by active endometrial implants. The pre- and post-treatment size of endometriomas did not change.[10]

The effect of pregnancy on endometriosis has more recently been reevalu-ated. An analysis of 24 cases from the world literature shows that endometriosis behaves in a variable way during pregnancy. The effect of pregnancy on both the clinical and histological manifestations of endometriosis is unpredictable when one patient is compared to another, when one trimester is compared to another in the same patient, and when successive pregnancies in the same patient are compared. Although endometriosis might clinically regress post partum, some endometriomas were noted to increase in size. No necrosis was observed post partum, and clinical regression of the lesions appeared to be the result of decreased tissue responsiveness to postpartum hormonal stimulation. The conclusion of the investigators was, "The impression that pregnancy exerts a consistent curative effect upon endometriosis is not supported by critical analysis of the reported cases and appears to be ill-founded."[11]

Few reports of the long-term effectiveness of progestogen therapy in treating the early lesions of endometriosis have appeared in the literature in recent years. This would seem to suggest a decrease in interest, perhaps based on decreased confidence in the real efficacy of the method. The drugs may play a useful role in the temporary alleviation of severe pelvic pain and dysmenorrhea, although this might be true whether endometriosis is present or not. The long-term administration of a progestogen to set the stage for conservative surgery by softening implants and rendering them more mobile remains a moot point for debate. The authors have not been impressed that such treatment renders surgery any easier or reduces the amount of surgery that must be done. Side-effects such as nausea and vomiting, water retention, and the functional suppression of other endocrine organs must be taken into consideration. The optimum time to perform surgery in the course of medical treatment is also difficult to assess.

Two other facets of medical management remain to be considered. The first concerns the continuous long-term use of progestogens following conservative surgery in order to produce necrosis in implants which could not be resected, in the hope of postponing recurrence of symptoms and enhancing fertility. No clear-cut evidence supports this, but implants which have been suppressed are known to recur, and it is doubtful that additional time can be gained beyond that provided by the dosage schedule. While treatment is in progress, pregnancy is, of course, impossible. Although its advantages are dubious, this form of treatment will probably continue to have its adherents.

Finally, estrogens may be used to treat symptoms which are the by-products of radical surgery. Although this is not a central issue in the treatment of endometriosis, it is quite important to give relief to women through their fifth decades who suffer the consequences of castration. There is some documentation of the fact that residual implants may be stimulated by exogenous estrogen administered for hot flashes or genital atrophy,[2] and there is abundant similar "hearsay" evidence. This is apparently a relatively rare phenomenon and the benefits of treatment seem to exceed the risks. If symptoms recur, the drug can be stopped and another remedy found. There are no data to indicate whether one steroidal or nonsteroidal estrogen in equivalent biological doses is more likely to cause recurrence than another. The cyclic use of estrogen-progesterone combinations might have a more deleterious effect than estrogen alone, and their continuous use for long intervals hardly seems justified.

Surgery should be performed in Stages I and II when culdoscopy or laparoscopy shows that adhesions interfere with the tubal or ovarian function needed for conception. Occasionally such adhesions can be released under laparoscopic visualization, but more frequently a laparotomy must be done, the implants resected, and the affected organs properly positioned.

Direct surgical intervention without delay is indicated in Stages III, IV, and V. Culdoscopy and laparoscopy have made nonintervention safe in Stages I and II because the diagnosis can be made with reasonable certainty with or without biopsy. Laparoscopy is to be preferred because of its more complete exposure of the pelvic peritoneum and because the distribution of the disease in the posterior cul-de-sac and rectovaginal septum may make culdoscopy technically more difficult and dangerous. When Stage III disease is present, correct laparoscopic diagnosis can usually be made, but the possibility of ovarian malignancy cannot be excluded, and laparotomy is indicated. Because of their tendency to adhere to the posterior surface of the broad ligaments, endometrial cysts rarely undergo torsion, and secondary infection is also uncommon. Acute rupture does occur, however, not necessarily preceded by trauma, and the diagnosis is usually made at the operating table. It has been alleged that the administration of progestogens may predispose cysts to rupture.

Conservative surgery should be attempted in the younger age group for Stages I, II, and III when fertility is an important factor. Some normal ovarian tissue near the hilum can nearly always be salvaged by resecting the entire distal wall of the cyst and the proximal cyst lining and folding together the remaining shell. Very small pieces of residual ovarian tissue can function satisfactorily. At the time of surgery all endometrial implants are resected when this is technically possible. In some instances, resection of large implants in inaccessible places or on vital organs may be too hazardous. Under such circumstances, fulguration may be a reasonable substitute, and cryosurgery may have a place in occasional cases. Reperitonealization of the raw areas left by resection will not halt the growth of residual disease but may prevent adhesions which interfere with reproductive function. Since the disease is often present in the posterior pelvis, it is sometimes advisable to perform a uterine suspension to prevent the retrograde fixation of the uterus and adnexa.

The fertility rate subsequent to conservative surgery has been variously reported as ranging from 26 to 81 per cent, with an average of 32 per cent.[3] Such differences in the figures indicate their fundamental unreliability aside from the fact that no cure rate can be considered valid when the rate of pregnancy in untreated endometriosis is unknown. The reoperation rate after conservative surgery has been estimated to be between 2 and 46 per cent.[3] Differences in the indications for surgery in different clinics may account for some of these variations. Unfortunately, the most meticulous operation with gross resection of all obvious disease does not necessarily relieve pain in every case. On this account, some surgeons prefer to perform presacral sympathectomy as an adjunctive procedure. If pain is the primary factor and the patient's condition permits, resection of the hypogastric nerves may provide relief which would otherwise be lacking, but this is strictly conjectural.

Hysterectomy with preservation of ovarian tissue has been recommended for young individuals with endometriosis for whom the preservation of reproductive capacity is not important. This is the procedure of choice only in young women who have completed their families, in whom the degree of endometriosis does not exceed Stage III, and whose pelves seem free of disease after resection. It often seems to provide relief of symptoms, and if retrograde menstruation is an important etiologic factor,[12] it should prevent the development of fresh implants.

Patients with Stage III disease too extensive to resect, who have completed their families, are best treated by total abdominal hysterectomy and bilateral salpingo-oophorectomy unless there are overwhelming psychiatric contraindications to such an operation. Stage IV disease involving the intestines can usually be treated by ovarian ablation if the extension into the bowel does not involve the mucosa and the scarring does not significantly narrow the lumen. Lesser degrees of narrowing of the lumen, especially in the colon, can usually be ignored after the ovaries have been removed, but symptomatic obstruction or mucosal bleeding requires bowel resection. Endometrial lesions invading the urinary bladder sometimes regress after castration. Possible persistence of these lesions can be monitored cystoscopically and fulgurated transurethrally if necessary. Obstruction of the ureters necessitates their mobilizaton and translocation. Castration should usually be a concomitant procedure. To temporize under these circumstances by resorting to medical or conservative surgical treatment places a heavy responsibility on the clinician.

To summarize the conclusions:

1. Cyclic or continuous progestogen therapy will often relieve the dysmenorrhea thought to be associated with endometriosis and also the dysmenorrhea not associated with endometriosis.

2. Continuous progestogen therapy will cause temporary regression of the implants of Stages I and II endometriosis but will not favorably affect Stages III and IV.

3. When ovarian masses are present, surgery is essential to rule out the possibility of ovarian malignancy. When fertility is a problem, conservative surgery is indicated.

4. The beneficial results of postoperative progestogens are hypothetical.

5. When childbearing is no longer desirable and the disease is extensive, total abdominal hysterectomy and bilateral salpingo-oophorectomy are in order.

6. When the disease affects the function of vital organs or is associated with malignancy, immediate surgery designed to restore function and remove the ovaries is indicated.

REFERENCES

1. Novak, E. R., and Woodruff, J. D.: Gynecologic and Obstetric Pathology. 6th Edition. Philadelphia, W. B. Saunders Co., 1967.
2. Ranney, B.: Endometriosis. III. Complete operations: reasons, sequelae, treatment. Amer. J. Obstet. Gynec. 109:1137, 1971.
3. Brewer, J. I., and Maher, F. M.: Conservatism in endometriosis. Amer. J. Obstet. Gynec. 68:549, 1954.
4. Meigs, J. V.: Endometriosis. Etiologic role of marriage, age and parity: conservative treatment. Obstet. Gynec. 2:46, 1953.
5. Kistner, R. W.: The use of newer progestins in the treatment of endometriosis. Amer. J. Obstet. Gynec. 75:264, 1958.
6. Andrews, M. C., Andrews, W. C., and Strauss, A. F.: Effects of progestin-induced pseudopregnancy on endometriosis: clinical and microscopic studies. Amer. J. Obstet. Gynec. 78:776, 1959.
7. Kistner, R. W.: The treatment of endometriosis by inducing pseudopregnancy with ovarian hormones: a report of fifty-eight cases. Fertil. Steril. 10:539, 1959.
8. Riva, H. L., Wilson, J. H., and Kawasaki, D. M.: Effect of norethynodrel on endometriosis. Amer. J. Obstet. Gynec. 82:109, 1961.
9. Riva, H. L., Kawasaki, D. M., and Messinger, A. J.: Further experience with norethynodrel in treatment of endometriosis. Obstet. Gynec. 19:111, 1962.
10. Scott, R. B., and Wharton, L. R.: Effects of progesterone and norethindrone on experimental endometriosis in monkeys. Amer. J. Obstet. Gynec. 84:867, 1962.
11. McArthur, J. W., and Ulfelder, H.: The effect of pregnancy upon endometriosis. Obstet. Gynec. Surv. 20:709, 1965.
12. Ridley, J. H.: The histogenesis of endometriosis: a review of facts and fancies. Obstet. Gynec. Surv. 23:1, 1968.

Medical Versus Surgical Management of Endometriosis

The Management of Endometriosis

Brooks Ranney

*University of South Dakota School of Medicine
and The Yankton Clinic*

Introduction

Endometriosis has been described by Gardner[22] as "heterotopic islands of uterine mucosa . . . found in many locations, [which are] most frequent in the pelvis. Histologically, they are identical to the mucosa which lines the body of the uterus, and they tend to respond to ovarian hormones in the same manner as it does."

When stimulated by cyclic estrogens, these heterotopic areas of glands and stroma (endometriomas) tend to proliferate. If this estrogen stimulation is punctuated periodically by progesterone stimulation, they tend to menstruate or bleed.[79] In the process of absorbing menstrual fluid and blood pigments, subjacent tissues produce inflammation, which results in the eventual development of variable amounts of dense, puckering scar surrounding the area. This scar may alter the blood supply which eventually reaches an individual endometrioma, thus modifying its physiologic response accordingly.[86]

During menstruation, the pressure within an endometrioma may cause it to break at its weakest point, either bursting and spilling bits of endometrium and blood into the abdominal cavity on to fresh peritoneal surfaces, or extravasating into adjacent subperitoneal tissues.

A logical consideration of the prevention, inhibition, or treatment of pelvic endometriosis should be based upon (1) knowledge and theories concerning its etiology (i.e., histogenesis and various factors which may stimulate growth of endometriosis), and (2) the gynecologist's observations concerning various patients who have this enigmatic disease.

Since there is not enough space here to summarize the vast literature relating to the causes of endometriosis, only a brief outline is presented, though such brevity carries with it the inherent danger of mixing facts and theories.

637

Histogenesis

"Theories concerning histogenesis may be divided into three general groups: (1) Those which imply that ectopic endometrial tissue is *transported* from the uterus to its pathological location, (2) those which imply that ectopic endometrial tissue develops *in situ* from local tissues, and (3) *combinations* of these two groups."[66]

Not only in experimental animals, but also in women, viable particles of endometrium may be deliberately or inadvertently transplanted from the uterus, during various operative procedures, and can grow in ectopic sites.[37,55,78] Such transplantation is enhanced by an adequate blood estrogen level,[37,55,79] and is somewhat inhibited by infection or inflammation.

During the past two decades, evidence has accumulated that tiny, menstrually discharged particles of endometrium can sometimes retain viability for about 24 to 48 hours after separating from underlying tissue,[6,7,46,72,80] and may be transported through the tubes in a retrograde direction.[75] It is not known how often this potential avenue for the development of pelvic endometriosis is actually utilized. Some writers consider it to be the main route.

Hematogenous spread of endometriosis has been postulated. Although endometriosis via venous metastasis has been produced experimentally in rabbits,[37,42] there is little evidence for its spontaneous occurrence in women.

Bits of endometriosis have been observed microscopically, apparently growing within lymphatics or pelvic lymph nodes.[31,43] However, lymphatic metastasis of endometriosis is relatively rare when compared with pelvic endometriosis which is found on or just beneath the serosal surface of the pelvic peritoneum.[22,63,86]

For many years, careful gynecologic pathologists[40,61,63] have theorized that the adult derivatives of the embryonic coelomic lining cells (particularly those in the female pelvis) will retain the potentiality of forming tissue which is histologically and functionally indistinguishable from endometrial tissue. Theoretically, this potentiality is triggered by the estrogen-progesterone stimulation of the menstrual cycle.[79] The embryologic basis for this theory was developed by Gruenwald.[30] Endometriosis is found most commonly on or near pelvic peritoneal surfaces which can most readily produce a decidual reaction in response to large doses of female hormones.[63] This "coelomic metaplasia" theory permits a physiologic explanation for spontaneously occurring endometriosis in *every* portion of the body in which it has been reported.[30] Unfortunately, this theory is not amenable to conclusive proof or disproof.

Years ago, Cullen demonstrated that the endometrium can extend projections outward through tissue spaces, between the muscle bundles of the myometrium.[8] This is the usual method of development of adenomyosis. Adenomyosis is usually found in somewhat older women, who generally have had more pregnancies than women in whom pelvic endometriosis is found.[16] Therefore, although adenomyosis is similar microscopically to pelvic endometriosis, its etiology is probably somewhat different.

The tendency to develop adenomyosis or endosalpingosis (the two different types of cells may be found in single microscopic sections) is most evident near the uterotubal junction in the cornual portion of the uterus.[15,65,77,87] Sampson demonstrated that cornual adenomyosis may extend directly beyond the serosal surface of the uterus into the abdominal cavity, producing adhesions and pain.[77]

Philipp and Huber theorized that bits of such tissue might also be squeezed out of the uterine tube to implant and grow on the pelvic peritoneum producing external endometriosis.[65]

Stimulating Factors

HORMONAL FACTORS

Endometriosis never occurs in premenarchal women.[17,33] Only occasionally is significant endometriosis found after the menopause,[19,62,70] and then its activity may be explained on the basis of fluctuating female hormones, either exogenous or endogenous.

Pregnancy seems to protect many women against the development of endometriosis, if the first pregnancy occurs not too many years after menarche, and if pregnancy is repeated frequently.[57,58] However, this protecting effect is not uniform, neither is it necessarily long-lasting.[32,68,69]

Women with anovulatory cycles seldom develop significant endometriosis during the anovulatory intervals, whether the lack of ovulation is spontaneous, or is induced by oral contraceptive progestins. When significant endometriosis does develop, it is usually during a two- to five-year interval of time when the woman is having regular, ovulatory cycles, each culminating in normal menstruation.[78,79]

Women who have endometriosis are less fertile than women who do not have endometriosis.[13,22,68]

All these observations accentuate the relationship between cyclic female hormonal function and the propagation of endometriosis.[79]

MECHANICAL FACTORS

As noted previously, any manipulation, examination, or obstruction which may propel, extrude, or transplant healthy bits of endometrium to an ectopic site can result in the development of endometriosis.[9,10,41,56,74] This is discussed more fully under *Prevention.*

HEREDITARY FACTORS

Why do some regularly menstruating women develop endometriosis, whereas many others do not? Also, why does endometriosis remain mild in some, but become severe in others? In answer to these questions, several authors[20,23,27,36,71,84] have implied that certain women have inherited a physiologic propensity to develop endometriosis whereas other women of similar age and habits do not have these inherited tendencies. The exact inherited factors (endocrinologic, enzymatic, or chemical) remain to be discovered.[46,59,80]

Prevention

The gynecologist may take, or avoid, certain actions in order *not* to initiate the development of endometriosis, nor to enhance his patient's potentiality of developing endometriosis. These actions will depend upon his theories concerning etiology.

"RETROGRADE" TRANSPORT OF ENDOMETRIAL PARTICLES

DURING MINOR GYNECOLOGIC PROCEDURES. It is probably important to perform any tubal insufflation or uterosalpingography carefully, and without prolonging the procedure unduly. Certainly, any such forceful retrograde insufflation should be avoided for at least three weeks *after* curettage, or after uterotubal surgery.[10,74]

It is probably wiser to perform bimanual pelvic examinations (under anesthesia) *before* curettage, rather than *after* curettage.

SECONDARY TO OBSTRUCTION OF NATURAL DRAINAGE. Some, but not all, young women with congenital anomalies of the paramesonephric ducts which interfere with natural menstrual drainage will develop endometriosis if the retrograde drainage is deposited on pelvic peritoneum.[2,41,56] These anomalies should be recognized and corrected early, preferably prior to regular, *ovulatory* cycles.

Acute anterior angulation of the uterus on the cervix may interfere with natural menstrual drainage.[9] Girls with such a condition usually also have dysmenorrhea, which may be treated with progestin contraceptive pills (see page 641, *Contraceptive Progestins*).

During cautery or cryosurgery of an "erosion," the treatment should not be carried up the cervical canal too high, in order to avoid scar stenosis during subsequent healing, which then could obstruct flow and cause retrograde menstruation.[71] In general, it is probably best to avoid treating such cervices until after the cervical canal has been dilated by the first delivery.

The careful gynecologist may wish to advise certain young girls with narrow introital openings that they should not "stopper" their vaginas with tampons during the heavy portions of menses, but should use perineal pads during those particular times.

NORMAL MENSTRUAL TRANSPORT OF ENDOMETRIAL PARTICLES

It is probably preferable that cautery or cryosurgical treatment of cervical "erosions," as well as other minor cervical, vaginal, or vulvar procedures, should be performed early enough during the cycle so that raw surfaces are well epithelialized prior to the next menses. This may reduce the incidence of endometriosis on the cervix, vagina, or vulva.[12,24,38,52,67] Since transplants of endometriosis do not grow well in the presence of infection or inflammation, the natural bacterial flora of the vagina may, incidentally, help prevent the implantation and growth of cervical, vaginal, or vulvar endometriosis.

INADVERTENT TRANSPLANT OF ENDOMETRIAL PARTICLES DURING ABDOMINAL GYNECOLOGIC OPERATIONS

Though the early literature contains numerous references to abdominal scar endometriosis following cesarean sections and hysterotomies, such occurrences are uncommon today.[11,25,34,60,85] Any gynecologic procedure which invades the nonpregnant endometrium (such as myomectomy or plastic repair of a double uterus) would seem to provide a greater potential for inadvertent transplantation endometriosis postoperatively, particularly if it is performed during the late proliferative phase of the cycle, when the blood estrogen level is high.[79]

Adenomyosis-endosalpingosis

Operations which involve the tube near the uterus, such as salpingectomy or tubal ligation close to the cornual portion of the uterus, were shown by Sampson[77] sometimes to result in subsequent, direct extension outgrowths of painful endosalpingosis, and in adhesions to surrounding viscera. We have seen a number of instances. This type of endometriosis, and the necessary second operations, may be avoided if a small wedge of the tubouterine cornu is resected along with the tube at the time of original salpingectomy. (After a few more years have passed, we may begin to see endosalpingosis developing following some instances of electrocoagulation of the uterine tubes for sterilization.)

Anovulation

Contraceptive Progestins.   The monthly use of contraceptive progestins, in small doses, results in a thin, relatively inactive endometrium which tends to slough and menstruate only slightly at the end of each cycle. In women who take oral contraceptives, neither the hormonal "climate" nor the "soil" is right for transplantation or propagation of endometriosis.[59,69] This protective side-effect of small-dose contraceptive progestins probably should be utilized by many young married women until they are ready to become pregnant. This is particularly true of girls with a family history of endometriosis (see page 639, *Hereditary Factors*).

Pregnancy.   Although pregnancy apparently loosens the muscle bundles of the uterus,[3] thus allowing the development of more adenomyosis than is usually found in nulliparous women,[16] the associated lack of cyclic hormonal changes and absence of periodic menstruation for nine months tend to protect against the development or progression of mild, external endometriosis.[57,58] (However, more extensive endometriosis may be aggravated by the tremendous hormone levels of pregnancy[32,69]—see page 642, *Complications from Progestational Endometriosis*.)

Inhibition

A young woman who has mild endometriosis and who does not wish to become pregnant should be advised to use contraceptive progestins in small doses. This will usually inhibit progression of the disease during the intervals of medication. Likewise, she should be urged to have her children as soon as she can, because both the severity of the disease and the infertility tend to become progressively worse with time, although there may be some ebb and flow of the disease at various times.[68] Stopping contraceptive progestins so that she may ovulate and attempt to conceive includes the hazard of more rapid progression of the endometriosis. If pregnancy does not occur within a reasonable time interval, one may consider a conservative operative procedure (see page 643, *Preservation of Reproductive Function*). If pregnancy does occur, progestin contraceptives may be used again after delivery, until another pregnancy is desired. If a woman has known endometriosis, she should be advised to choose a short interval between pregnancies (assuming that she is fortunate enough to conceive without further treatment) because her fertile years probably are limited.

Treatment

NO TREATMENT

Patients with endometriosis who have few or no symptoms and minimal changes may need *no treatment*, particularly if they do not desire progeny, or if they happen to be fertile without treatment. Because endometriosis can change its course abruptly, such patients should be examined every six to 12 months.

PALLIATION FOR ENDOMETRIOSIS

HORMONE THERAPY. Our experience indicates that hormone therapy for endometriosis may be palliative, but that it does not eliminate endometriosis. In most instances, the endometriosis worsens within one to six months after discontinuing therapy.[69,81]

Years ago we used large doses of estrogens to inhibit ovulation; however, side reactions made many of these women more miserable than the endometriosis did.

Later, we used small, daily oral doses of testosterone—about one-half the amount which might be calculated to produce minimally masculinizing symptoms. Four such patients actually conceived while taking testosterone. These are the only endometriosis patients treated by the author who have conceived during or soon after palliative hormone therapy. However, our success with operative treatment of endometriosis-infertility patients was considerably better (see page 643, *Conservative Operations*).

Many years ago, Meigs[57,58] called attention to the palliative effects which the more fertile patients with endometriosis could derive from pregnancy. During recent years, these hormonal effects have been imitated by giving endometriosis patients progressively larger doses of progestins for several months.[1,47,48,49,51,53,73] The resulting anovulation and amenorrhea simulate the effects of pregnancy. The major side reactions of this therapy likewise simulate or exaggerate those noted during pregnancy (nausea, weight gain, edema, depressions, modified libido and vaginal discharge). The first ovulation will frequently occur within two or three months after hormone administration has been stopped. About 30 per cent of these patients are reported to achieve pregnancies sometime following hormone treatment.[50]

However, our experience has been that infertility patients have not become pregnant following progestin-pseudopregnancy therapy, and the complications associated with the therapy have been very annoying.[53,69] Therefore, we reserve this palliative therapy for the occasional patient with moderate endometriosis who has rather severe dysmenorrhea, and who has good reasons for postponing operations for a few months—i.e., the schoolteacher who wishes to have her operation during the summer vacation.

COMPLICATIONS FROM PROGESTATIONAL ENDOMETRIOSIS. Among 350 patients with endometriosis who were operated upon by us during a 20-year

interval,[68] 13 (3.7 per cent) required *emergency* operations because of hemoperitoneum owing to spontaneous avulsions of pelvic endometriosis.[29,39,69] All of
these occurred during *progestational* phases of the endometriosis (premenstrual,
menstrual or decidual)—some caused by exogenous progestins. The softening
effect of endogenous or exogenous progesterone allowed adherent endometriotic
surfaces to separate spontaneously, resulting in massive intra-abdominal hemorrhage, pain, shock, fever, extensive emergency operations, and transfusions.[69]

Among eight married women in this group whose husbands were fertile,
who avoided contraception, who wanted to become pregnant, and from whom
pelvic endometriosis was resected, only two subsequently conceived; six did *not*
conceive. Three others required a subsequent operation specifically for resection
of endometriosis and hysterectomy. Because of these experiences, we have
deduced that there is an inherent danger during the progestational phase, or during progestin-pseudopregnancy therapy, among women who have moderate to
severe pelvic endometriosis. Likewise, postoperative results among such patients
are much worse than among all other endometriosis patients who were treated
by operation (see next section, *Preservation of Reproductive Function*).

Furthermore, the vaunted beneficial effects of pregnancy[57,58] on pelvic
endometriosis are not necessarily uniform or permanent.[32,69,81] We have palpated
cul-de-sac endometriomas which enlarged each month during pregnancy. Two
such patients had soft tissue dystocia from endometriomas during labor. Another
patient developed intestinal obstruction requiring cesarean section and resection
of endometriosis two weeks before term. Other authors have reported similar
results.[32] Likewise, we have observed recurrence of symptoms of endometriosis
during first postpartum menses.[69]

OPERATIONS FOR ENDOMETRIOSIS

CONSERVATIVE OPERATIONS

Preservation of Reproductive Function. Persistent infertility is often the
presenting complaint of otherwise healthy young married women, in whom the
gynecologist then discovers palpable evidence of endometriosis during pelvic
examination.[13,21,68] The patient may have no symptoms, or may have variably
severe symptoms. Symptoms from endometriosis do not always correlate well with
the severity of the disease. An old, small, scarred, sclerotic, but barely palpable
endometrioma may impinge on more nerve endings than a younger, larger,
actively proliferating, readily palpable endometrioma.[86] Sometimes, in questionable instances, examination during menses will help to confirm a diagnosis.

When endometriosis is the likely cause of infertility, this infertility usually
will have persisted for two, three, or more years.[68] The infertility study of the
couple over several months must make certain there is no other ascertainable
cause for the infertility than endometriosis. Incidentally, this allows time and
opportunity for repeated evaluation of the pelvic findings.

Since meticulous resection of endometriosis is often difficult and time consuming, the gynecologist must judge what advantages will accrue to each individual patient. He must consider:

  1. The couple's desire for progeny.
  2. The age of the patient.
  3. The duration of infertility.

4. The location and extent of endometriosis.

5. The severity of the symptoms.

6. Associated pelvic pathology.

7. The possibility of preserving uninvolved ovarian tissue with a good blood supply.

8. The possibility that a subsequent pelvic operation may be needed.

It is apparent that some of these judgments must be made in consultation with the couple, but others can only be made by the gynecologist at the operating table. If the collective judgment favors preservation of reproductive function, then the uterus, one or both tubes, and all healthy ovarian tissue are preserved.

We prefer not to administer exogenous progestins prior to an operation for endometriosis, because (1) resultant softening that may occur will obscure true boundaries, (2) the resultant friability increases tissue fragmentation, and (3) the enhanced vascularity increases blood loss—all of which make the procedure more difficult and the resection less meticulous.[69,86]

We have reported that 60 per cent of previously infertile, married women conceived and delivered viable babies after resection of endometriosis.[68] Twenty-two of these couples were using contraception postoperatively or had infertility problems from some other cause than the endometriosis. There remained 48 married patients with endometriosis, with fertile husbands, who did not use contraception. Of this group, 42 (87.5 per cent) conceived and were delivered of 71 babies after resection of endometriosis. Only six of this group did not conceive (see page 642, *Complications from Progestational Endometriosis*).

Other authors have noted similar success following operations for endometriosis-infertility patients.[13,22,28,29,39,45,64,83]

In general, women who are under the age of 30, and who have been infertile for less than five to seven years, are more likely to conceive postoperatively than are older women or those with longer histories of infertility.

Most infertility patients with endometriosis ovulate regularly, and have patent, functional tubes.[68] Therefore, it seems illogical to indict ovarian or tubal dysfunction as a cause of infertility among these patients. One might postulate the existence of an enzymatic, chemical, or hormonal disorientation resulting from heterotopic endometriomas which bleed cyclically, and which are surrounded by inflammation. Resection of these areas might favor subsequent fertility. Our only basis for such a theory is the simple fact that six of our infertility patients conceived during the *first* ovulation after resection of endometriosis, and half had conceived within six months postoperatively.

Among 77 patients who had resection of endometriosis, 16 needed second pelvic operations an average of about 10 years later. However, 13 of these operations were performed to treat uterine myomas, adenomyosis, endometrial hyperplasia (tumors which are sometimes called "associated pelvic pathology" because their growth is estrogen dependent).[68,70] Only three subsequent operations were needed specifically because of recurring pelvic endometriosis (see page 642, *Complications from Progestational Endometriosis*).

Preservation of Ovarian Function. About 36 per cent of endometriosis patients may be treated by hysterectomy, plus resection of endometriosis, preserving healthy ovarian tissue which has a good blood supply.[4,13,28,64,68,83] Certainly it would be easier merely to castrate such women, and not attempt to resect all of the endometriosis. This would eliminate the usual source of fluctuating female hormones—the "generator" and stimulator of endometriosis. The patient's pelvic endometriosis would gradually resolve into quiescent glands and stroma surrounded by scar.

However, any subsequent attempt to treat the patient's surgically produced menopausal symptoms or physiologic problems with estrogens would tend to restimulate the quiescent endometriosis, producing pain or tumor[18,70] (see below, *Symptomatic Endometriosis in Postmenopausal Patients*). Therefore, hysterectomy and resection of endometriosis and retention of ovarian function is preferable where future childbearing is not a consideration.

Most of these patients will retain good ovarian hormonal function for years without needing exogenous estrogen therapy for menopausal symptoms.[68]

Also, if the endometriosis is resected meticulously during the initial operation (particularly from the ovarian region), the need for subsequent pelvic operations will be rare (less than 1 per cent).

COMPLETE OPERATIONS

In Patients Before the Menopause. Many middle-aged women with painful endometriosis, and a few younger women with severe disease, are better treated by more complete operations.[5,22,28,39,70] In one reported series,[70] about 41 per cent of patients were treated at operation by removal of the uterus and adnexa, and usually by resection of endometriosis (see page 646, *Estrogen Therapy for Postoperative Menopausal Symptoms*). This was done for one or several of the following reasons:

1. The severity of the endometriosis.
2. The extent of other pelvic pathology.
3. The patient's age.
4. The evidence that future fertility was most improbable.
5. The probability that a lesser operation would be followed by increasing pelvic pain.

At the times of their operations these patients had reached an average age of 44.4 years. Only eight were under 35 years of age.

The *key location* of endometriosis is in the hilar region of the ovaries. The blood supply to such ovaries is jeopardized by *deep* involvement, particularly just underneath the ovary. If such deep endometriosis is resected, the blood supply is transected. If such endometriosis is left in situ, it will usually proliferate actively. If *both* ovaries are thus severely damaged, the adnexa and uterus should be removed and other endometriosis should be resected, if feasible.

Also, in some instances, severe endometriosis of the sigmoid, ureters, or bladder, or other pelvic pathology may dictate that the complete type of operation should be performed.

Symptomatic Endometriosis in Postmenopausal Patients. Endometriosis was found in 17 patients who required operations one to 20 years after the menopause.[19,70] In seven of these, the operation was performed primarily because of other pelvic pathology. However, endometriosis caused the major symptoms and findings in the other 10 patients (2.9 per cent of all endometriosis patients treated by operation).

Eight of these had some endogenous resurgence of estrogen function one to 11 years after the menopause, which restimulated quiescent endometriosis, causing pelvic pain or tumor. However, in two instances, quiescent endometriosis was stimulated to produce severe pain and tumor by the injudicious use of exogenous estrogens, eight and 12 years after the menopause, respectively.

ESTROGEN THERAPY FOR POSTOPERATIVE MENOPAUSAL SYMPTOMS

Since particles or endometrium can be most readily transplanted into tissues with an adequate blood supply containing sufficient quantities of estrogen,[79] one can deduce that estrogens tend to stimulate hyperplasia in plaques of endometriosis which have adequate blood supplies. Therefore, even when removing the uterus and adnexa, there is logical reason also to remove all resectable endometriosis if one plans to treat postoperative menopausal symptoms with oral estrogens.[70]

After removal of the uterus, tubes, ovaries, and endometriosis tissues, some patients are free of menopausal symptoms and will not require estrogen therapy. However, in most instances, oral estrogen therapy is very beneficial for these patients. Rarely, recurring pelvic pain or palpable pelvic nodulation may force the gynecologist to stop postmenopausal estrogen therapy.

Such estrogen therapy for menopausal symptoms should not be started if the prior operation revealed severe, unresectable endometriosis involving bowel or ureters or if the patient had malignancy of the breast, endometrium, or ovary.

Malignancy

In three of our reported patients (0.85 per cent), endometrioid carcinoma of the ovary was found adjacent to extensive endometriosis.[14,70,76,88] This type of cancer is reported to have a better than average prognosis among ovarian cancers.[54,82] Likewise, we have noted an instance of "stromatosis," with its worm-like projections of "stromal adenomyosis" out through pelvic lymphatics. These are reported to be sarcomatous in varying degrees.[35,44] All four of these patients are alive and well some years after their respective operations.

The occasional possibility of cancer occurring in or around endometriosis, and the more frequently encountered difficulty in differentiating between adnexal endometriosis and adnexal cancer during pelvic examination, are additional reasons for utilizing the operative approach in the management of certain patients who are thought to have endometriosis.

Summary

1. While caring for young women, the gynecologist should take reasonable precautions to avoid actions which might enhance the patient's propensity to develop or propagate endometriosis.

2. Management of patients with endometriosis must be based upon one's knowledge and theories concerning etiology, and upon one's experience with other endometriosis patients.

3. Small-dose contraceptive progestins may inhibit early development or propagation of endometriosis.

4. Large-dose, pseudopregnancy progestins may be used as palliative therapy for patients with moderate endometriosis who have good reasons to postpone operative treatment. However, the strong progestational effect can

cause softening of pelvic endometriotic adhesions, resulting in spontaneous avulsion, producing intra-abdominal hemorrhage, and requiring emergency operations. Other side-effects of pseudopregnancy progestins may be annoying and unacceptable to the patient.

5. At least 60 per cent of previously infertile married women who have pelvic endometriosis will conceive after meticulous resection of the endometriosis. Although about 15 per cent of these patients may need subsequent operations, an average of 10 years later, to remove tumors such as fibromyomas, adenomyosis, endometrial hyperplasia, or cancer, fewer than 4 per cent will need subsequent operations specifically to remove endometriosis.

6. Mature women with symptomatic endometriosis (about age 35), and those who have finished having their families, may best be treated by hysterectomy and resection of endometriosis, when it is feasible to do so and retain good ovarian tissue. Endogenous ovarian hormones will be secreted until the natural menopause occurs. Subsequent pelvic operations are rare—less than 1 per cent.

7. More mature women with symptomatic endometriosis, and those with very severe endometriosis, should be treated by removal of the uterus, tubes, and ovaries, and, if feasible, by resection of the endometriosis. If all or most of the endometriosis was resected, postmenopausal symptoms may be treated with oral estrogens. However, estrogens should not be used if remaining endometriosis deeply involves bowel or ureters.

8. Occasionally, in women who are already past the menopause, exogenous hormones or resurging endogenous hormones may cause quiescent pelvic endometriosis to become active and produce tumor and pain, requiring major operation.

9. Very rarely, either carcinoma or sarcoma may occur in close association with endometriosis (about 1 per cent).

10. Specific studies are needed to determine the basic physiologic reasons why women in certain families seem to *inherit a propensity* to develop endometriosis, whereas women in many other families seldom exhibit this enigmatic disease.

REFERENCES

1. Andrews, M. C., Andrews, W. C., and Strauss, A. F.: Effects of progestin-induced pseudopregnancy on endometriosis. Amer. J. Obstet. Gynec. 78:776, 1959.
2. Bernstein, P., and Walter, R.: Hematometra. Amer. J. Obstet. Gynec. 37:126, 1939.
3. Bloom, W., and Fawcett, D. W.: Textbook of Histology. 3rd Ed. Philadelphia, W. B. Saunders Company, pp. 525–563, 1938.
4. Cashman, B. Z.: Hysterectomy with preservation of ovarian function in the treatment of endometriosis. Amer. J. Obstet. Gynec. 49:484, 1945.
5. Counseller, V. S.: Endometriosis. Amer. J. Obstet. Gynec. 36:877, 1938.
6. Craig, G.: Discussion of Watkin's paper on retroversion and endometriosis. Trans. Pac. Coast Obstet. Gynec. Soc. 7:129, 1937.
7. Cron, R. S., and Gey, B. S.: The viability of cast-off menstrual endometrium. Amer. J. Obstet. Gynec. 13:645, 1927.
8. Cullen, T. S.: Adenomyosis of the uterus. W. B. Saunders Co., Philadelphia, 1908.
9. Curtis, A. H.: Stricture of the uterine cervix. J.A.M.A. 98:861, 1932.
10. Curtis, A. H.: Textbook of Gynecology. 5th Ed. 1946. Philadelphia, W. B. Saunders Co., 1946, p. 237.
11. Danforth, W. C. Adenomyoma of the abdominal wall. Amer. J. Obstet. Gynec. 10:630, 1925.
12. Dason, C. K., and Zelenik, J. S.: Vulvar endometriosis. Obstet. Gynec. 3:76, 1954.
13. Devereaux, W. P.: Endometriosis: long-term observations with particular reference to incidence of pregnancy. Obstet. Gynec. 22:444, 1963.

14. Dockerty, M. B.: Malignancy complicating endometriosis. Amer. J. Obstet. Gynec. 83:175, 1962.
15. Everett, H. S.: Probable tubal origin of endometriosis. Amer. J. Obstet. Gynec. 22:1, 1930.
16. Fallas, R., and Rosenblum, G.: Endometriosis. Amer. J. Obstet. Gynec. 39:964, 1940.
17. Fallon, J. Endometriosis in youth. J.A.M.A. 131:1405, 1946.
18. Faulkner, R. L., and Reimenschneider, E. A.: Reactivation of endometriosis by stilbestrol therapy. Amer. J. Obstet. Gynec. 50:560, 1945.
19. Frank, I. L., and Geist, S. H.: Postmenopausal endometriosis. Amer. J. Obstet. Gynec. 44:652, 1942.
20. Frey, G. H.: The familial occurrence of endometriosis. Amer. J. Obstet. Gynec. 73:418, 1957.
21. Gardner, G. H.: Pelvic endometriosis. Northwest. Med. 38:367, 1939.
22. Gardner, G. H.: Endometriosis: comments on its pathology. Transactions of the 5th American Congress of Obstetrics and Gynecology, p. 378, 1952.
23. Gardner, G. H., Greene, R. R., and Ranney, B.: The histogenesis of endometriosis. Obstet. Gynec. 1:615, 1953.
24. Gardner, H. L.: Cervical and vaginal endometriosis. Clin. Obstet. Gynec. 9:358, 1966.
25. German, W. J.: Endometrial adenomata in abdominal scar following cesarean section. Surg. Gynec. Obstet. 47:710, 1928.
26. Goldzieher: Homotransplant of endometrium into anterior chamber of rabbit's eye. Path. u. Pharmakol. 2:387, 1874.
27. Goodall, J. R.: Endometriosis. Philadelphia, J. B. Lippincott, 1943.
28. Gray, L. A.: Endometriosis. Clin. Obstet. Gynec. 3:472, 1960.
29. Green, T. H.: Conservative surgical treatment of endometriosis. Clin. Obstet. Gynec. 9:293, 1966.
30. Gruenwald, P.: Origin of endometriosis from the mesenchyme of the coelomic walls. Amer. J. Obstet. Gynec. 44:470, 1942.
31. Halban, J.: The lymphatic origin of endometriosis. Arch. für Gynäkologie 74:457, 1925.
32. Hanton, E. M., Malkasian, G. D., Dockerty, M. B., and Pratt, J. H.: Endometriosis symptomatic during pregnancy. Amer. J. Obstet. Gynec. 95:1165, 1966.
33. Hanton, E. M., Malkasian, G. D., Dockerty, M. B., and Pratt, J. H.: Endometriosis in young women. Amer. J. Obstet. Gynec. 98:116, 1967.
34. Heaney, N. S.: Adenomas of endometrial origin in laparotomy scar following incision of pregnant uterus. Amer. J. Obstet. Gynec. 10:625, 1925.
35. Henderson, D. N.: Endolymphatic stromal myosis. Amer. J. Obstet. Gynec. 52:1000, 1946.
36. Henricksen, E.: Discussion of Scott, R. B., TeLinde, R. W., and Wharton, L. R., Jr.: Further studies on experimental endometriosis. Amer. J. Obstet. Gynec. 66:1101, 1953.
37. Hobbs, J. E., and Bortnick, A. R.: Endometriosis of the lungs. Amer. J. Obstet. Gynec. 40:832, 1940.
38. Hobbs, J. E., and Lazar, M. R.: Primary endometriosis of the cervix uteri. Amer. J. Obstet. Gynec. 42:509, 1941.
39. Huffman, J. W.: External endometriosis. Amer. J. Obstet. Gynec. 62:1243, 1951.
40. Iwanoff: Metaplasia from peritoneal layer of uterus. Monatschr. f. Geburtsch. u. Gynäk. 7:295, 1898.
41. Jackson, R. A.: Hematometra with endometrial cyst. Amer. J. Surg. 4:43, 1928.
42. Jacobsen, V. C.: Experimental endometrial embolism in rabbits. Arch. Path. 15:1, 1933.
43. Javert, C. T.: Observations on the pathology and spread of endometriosis based on the theory of benign metastasis. Amer. J. Obstet. Gynec. 62:477, 1951.
44. Jensen, P. A., Dockerty, M. B., Symmonds, R. E., and Wilson, R. B.: Stromal endometriosis. Amer. J. Obstet. Gynec. 95:79, 1966.
45. Jones, H. W., Jr.: Editorial comment concerning endometriosis. Obstet. Gynec. Surv. 18:481, 1963.
46. Keettel, W. C., and Stein, R. J.: The viability of cast-off menstrual endometrium. Amer. J. Obstet. Gynec. 61:440, 1951.
47. Kistner, R. W.: The use of newer progestins in the treatment of endometriosis. Amer. J. Obstet. Gynec. 75:264, 1958.
48. Kistner, R. W.: Infertility with endometriosis—a plan of therapy. Fert. Steril. 13:237, 1962.
49. Kistner, R. W.: Current status of hormonal treatment of endometriosis. Clin. Obstet. Gynec. 9:271, 1966.
50. Kistner, R. W. In Behrman, S. J., and Kistner, R. W., Eds.: Progress in infertility. Boston, Little, Brown & Co., 1968.
51. Kourides, I. A., and Kistner, R. W.: Three new synthetic progestins in the treatment of endometriosis. Obstet. Gynec. 31:821, 1968.
52. Lash, A. F., and Rappaport, H.: Primary endometriosis of the cervix uteri. Surg. Gynec. Obstet. 77:576, 1943.

53. Lebherz, T. B., and Forbes, C. D.: Management of endometriosis with norprogesterone. Amer. J. Obstet. Gynec. *81*:102, 1961.

54. Long, M. E., and Taylor, H. C., Jr.: Endometrioid carcinoma of the ovary. Amer. J. Obstet. Gynec. *90*:936, 1964.

55. Markee, J. E.: Menstruation in intraocular transplants in the rhesus monkey. Contrib. Embryol. *28*:221, 1940.

56. McDonald, R. E.: Uterus didelphis with endometriosis. Amer. J. Obstet. Gynec. *45*:1038, 1943.

57. Meigs, J. V.: Endometriosis—a possible etiologic factor. Surg. Gynec. Obstet. *67*:253, 1938.

58. Meigs, J. V.: An interest in endometriosis and its consequences. Amer. J. Obstet. Gynec. *79*:625, 1960.

59. Merrill, J. A.: Endometrial induction of endometriosis across millipore filters. Amer. J. Obstet. Gynec. *94*:780, 1966.

60. Meyer, R.: A hitherto unknown type of adenomyoma of the uterus. Ztschr. f. Geburtsch. u. Gynäk. *49*:32, 1903.

61. Meyer, R.: Metaplasia theory, with inflammation as primary inducing factor. Adenomyosis, adenofibrosis and adenomyoma. München, Viet-Stoekel Handbuch der Gynäkologie, 1930.

62. Montes, M., Beautyman, W., and Haidak, G. L.: Postmenopausal endometriosis. Amer. J. Obstet. Gynec. *82*:119, 1961.

63. Novak, E.: Pelvic endometriosis. Amer. J. Obstet. Gynec. *22*:826, 1931.

64. Parsons, L.: Conservative surgical management of external endometriosis. Obstet. Gynec. *32*:576, 1968.

65. Philipp, E., and Huber, H.: Endometriosis. Zentralbl. für Gynäk. *63*:7, 482, 760, 2153, 2448; 1939.

66. Ranney, B.: Etiology of endometriosis. Surg. Gynec. Obst. (Internat. Abstracts. Surg.) *86*:313, 1948.

67. Ranney, B., and Chung, J. T.: Endometriosis of the cervix uteri. Amer. J. Obstet. Gynec. *64*:1333, 1952.

68. Ranney, B.: Endometriosis: I. Conservative operations. Amer. J. Obstet. Gynec. *107*:743, 1970.

69. Ranney, B.: Endometriosis: II. Emergency operations due to hemoperitoneum. Obstet. Gynec. *36*:437, 1970.

70. Ranney, B.: Endometriosis: III. Complete operations. Amer. J. Obstet. Gynec. *109*:1137, 1971.

71. Ranney, B.: Endometriosis: IV. Hereditary tendencies. Obstet. Gynec. *37*:734, 1971.

72. Ridley, J. H., and Edwards, I. K.: Experimental endometriosis in the human. Amer. J. Obstet. Gynec. *76*:783, 1958.

73. Riva, H. L., Kawasaki, D. M., and Messinger, A. J.: Further experience with norethynodrel in treatment of endometriosis. Obstet. Gynec. *19*:111, 1962.

74. Rubin, I. C.: Most favorable time for transuterine insufflation. J.A.M.A. *84*:486, 1925.

75. Sampson, J. A.: Life history of ovarian hematomas. Amer. J. Obstet. Gynec. *4*:451, 1922.

76. Sampson, J. A.: Carcinoma in endometriosis. Arch. Surg. *10*:1, 1925.

77. Sampson, J. A.: Postsalpingectomy endosalpingosis. Amer. J. Obstet. Gynec. *20*:443, 1930.

78. Scott, R. B., TeLinde, R. W., and Wharton, L. R., Jr.: Further studies on experimental endometriosis. Amer. J. Obstet. Gynec. *66*:1082, 1953.

79. Scott, R. B., and Wharton, L. R., Jr.: The effect of estrone and progesterone on the growth of experimental endometriosis in rhesus monkeys. Amer. J. Obstet. Gynec. *74*:852, 1957.

80. Scott, R. B., Nowak, R. J., and Mannerelli, V. T.: Viability of endometrial transplants within millipore filters. Amer. J. Obstet. Gynec. *84*:1010, 1962.

81. Scott, R. B., and Wharton, L. R., Jr.: Effects of progesterone and norethindrone on experimental endometriosis in monkeys. Amer. J. Obstet. Gynec. *84*:867, 1962.

82. Scully, R. E., Richardson, G. S., and Barlow, J. F.: The development of malignancy in endometriosis. Clin. Obstet. Gynec. *9*:384, 1966.

83. Sheets, J. L., Symmonds, R. E., and Banner, E. A.: Conservative surgical management of endometriosis. Obstet. Gynec. *23*:625, 1964.

84. Stevenson, C. S.: Some general and specific considerations of endometriosis. Clin. Obstet. Gynec. *3*:501, 1960.

85. Stock, W. D., and Helwig, E. B.: Cutaneous endometriosis. Clin. Obstet. Gynec. *9*:373, 1966.

86. Sturgis, S. H., and Call, B. J.: Endometriosis peritonei—relationship of pain to functional activity. Amer. J. Obstet. Gynec. *68*:1421, 1954.

87. Wrork, D. H., and Broders, A. C.: Adenomyosis of the fallopian tube. Amer. J. Obstet. Gynec. *44*:412, 1942.

88. Zussman, W. V., and Hollander, J. S. Unilateral carcinoma arising in bilateral ovarian endometriosis. Amer. J. Obstet. Gynec. *101*:261, 1968.

Medical Versus Surgical Management of Endometriosis

E. J. WILKINSON and R. F. MATTINGLY

Medical College of Wisconsin

Treatment of the symptomatic woman with endometriosis challenges the gynecologist with a medical and surgical dilemma. The patient may be benefited by either hormonal suppression or surgical resection of her disease. The objectives of therapy are primarily to relieve pain and to improve fertility. Although approximately 25 per cent of women with known endometriosis have few or no symptoms of the disease, the most common clinical problem is pelvic pain, which is usually associated with progressive secondary dysmenorrhea and dyspareunia. Abnormal vaginal bleeding is occasionally seen but usually results from anovulatory dysfunction, unrelated to endometriosis. Infertility is the primary complaint in 6 to 15 per cent of patients with documented endometriosis, although it is estimated that 30 to 40 per cent of patients with endometriosis are infertile. It is obvious, therefore, that infertility and pelvic pain constitute the major clinical problems related to this disease. The patient's symptoms, however, are not necessarily proportional to the extent of her disease; for example, the smallest endometrial implant may cause the most severe symptoms.

To the experienced gynecologist, the physical findings alone may be adequate for the clinical diagnosis. Reportedly, a correct clinical diagnosis by history and physical examination alone can be made in approximately 60 to 80 per cent of patients. The classic clinical findings of adnexal masses, nodularity of the utero-sacral ligaments, and a fixed retroverted uterus are well established, although these are not unique to endometriosis. The ease of diagnosis by current endoscopic techniques, including culdoscopy and laparoscopy, has greatly enhanced the diagnostic accuracy of this disease process. The current use of laparoscopy not only increases the acuity of the examiner where small foci of pelvic disease are concerned and improves the diagnostic accuracy of this disease but also eliminates the necessity to gain entrance to the peritoneal cavity through the cul-de-sac, where endometriomas or adherent bowel or uterus may be located. Our experience, as well as that of Gray and others, recognizes the fact that the cul-de-sac and rectal wall are involved in approximately 75 per cent of the cases. At least one ovary is involved in over 75 per cent of patients, while tubal involvement is somewhat less common and is usually superficial, invading primarily the serosal surfaces (Figure 19–1).

650

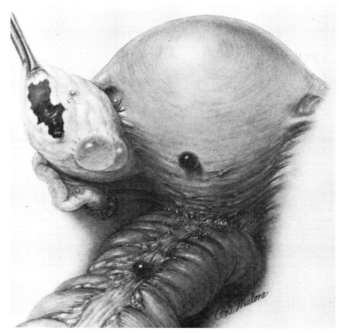

Figure 19-1   Pelvic endometriosis with a "chocolate" ovarian cyst. This is a typical picture often seen at operation. The cul-de-sac is obliterated by dense adhesions. There is a large endometrial implant on the posterior surface of the uterus and the anterior surface of the rectum. (From TeLinde, R. W., and Mattingly, R. F.: Operative Gynecology. 4th Ed. Philadelphia, J. B. Lippincott Co., 1970.)

The therapeutic approach to endometriosis should be based on the anatomic extent of the disease. For the patient with pelvic pain who has minimal pelvic findings of endometriosis, without adnexal masses, a course of progestin therapy for a period of six months or longer is the logical initial therapy. In those patients who demonstrate beneficial response to hormone therapy, treatment is usually continued for six to nine months for maximum biologic effect of the progestin on the disease process. Whereas many theories are advanced regarding the mechanism of action of progestins, the best data to the present time demonstrate a necrobiosis effect on both the endometrial glands and the stroma as a result of the catabolic effect of the progestins. Direct histologic evidence supports this thesis and demonstrates gradual regression and atrophy of the lining epithelium of the glands as well as edema and graded decidual reaction of the stroma. After prolonged hormonal therapy, the endometrial tissue, both in the endometrial cavity as well as in ectopic sites, demonstrates a degree of atrophy that parallels the therapeutic response. Although historically, estrogen was the first endocrine preparation to be used, the biologic effect on the endometrium from this hormone is stimulatory rather than suppressive and may produce breakthrough bleeding and endometrial hyperplasia, as well as stimulation of other estrogen target organs. Although diethylstilbestrol in doses to 100 mg. daily has been championed by some advocates of this drug, the current association of this nonsteroidal estrogen with reproductive tract neoplasia in the offspring of mothers who were given the agent in pregnancy strongly suggests that this drug is not appropriate for current use.

Methyltestosterone linguettes daily in 5 mg. doses for periods of six months or longer have been used effectively by some investigators. However, prolonged use of androgens is not advised because of their virilizing effects. Progestins or combinations of estrogen and progestin are currently favored in preference to androgens in view of the fact that the biologic effect of testosterone and related compounds is unclear, except for its suppressive effect on ovulation through the hypothalamic circuit. The choice of hormone therapy in endometriosis is currently divided between the combination estrogen-progestin compounds and progestin alone. As outlined in Table 19–1, a variety of combination compounds and progestins have been used during the past decade. In assessing the clinical efficacy of these hormones, the clinician is handicapped by the existence of a variety of drugs, with lack of consistent information. Unfortunately, the various clinical studies to date lack uniformity and consequently correlative data on the biologic effect of the drug are difficult to interpret. Although there is general agreement that approximately 80 per cent of the patients on hormonal therapy obtain some relief of pelvic symptoms, the duration of this effect is extremely variable, and in some reports this information is unavailable. More distressing is the fact that some of the most recent studies fail to document the recurrence rate of the disease process after full hormonal therapy has been given for six months to one year. Although Kistner reports an 83 per cent response for symptoms for a follow-up period of six to 52 months, other studies often fail to document the duration of clinical response. Riva's experience is particularly pertinent in identifying that approximately 11.8 per cent of the cases treated with hormonal therapy had clinical recurrence and required either secondary hormonal treatment or pelvic surgery.

The major side-effects of combination drug therapy include weight gain, fluid retention, nausea, breakthrough bleeding, and breast tenderness. In addition, irritability, depression, nervousness, headaches, vaginal discharge, superficial vulvitis, and acne have been noted with the use of these compounds. A particularly distressing complication of the use of combination drugs and progestins observed during the past 10 years is the occurrence of oversuppression with secondary amenorrhea and occasionally galactorrhea. When progestins alone are used, less nausea and breast tenderness is noted. Progestins have the advantage of not stimulating the growth of uterine leiomyomas when these are present.

Unfortunately, progestins alone have the disadvantage of producing breakthrough bleeding with prolonged therapy and may require supplemental estrogen. The most commonly used progestins include 17 α-hydroxyprogesterone, caproate (Delalutin), medroxyprogesterone acetate (Depo-Provera), and oral medroxyprogesterone (Provera). In order to avoid troublesome breakthrough bleeding, combined drug therapy has been most popular, and the most commonly used combinations are norethynodrel and mestranol (Enovid) and norethindrone acetate and ethinyl estradiol (Norlestrin).

One limitation of endocrine therapy for endometriosis concerns the period of time required for the hormonal treatment and the recovery of ovulatory function following cessation of the hormonal treatment. Since the method of therapy and time of ovulation recovery requires more than one year of clinical observation, this time factor must be balanced with the duration of infertility and the age of the patient, taking into account as well the recognized incidence of recurrent

TABLE 19–1.

AUTHOR	DRUG	DOSAGE AND SCHEDULE	TOTAL PATIENTS	SYMPTO- MATIC RESPONSE	CORRECTED CONCEPTION RATE
Andrews et al.[1]	17 α-hydroxy- progesterone caproate (D) and conjugated estrogen (Pr) or stilbestrol (S)	250 mg. (D) I.M. q 7, or 10 days + 5 mg. (Pr) qd, or 2 mg. (S) qd	24	46.6% well, 46.6% improved (of 15 patients)	NR
	Norethynodrel and mestranol (E)	30 mg. qd 14–22 wks.			
Chambers[5]	Norethisterone acetate ethinylestradiol (A)	2 tab./day 4–9 mo.	55	75%	26.5% (12 patients)
Gunning and Moyer[12]	Medroxyprogesterone acetate (DP) and conjugated estrogen (Pr) or Estinyl or depo-estradiol	100 mg. (DP) I.M. q 2 wks.	14	78.5% (follow-up, 4–7 mo.)	28.5% (2 patients)
Kistner[16]	Norethynodrel and mestranol (E) or norethindrone and ethinylestradiol (N)	2 mg. qd 12–36 mo. 7.5–10 mg. qd 12–36 mo.	110	83% (follow-up, 6–52 mo.)	47%
	17 α-hydroxy- progesterone caproate and estradiol valerate (DL2X)	250 mg. (1 ml.) q wk. I.M. 12–36 mo.			
	Medroxyprogesterone acetate with ethinyl- estradiol (P)	20 mg. qd 12–36 mo.			
Kourides and Kistner[18]	Norethindrone acetate and ethinylestradiol (N)	1–3 tabs./day 3 mo.–1 yr.	22	72.7%	63% (7 patients)
	Lynestrenol and mestranol	1–2 tabs./day 3 mo.–11 mo.	19	87.3%	45% (5 patients)
	Norgestrel and ethinyl estradiol (NG)	1–2 tabs./day 3 mo.–6 mo.	19	87.3%	30% (6 patients)
Riva et al.[33]	Norethynodrel and mestranol (E)	2.5–40 mg. qd. 1–12 mo.	132	72% (follow-up, 6 mo.)	72% (8 patients)
Snaith[42]	Noresthisterone acetate or allyl estrinol or norethynodrel and mestranol (A) or (E)	1 tab./day 2–7 mo.	28	78.7%	25% (1 patient)
Timonen and Johansson[47]	Lynestrenol (O)	5 mg. qd to 7.5 mg. qd 1½ to 29 mo.	20	60%	5% (1 patient)
Williams[49]	Norethynodrel and mestranol (E)	20 mg. qd 60–120 days	44	93% (follow-up, 3 mo.)	72% (11 patients)

A—Anovlar
D—Delalutin
DL2X—Deluteval 2X
DP—DepoProvera
E—Enovid
Ng—Norgestril

N—Norlestrin
O—Organon
P—Provest
Pr—Premarin
S—Stilbestrol
NR—Not reported

endometriosis following cessation of full therapy. Should re-treatment be required, a significant therapeutic interval is required for the beneficial effects of hormonal therapy to be felt. For those patients who fail to respond to this treatment and remain symptomatic, operative intervention becomes mandatory. It is important to stress the fact that low-dose hormonal therapy or cyclic hormonal therapy with oral contraceptives has no significant therapeutic effect on pelvic endometriosis and should not be used.

Indications for Surgery

The primary surgical approach to the treatment of pelvic endometriosis provides specific diagnostic and therapeutic advantages that are unattainable by other, nonoperative methods. The ability to accurately define the anatomic extent and histologic characteristics of this disease at the time of surgery avoids errors in clinical judgment and management of this benign process. Of major therapeutic advantage is the documentation of the anatomic limits of the pathologic condition while excluding the possibility of a neoplastic process in an enlarged ovarian cyst. Restoration of reproductive function to the oviduct by surgical excision of fibrous adhesions is an important advantage of surgery. The immediate control of pelvic pain, characteristic of this disease, by the resection of the presacral (hypogastric) nerves is an added advantage of the surgical treatment of endometriosis. In addition, the opportunity to remove other pelvic disease processes which may interfere with future reproductive function, such as myoma uteri, is provided in this modality of treatment.

The extent of the surgical treatment is dependent on the age of the patient and her reproductive interests. The major goal of conservative surgery for this disease is to preserve the patient's reproductive capability. Excision and fulguration of endometrial implants within the pelvis, including removal of ovarian endometriomas, lysis of adhesion, and removal of cul-de-sac nodules, as well as of endometriomas of the bowel, constitute the conservative surgical approach to this disease. Fulguration of the characteristic "powder-burn" implants in the pelvic peritoneum is important in avoiding recurrence of the disease. Occasionally, cul-de-sac implants extend through the posterior vaginal fornix and produce not only dyspareunia but also postcoital bleeding. Such vaginal lesions should be excised surgically, with removal of the mucosal lesion. A major surgical effort should be to conserve ovarian function while excising the ovarian endometrial implants. While many cases of advanced ovarian endometriosis with chocolate cyst formation suggest complete destruction of the ovary, in general the cyst can be excised and the lining removed from the ovarian tissue with preservation of ovarian cortical tissue and ovarian function. If the patient is menstruating regularly, there is physiologic evidence of ovarian function, which should be preserved. The incidence of conception following conservative surgery for endometriosis is between 31 and 87 per cent and depends upon the extent of the disease at the time of surgery and the skill of the surgeon in restoring reproductive function (Figure 19–2).

The conception rate following conservative surgery is mainly related to the extent of tubal involvement in the disease process. If the disease is limited to the ovary without involvement of the oviducts, the conception rate is far better

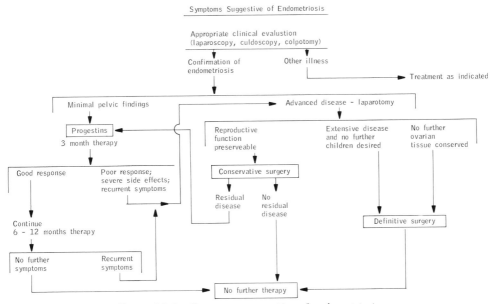

Figure 19-2. Symptoms suggestive of endometriosis.

than when extensive resection of peritubal adhesions is required. Contrary to the popular belief that surgery should be delayed until either the disease has advanced clinically or all other therapeutic modalities have failed, the reproductive potential is far greater when surgery is utilized early in the disease. The spontaneous rupture of an ovarian endometrioma has a worsening effect on prognosis for fertility and increases the risk of reoperation by 33 per cent. Whereas conservative surgery is possible in 22 to 40 per cent of patients with pelvic endometriosis, the reoperation rate is approximately 12 per cent in patients initially treated with conservative surgery.

The extent of the disease, particularly its involvement of the ovaries, serves as the most important guide for choosing among conservative, semiconservative, or definitive surgery. For the young patient with advanced pelvic disease, the major question concerns the advisability of conserving the ovary when the extent of the endometriosis requires hysterectomy. Conservation of some ovarian function in the younger women is desirable, provided that all visible endometriosis is removed. This semiconservative surgical approach is particularly indicated when the patient approaches the age of 40 and reproduction is no longer a serious consideration. The semiconservative approach towards maintaining ovarian function while removing the uterus and pelvic endometriosis effectively eliminates the symptoms of dysmenorrhea and uterine bleeding while avoiding premature castration and preventing development of menopausal symptoms. It is important that the retained ovarian tissue be free of endometriosis in order to avoid the necessity for further surgery. Repeat surgery was reported by Scott and TeLinde to be required in 4.1 per cent of such patients. Bilateral ovarian cysts are not a contraindication to ovarian conservation but require a vigorous effort on the part of the surgeon to completely remove all of the endometrial implants in the ovary. It has been demonstrated that only a small portion of viable ovarian cortex can provide long periods of continued ovarian function. However, when both ovaries are completely destroyed by ovarian cysts, a definitive operative procedure is required, with complete removal of the uterus and adnexa on both sides. Occasionally, the extent of the cul-de-sac disease is so great that a subtotal hysterectomy is considered advisable to avoid complications of the adherent rectosigmoid. Although many authors consider involvement of the serosal surface of the large or small bowel to contraindicate conservative treatment, Gray and others have demonstrated that when reproductive function is the primary objective of the treatment, such lesions can be adequately excised, with preservation of a functioning reproductive tract. When bowel lesions do occur, they appear on the serosal surface and occasionally extend into the muscularis and submucosa but rarely extend through the mucosa proper. Therefore, bowel obstruction from endometriosis, secondary to intrinsic lesions, is infrequent, as the disease usually involves the antimesenteric surface of the bowel rather than producing an annular constrictive process. When endometriosis of the bowel is encountered, it can usually be removed by serosal excision of the endometrioma and repair of the bowel. Only rarely is bowel resection and end-to-end anastomosis required. Involvement of the pelvic ureter by endometriosis and resultant scar tissue may produce progressive hydronephrosis and compromise the upper urinary tract. In such instances, the disease should be excised from the course of the ureter without damage to its blood supply. Rarely, reimplantation of the ureter into the bladder is necessary, as well as resection of a bladder endometrioma adjacent to the lower uterine segment. Clinical experience has demonstrated that only 40 per cent of the patients with pelvic endometriosis require definitive, complete surgical treatment; the remainder of the cases may be managed with hormonal therapy or conservative surgical methods.

The benefit of progestational therapy for two to three months prior to surgery has been both challenged and championed by many experienced gynecologists. Although the reported advantages of preoperative progestin therapy include softening of the endometrial implants, which would facilitate surgical dissection of the disease, more serious clinical objections to this approach have limited their preoperative use. The major concern, particularly in cases of ovarian enlargement, is the real possibility of delaying therapy of an obscure ovarian malignancy. Additionally, endometriomas of the ovary have been known to rupture spontaneously when treated with progestins. Where the surgical approach is concerned, the major disadvantage of progestin therapy is its documented effect of increasing pelvic vascularity. Additionally, many surgeons recognize the difficulty in identifying the extent of the disease process, especially the small peritoneal implants, which may be masked but not eliminated by the progestin therapy. In our experience, the preferable time for the augmentation of surgery with hormonal therapy is in the postoperative period. In cases of advanced disease, in which recognized foci of viable endometrial implants cannot be totally removed, the use of progestins for six to 12 months has proved to be therapeutically effective when combined with surgery. We have not found the routine prophylactic use of postoperative progestins to be particularly beneficial. The therapeutic value of postoperative hormonal therapy is limited to those cases with residual or recurrent disease. While the primary surgical treatment of endometriosis has the distinct advantage of identification and removal of carcinoma developing in endometriosis, this rare pathologic finding occurs in less than 1 per cent of all cases. Fortunately, the most prevalent site of benign endometriosis, as well as the most frequent site of origin of carcinoma arising in endometriosis, is the ovary, the enlargement of which should lead to primary surgery, at which identification of this occult lesion can be accomplished and definitive therapy carried out.

Endometriosis with associated symptomatic adenomyosis is a clear example of the location of disease as a guide to the method of therapy. Adenomyosis is a fairly common pathologic finding, occurring in 30 to 35 per cent of cases of pelvic endometriosis. While minimal histologic involvement of the myometrium may produce maximum clinical symptoms of severe dysmenorrhea and menorrhagia, hormonal therapy has proved ineffective in arresting and resolving this intramural disease. Consequently, primary surgery remains the most effective and definitive method of treatment for such cases, although the diagnosis of this entity is frequently obscured by the extrauterine disease and it is identified only in the operative specimen.

The primary method of treatment of pelvic endometriosis therefore seems clear. On the basis of the anatomic extent of the disease, one can define the early, limited disease process which has not involved the ovaries or significantly distorted pelvic anatomy. Of paramount importance in defining this early disease is the verification of normal tubal function by endoscopic techniques. In these early cases, the primary use of hormonal therapy for a period of six to 12 months is reasonable and therapeutically justifiable. However, when reactive fibrosis has impaired the tubal motility, the process is advanced and cannot be reversed by hormonal therapy alone. For more advanced disease, the primary method of treatment is surgical. The unpredictable hormonal response of advanced ovarian endometriosis provides a clear indication for surgical treatment. More important is the fact that advanced pelvic endometriosis and ovarian carcinoma may exhibit identical clinical findings, including ovarian enlargement, pelvic pain, and cul-de-sac nodularity. The extent of the surgery must be balanced with the severity of the disease and symptoms, the age of the patient, and the desire for future reproduction. There is no surgical formula that can be utilized in all cases because of the variability of these basic clinical factors. However, when the extent of the disease process is used as the major therapeutic guide, most cases of pelvic endometriosis can be easily assessed where the therapeutic advantages of either hormone therapy or surgical intervention are concerned.

REFERENCES

1. Andrews, M. C., Andrews, W. C., and Strauss, A. F.: Effects of progestin induced pseudopregnancy on endometriosis. Clinical and microscopic studies. Amer. J. Obstet. Gynec. 78:776, 1959.
2. Bates, J. S., and Beecham, C. T.: Retroperitoneal endometriosis with ureteral obstruction. Obstet. Gynec. 34:242, 1969.
3. Beller, F. K., and Porges, R. F.: Blood coagulation and fibrinolytic enzyme studies during cyclic and continuous application of progestational agents. Amer. J. Obstet. Gynec. 97:448, 1967.
4. Cavanagh, W. V.: Fertility in the etiology of endometriosis. Amer. J. Obstet. Gynec. 61:539, 1951.
5. Chambers, I. A.: Conservative management of endometriosis. Proc. Roy. Soc. Med. 61:360, 1968.
6. Chang, S. H., and Maddox, W. A.: Adenocarcinoma arising within cervical endometriosis and invading the adjacent vagina. Amer. J. Obstet. Gynec. 110:1015, 1971.

7. Cutler, B. S., Forbes, A. P., Ingersoll, F. M., *et al.*: Endometrial carcinoma after stilbestrol therapy in gonadal dysgenesis. New Eng. J. Med. 287:628, 1972.
8. Fathalla, M. F.: Malignant transformation in ovarian endometriosis. J. Obstet. Gynaec. Brit. Comm. 75:85, 1967.
9. Gray, L. A.: Surgical treatment of endometriosis. Clin. Obstet. Gynec. 3:472, 1960.
10. Gray, L.: The management of endometriosis involving the bowel. Clin. Obstet. Gynec. 9:309, 1966.
11. Green, T. H.: Conservative surgical treatment of endometriosis. Clin. Obstet. Gynec. 9:293, 1966.
12. Gunning, J. E., and Moyer, D.: The effect of medroxyprogesterone acetate on endometriosis in the human female. Fertil. Steril. 18:759, 1967.
13. Herbst, A. L., Ulfelder, H., and Poskanzer, D. C.: Adenocarcinoma of the vagina—association of maternal stilbestrol therapy with tumor appearance in young women. New Eng. J. Med. 284:878, 1971.
14. Hughes, P., Gillespie, A., and Dewhurst, J.: Amenorrhea and galactorrhea. Obstet. Gynec. 40:147, 1972.
15. Karnaky, K. J.: Treatment of endometriosis with stilbestrol, an antiestrogen, plus the B complex vitamins in man: a therapy record proved effective over the last 32 years. Southwest. Med. 12:205, 1968.
16. Kistner, R. W.: Current status of the hormonal treatment of endometriosis. Clin. Obstet. Gynec. 9:271, 1966.
17. Kistner, R. W.: Gynecology Principles and Practice. 2nd Ed. Chicago, Year Book Medical Publishers, 1971.
18. Kourides, I. A., and Kistner, R. W.: Three synthetic progestins in the treatment of endometriosis. Obstet. Gynec. 31:821, 1968.
19. Lamb, E. J., Guderian, A. M., and Cruz, A. L.: Culdoscopy in infertility. Obstet. Gynec. 33:822, 1969.
20. Mattingly, R. F., and Patillo, R. A.: Carcinogenic side effects associated with steroid hormone intervention in the treatment of the menopause and postmenopause. (Unpublished.)
21. McArthur, J. W., and Ulfelder, H.: The effect of pregnancy upon endometriosis. Obstet. Gynec. Surv. 20:706, 1965.
22. McCoy, J. B., and Braford, W. Z.: Surgical treatment of endometriosis with conservation of reproductive potential. Amer. J. Obstet. Gynec. 87:394, 1963.
23. Meigs, J. V.: An interest in endometriosis and its consequences. Amer. J. Obstet. Gynec. 79:625, 1960.
24. Molitor, J. J.: Adenomyosis: a clinical and pathological appraisal. Amer. J. Obstet. Gynec. 110:275, 1971.
25. Norwood, G. D.: Sterility and fertility in women with pelvic endometriosis. Clin. Obstet. Gynec. 3:456, 1960.
26. Parsons, L.: Conservative surgical management of external endometriosis. Obstet. Gynec. 32:576, 1968.
27. Parsons, L., and Sommers, S. C.: Gynecology. Philadelphia, W. B. Saunders Co., 1962.
28. Petersohn, L.: Fertility in patients with ovarian endometriosis before and after treatment. Acta Obstet. Gynec. Scand. 49:331, 1970.
29. Ranney, B.: Endometriosis. II. Emergency operations due to hemoperitoneum. Obstet. Gynec. 36:437, 1970.
30. Ranney, B. Endometriosis. I. Conservative operations. Amer. J. Obstet. Gynec. 107:743, 1970.
31. Ranney, B.: Endometriosis. III. Complete operations. Amer. J. Obstet. Gynec. 109:1137, 1971.
32. Ridley, J. H., and Edwards, I. K.: Experimental endometriosis in the human. Amer. J. Obstet. Gynec. 76:783, 1958.
33. Riva, H. L., Kawasaki, D. M., and Messinger, A. J.: Further experience with norethynodrel in treatment of endometriosis. Obstet. Gynec. 19:111, 1962.
34. Rogers, S. F., and Jacobs, W. M.: Infertility and endometriosis. Conservative surgical approach. Fertil. Steril. 19:529, 1968.
35. Sampson, J. A.: Perforating hemorrhagia (chocolate cysts of the ovary) their importance and especially their relation to pelvic adenomas of endometrial type. Arch. Surg. 3:245, 1921.
36. Sampson, J. A.: Intestinal adenomas of endometrial type. Arch. Surg. 5:217, 1922.
37. Sampson, J. A.: Peritoneal endometriosis, due to menstrual dissemination of endometrial tissue into the peritoneal cavity. Amer. J. Obstet. Gynec. 14:422, 1927.
38. Sampson, J. A.: Endometrial carcinoma of ovary arising in endometrial tissue in that organ. Arch. Surg. 10:1, 1925.

39. Scott, R. B., and Wharton, R. J.: The effect of testosterone on experimental endometriosis in monkeys. Amer. J. Obstet. Gynec. 78:867, 1959.
40. Scully, R. E., Richardson, G. S., and Barlow, J. F.: The development of malignancy in endometriosis. Clin. Obstet. Gynec. 9:384, 1966.
41. Sheldon, R. S., Wilson, R. B., and Dockerty, M. B.: Serosal endometriosis of fallopian tubes. Amer. J. Obstet. Gynec. 99:882, 1967.
42. Snaith, L.: The treatment of endometriosis by oral progestogens. Proc. Roy. Soc. Med. 61:358, 1968.
43. Spangler, D. B., Jones, G. S., and Jones, H. W.: Infertility due to endometriosis. Amer. J. Obstet. Gynec. 109:850, 1971.
44. Sulter, M. R.: Endometriosis of the intestinal tract. Surgery 22:801, 1947.
45. Stevenson, C. S.: Malignant transformation of ovarian endometriosis—nature, treatment, and report of two cases. Obstet. Gynec. 36:443, 1970.
46. TeLinde, R. W., and Mattingly, R. F.: Operative Gynecology. 4th Ed. Philadelphia, J. B. Lippincott Co., 1970.
47. Timonen, S., and Johansson, C. J.: Endometriosis treated with lynestrenol. Ann. Chir. Gynecol. Fenn. 57:144, 1968.
48. Wilkinson, E. J., Friedrich, E. G., Mattingly, R. F., et al.: Turner's syndrome with endometrial carcinoma associated with diethylstilbestrol therapy. Obstet. Gynec. 42:193, 1973.
49. Williams, B. F. P.: Conservative management of endometriosis: follow-up observations of progestin therapy. Obstet. Gynec. 30:76, 1967.

Medical Versus Surgical Management of Endometriosis

Editorial Comment

The subject of endometriosis has been covered in some detail by the collected efforts of the contributors to this chapter. The desirability of a classification system, as proposed by Dr. Mitchell, would appear basic to the ultimate management of the patient. Specifically, a description of the extent of the endometriosis when the patient is seen initially not only is imperative for any contemplated immediate therapy but would also appear to be a requirement in assessing the possible spread of the disease and the influence of therapy.

Besides discussions of theories of etiology there is general comment that the symptoms or lack of symptoms are often difficult to explain. It is a universal experience that a patient may have extensive endometriosis, with literally a "frozen pelvis," and be free of complaints. Contrariwise, the disease may be minimal on both pelvic and laparoscopic examination, and yet the patient may have a multitude of symptoms. Pelvic discomfort in endometriosis is compounded by laparoscopic examination. It has been suggested that pain in association with endometriosis may occur throughout the menstrual cycle (see Chapter 18).

The question has been raised concerning the cause of dysmenorrhea in patients with endometriosis. If prostaglandin being secreted by the endometrium were a factor, one would expect all patients with adenomyosis to be afflicted with dysmenorrhea.

Although presacral neurectomy is considered a useful procedure in the control of pain associated with endometriosis, the limitations of the procedure are rarely mentioned. If, indeed, presacral neurectomy has therapeutic merit in endometriosis, careful documentation of the extent of the disease at the time of the procedure is needed. This is because the areas served by the presacral nerves are mainly the uterus and the midportion of the oviducts. It is reassuring that large bowel involvement is not liable to cause intestinal obstruction. Hence, unless the small bowel is involved, ovarian conservation is permissible at the time of laparotomy for endometriosis.

A polite bow is made to hormonal therapy possibly because endometriosis is a disease whose treatment is predicated on relief of symptoms rather than on cure of the disease. There seems to be general acceptance of use of hormonal therapy for short periods to relieve symptoms, especially in patients whose disease is not extensive or is minimal. With this type of treatment, the symptoms may be held in abeyance but can quickly return with cessation of therapy. The side-effects of hormonal therapy are definite and, as one author states, in some patients apparently they compare to the discomfort of the disease itself. The debate continues as to whether or not endocrine therapy can cause the disease to regress with any degree of permanency. Morover, adenomyosis apparently is not influenced by hormone therapy, and it is entirely possible that the uterus may actually enlarge. The use of hormone therapy preoperatively, supposedly to enhance the surgical dissection of the endometriosis, has not been found to be of value in the experience of many gynecologists. Rather, the outlining of the borders of the endometriotic implants by such therapy is made more difficult, and the increase in vascularity adds to the blood loss. Also, the pseudopregnancy reaction within the endometriosis can on rare occasion lead to avulsion and serious hemoperitoneum.

Moreover, if ovarian conservation is desirable, and most gynecologists believe that it is in women 35 years or younger, it seems unlikely that prolonged hormone therapy is the proper approach. Indeed, a decision must be made at the time of laparotomy, when conservative surgery for endometriosis is first contemplated, as to whether the uterus should be removed in order to preserve healthy tissue and endocrine function if the disease is found to be more extensive than anticipated. If the uterus is left in situ and conception fails, the endometriosis may involve or destroy the entire ovary in a year or two, so that ovarian conservation is no longer possible. In passing, the same principle is at stake in recurrent gonorrhea infection. In patients in whom tubal involvement is such that the ability to conceive is at best only remote, the question must be answered whether medical management of the infection should be discarded in favor of surgery with hysterectomy and salpingectomy before there is total ovarian destruction from recurrent infection, and ovarian conservation is no longer possible.

In summary, the medical management of endometriosis has limited value and is not without adverse effects. Rather, patients must be followed carefully to determine the extent of the endometriosis as determined by laparoscopic evaluation. With due regard to the conservative approach, if the disease is progressive, surgery appears preferable when there is hope that ovarian conservation is still feasible, at least in women under 35 to 40 years of age.

20

When Is Chromosomal Analysis Indicated in Obstetrical and Gynecological Practice?

Alternative Points of View:

By Kurt Benirschke

By Arthur C. Christakos and Harlan R. Giles

By Morton A. Stenchever

Editorial Comment

When Is Chromosomal Analysis Indicated in Obstetrical and Gynecological Practice?

KURT BENIRSCHKE

University of California at San Diego

The emphasis of this discussion is placed on what is useful for the *practice* of obstetrics and gynecology. Nevertheless, it must be borne in mind that some aspects that are currently being explored by investigators are likely to become tomorrow's daily procedures. To make a clear distinction, then, of *practice versus research* procedures is not altogether feasible, nor is it desirable, from my point of view. Probably more important is a discussion that is comprehensible to the clinician of the current state of the art of cytogenetics so that he can make a personal choice of when to ask for the help in this area, and also whom to call upon.

Types of Study

Recent years have brought significant new tools in cytogenetics whose application to clinical problems is now under way (Jones[1]). In addition to the usual Barr body study from buccal and vaginal smears, hair roots, or tissue sections, and the lymphocyte chromosome analysis with which we are all familiar, it has now become possible to assess the chromosome complement more precisely. The preferential affinity of certain segments of chromosomes for fluorescent dyes and Giemsa stain allow precise definition of each chromosome, in man and in other species. Special other techniques have given further insight into the structure of chromosomes, providing evidence to indicate that heterochromatin and euchromatin have a very specific distribution along the chromosomes that allows more precision in karyotyping. This requires special instrumentation (ultraviolet microscopy as for the Coons antibody technique), and greater knowledge and experience by the person undertaking the chromosome study. Without these, modern cytogenetics cannot yield optimal results, and it is thus imperative that the practitioner know whether or not the analysis will be carried out in competent hands.

To a large extent, these methods have replaced the more cumbersome autoradiography, with the possible exception of the study of sex chromosomes. A standard, internationally prepared nomenclature is now available.[2] Likely, new techniques will further define the human chromosomes in the future.

Man and gorilla, and only these, have accumulated on the Y chromosome a substantial amount of heterochromatin with special affinity for fluorochromes.[3] This heterochromatin is located on the long arms. In interphase cells, e.g., the cells scraped from the buccal mucosa, this "Y fluorescence" is seen as a small dot called the Y body or F body. It is also evident in about one-half of mature spermatozoa. (Parenthetically, it might be said here that buccal cells are *not* used or useful in attempts to analyze the karyotype. They do not undergo mitosis, which is not commonly understood by practitioners.) The F body is quite characteristic and, in experienced hands, it can be useful for the rapid diagnosis of an XY complement. Two F bodies indicate two YY chromosomes. Inasmuch as such preparations can subsequently be stained with the Feulgen stain (or other dyes) it is practical to ascertain the number of X chromosomes as well. Thus, a cell with XXXYY sex chromosomes would contain two F bodies and two Barr bodies. The F body differs in size with the length of the Y chromosome, and considerable variation exists in this respect. A diminutive Y may be functionally quite normal as male determinator and still have only a very small amount or no specific fluorescence.[4] Moreover, some other regions of the karyotype (the satellites of the acrocentrics, the centromere of chromosome No. 3) have variable amounts of heterochromatin stainable by quinacrine, and this may lead to occasional confusion. Here, experience and judicious evaluation come in. Finally, in XO/XY mosaics the Y occasionally fails to stain, for as yet unknown reasons.[5] The technique can be employed in frozen sections of tissue[6] (not in formalin-fixed material), touch preparations of tumors, and amniotic fluid and cell cultures. It is a *sine qua non* for all chromosome studies as an adjunct procedure. This technique is rapid and the recommendation has been made that it be carried out in the anteroom at amniocentesis to maximize therapy.[7]

When are these procedures necessary, when are they desirable, and when are they a luxury[8]? Answers to these questions will be attempted in the subsequent paragraphs, but it should be borne in mind that they cannot be painted in black and white. Moreover, often the practicality is determined in part by economic feasibility, religious attitudes, and other factors.

Abnormal Phenotype of Newborn

SEXUAL ABERRATIONS

When the external genitalia are significantly abnormal, clarification of the underlying mechanism is mandatory, and it should be done as quickly as possible. Although often the study of buccal smears for Barr and F bodies is sufficient, particularly when the adrenogenital syndrome is suspected, a complete cytogenetic assessment is recommended. In this way, the possible cause of hermaphroditism can be more completely assessed. Thus, many patients now coming to attention because of problems developing in later life had had ambiguous genitalia at birth. True hermaphrodites with chimerism (e.g., XY/XX) may be diagnosed confidently when the condition is suspected. Sophisticated blood grouping study, executed in knowledgeable laboratories, is extremely helpful, but the suspicion of chimerism must be indicated in the request.[9] Not all true hermaphrodites, however, have two populations of cells, and by itself cytogenetic study is not always diagnostic.

Infants suspected of having Turner's syndrome at birth benefit from cytogenetic studies, as a significant number of those found to be XO/XY mosaics, and occasionally an XO/XX mosaic, will develop gonadal tumors.[10] Similarly, women with XY gonadal dysgenesis are more prone to develop germ cell tumors[11] and can be identified when studied for primary amenorrhea.

NONGENITAL MALFORMATIONS

A few classical syndromes are clinically apparent without cytogenetic study. Nevertheless, if doubt exists, even children who are suspected to have Down's syndrome (mongolism, or trisomy 21) should have chromosome study. Here, and in the trisomy 13 syndrome as well, a certain number of translocations will be uncovered, in which case subsequent genetic counseling of the parents will be important.[12] Similarly, in children with suspected cri-du-chat syndrome (5p-, a deletion of the short arm [p] of chromosome 5), a precise diagnosis can be of great importance to the pediatrician and the family. In other congenital anomalies, by and large, cytogenetic study has not frequently yielded evidence of significant chromosomal errors. To be sure, chromosome anomalies are occasionally found (e.g., in some cases of cyclopia) but the more common teratologic events (e.g., anencephaly, cleft palate, renal dysplasia, congenital heart diseases) usually occur in the face of a normal chromosomal complement. Perhaps new techniques will improve our diagnostic acumen in such cases, but I doubt this. These infants will be investigated cytogenetically only for research purposes, and routine screening cannot be advised.

OTHER ANOMALIES

A possibly fruitful area for study is infants with unexplained "growth retardation" and also stillborns.[24] Again, this is for research purposes or when special family circumstances dictate such a procedure. A special category is perhaps anomalies occurring repetitively in the siblings. While few can be traced to structural chromosomal errors, now and then such events are uncovered, and cytogenetic study may be important for counseling if, for instance, translocations are detected. It should be mentioned here that it is entirely feasible to obtain tissue culture growth sufficient for cytogenetic analysis from postmortem material and, in the case of macerated stillborns, it can often be obtained from the chorionic tissue of the placenta. We have recently karyotyped the amnion of a stillborn infant in whom growth retardation and hypospadias were the only findings. An XX complement was identified, much to our surprise. Similar findings have been reported sporadically by others; however, no systematic study has yet been undertaken.

Amenorrhea

Patients with primary *and* with secondary amenorrhea should be considered as candidates for cytogenetic study, particularly when no underlying structural anomaly has been identified. At times, such patients will be found to have amenorrhea because of their XY chromosome constitution, and the diagnosis of testicular feminization can be made.[13] This precise diagnosis is of importance because gonadectomy is advisable in postpubertal patients, since the incidence of gonadal tumors is high. Some of these are malignant. When the syndrome is diagnosed prepubertally in girls with inguinal hernias, preoperative F body study will anticipate the finding of an XY chromosome constitution and prevent undesirable gonadectomy before full sexual development has been attained. It should be stressed that the F body analysis takes but a few minutes and should be widely practiced preoperatively. Not all women lacking a uterus have testicular feminization with XY karyotype. Some have enzymatic errors and are of special interest to investigators. Also, most patients with vaginal agenesis and Müllerian tract anomalies have a normal female sex chromosome complement.

Of particular concern are patients with amenorrhea and stigmata of Turner's syndrome. These stigmata may be minimal and cytogenetic study is necessary. In fact, we now perform a minimal buccal smear analysis for Barr and F body assessment on *all* patients coming for infertility or any type of amenorrhea. The XO karyotype, representing the commonest chromosomal error in man, is lethal to over 90 per cent of its bearers, who form an important segment of spontaneous abortuses.[14] Perhaps expectedly, the survivors of this prenatal selective event are not infrequently mosaics. That is to say, they have more than one population of cells (XO/XY, XO/XX, and so forth).[15] The clones of such mosaic populations can be very irregularly distributed. At times, partial or time-limited ovarian function is perhaps the sequel to this irregular distribution. The practicing physician should be aware, however, that such mosaicism may be causally related to the development of gonadal tumors. Gonadoblastomas, dysgerminomas, and embryonal carcinomas are much more frequent when an XY line is also present, and we practice preventive gonadectomy when it is identified. Very recently, it has been reported that such a tumor may develop in XO/XX mosaics also.[10] The search for an XY clone of cells is much eased by the quinacrine technique[9] and, in my opinion, this is a mandatory study in all patients with Turner stigmata, including males. It has now been recognized that occasionally the Y chromosome in XO/XY mosaics fails to fluoresce "normally" for as yet unknown reasons.[6] The father, whose Y is responsible for the male sex of these patients, has repeatedly been found to possess normal Y fluorescence.

Patients with unexplained infertility (from other factors than pituitary destruction, testicular feminization, postinflammatory events) benefit from cytogenetic study as well. Not only will mosaics come to light but also structural anomalies of chromosomes, including X anomalies, are discovered that are of causal significance. Study of the husband must be considered, as discussed in more detail below.

The physician ordering these studies must be aware of the limitations and the competence of the laboratory that undertakes these tests and it cannot be stressed enough that he supply complete information of the clinical findings to the laboratory. Often such information dictates more specific study than would routinely be done.

Habitual Abortion

Patients with primary sterility and repeat abortions should be considered for cytogenetic study, particularly, of course, when clinical examination does not uncover a potential cause of the reproductive failure. The yield is not high, but published data of prospective case analyses are insufficient to express a valid opinion at this time. It may be as low as 10 per cent[16] or, when various series are pooled, even 6 per cent. Conversely, numerous pedigrees have been described when habitual abortion has occurred because of structural chromosomal anomalies, and several new types are currently under study.[17]

Translocations among chromosomes of almost all major chromosome groups have been found in such patients, and more complicated exchanges, such as insertions or deletions, are seen on occasion. Banding as well as fluorochrome techniques will aid in the precise definition of such interchanges and perhaps enable us to uncover a higher percentage of abnormal individuals in the future in patients now considered to possess normal chromosomes. It is imperative to understand that both husband and wife may be affected and, therefore, both should have the benefit of cytogenetic study. Very rarely has the aborted conceptus of a chromosomally abnormal habitual aborter been examined by this technique. Presumably it is aneuploid because of a parental rearrangement, but studies are needed to verify this hypothesis.

Prenatal Diagnosis

The advisability of chromosomal study of the embryo in utero is much more controversial.[7,8] It is feasible to do tissue culture of the free cells in amniotic fluid after the twelfth week of pregnancy. The procedure has some—but few—complications; occasionally the needle puncture has led to fetal death. Amniotic fluid study should be considered *only* if both the physician and the family are willing to accept therapeutic abortion in the event of positive findings. Cytogenetic analysis of fetal cells has been advocated for the following reasons: (1) To determine fetal sex in lethal or undesirable familial sex-linked diseases—e.g., hemophilia. (Sex can now be determined within minutes by staining amniotic cells with fluorochromes to be followed by conventional stains.) (2) In families with parental balanced translocations, largely those involving chromosome 21. In effect this is practiced in order to prevent the development to term of fetuses with Down's syndrome. In translocations of the 21/21 type, the risk is 100 per cent. Similar problems are encountered with other translocations, as shown in Figure 20–1. (3) To diagnose Down's syndrome in infants of women over the age of 35 to 40 years, for whom there is a much increased risk.[1] (4) To diagnose fetal sex merely because of parental whims, which is a practice to be discouraged.

This procedure requires skill on the part of the obstetrician, full understanding of the consequences, and the availability of a capable laboratory. In general, the diagnosis cannot be expected until 2 to 3 weeks after amniocentesis, but it must be understood that not many laboratories are set up to accomplish this more difficult tissue culture procedure. Edwards[7] has given some very specific recommendations in this respect, to which I subscribe. For example, the laboratory must have successfully analyzed previously at least six amniotic fluid specimens.

The indications for prenatal diagnosis have to be clearly thought through by the obstetrician, because unforeseen problems will often arise. With an increasingly sophisticated clientele patients have begun to request prenatal studies to alleviate fear of a child with Down's syndrome. When through this means the sex of the anticipated child, which was normal, became known and it was deemed undesirable, requests were sometimes made to secure an abortion.[19]

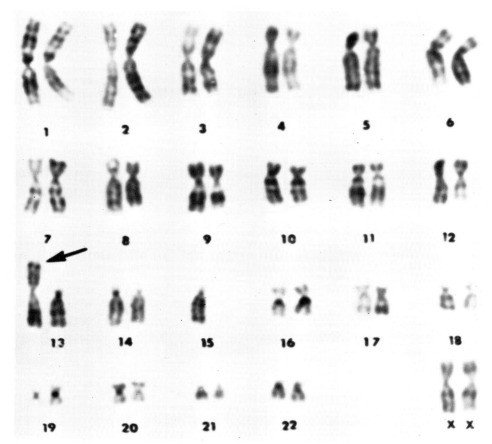

Figure 20–1. Karyotype prepared with the Giemsa technique to show "G-bands." Each chromosome is identifiable by its characteristic staining pattern. This woman has a translocation ("fusion") between a No. 13 and a No. 15 chromosome, indicated by arrow [45,XX,t(13,15)]. The importance of diagnosing translocation 13/15 as opposed to translocation 13/13, 14/14, or 15/15 lies in the fact that some normal offspring can be expected, in addition to some unbalanced offspring or abortions. If one of the latter three types of translocation is present, no normal pregnancies can result. Prenatal chromosome study in this patient will allow precise anticipation of the normality or abnormality of the conceptus.

One can envisage that in societies in which one sex or the other is less favored, this procedure could eventually result in a skewed sex ratio. Perhaps this is the ultimate effect of planned parenthood. To the writer and others[7] this is not a desirable prospect. Groups of individuals have formed to deliberate upon these ethical issues, including whether negative selection of unwanted genotypes by abortion is actually ultimately beneficial to society.[20]

Cost

In most laboratories, complete lymphocyte cytogenetic study is priced between $100 and $150, and usually one week must be allowed for completion (longer for amniotic fluid). For special purposes only, specific grant support is available to defray the cost, and such support must be individually negotiated.

There are some 200 laboratories listed by the National Foundation[21] that perform cytogenetic study, and the Foundation can be contacted to give the most up-to-date information on all ramifications of these studies and on location of laboratories. Contacting this organization is strongly encouraged.

Research

The practitioner has an obligation to make available some clinical material for research purposes. Although he may question how cytogenetic study in some circumstances benefits this particular patient, he should realize that increased knowledge will eventually be useful in therapy and prevention of disease in others. Some examples have been mentioned—e.g., the abortus from a balanced translocation carrier. Abortuses, including ectopic conceptuses, continue to be of investigative interest, as are growth retarded and stillborn babies. Twins form a special group, especially those with malformations.[22] In recent years the understanding of the pathogenesis of teratomas (dermoid cysts) has been advanced through genetic study,[23] and these tissues need to be submitted before fixation. An even stronger case can be made for the less well understood gonadoblastomas. Other special situations can be anticipated, but it suffices to draw attention to the need for cooperative efforts. Often animal studies cannot substitute for studies of human illnesses, and conservation of tissues (before fixation or contamination) is an obligation of the intelligent practitioner.

Summary

In my view, the indications for cytogenetic analysis in the practice of obstetrics and gynecology can best be summarized as follows:

MANDATORY

1. Young parents of a child or children with Down's syndrome.
2. Parents of more than one child with Down's syndrome.
3. Couples with infertility and habitual abortion who lack a specific other cause, such as pelvic inflammatory disease, tuberculosis, and so forth.
4. Prenatal diagnosis in families with destructive sex-linked disease (e.g., hemophilia) or structural chromosome errors (translocations).
5. Patients with amenorrhea and Turner's syndrome.
6. All hermaphrodites.

DESIRABLE

1. Prenatal diagnosis in families to reassure nonrecurrence of such diseases as Down's syndrome.
2. Pregnant women over 40 years of age.
3. Conceptuses (abortions) of patients with known translocations.
4. Stillborns and growth retarded newborns.[24]

OPTIONAL

1. Neonates with congenital anomalies.
2. Twins with anomalies.
3. Gonadoblastoma and other unusual tumors.
4. Special request—e.g., suspicion of XYY karyotype.
5. Routine neonatal "sexing."[25]

UNDESIRABLE

1. Prenatal sex determination for family planning.

REFERENCES

1. Jones, O. W.: A new era for cytogenetics. Curr. Probl. Pediatr. *11*:1, 1972.
2. The National Foundation, New York. Results of deliberations by a group of cytogeneticists meeting in Paris, 1971. Birth Def. 8:1, 1972.
3. Pearson, P. L., Bobrow, M., Vosa, C. G., and Barlow, P. W.: Quinacrine fluorescence in mammalian chromosomes. Nature *231*:326, 1971.
4. Retief, A. E., and Van Niekerk, W. A.: Non-fluorescence of Y chromosome. Lancet *1*:270, 1971.
5. Curto, F. L., Scappaticci, S., Zuffardi, O., Chierichetti, G., and Fraccaro, M.: Non-fluorescent Y chromosome in a 45,X/46,XY mosaic. Ann. Génét. *15*:107, 1972.
6. Kegel, J., and Conen, P. E.: Nuclear sex identification in human tissues: a histologic study using quinacrine fluorescence. Amer. J. Clin. Path. *57*:425, 1972.
7. Edwards, J. H.: Uses of amniocentesis. Lancet *1*:608, 1970.
8. Freeman, M. V. R., and Niles, P. A.: Cytogenetic evaluation: luxury or necessity? Milit. Med. *136*:851, 1971.
9. Benirschke, K., Naftolin, F., Gittes, R., Khudr, G., Yen, S. S. C., and Allen, F. H.: True hermaphroditism and chimerism. Amer. J. Obstet. Gynec. *113*:449, 1972.
10. Patel, S. K., and Prentice, R. S.: Gonadoblastoma. Distinctive ovarian tumor. Arch. Path. *94*:165, 1972.
11. Schellhas, H. F., Trujillo, J. M., Rutledge, F. N., and Cork, A.: Germ cell tumors associated with XY gonadal dysgenesis. Amer. J. Obstet. Gynec. *109*:1197, 1971.
12. Hamerton, J. L.: Human Cytogenetics. Vol. II. New York, Academic Press, 1971.
13. Naftolin, F., and Judd, H. L.: Testicular feminization. *In* R. M. Wynn, Ed.: Obstetrics and Gynecology Annual: 1973. New York, Appleton-Century-Crofts, 1973.
14. Carr, D. H.: Genetic basis of abortion. Ann. Rev. Genet. *5*:65, 1971.
15. Dahl, G., and Andersen, H.: Chromosome studies in 30 children with Turner's syndrome. Acta Paed. Scand. *61*:17, 1972.
16. Stenchever, M. A., and Jarvis, J. A.: Cytogenetic studies in reproductive failure. Obstet. Gynec. *37*:83, 1971.
17. Khudr, G.: Personal communication.
18. Dorfman, A. (ed.): Antenatal Diagnosis: Mental Retardation Centers Series. Chicago, University of Chicago Press, 1972.
19. Stenchever, M. A.: An abuse of prenatal diganosis. J.A.M.A. *221*:408, 1972.
20. Lappé, M., Gustafson, J. M., and Roblin, R.: Ethical and social issues in screening for genetic disease. New Eng. J. Med. *286*:1129, 1972. (See also Letters to the Editor, New Eng. J. Med. *287*:204, 1972.)
21. International Directory. 3rd Ed. Genetic Services. New York, The National Foundation, 1971.
22. Kim, C. K., Barr, R. J., and Benirschke, K.: Cytogenetic studies of conjoined twins. Obstet. Gynec. *38*:877, 1971.
23. Linder, D., and Power, J.: Further evidence for post-meiotic origin of teratomas in the human female. Ann. Hum. Genet. *34*:21, 1970.
24. Chen, A. T. L., Sergovich, F. R., McKim, J. S., Barr, M. L., and Gruber, D.: Chromosome studies in full-term, low-birth-weight, mentally retarded patients. J. Pediatr. *76*:393, 1970.
25. Harris, J. S., and Robinson, A.: X-chromosome abnormalities and the obstetrician. Amer. J. Obstet. Gynec. *109*:574, 1971.

When Is Chromosomal Analysis Indicated in Obstetrical and Gynecological Practice?

ARTHUR C. CHRISTAKOS

Duke University Medical Center

HARLAN R. GILES

University of Arizona Hospital and Medical Center

As the title would suggest, technological advances over the past decade have made the detection of certain genetic disorders in utero a reality. Recent legal and social advances have provided for practical applications of our newly acquired antenatal research tools. Until recently, the diagnosis of a genetically defective fetus would have been merely academic because most states proscribed interruption of pregnancy on fetal grounds. The Supreme Court in 1973 ruled that it was unconstitutional to deny an abortion at any time of pregnancy and in effect did away with all restrictions that heretofore existed.

A realistic appraisal of the subject of prenatal diagnosis, however, will reveal definite limitations in the scope of this recent addition to the clinician's armamentarium in combating human genetic disorders. There has been considerable exaggeration and dramatization in the lay press of the techniques used in the prenatal diagnosis of genetic disease. Busy clinicians fall into the trap of relying on these overly optimistic reports, which are not necessarily confined to lay publications. Many enthusiastic investigators report results of their research work before the results can be confirmed or found to be reliably reproduced in other laboratories and clinics. The clinician is left with the impression that such techniques are readily available in all medical centers, if not in the community hospital. In addition, although there are literally hundreds of genetic diseases recognized as such in humans, to date only a small percentage have been consistently detected accurately prenatally. Of those conditions which have hereditary implications, few practicing physicians are aware of their significance. Moreover, offers of prenatal diagnosis often give false hope to potential parents, when indeed no method is available for accurate detection of a specific genetic disease in utero.

In the following discussion, an attempt will be made to delineate some of the problems confronting antenatal genetic diagnosis today. Second, those cate-

673

gories of individuals who should be proffered antenatal diagnostic efforts through amniocentesis will be identified. Third, a realistic assessment of the available studies on amniotic fluid will be presented. Finally, caution in interpretation of results of the studies on amniotic fluid will be stressed.

The Problems

It is generally accepted that 1 in 40, or 2.5 per cent, of all live births are associated with significant birth defects. According to Carter,[1] roughly 10 in 1000 live births have serious defects resulting from mutant genes expressed as hetero-zygotes (dominant traits), homozygotes (recessive traits), or as hemizygotes (X-linked traits). Court-Brown and Smith[2] estimate the frequency of chromosomal abnormalities at 4 per 1000 live births, while Lubs and Ruddle[3] estimate the frequency at 1 in 100 births if stillbirths are also considered. Carr[4] reports that the frequency of chromosomal abnormalities in instances of fetal wastage may reach as high as 33 per cent when only spontaneous abortuses are studied.

The occurrence of an autosomal dominant trait in an individual empiri-cally carries with it a 50 per cent recurrence rate for all subsequent siblings. On the other hand, only a 25 per cent risk is expected for the siblings of an individual with an autosomal recessive condition. Proband males with X-linked (hemi-zygous) traits indicate that all male siblings run a 50 per cent risk; one-half of all female siblings become carriers of the mutant gene with no manifestation of the trait, while the male offspring of the "carrier females" have a 50 per cent risk of being affected.

Chromosomal disorders result mainly from errors in division during gametogenesis, especially oogenesis, that yield abnormal numbers of chromo-somes. These mistakes are generally considered a function of the aging ovary and, as such, are more likely to occur in conceptions occurring in older women. Indeed, there is a definite increase in the risks for chromosomal abnormalities once a specific chromosomal abnormality has occurred in a sibship. For example, once the standard variety of Down's syndrome has occurred (with 47 chromo-somes as a result of G trisomy), there is a threefold increase in the risk that this condition may recur in that family, regardless of the maternal age group. The older the mother, the greater the initial risk, and consequently, the greater the recurrence risk (see Table 20–1). The greatest risks for Down's syndrome and most other aneuploidies seem to occur after the age of 35 years.

TABLE 20–1.   *Risk of Down's Syndrome**

MATERNAL AGE	ANY PREGNANCY	AFTER BIRTH OF AN AFFECTED CHILD
Under 30	1/3000	1/1000
30–34	1/600	1/200
35–39	1/200	1/100
40–44	1/70	1/25
45–49	1/40	1/15
All ages	1/665	1/200

* Courtesy of J. Hijmans (personal communication).

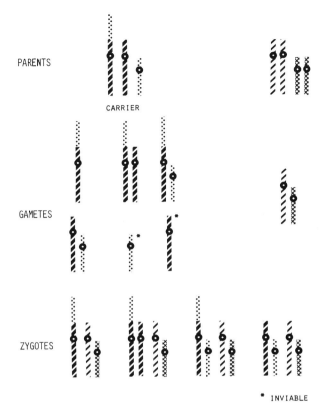

Figure 20-2. Gametic and zygotic possibilities in translocation matings.

Congenital anomalies associated with translocated chromosomes contributed by carrier parents present much more serious recurrence risks. Theoretically, gametes produced by carrier parents may be one of six combinations. Two possible combinations will be lethal because of the lack of one or the other entire chromosome. The other four possible gametes are capable of fertilization and can result in zygotes which are either (1) totally normal, having a pair of each of the chromosomes in question (1:4); (2) abnormal, being translocation "carriers" identical to the "carrier" parent (1:4), or (3) abnormal, having translocated chromosomes associated with one or the other representatives of those chromosomes not actually translocated to one another (2:4). Risks for subsequent siblings, therefore, are considerably higher than the empiric risks of recurrence seen with trisomies (Figure 20–2).

Candidates for Antenatal Diagnosis

Ideally, all pregnancies which run a risk of 25 to 50 per cent recurrence for serious genetic disease would be candidates for the antenatal detection of these disorders through amniocentesis. In addition, aside from those with high recurrence risks, all other pregnancies at risk for a serious defect could be candidates for prenatal diagnosis, depending upon maternal age and the condition under study. The questions of performing therapeutic abortion if studies so indicate should always be raised; otherwise, the studies are of little practical value.

Theoretically, all patients suspected of carrying fetuses with autosomal dominant traits which are potentially serious should be offered prenatal diagnosis if possible. Because of the 50 per cent recurrence figure, most families with a child already affected with an autosomal dominant defect would prefer to abandon further attempts at childbearing than to run the risk of delivering another, similarly affected infant. On the other hand, half of the pregnancies terminated therapeutically in such marriages could be expected to represent potentially normal siblings. To date, with the possible exception of Marfan's syndrome and Gaucher's disease (adult form), no autosomal dominant diseases considered serious are amenable to available techniques in antenatal detection.

Early investigation of the potential for genetic counseling in congenital metabolic disorders was initially focused on the X-linked diseases, such as the hemophilias (A and B), Hunter's syndrome (mucopolysaccharidosis), or the Duchenne type of muscular dystrophy. With the advent of antenatal determination of fetal sex, abortion could be considered if the fetus were male; female fetuses, although they are potential carriers, could be allowed to progress to term with no greater risk of abnormality than the population at large. The recognition of the unaffected male fetus in individual X-linked disorders has thus become the objective of multiple research units in antenatal diagnosis across the nation and, indeed, around the world.

The great majority of inborn errors of metabolism, however, follow an autosomal recessive pattern of inheritance. In this situation, both parents are unaffected carriers; unfortunately, the birth of an affected proband is necessary before such a carrier state can be recognized. Mass screening of the population is generally prohibitive both because of limited available laboratory facilities and because of sheer cost alone. Moreover, almost everyone in the population carries mutant genetic material for one or more metabolic disorders. It is only the marriage of two individuals who are born carriers for the *same* recessive trait that is likely to produce affected offspring, and even then the observed risk of occurrence in such a setting approximates the theoretical 25 per cent. Examples of metabolic disorders which follow an autosomal recessive pattern of inheritance include the glycogen storage diseases (Types I to IV), congenital adrenal hyperplasia, Hurler's syndrome, cystinuria, Morquio's syndrome, and Niemann-Pick disease. Inherited in a similar fashion are such serious disorders as sickle cell disease, thalassemia major, cystic fibrosis, and even diabetes mellitus.

Those couples who should be considered candidates for prenatal chromosomal analysis fall into several categories:

1. Family history of, or previous progeny with, aneuploidy.
2. Previous progeny with translocation.
3. Maternal age of 35 years or over.

It would be worthwhile to provide such families with fetal karyotypes if for no other reason than to assure them that chromosomes are "normal."

In addition, the investigator involved in prenatal chromosomal analysis may find himself in the awkward position of performing amniocenteses to reassure anxious patients and anxious physicians when, indeed, no bona fide indication exists.

For those couples who have already had a child with aneuploidy there is a definite increased risk that another aneuploidic child will be conceived. As pointed out above, the risk for recurrence of G trisomy Down's syndrome is tripled. Risk figures for other aneuploid conditions are not as yet available. However, it has been shown that repeated fetal wastage in some pedigrees is associated with more than the usually expected aneuploidies in those fetuses that survive gestation—e.g., families with one type of aneuploidy may have other types of aneuploidies [predilection for nondisjunction (?)] and many spontaneous abortions.

Whenever a translocation is found associated with congenital disease, the parents should be advised to consider the possibility of sterilization. If the proper emphasis is not expressed by the physician, or if the advice is not accepted and another pregnancy occurs, amniocentesis is unquestionably in order. If the one in four chance of "normal" is found to have eventualized, the pregnancy could be allowed to proceed, with the expectation that an unaffected baby will be born. If the carrier state for translocation is discovered, the parents should be given the opportunity to consider induced abortion. If an affected fetus is seen on karyotype, the parents should be made to understand that an abnormal baby can be expected if they choose not to have an induced abortion.

Because chromosomal abnormalities occur with greater frequency in babies born to mothers over 35 years of age, it is becoming increasingly common for women in their latter years of childbearing to request amniocentesis to rule out chromosomal abnormalities.

The risks of amniocentesis have been amply reviewed in the literature. Although complications such as hemorrhage, infection, and fetal puncture have been reported, their overall incidence has been shown to be quite low.[5] Whenever any procedure is performed that can possibly produce morbidity or mortality, the physician should compare the risk of the procedure with the advantages anticipated and with the risks involved if the procedure is not undertaken. Although the risks of amniocentesis to the mother and fetus are minimal in selected study groups, the morbidity and mortality figures may become significant when applied to mass screening programs.

Methodology

Perhaps the simplest (albeit indirect) approach to the antenatal detection of genetic disorders involves the screening of maternal urine for metabolites. For example, the presence of a fetus with methylmalonic aciduria has been shown to be associated with increased maternal urinary excretion of methylmalonyl coenzyme A.[6] The adrenogenital syndrome was similarly noted to be associated with excessive quantities of maternal urinary estriol. The accuracy of such diagnoses, however, was frequently impaired, by both a wide range of "normal" excretion patterns as well as the interference created by the presence of maternal precursors and metabolites. Urinary assays have thus largely been abandoned in favor of more direct methods.

Certain disorders which produce no readily detectable metabolite or enzyme deficiency per se may be indirectly diagnosed by their genetic proximity to loci for other traits (linkage studies). For example, the factor VIII deficiency of classic hemophilia may be assessed by its linkage with the glucose-6-phosphate dehydrogenase (G6PD) locus; in the Negro population, these G6PD variants are frequently detectable in cultured amniotic fluid cells.

Yet another indirect approach which has enjoyed limited success involves metachromatic staining properties of affected cells with toluidine blue. Multiple studies have shown the method to be nonspecific; in attempting to diagnose cystic fibrosis antenatally, for example, not only did a significant number of cultures from affected cystic fibrosis subjects prove to be nonmetachromatic but also a significant number of normal cell lines showed metachromasia.[7]

Evaluation of the uptake and metabolism of radioactively labeled substances has been used to diagnose such disorders as cystinosis, mucopolysaccharidosis, and the Lesch-Nyhan Syndrome. The reliability of such assay techniques, however, is far from absolute. Difficulty still exists in distinguishing between the affected homozygote and the "normal" carrier.

Amniotic fluid assays for metabolites have been used with some degree of success to predict errors of amino acid and organic acid metabolism. Various workers disagree as to whether amniotic fluid pregnanetriol levels are of value in the antenatal detection of the adrenogenital syndrome. Such disorders as Tay-Sachs disease have been correctly identified in utero by the demonstration of decreased amniotic fluid concentration of hexoseaminidase A. Differences in enzyme concentration between normal and affected fetuses have been shown to be greater in cultured amniotic fluid cells than in the fluid alone; therefore, the use of cultured cells is considered to be the more accurate technique by most workers. In the fetus affected with Pompe's disease (Type II glycogen storage disease), amniotic fluid concentrations of the enzyme acid α1,4-glucosidase approached normal levels while the same enzyme was undetectable in cultured cells from the same fluid. Thus the accurate diagnosis of this disorder rests solely upon the assay of cultured amniotic fluid cells.

Successful culture of amniotic fluid cells poses many serious technical problems. In order to avoid confusing the homozygous affected fetus with the heterozygous (carrier) fetus, it is necessary to establish "control" cell lines for comparison; this difficult project is presently being spearheaded by the National Institute of Child Health and Human Development, but it is far from complete. Another difficult aspect of amniotic fluid cell culture is the recognition and elimination of contamination by cells of maternal origin. This can be reduced significantly by discarding the initial portion of fluid obtained during amniocentesis. The only *positive* identification of fetal cells to date is a *male karyotype*. Enzymatic differences between epithelioid and fibroblastic cell types must be appreciated. Bacterial, fungal, and even PPLO-form invasion of cultures must be eliminated to insure accurate and meaningful results. Finally, human error in technique or interpretation of results must not be overlooked. This can be minimized if each research laboratory "specializes" in one or several enzymatic defects. Amniotic fluid samples could easily be shipped by air to the appropriate center for the particular disorder in question.

Conclusion

Today, impressive lists of disorders amenable to antenatal diagnosis are figuring prominently in the obstetrical, pediatric, and metabolic literature.[8] What is so often omitted from such articles, however, is the fact that at present these techniques may be time-consuming, difficult to perform, and, in some cases, prohibitively expensive when applied to mass screening techniques. Furthermore, results often cannot be reproduced from one laboratory to another. On the other hand, there is also ample evidence in the literature for reduplication of effort by some diagnostic centers.

Even when genetic counseling is restricted to those couples with an already affected proband, few individuals today are able to avail themselves of such potentially beneficial information. This may result, in part, from the fact that the number of genetic counselors is grossly inadequate to the task of providing such information to every family in need of it. Clearly, this burden can and must be alleviated by greater participation on the part of the private practitioner. Lack of communication between various research centers can also drastically reduce the availability of genetic counseling services. Perhaps a central counseling service could provide specific information to individual practitioners and, at the same time, enhance cooperative efforts in the monumental task before us all—that is, to prevent genetically determined birth defects and to reassure the concerned parents when there is a normal fetus in utero.

While great strides are being made in the antenatal diagnosis of heritable diseases, equal attention must be given to the care of those individuals whose disorders could not be detected before birth.

REFERENCES

1. Carter, C. O.: Practical aspects of early diagnosis of human genetic defects. *Fogarty International Center Proceedings* No. 6, 1970.
2. Court-Brown, W. M., and Smith, P. G.: Human population cytogenetics. Brit. Med. Bull. 25:74, 1969.
3. Lubs, H. A., and Ruddle, F. H.: Chromosomal abnormalities in the human population: estimation of rates based on New Haven Newborn Study. Science 169:495, 1970.
4. Carr, D. H.: Cytogenetic aspects of induced and spontaneous abortions. Clin. Obstet. Gynec. 15:203, 1972.
5. Burnett, R. G., and Anderson, W. R.: The hazards of amniocentesis. J. Iowa Med. Soc. 58:130, 1958.
6. Schulman, J. D.: Present status and future trends in prenatal diagnosis of metabolic disorders. Clin. Obstet. Gynec. 15:249, 1972.
7. Schulman, J. D.: Present status and future trends in prenatal diagnosis of metabolic disorders. Clin. Obstet. Gynec. 15:249, 1972.
8. Townes, P. L.: Preventive genetics and early therapeutic procedures in the control of birth defects. Birth Defects 6:42, 1970.

When Is Chromosomal Analysis Indicated in Obstetrical and Gynecological Practice?

MORTON A. STENCHEVER

University of Utah College of Medicine

In 1949, Barr and Bertram described the sex chromatin body in the nerve cell of the female cat. Since that time, the sex chromatin body has been identified as the constricted, nonfunctioning X chromosome in a mammalian cell which has more than one X chromosome. In general, it may be stated that only one X chromosome functions in a cell at a given time and that all other X chromosomes are present in the form of a sex chromatin body. Thus, if the number of sex chromatin bodies is known, the number of X chromosomes the cell has can be found by adding one. If the number of X chromosomes the cell has is known, the number of sex chromatin bodies can be determined by subtracting one.

In the mid-1950's, techniques became available which made it possible to swell mammalian cells in mitosis and produce chromosome plates which lend themselves to karyotyping. The human chromosome complement at this time was found to be 46, consisting of 22 pairs of autosomes and two sex chromosomes. Conferences held in Denver, London, and Chicago in 1960, 1963, and 1965, respectively, labored to standardize the nomenclature of human chromosomes. A composite of agreements recorded at these meetings provides for all autosomal pairs to be numbered in order of descending size from 1 to 22. Autosomes are divided into seven groups on the basis of their morphology (size, location of centromere, and so forth) and these groups are labeled by the letters A through G. The A group is comprised of pairs 1 through 3; the B group of pairs 4 and 5; the C groups of pairs 6 through 12; the D group of pairs 13 through 15; the E group of pairs 16 through 18; the F group of pairs 19 and 20; and the G group of pairs 21 and 22. The sex chromosomes are labeled X and Y. The X chromosome is similar in size and morphology to the No. 7 pair, and thus it is frequently included in the C group (C-X), and the Y chromosome is similar in morphology and size to the G group (G-Y) (Figure 20–3).

The short arm of a chromosome is labeled "p" and the long arm "q." If a translocation occurs in which the short arm of a chromosome is added to another chromosome, it is written "p+." If the short arm is lost, it is written "p−." The same can be said for the long arm ("q+" and "q−").

680

KARYOTYPE

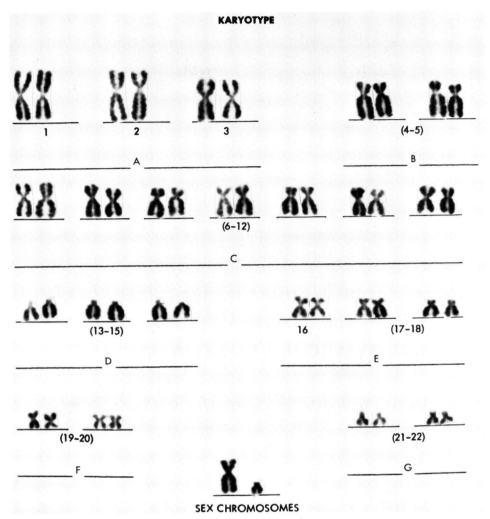

SEX CHROMOSOMES

Figure 20-3. A normal male karyotype.

On a morphologic basis alone, many chromosomes can not be differentiated from others of their group. However, by using techniques of radioactive thymidine labeling (autoradiography) or by studying the banding patterns of the chromosome, using either fluorescent techniques or special digestion and staining processes, it is now possible to define each chromosome in the karyotype.

Using fluorescent techniques on interphase nuclei, it is possible to identify the Y chromosome, since a large portion of the long arm of the Y chromosome is inert and takes a bright fluorescent stain. Thus, it is possible to count the number of Y chromosomes in a cell with this technique.

Who Should Have Chromosome Analysis?

The following is a list of indications for suggesting that a chromosome study be carried out:

1. Ambiguity of sex organs.
2. Mental retardation.

3. Low birth weight at full term.
4. Failure to thrive.
5. Congenital heart disease.
6. Abnormal dermatoglyphics.
7. Abnormal ears.
8. Limb anomalies.
9. Multiple anomalies.
10. Persistent fetal hemoglobin.
11. Habitual abortion.
12. Infertility.
13. Azoospermia.
14. Primary amenorrhea.
15. Reproductive wastage.
16. Family history of chromosome abnormalities.

Ambiguity of sex organs can be considered the one true cytogenetic emergency. A baby born that can not be properly sexed represents a traumatic experience for both mother and father, as society expects them to announce the sex of the child and bestow a proper name upon it. The problem is critical for the infant as well, since assigning the wrong sex may lead to difficulties when the child learns certain behavior patterns which may of necessity have to be changed in later life. For the purpose of establishing sex, frequently sex chromatin body or fluorescent staining for the Y chromosome is all that is necessary, but in each case a chromosome analysis should be carried out as a back-up procedure to make absolutely certain that the individual has been sexed properly. Occasionally the individual may be an hermaphrodite, at which time the physician must, after assembling all the facts, including the results of chromosome analysis, decide upon a course of action to establish the sex in which the individual will be raised. Pseudohermaphroditism of both the male and the female type poses special problems, which can be aided occasionally by proper sexing. The female pseudohermaphrodite, masculinized because of an endocrine problem, should be identified as such as soon as possible and the condition corrected to prevent difficulty in development in later life. The male pseudohermaphrodite, which frequently is encountered as the testicular feminization syndrome or related syndromes, poses a different problem. Most of these infants would not be identified by the usual physical examination at birth since they are phenotypic females. When they are discovered in later life, as a result of amenorrhea, to be 46,XY males genetically, they must be protected from this information and continue to be raised as females, since there is no way in which they can be converted into males, and they are usually psychologically and physically female.

Although many syndromes involving *mental retardation* are not associated with chromosome abnormalities, a good number are. In fact, so many are that probably all mentally retarded individuals should be subjected to chromosome analysis for proper diagnosis. The most common type of mental retardation associated with a chromosome abnormality is Down's syndrome. Here the individual has an extra chromosome 21 (trisomy 21) or an extra chromosome 21 translocated to some other chromosome. It is extremely important that the diagnosis be made correctly as the risks for other members of the family and for future siblings are greater should a translocation be the problem. In addition, it is good to have a definite diagnosis for the individual so that appropriate care can be planned. Other chromosome abnormalities are commonly associated with mental retarda-

2

5663

83

tion. Several of these involve a sex chromosome (for example XXY and XYY) or other autosomal trisomies, and most unbalanced translocations will also be associated with mental retardation.

Many chromosome anomalies, particularly the trisomies, are associated with *low birth weight at term*. In addition, the typical Turner's syndrome child (a female with 45, XO or some mosaic variation) is frequently small at birth, with the usual birth weight being under five pounds, and continues to be small throughout her life. A small baby at term who is a female should certainly be suspected of being a potential victim of Turner's syndrome.

Failure to thrive, that is, the chronically wasted child who does not grow or gain weight, should be suspected of having an unusual chromosome abnormality, usually an unbalanced translocation, and should undergo chromosomal analysis.

Individuals with *congenital heart disease, abnormally formed and positioned ears, limb abnormalities*, or *multiple congenital malformations* should be studied for possible chromosome anomalies. This is particularly true if there is a family history of congenital malformations, stillbirths, or abortions.

Individuals who are noted to have *abnormal dermatoglyphics* as part of the genetics evaluation certainly warrant a chromosome study, since many individuals with chromosome abnormalities have abnormal skin patterns.

It has been noted that persistence of *fetal hemoglobin* occurs in association with many chromosome abnormalities and should such a circumstance be noted in hematologic studies, an analysis is probably warranted.

Infertility, particularly involving the male in whom azoospermia is noted, is reason to do chromosome analysis. Individuals suffering from Klinefelter's syndrome (47, XXY pattern or variations) will be azoospermic. Occasionally, females with a history of *habitual abortion* will prove to have chromosome abnormalities, usually of the translocation type. The most common one seen in otherwise normal females is the heterologous D/D translocation carrier state. Infertility in a couple in which the female is apparently normal and there is a normal semen analysis in the male will rarely prove to be associated with a chromosome abnormality. Nonetheless, some infertile females are 47, XXX or variations thereof, and chromosome analysis is probably worth doing.

Certainly all females with *primary amenorrhea* should be studied, since a variety of chromosome abnormalities, e.g., testicular feminization syndrome, may be associated with primary amenorrhea. *Chronic pregnancy wastage* involving a variety of reproductive problems warrants study, because chromosome anomalies may be associated with these, the most common occurring with balanced translocation carriers.

Certainly where there is a *family history* of a chromosome abnormality, it is worthwhile to study individuals who are in the reproductive years to help them in planning their families.

Who Should Have Prenatal Diagnosis?

In 1955, Fuchs demonstrated that cells from amniotic fluid obtained by amniocentesis could be stained for sex chromatin. Thus, it became possible to diagnose sex prenatally. This gave physicians the option of counseling patients who were carriers of known sex-linked diseases to consider therapeutic abortion when a male fetus was found to be present.

In 1964, several laboratories at about the same time succeeded in culturing amniotic fluid cells and producing fetal karyotypes. It was possible to do this at about 14 to 15 weeks' gestation, and thus the doctor had another diagnostic tool for counseling.

This technique can be applied in the following instances:

1. One parent is a known carrier of a chromosome translocation.
2. The couple has had a previous trisomic child.
3. The mother is over 40 years of age.
4. There is a family history of a metabolic disease which lends itself to prenatal diagnosis.
5. A sex-linked recessive trait exists and amniocentesis is carried out for sex determination.

When a parent is a known carrier of a chromosome translocation, the risk of producing an abnormal child is great. The risk varies from 100 per cent where a homologous translocation exists (translocation between two members of the same pair) to one in four where a balanced translocation between two different chromosomes exists. At any rate, a high degree of risk exists in such circumstances and, depending on the chromosomes involved, infants with severe abnormalities may be produced. Prenatal diagnosis allows the parents to continue pregnancies which involve fetuses who are either normal or carriers of the chromosome translocation and to elect therapeutic abortion when fetuses with unbalanced translocations are being carried. Thus, individuals with very high risk who might have elected not to become pregnant at all, are now afforded the opportunity of bearing a phenotypically normal child.

Where the couple has had a previous trisomic child, such as one with trisomy 21 Down's syndrome, the risk of repeating is much greater than for that of the normal population, but it is not as high as in the translocation carrier group. Overall, the risk of repeating a trisomy 21 Down's syndrome is about one in 30. Nonetheless, the couple that has produced such a child generally does not want to produce a second one, and amniocentesis allows them the options of therapeutic abortion when a fetus with a trisomy 21 is discovered or of continuing the pregnancy when the fetus is chromosomally normal, with peace of mind, knowing that they are not repeating their problem.

In the case of the mother who is over the age of 40, the risk of producing fetuses with trisomic states is greater than for the usual population. As an example, the risk of producing a trisomy 21 Down's syndrome infant is about 1 in 2500 in a 20 year old female, whereas at age 40 it is 1 in 100, and at age 45 it is 1 in 40. Although such risks are not terribly great, most women in this age group welcome the opportunity of having a test performed which will allow them to continue normal pregnancies while using therapeutic abortion as a means of ending abnormal ones.

Where there is a family history of a metabolic disease which can be diagnosed prenatally, such diagnosis allows individuals who are known carriers of these diseases to continue pregnancies if the fetus is normal or a carrier and consider therapeutic abortion when homozygous recessive fetuses are discovered. To date, a number of hereditary diseases have been diagnosed prenatally. These include at least seven lipoidoses (e.g., Gaucher's, Tay-Sachs, Fabrey's, and so forth); at least six mucopolysaccharidoses (Hurler's and Hunter's syndromes); at least 11 amino-acidurias (cystinosis, homocystinuria, maple syrup urine disease, and so forth); at least eight diseases of carbohydrate metabolism (glucose-6-phosphate dehydrogenase deficiency, glycogen storage disease, and so forth); and a variety of other diseases including adrenogenital syndrome, Lesch-Nyhan syndrome, and others.

Where a sex-linked recessive trait exists, amniocentesis may be carried out. A male fetus has a 50 per cent risk of being affected. If there is no other prenatal diagnosis available for the particular trait, the parents may desire therapeutic abortion for male fetuses, and spare the female fetuses.

A number of laboratories in the United States are capable of performing chromosome analysis prenatally. In the case of syndromes involving metabolic disorders, certain laboratories are proficient in doing certain tests. However, most laboratories keep a list of where tests can be performed most successfully and will refer fluid from patients who are at risk for these to the appropriate institution.

In 1971, the author undertook a survey of a number of laboratories which undertook prenatal diagnosis of genetic diseases and compiled the accompanying table of data (Table 20-2). Inspection of these data accentuates the fact that the vast majority of babies exposed to this diagnostic test are actually saved. It can be assumed that many of these pregnancies would have ended in therapeutic abortion had the parents not had the option of prenatal diagnosis before undertaking such an endeavor.

These are the two major points to be made: first, individuals who are known carriers of genetic disease are afforded the opportunity of having normal children, whereas they might have been afraid to chance pregnancy before this diagnostic tool became available; second, once a pregnancy is conceived in known carriers, a number of babies are saved who ordinarily would have been subjected to therapeutic abortion had the family not had the advantage of prenatal diagnosis.

Technically amniocentesis is best carried out between the fourteenth and fifteenth weeks of gestation, which is the time at which there is enough fluid to obtain cells which can be grown in tissue culture. Between 10 and 40 cc. of fluid is removed in a sterile fashion transabdominally. This fluid is taken immediately to the laboratory. It is not frozen, since freezing kills cells. Of course, the sample is maintained in a sterile state. The first few cubic centimeters obtained after

TABLE 20–2. *Experience with Prenatal Diagnosis in Selected Laboratories**

REASON FOR EVALUATION	TOTAL CASES	BABIES SAVED (NORMAL OR CARRIER)	ABORTED (THERAPEUTIC OR SPONTANEOUS)	BORN AFFECTED
D/G or G/G translocation carrier parent	48	34	14	0
Other translocation carrier parent	11	7	3	1†
Previous nondisjunctional trisomic child	195	189	5	1‡
Maternal age	175	167	8	0
Metabolic disease	81	60	19	2§

* Data contributed by: M. N. Macintyre, C. Valenti, C. B. Jacobsen, H. Nadler, K. Hirschhorn, J. W. Littlefield, and M. A. Stenchever.
† Cri-du-chat.
‡ Down's syndrome.
§ 1 hemophilia, 1 Hurler's syndrome.

amniocentesis are generally discarded because every effort should be made to avoid contamination with maternal cells.

At the laboratory, several cultures are begun, using any one of a variety of techniques now acceptable. It generally takes about three weeks for cells to grow in tissue culture sufficiently to allow for cytogenetic evaluation or for analysis for metabolic defects. There are several risks in this method. The first is that maternal cells may be cultured, giving a false diagnosis. There is a particular risk of this occurring when the karyotype of the child proves to be the same as that of the mother. Attempts are made to avoid this risk by reporting observations from several different cultures. The second risk is that of contamination. Bacterial and viral contaminations are quite common in tissue culture laboratories and may cause the destruction of the cultures.

Even with these risks, the diagnosis is generally accurate, and success in culturing in most laboratories is well above 80 per cent at the present time.

It is not specifically known what the magnitude of risk of amniocentesis is to either the mother or fetus. Potential risks to the mother include infection, amniotic fluid embolus, perforation of an abdominal wall blood vessel with hematoma formation, isoimmunization, initiation of a coagulopathy, perforation of an abdominal viscus, peritonitis, and vaginal hemorrhage owing to abruptio placentae. Risks to the fetus include damage to the placenta from infection, initiation of rupture of membranes and abortion, and direct trauma, leading to death or congenital anomaly. In actual experience, all of these possibilities have been extremely rare, and the procedure has been surprisingly free of obvious hazard. Still more data are needed to assess the real risks, and the procedure should be performed only when the physician and the patient fully understand that there is potential risk and weigh this against the importance of the information to be gained.

What is the Place in Diagnosis of Buccal Smear for Sex Chromatin Body or Fluorescence for Y Chromosome?

Use of a buccal smear to diagnose genetic sex is of great help, particularly in screening studies, or in situations in which sex must be known and a diagnosis made rapidly. Nevertheless, at no time is a study of cells for sex chromatin or fluorescent Y superior to a chromosome karyotype. In the case of sex chromatin body studies, there is a certain amount of error brought about by the presence of more than one X chromosome in the cells of a male (XXY, XXXY), and the absence of a chromatin body in the chromatin negative female who has Turner's syndrome (XO).

Still, these studies have their place in large screening situations and in the rapid diagnosis of sex when ambiguity exists. Any mammalian cells, from any tissue, in which there are interphase nuclei can be used for sex chromatin studies or for tests for fluorescent Y chromosome. Occasionally an individual with a group C/X trisomy is encountered, and one wonders whether the extra chromosome is a member of the X group. Here staining for sex chromatin bodies is helpful in making the differential diagnosis. This is particularly important in prenatal diagnosis, as a tri-X individual would be allowed to carry to term, being expected to be phenotypically normal, whereas a trisomy of one of the members of the C group would probably cause consideration of therapeutic abortion.

What is the Place for Study of Chromosome Banding Patterns?

The advent of methods to differentiate specific chromosomes of the karyotype is of help primarily in counseling people with chromosome translocations or as a research tool. Nonetheless, these techniques are extremely valuable to the cytogeneticist and have made it possible to redefine several syndromes which were only poorly defined by previous methods. They are not necessarily important for the usual chromosome analysis unless a chromosome abnormality is found and identification of the particular chromosome is important.

REFERENCES

1. Nadler, H. L., and Gerbie, A. B.: Role of amniocentesis in intrauterine detection of genetic disorders. New Eng. J. Med. 282:596, 1950.
2. Milunsky, A., Littlefield, J. W., Kanfer, J. N., Kolodny, E. H., Shih, V. E., and Atkins, L.: Prenatal genetic diagnosis. New Eng. J. Med. 283:1370, 1441, 1498; 1970.
3. Stenchever, M. A., Jarvis, J. A., and Macintyre, M. N.: Cytogenetics of habitual abortion. Obstet. Gynec. 32:548, 1968.
4. Stenchever, M. A., and Jarvis, J. A.: Cytogenetic studies in reproductive failure. Obstet. Gynec. 37:83, 1971.
5. Stenchever, M. A., Macintyre, M. N., Jarvis, J. A., and Hempel, J. M.: Cytogenetic studies in 32 infertile couples. Obstet. Gynec. 33:380, 1969.

When Is Chromosomal Analysis Indicated in Obstetrical and Gynecological Practice?

Editorial Comment

The obstetrician-gynecologist is being confronted with increasing frequency with patients or their offspring who may require cytogenetic studies. Whether or not he chooses to indulge in genetic counseling, he must be familiar with the various conditions for which cytogenetic investigations are indicated or mandatory and with their identification. The rapid expanse of genetic information is to be admired, but how to relate much of the new knowledge to patient management poses problems and difficulties. As one contributor emphasizes, there are many conditions that must still be approached as a research effort, and clinicians are reminded that they have a responsibility to furnish whatever material they have to the cytogeneticist in order that he may unravel the many genetic conditions that are now poorly understood. However, these studies are time consuming and expensive to perform. For this reason the clinician must decide from among a rather large maze of cytogenetic information what indeed has clinical relevance.

In addition, the obstetrician-gynecologist must be prepared to carry through any procedure, including a medical abortion, if it appears that the fetus may be afflicted with a serious genetic condition. Until the various methods of identification of genetic disease are universally available the limitations of statistics where decision making is concerned are vividly illustrated. It might be relevant to the prospective mother whether the incidence of a particular condition that might affect the fetus is 5 or 25 per cent of instances, but it certainly is not to the physician. If the physician would be hesitant to perform an abortion when the chance that the fetus will be afflicted is 5 per cent or less, rather than 25 per cent, he should not become involved in the patient's problem. Rather, he should ask himself what his attitude might be if it were his wife who was faced with the problem. Moreover, the argument that the patient might not have another pregnancy because of age if the current one is terminated is a specious one, because age alone may well increase the genetic risk. In contrast, experience will testify that many patients may choose to continue the pregnancy, regardless of percentage of risk of fetal involvement.

In the overall management of the patient hopefully there will be obstetricians and gynecologists who because of special training and interest will be prepared to give genetic counseling of high quality. Certainly obstetrics and gynecology must play a greater role in this area if the primary objective of quality of life is to be attained and protected.

21

Diagnosis
and Management
of Ambiguous
Sexual Development

Alternative Points of View:

By Vincent J. Capraro

By John F. Crigler, Jr.

By John W. Huffman

Editorial Comment

Diagnosis and Management
of Ambiguous Sexual Development

Vincent J. Capraro

State University of New York at Buffalo and Buffalo Children's Hospital

Ambiguity of genitalia results from any of the following:
1. Virilization.
2. Absence of development.
3. Duplication of development.
4. Abnormal development.
5. Genetic influences.

These factors may be operative antenatally or postnatally. Ambiguity owing to antenatal factors may continue after birth if the disease is inherent in the child, such as the adrenogenital syndrome. If the genital abnormality was caused by exogenous factors in pregnancy, such as androgens administered to the mother or presence of a tumor in the mother, the condition does not progress after birth. Some types of ambiguity of the genitalia will be found to have a familial incidence, in particular certain forms of male hermaphroditism and the adrenogenital syndrome.

Anomalies of the genitalia can be divided into three categories: (1) those limited to the genitalia only, (2) those involving both the genitalia and other, local structures, such as the urinary tract or rectum, and (3) those involving the genitalia and associated with distant anomalies.

When all is said and done, regardless of etiology or classification, the most important problem confronting the physician and the parents is the determination of the sex for rearing. This must be done early if we hope to give the child a fair opportunity for normal psychosexual development. By "early," I mean the first few weeks or preferably the first few days of life.

Criteria for Sex

At the present time, there are eight factors (Table 21-1) which can be used in the sexing of an individual. If all of these factors are in proper relationship,

TABLE 21–1.   *The Criteria for Sex*

Nuclear:
    Sex Chromatin (Barr body)
    Sex Chromosomes (XX, XY)
Anatomic Sex:
    Gonads
    Morphology of external genitalia
    Morphology of internal genitalia
Hormonal:
    Estrogen vs. androgen
Psychologic:
    Sex of rearing
    Gender role

supposedly we are dealing with a normal individual. It must be remembered that not all patients with ambiguity of the genitalia have intersex problems.

Classification of Problems of Intersexuality

Our clinic no longer use the term "pseudohermaphroditism," believing it causes confusion. We prefer the simpler terms *male hermaphroditism* (male intersexuality), *female hermaphroditism* (female intersexuality), and *true hermaphroditism*. In this clinic, we have found it convenient to use the very practical classification proposed by Jones and Scott:[1]

1. Gonadal aplasia and dysplasia.
2. Male intersexuality (nonfamilial and masculinizing).
3. Male intersexuality (familial, feminizing, masculinizing, or mixed).
4. Klinefelter's syndrome.
5. Other syndromes of male intersexuality.
6. Female intersexuality associated with adrenal hyperplasia.
7. Female intersexuality not resulting from adrenal hyperplasia.
8. Other syndromes of female intersexuality.
9. True hermaphroditism.

Anatomic Deviations

Female anatomic deviations from the normal which are not really problems of intersexuality, but cause confusion by altering the appearance of the vulva, include: (1) polyps of the hymen, (2) cysts of the hymen, (3) ectopic ureter, (4) imperforate hymen, (5) microperforate hymen, and (6) vaginal septa, which may be longitudinal or transverse. Management of some of these will be discussed later in this presentation. The important significance of these lesions is to know they exist and can be easily treated so as to spare the parents any unnecessary anguish.

Recognition Time of Genital Anomalies

Most patients with ambiguous genitalia have problems of intersexuality, but this is by no means the only cause for ambiguity of the genitalia. Depending on what the lesion is, such problems arise and confront us at varying times in the life of the patient.

1. At *birth* most intersex problems are discovered—or should be.

2. In *childhood* adhesions of the labia minora which obscure the normal female vulva are found.

3. At *puberty*, amenorrhea brings our attention to those patients with absence of the vagina or uterus.

4. In the *young adult*, coital activity may reveal the septate and the short vagina.

5. At the time of *childbearing*, one is alerted to abnormality involving uterine septal defects.

Problems Involving the Parents

Naturally the parents of a child with ambiguity of the genitalia are usually quite distressed. Many of these parents may have guilt feelings and feel they are being punished by having a child with ambiguous genitalia because of their own sexual practices. They may recall the biblical verse—"but punishing children and grandchildren to the third and fourth generation for their fathers' wickedness" (Exodus 34:7). It is important to erase such myths from the minds of the parents. Whether or not a couple's marriage will survive the psychic trauma associated with raising a child with ambiguous genitalia depends on their interpersonal relationship and understanding.

We may help the parents face the community by suggesting a name which is also ambiguous. Name changing can cause considerable upheaval within the family circle and possibly within the community. Hence, if the child is given a name that is applicable to both male or female, such as Francis(ces), there is no need to change the name when the final sex of rearing is determined. Some may disagree with this concept, feeling that the parents must have a strongly positive attitude toward the sex of the child and giving an ambiguous name does not help. However, I feel that it is less traumatic not to have to change the name after several weeks or several months, and the parents could just as well work to reinforce the sex of the baby in other ways.

We should not use the term "sex chromatin" in talking to parents or patients. A statement that the female patient is sex chromatin negative, may be misinterpreted as absence of some part of normal female sexuality. On the other hand, if we use the term "Barr body," we can easily say that a patient is Barr body positive or Barr body negative without any implication of sexuality whatsoever. We have found this to be of considerable help in talking to both patients and parents.

One should also use terms which are easily comprehended by lay people and are not likely to cause anxiety. For example, if the clitoris is enlarged, we do not refer to it as a penis-like structure, but rather as an overdeveloped clitoris. If the ovaries are not producing hormones properly or if mixed gonads are present, we do not tell the patient or her parents that she is without ovaries. This also is misunderstood as a lack of femaleness. Hence, we use the term "underdeveloped gonads." If an ovary is present, we of course emphasize the fact. However, if a normal ovary is not present, or if we are dealing with a patient to be reared as female, we do not use the word "testis," but in both cases the term "gonad" will suffice. Therefore, using "underdeveloped," "overdeveloped," or "incompletely developed gonads" serves as well and thus avoids damaging the patient or her parents.

Experience has also taught us that in working with parents, it is best to designate one physician to be the sole contact. If several physicians talk to the parents, they frequently become confused. We may all be saying the same thing but using different words. In general, it has worked out well for either the pediatrician, the endocrinologist, or the gynecologist to be the spokesman for the group. Above all, we must not harm or frighten the patient or parents by ill-chosen words. The classic dictum, in the words of one of my early teachers, always comes to mind—"Don't do anything to harm your patient either by word or by deed."

In helping these parents, it is important to have a positive approach. The sex of rearing should be determined as soon as possible and from that point on we must be positive in our discussion and our attitude. The mother and father must be made to feel certain they are dealing with a girl or a boy. An attitude of uncertainty is detrimental to the child's future gender identity.

We rely heavily upon teamwork by the gynecologist, endocrinologist, pediatrician, geneticist, urologist, pathologist, and whatever other specialist is needed. In some situations, we find that psychiatric and psychologic evaluation and therapy of the parents or the child or both may be necessary, for, as mentioned earlier, some parents can stand up to the psychic trauma involved and others cannot.

Sex of Rearing

The approach to studies on the newborn with ambiguous genitalia, as described in Figure 21-1, begins with a buccal smear and with chromosome karyotyping. However, the sex of rearing does not depend exclusively on presence or absence of gonads or sex chromatin. It depends primarily on the answer to one question—how can this child best function sexually? Will this child be able to perform sexually as a male or as a female? In general, we prefer to keep the baby within its own chromosomal sex. However, if the appropriate structures of the external genitals are not present we must then consider sex conversion.

In the case of the male hermaphrodite with inadequate development of the genitalia, the size of the phallus is the one single important factor in determining the sex of rearing. If the child does not have an adequate phallus which will function sexually as a male organ, a sex conversion operation should be performed and the patient should be reared as a female.

It is difficult at times to determine how much penile growth will occur over the first few weeks of life. During the last several years, a therapeutic trial with local testosterone cream in several of these children has been of great help in determining whether or not the penis will grow and enlarge.

The penile tissue may fail to respond to testosterone cream (end organ failure), in which case hormone therapy at birth or at adolescence will not succeed in enlarging the phallus (Group B, Table 21-2). These children should be reared as females and corrective surgery should be performed early in life. On the other hand, if the small phallus results from lack of androgen, either quantitatively or

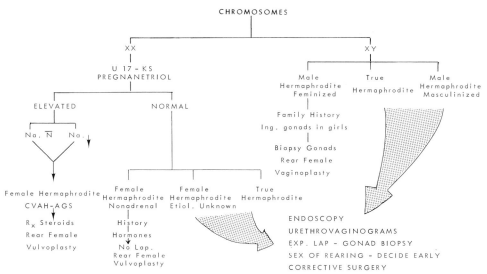

Figure 21-1. Flowsheet showing pattern of diagnostic studies to arrive at correct diagnosis and management of newborn with ambiguous genitalia.

TABLE 21–2. *Sex Assignment in Cases of Micropenis*

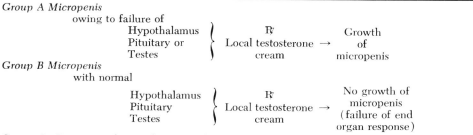

Group A Micropenis
 owing to failure of

| Hypothalamus Pituitary or Testes | ℞ Local testosterone cream | Growth of micropenis |

Group B Micropenis
 with normal

| Hypothalamus Pituitary Testes | ℞ Local testosterone cream | No growth of micropenis (failure of end organ response) |

Group A: Rear as male. We know phallus *does* respond to androgen. Treat with androgen at puberty.

Group B: Rear as female with necessary sex conversion surgery early in life. We know phallus *does not* respond to androgen, and therapy at puberty will be futile.

qualitatively, local application of testosterone cream will show some growth in the size of the phallus (Group A, Table 21-2). We feel that these children should be reared as males, with the intention of giving them hormone therapy in later life for the growth of the phallus and for development of secondary sexual characteristics.

Females born with virilization of the genitalia owing to congenital adrenal hyperplasia are reared as females regardless of the degree of masculinization of the external genitalia. The internal genitalia are normal for a female and require no treatment; the external genitalia can be corrected surgically. The time of repair will be discussed later.

Male hermaphrodites with androgen insensitivity (testicular feminization syndrome) are reared as females. The body contour at puberty is female. The external genitalia are female in appearance and a vagina, although usually short, is present.

True hermaphrodites are reared according to what structures are present in the external genitalia.

The Diagnostic Approach

The diagnostic workup of children with ambiguous genitalia requires a logical planned approach. We proceed through the following steps, but not necessarily in the order listed.

A. History.
B. Physical examination.
C. Vaginoscopy.
D. Cystoscopy.
E. Buccal smear.
F. Chromosome karyotype.
G. X-rays for bone age, vaginogram, hysterogram, cystogram, intravenous pyelogram, and gynecography.
H. Hormone studies.
I. Laparoscopy-laparotomy.
J. Psychiatric and psychologic evaluation.

HISTORY

A family history is obtained. A female born with virilization may have congenital virilizing adrenal hyperplasia (CVAH). Obtaining the family history of CVAH in siblings will aid in making a diagnosis. In the testicular feminization syndrome, one may obtain the history that other relatives have had abnormalities of their "ovaries" and have had them removed. There will be an occasional case of male hermaphroditism of the masculizing type that has a familial pattern.

In the older patient, the history of menses or of amenorrhea is of importance in arriving at the diagnosis. Also, the development of the other secondary sexual characteristics should be investigated thoroughly in the patient and in members of her family.

The exposure to androgenic hormone must be investigated. If the infant is born with evidence of virilization, one must check the prenatal record to be sure that the mother had not been given hormone therapy which might have caused the virilization. One must also rule out an ovarian tumor or an adrenal tumor in the mother which may have produced androgens, causing virilization in the baby. The older child may be virilized because of exogenous androgen, administered in error or in contaminated medication.

PHYSICAL EXAMINATION

A general physical examination is performed. The structures of the vulva are then inspected and palpated to be sure each and every structure is present, located correctly, and giving the appearance that it will function normally. The vagina and cervix should be visualized if there is any question of ambiguity of the external genitalia. This can be done readily with the use of a vaginoscope. A recto-abdominal, or, in the older patient, a vaginal-abdominal bimanual examination is performed to palpate for masses and to confirm the presence or absence of the uterus. The extrapelvic sex areas are then examined for evidence of abnormalities. This includes the breasts, the axillae, and the face for evidence of acne and distribution of body hair. The details of a complete gynecologic examination in children have been described elsewhere.[2,3]

VAGINOSCOPY

Vaginoscopy should be performed whenever there is a question of ambiguity of the genitalia. One may sometimes visualize the vaginal canal simply by separating the labia and depressing the perineum downward. One may also probe the vagina. However, in order to be sure a cervix is present, the structure must be visualized directly with a vaginoscope in a small child, or with a Huffman vaginal speculum[3] in the older child. Usually vaginoscopy can be performed without anesthesia. However, if the child has been traumatized by previous blunt attempts at examination, she will need analgesia in some form—such as a tranquilizer. Those patients who cannot be properly examined in the office or clinic should be examined under anesthesia.

CYSTOSCOPY

There is a high incidence of urologic abnormalities in patients with genital abnormalities.[4] Hence, any patient with abnormalities of the development of the Müllerian duct system may very well have abnormalities of the bladder, urethra, ureter, or kidney. We frequently work with the urologist and perform vaginoscopy in conjunction with the urologic studies, thus requiring anesthesia only once.

THE BUCCAL SMEAR

The buccal smear shows the presence or absence of Barr bodies (sex chromatin). In the normal female, the buccal smear will show Barr bodies in 20 to 40 per cent of the cells, whereas in the male none are present. There is a question as to whether this is an accurate test in the first few days of life. It appears that a greater percentage of Barr bodies are visualized after the first several days of life. However, enough are present early so that we can utilize this as a reliable test. Lucas, Dewhurst, and Hurly and others found that the mean Barr body count taken on the first day of life was 7.4 per cent; on the second day, 8.1 per cent; and on the fourth and subsequent days, 10.9 per cent. We have not had any difficulty with buccal smears taken during the first few days of life, although others do report difficulty. As we have already indicated, in talking to the parents, we do not use the term "sex chromatin," but rather "Barr bodies."

CHROMOSOME KARYOTYPE

Chromosome karyotyping is a rather expensive and time-consuming procedure and is not done as a matter of routine, as is the buccal smear. However, we feel that it should be done in patients with ambiguous genitalia.

Some patients are mosaics—i.e., they have more than one type of cell line genetically. In addition to blood samples, it may be necessary to study other tissues, such as skin or gonads.

X-RAYS

X-ray examinations can be very helpful in arriving at a diagnosis and we use these in determining the patient's bone age. If the bone age is advanced, it may be a result of excessive steroids, as in adrenogenital syndrome. X-ray examinations can also be used to follow the patient with the adrenogenital syndrome. If the bone age advances too rapidly, we are made aware that the patient's adrenal androgen production is not being adequately suppressed.

Vaginograms and hysterograms are a great help when the labioscrotal folds are fused (Figure 21-2). We can assume, for example, in the adrenogenital syndrome that the patient has a normal vagina and uterus. However, the parents will not accept this when it is only a statement of probability. They want to know for sure—does our daughter have a vagina? Does our daughter have a uterus? The only way we can answer this question completely and with absolute certainty is by vaginoscopy. If the degree of labioscrotal fusion is severe, it is easier to perform x-ray studies in the young patient. If a urogenital sinus is present, a urethrovaginogram (Figures 21–3 and 21–4) can be performed and we can describe to the parents exactly what structures lie behind the fused perineum. The knowledge that the child does indeed have a vagina and uterus reinforces the image of femaleness.

Gynecography can also be used to outline the pelvic organs.

ENDOCRINE STUDIES

In the patient with congenital virilizing adrenal hyperplasia, the 24 hour urinary excretion of 17-ketosteroids and pregnanetriol is elevated. The administration of cortisone to the child will cause a drop in both these values, thereby

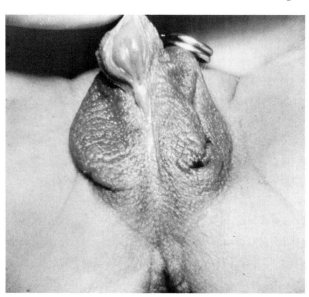

Figure 21-2. Newborn female with congenital virilizing adrenal hyperplasia, showing severe degree of fusion of labioscrotal folds and a single urogenital sinus opening in midportion of the enlarged phallus (clitoris). Note marked pigmentation and rugae of labial folds, which give appearance of scrotal sac.

Step 1

Step 2

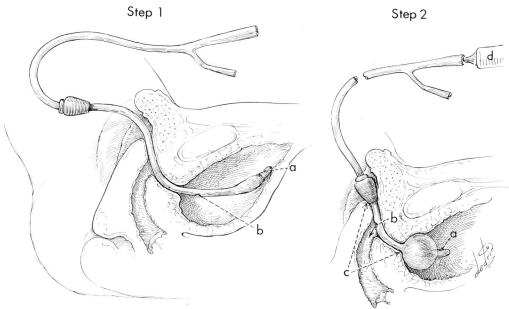

Figure 21-3. Double contrast x-ray of bladder, urogenital sinus, and vagina with modified Foley catheter. *Step 1:* Air cystogram. *a,* Normal opening of Foley catheter sealed off with silastic cement. *b,* Special opening cut into lumen of Foley catheter used to drain out urine and then to fill bladder with air for contrast. *Step 2:* Outlining urogenital sinus. *c,* Catheter now withdrawn, with inflated balloon held tightly against internal urethral meatus and soft rubber olive tip slid tightly against external urogenital sinus opening. *d,* Injection of radiopaque dye under pressure. Dye enters urogenital sinus through special opening (*b*) cut into lumen of Foley catheter.

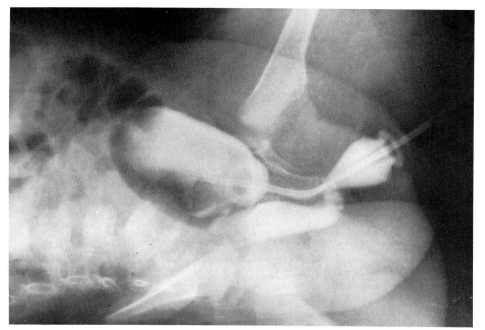

Figure 21-4. Double contrast x-ray demonstrating urogenital sinus, vagina, urethra, and bladder. In this patient, there is some dye spillage into bladder because inflated Foley balloon was not held tightly against internal urethral orifice. This patient's external genitalia were similar in appearance to those in Figure 21-2.

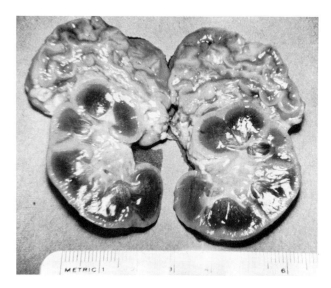

Figure 21-5. Massive adrenal hypertrophy in female infant with salt-losing type of congenital virilizing adrenal hyperplasia. This infant died shortly after hospital admission. Erroneous diagnosis at birth was male with cryptorchidism and hypospadias.

confirming the diagnosis of congenital virilizing adrenal hyperplasia. Some forms of this disease also are associated with sodium loss. The resulting hyponatremia, if not diagnosed, can cause death (Figure 21-5). Administration of deoxycorticosterone acetate (DOCA) corrects the salt loss. In early life, DOCA is given by injection. It may later be administered yearly in subcutaneous DOCA pellet implants.

In some instances, we may wish to know if estrogen is being produced. This can be studied in 24 hour urinary excretion specimens. If the patient has a vagina, vaginal cytology will reflect the presence or absence of estrogen production. Cells in the urinary sediment will also reflect estrogen production.

Some preliminary research by our service appears to indicate that axillary pH may also reflect estrogen production.

In gonadal dysgenesis, the estrogen levels are low and pituitary gonadotropin excretion levels are high.

LAPAROSCOPY AND LAPAROTOMY

At the present time, our experience with laparoscopy in children with ambiguous genitalia is rather limited. My feeling at this point, when dealing with an intersex problem, is that we may have difficulty enough with the abdomen opened in determining whether the oviducts, round ligaments, uterus, and gonads are normal or abnormal. We sometimes must follow the gonadal vessels to determine if gonads are present. As a matter of fact, in some patients, we never do find the gonads. If the physician is concerned about intersexuality, and so long as he accepts the risk of administering anesthesia to the child, I believe that he must go all the way and perform an exploratory laparotomy.

In the patient who has clear-cut gonadal dysgenesis clinically, I believe that laparoscopy with biopsy of the streaks will suffice in making the diagnosis. However, with the other types of intersexuality, it is my belief that one must actually palpate, biopsy, and do frozen sections in order to know exactly what one is dealing with.

When do we do an exploratory laparotomy? If we cannot completely explain all the findings in terms of the anatomic abnormality, the genetic component, and the hormonal deviations, one must do a laparotomy to rule out the possibility of true hermaphroditism. Also, the phenotypic female with XY sex chromosomes should also be operated on because of the high incidence of malignancy in dysgenetic gonads.

In general, if one is dealing with intraperitoneal gonads which are not normal ovaries, gonadectomy should be performed.

PSYCHOLOGIC AND PSYCHIATRIC EVALUATION

Psychologic and psychiatric evaluation of the patient may be necessary, particularly when the parents are confused. As a matter of fact, many times the parents themselves will need psychiatric evaluation and guidance.

The best assurance for avoiding psychiatric problems is to arrive at the sex of rearing early—in the first few days. Corrective surgery should also be done early—in the first few years of life and preferably in the first few months. There must be no ambivalent feelings by the parents about the child's sex if normal psychosexual development and normal sexual identity is to be accomplished.

Treatment for Genital Abnormalities

Some genital anomalies require *no treatment*. The baby with slight enlargement of the clitoris resulting from androgens given to the mother during pregnancy is only kept under observation. Since she is no longer exposed to androgens postnatally, there will be no further clitoral growth. The baby will "grow around" the slightly enlarged clitoris and in time, the vulva will appear normal.

Physical therapy in the form of dilatation is indicated in patients with an inadequate vagina. Several of our patients with adrenogenital syndrome, who had stenosis of the vagina, responded well to the use of graduated dilators (Figure 21–6). Another group of patients, those with a short vagina, such as testicular feminization patients, may develop a vagina of adequate depth by the use of dilators.

Medical therapy is indicated in many patients. Patients with adrenogenital syndrome must be treated with cortisone, and those with the salt-losing syndrome with DOCA tablets. Patients whose gonads do not produce estrogen (gonadal dysgenesis and male hermaphrodites) are given estrogens.

Surgery is required in some patients. This must be done with care, and it must be properly timed.

Surgery of the Ambiguous Genitalia

The aim of surgery—and indeed all therapy in patients with ambiguous genitalia—is to achieve the following:

1. To restore anatomic and sexual function.
2. To make the patient appear socially acceptable among her peers.
3. To make the appearance of the genitalia psychologically acceptable to the patient and her family.

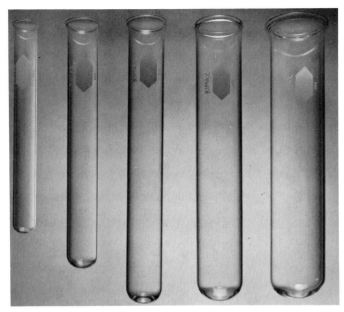

Figure 21-6. Vaginal dilators: Test tubes in graduated sizes, with outside diameter ranging from 1.8 to 3.7 cm.

4. Most important of all—*DO NO HARM* to the patient.

The surgery itself may be reconstructive (vaginoplasty), ablative (gonadectomy or phallectomy), or curative (adrenalectomy, gonadectomy).

When to Operate

The age of the patient influences the extent of surgery and the type of surgery indicated. Given the severely virilized patient with a complete urogenital sinus, labioscrotal fusion, and enlarged clitoris (Figure 21–2), we proceed as follows:

INFANCY.   Clitoridectomy is performed for cosmetic reasons, with enlargement of the urogenital sinus opening sufficiently to permit free flow of urine. The exteriorization of the vagina, I believe, should wait until the child is a bit larger and there is more tissue to work with.

PREPUBERTY.   In addition to the cosmetic need for a normal appearing vulva and the anatomic need for free flow of urine, we must now prepare the genitalia to permit free egress of menstrual flow.

MATURITY.   In the sexually mature patient, we are concerned not only with the cosmetic appearance and the free flow of urine and menstrual fluid, but in addition, the vagina must be of adequate depth and caliber for coitus.

Clitoris

Surgical treatment of the clitoris may involve complete amputation or partial resection. Various ingenious operations have been devised for resecting the enlarged clitoris. In my opinion, if the clitoris must be operated on owing to excessive enlargement, it should be amputated in toto rather than using any of the surgical procedures which leave portions of the corpora or the glans behind. In the presence of persistent androgen exposure, the remaining structures continue to grow.

The question of the need of the clitoris for orgasm is not completely settled. It is my impression that well adjusted females do not lose their libido or their ability to achieve orgasm following clitoridectomy. Adult patients in whom vulvectomy has been performed for leukoplakia or malignancy usually lose the clitoris. In these patients, if they are properly adjusted to the radical surgery, there is no loss of orgasm.

The babies born with an enlarged phallus after virilizing hormones were given to the mother need not necessarily be operated on at birth. If the clitoris is not extremely large, one does nothing but wait. In the absence of further androgenic stimulation, there will be very little further growth in the clitoris. However, if the clitoris is extremely large, it should be amputated early. In most cases, the vulva and the baby "grow around" the clitoris and in this manner, the structure becomes less prominent, and less and less out of proportion as the patient reaches full body size.

Management of Problems of the Vagina

Absence of the vagina may be either complete or incomplete. If there is complete absence, generally the uterus is absent as well. A few patients in whom a functioning uterus is present will develop hematometra, which requires prompt intervention at the time of adolescence. In the absence of the uterus and vagina one need only perform a vaginoplasty to give the patient a vaginal canal for coitus. The big question is, when should it be done? First, it should not be done until the patient reaches full body size, since the artificial vagina will not grow with the patient. Even more important, it should be performed only after the patient feels the need for it and is motivated to cooperate in the postoperative management. She must use vaginal dilators until regular coitus occurs, or the new canal will become stenotic.

Some authorities advocate waiting until just prior to marriage. However, if the result is unsatisfactory, a tragedy can result, since there is no time for a second procedure before the marriage.

There are various techniques for this operation—the Frank nonoperative technique, the McIndoe technique, the Wharton technique, and the Pratt technique. Recently, we have reported on the use of a simplified vulvovaginoplasty[6] producing a well functioning vagina. which is associated with considerably less blood loss and less hospitalization time.

Some patients, such as those with adrenogenital syndrome or some male hermaphrodites, who are reared as females, will have a vagina of small caliber. This can be corrected with the use of dilators (Figure 21–6). The administration of oral estrogen or use of estrogen cream locally helps to keep the vagina moist and supple during the dilating procedure. At times, a perineoplasty, incising the perineum in the sagittal plane and closing the incision transversely, is necessary.

A septum of the vagina may be either longitudinal or transverse and the type of repair varies accordingly. In the case of the longitudinal septum, usually one side of the vagina is larger than the other, so that there should be no difficulty with coitus. I believe the only indication for excision of a longitudinal septum is difficulty with coitus. The transverse annular vaginal septum also may be a hindrance to coitus. If the septum is high in the vagina, coitus is possible, but the sperm may have difficulty in reaching the cervix. Under these circumstances, and if pregnancy is desired, I believe that the transverse annular septum should be excised. It is necessary that the fibrous ring be excised as well,[7] otherwise the obstruction will recur. I have seen patients with a transverse annular septum who have become pregnant and had to be delivered by cesarean section because obstruction of the head by the transverse constriction prevented descent.

Microperforate Hymen

The microperforate hymen may at first glance appear to be an imperforate hymen; however, with pressure on the hymen at the posterior fourchette, one can usually discern a small opening beneath the urethra. This usually is sufficient to permit the flow of menstrual blood, so that the patient is unaware that there is anything wrong. When the young child voids, urine spills into the vagina (this is normal for young girls). However, in microperforation of the hymen, the urine does not drain out readily. These children tend to have recurrent episodes of vulvovaginitis. In the older patient, it may be difficult to penetrate the hymen at the time of first coitus. The treatment is to incise the hymen longitudinally in the sagittal plane from the 12 o'clock position down to 6 o'clock position and then to close the wound transversely.[7] I do not remove any hymenal tissue because less scar tissue is formed with this simple slitting technique.

Adhesions of the Labia Minora

The microperforate hymen may sometimes be confused with adhesions of the labia minora,[8] which is more likely to occur in the younger patient who has low estrogen levels. It results from local inflammation of the labia minora, which then fuse together in the midline and cover the hymenal opening. The vulva in these children gives the appearance of congenital absence of the vagina. However, on close inspection, one will note that the vulva is flat, there is a raphe in the midline, and there is a tiny opening beneath the clitoris from which urine escapes. In these patients, there is no free flow of urine. Urine remains in the vagina and recurrently becomes infected, and the situation may be comparable to a cesspool.

Therapy for adhesions of the labia minor in children is local application of estrogen cream. It is cruel to forcefully separate the labia manually. This is not only physically painful, but also psychologically traumatic.

Unfortunately sometimes these patients are taken to the operating room by the inexperienced and surgery (separation) is done under anesthesia. This is an unwarranted anesthetic risk, since application of estrogen cream locally accomplishes the same thing very nicely. Many of these children will have recurrences and the estrogen cream therapy must be repeated anyway. Corticosteroid creams may be used, but I do not feel they give any better results than estrogen cream.

REFERENCES

1. Jones, H. W., and Scott, W. W.: Hermaphroditism, Genital Anomalies, and Related Endocrine Disorders. 2nd Ed. Baltimore, Williams & Wilkins Co., 1971.
2. Capraro, V. J.: Gynecologic examination in children and adolescents. Pediat. Clin. North Am. *19*:511, 1972.
3. Huffman, J. W.: The Gynecology of Childhood and Adolescence. Philadelphia, W. B. Saunders Company, 1968.
4. Dewhurst, C. J., and Gordon, R. R.: The Intersexual Disorders. Baltimore, Williams & Wilkins, 1969.
5. Lucas, M. Dewhurst, C. J., Hurly, R., Anderson, S., and Blunt, S.: A search for triple X females in a fertile population. J. Obstet. Gynaec. Brit. Comm. 78:1087, 1971.
6. Capraro, V. J., and Capraro, E. J.: Creation of a neovagina—a simplified technique. Obstet. Gynec. *39*:544, 1972.
7. Capraro, V. J.: Surgical Correction of Genital Anomalies. *In* Davis' Gynecology and Obstetrics. Chapter 27, Vol. 2. Hagerstown, Md., Harper & Row Publishers, 1968.
8. Capraro, V. J., and Greenberg, H.: Adhesions of the labia minora. Obstet. Gynec. *39*:65, 1972.

Diagnosis and Management
of Ambiguous Sexual Development

JOHN F. CRIGLER, JR.

Harvard Medical School,
The Children's Hospital Medical Center

INTRODUCTION—THE PROBLEM

Variations of external genitals (ambiguous sexual development) from "almost normal" male to normal female can be seen in patients with any of the causes of abnormal genital development. Patient 1 (Figure 21–7), who had slight enlargement of the genital tubercle and minimal fusion of the posterior labio-scrotal folds, had palpable masses in the inguinal canal, a chromatin negative buccal smear, and a leukocyte karyotype with a 46,XY chromosomal complement. Retrograde contrast studies revealed a shallow, V-shaped vagina but no cervix or uterus. Two testes, each with a vas deferens, were found in the inguinal canals at surgery, with no internal female genital structures being seen (regression of

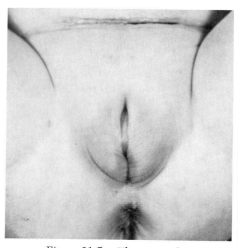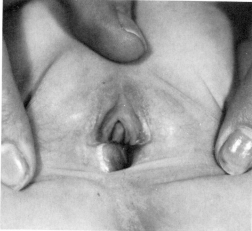

Figure 21-7. The external genitalia of an infant with a 46,XY leukocyte karyotype and normal testis (male pseudohermaphrodite).

Müllerian ducts). This infant, therefore, is phenotypically female but genetically and gonadally male. Sex assignment should be female, since masculinization of the external genitals is minimal, in spite of the presence of testis, and reconstruction of normal male genitals (a surgical decision) is virtually impossible. The patient is a male pseudohermaphrodite (an individual with ambiguous genital development and testes) who, presumably, has a cellular defect in the metabolism of testosterone (deficiency of 5α-reductase) in genital tissues (the external genitals), which made him unresponsive to normal concentrations of testicular androgens during fetal life. For this reason, the patient would not be expected to undergo normal masculinization at adolescence, another reason for the female sex assignment.

In contrast, the patient whose genitalia are shown in Figure 21–8 is obviously a phenotypic male, having a well-developed phallus with a slight cordee but with total fusion of the labioscrotal folds and a penile urethra, although there are no palpable gonads. The buccal smear was chromatin positive and leukocyte karyotype was 46,XX. Retrograde contrast studies revealed a male-type urethra without evidence of a urogenital sinus, vagina, or other Müllerian duct structures (uterus or tubes). Urinary 17-ketosteroid levels were elevated, and the infant showed salt-losing at the end of the second week of life, thus establishing a diagnosis of congenital adrenocortical hyperplasia in an otherwise normal female infant. This infant, therefore, is a female pseudohermaphrodite, with ambiguous external genitals and ovaries. A female sex assignment, with surgical correction of the external genitals (removal of phallus, protecting the urethral sphincter, and a vaginoplasty) is indicated, since she has the potential for an entirely normal life in this sex role.

These two patients have been chosen to introduce a discussion of the diagnosis and management of infants with ambiguous genital development, since they illustrate the importance of a systematic approach to the problem based on an understanding of the factors that determine differentiation of the gonads, genital ducts, and external genitalia in fetal life. Such a definition of the pathophysiology

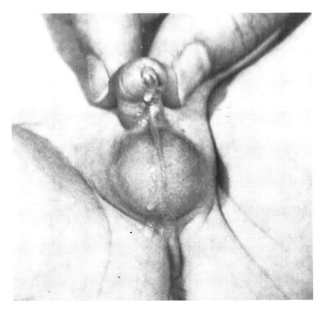

Figure 21-8. The external genitalia of an infant with a 46,XX leukocyte karyotype and normal ovaries and internal female genitalia (female pseudohermaphrodite with congenital adrenocortical hyperplasia).

of these disorders takes advantage of the infant's own fetal hormonal function (e.g., inadequate masculinization of the external genitals in the first patient or abnormal masculinization in the second) not only to establish a cause for the disorder but also to predict subsequent function in adult life, often a most important consideration in patients in whom no ideal solution may be evident.

DIAGNOSIS: AN ETIOLOGIC CLASSIFICATION OF THE CAUSES OF ABNORMAL SEXUAL DEVELOPMENT

The classic studies of geneticists and experimental embryologists on the roles of the sex chromosomes in the differentiation of gonads and of fetal gonadal function on the development of genital ducts and external genitalia serve as a basis for a diagnostic classification of the cause of abnormal sexual development in infants (Table 21–3).

It is postulated currently that sex-determining genes on the X and Y chromosomes are responsible, through their effects on cellular function of the primitive gonads, for differentiation of the tissues into either a testis or an ovary.

TABLE 21–3.   *An Etiologic Classification of Causes of Ambiguous Genital Development*

PRIMARY ABNORMALITY	PHENOTYPE	BUCCAL SMEAR
I. Gonadal		
A. Structural		
1. Gonadal dysgenesis or destruction	Male, female, or ambiguous	±
2. True hermaphroditism	Ambiguous	±
3. Tubular fibrosis (Klinefelter's) or atrophy (Reifenstein's) and germinal aplasia	Male or ambiguous	±
4. Secondary to neuroendocrine dysfunction (hypopituitarism, Kallman's)	Male (micropenis, small testes)	–
B. Functional*		
1. Male pseudohermaphroditism (including feminizing testicular syndrome and CAH† due to 3β-ol-dehydrogenase deficiency)	Ambiguous, female	–
2. Female pseudohermaphroditism? (cystic ovaries of newborn—Stein-Leventhal syndrome?)	Ambiguous	+
II. Extragonadal (female pseudohermaphroditism)		
A. Congenital adrenocortical hyperplasia	Ambiguous	+
B. Maternal ingestion of virilizing hormones	Ambiguous	+
C. Maternal virilizing lesions (e.g., arrhenoblastoma)	Ambiguous	+
III. End organ: defects of the external genitals without an apparent gonadal abnormality (e.g., extrophy of the bladder, cleft scrotum, etc.). Often associated with urinary tract abnormalities.	Ambiguous	±

* Includes patients who may have a defect in gonadal steroid synthesis or an end-organ insensitivity owing to an abnormality of extragonadal steroid hormone metabolism or some other factor. This fact must be kept in mind when assigning the sex of the patient.
    † Congenital adrenocortical hyperplasia.

Embryologic studies have indicated that (1) normal fetal testicular function (production of a Müllerian inhibition factor and an androgen) is required for masculine differentiation of genital ducts (i.e., Wolffian duct development with regression of the Müllerian duct) and external genitals; (2) female differentiation of genital ducts and external genitalia will occur when gonadal tissue fails to develop or is destroyed before genital duct development begins; (3) androgenic steroid hormones (e.g., testosterone) can substitute in part for the loss of testicular androgens in the castrated male fetus (development of the Wolffian duct and external genitals) and will produce varying degrees of masculinization of the genital system, principally external genitalia, of normal female fetuses.

Diagnostic information concerning these factors which determine genital development are gained from the following clinical procedures: (1) a genetic history, with a buccal smear and cytogenetic study; (2) serum or urinary steroid hormone analysis (17-hydroxyprogesterone in serum or urinary 17-ketosteroids usually suffice); (3) retrograde contrast x-ray studies to define the urogenital abnormalities; (4) clinical follow-up for evidence of a salt-losing state; and (5) a surgical exploration if extragonadal causes of the ambiguous genitalia are excluded (Table 21–3).

MANAGEMENT

SEX ASSIGNMENT. When inappropriate sex assignments are made in the neonatal period, the problems arising may indeed be difficult ones. It is imperative, therefore, to make a workable decision at the earliest possible age.

GONADAL OR END-ORGAN ABNORMALITIES (GROUPS I AND III). In patients with these disorders, sex assignments are largely made on the basis of the appearance of the external genitals and the problems in surgical reconstruction which they present. Such an important decision, however, should not be made until the probable cause of the abnormality is known from genetic studies, physical examination, x-ray retrograde contrast investigations, and surgical exploration, the latter two procedures carried out when other studies are insufficient to define the total anomaly. Buccal smears, which are very helpful in excluding extragonadal masculinization of females (excluded by a chromatin negative smear), most often do not differentiate between the gonadal and end-organ causes of abnormal genitalia, since both groups of patients may have either chromatin positive or chromatin negative cells. Cytogenetic studies, however, may differentiate between those patients with structural defects (e.g., gonadal or mixed gonadal dysgenesis, true hermaphroditism, and so forth) and those with structurally normal gonads (functional gonadal abnormalities, end-organ defects), the former showing abnormal sex chromosomes and the latter normal male or female karyotypes.

Patients with *structural defects of gonads* and ambiguous development (see Table 21–3) are most often reared as females since they have little, if any, potential for male fertility and often have inadequate male external genitalia, making surgical correction difficult or impossible. True hermaphrodites, after removal of testicular tissue and inappropriate male organs, may be able to fulfill the role of a normal adult female without hormonal therapy. The greatest problem arises in this group of patients when an infant has a small and probably inadequate phallus with a penile urethra. In such patients, a sex assignment is made only after a careful radiological and surgical evaluation of the entire genital system. If gonads are absent, a female sex assignment is usually made, especially if retrograde studies show a rudimentary vagina. If a micropenis and small testes exist, the decision on sex assignment is difficult. In general, a male sex assignment is made if the penis increases in size with the administration of human chorionic gonadotropin (HCG) or testosterone for 1 to 3 months, the response of the testes to HCG being determined by following changes in serum testosterone levels.

A diagnosis of *male pseudohermaphroditism* is established essentially when the patient has a chromatin negative buccal smear and gonads which are normal in size for age are palpable in the inguinal canal or scrotum. A genetic history may reveal other affected individuals in the family, as some forms of the syndrome are inherited as either a sex-limited recessive or a sex-limited autosomal dominant trait. In male pseudohermaphrodites, however, there may be a paradoxical relationship between the appearance of the external genitals and type of secondary sexual development at adolescence on the one hand, and the development of the genital ducts on the other. This fact is illustrated by the adult male pseudohermaphrodite who is completely feminized externally but who has a blind vaginal pouch without an upper vagina, cervix, uterus, or fallopian tubes (feminizing testicular syndrome). In contrast, male pseudohermaphrodites with external genitals that are ambiguous or resemble the hypospadiac male and who undergoes masculinization at puberty may show, at surgical exploration, extensive development of female genital ducts (urogenital sinus with vagina, uterus, and tubes). These individuals presumably have testes which do not produce the Müllerian inhibition factor. In addition, testes of adult male pseudohermaphrodites are reported to show undeveloped tubules composed mostly of Sertoli cells and undifferentiated germinal epithelium. For these reasons, it is most often advisable to recommend that male pseudohermaphrodites be reared as females in spite of their genetic sex and the structurally normal-appearing testes in childhood. Such a decision is especially appropriate if there is minimal masculinization of the external genitals in the newborn, suggesting end-organ insensitivity to androgens.

EXTRAGONADAL ABNORMALITIES (FEMALE PSEUDOHERMAPHRODITES)

An early diagnosis of these disorders, important at times to the survival of the patient (for example, in infants with salt-losing congenital adrenocortical hyperplasia), eliminates a problem in sex assignment even though the external genitalia may be totally masculinized (Figure 21–8). The genital abnormality in almost all of these infants (or children, if the condition is overlooked in the neonatal period) is associated with either congenital adrenocortical hyperplasia or maternal ingestion of sex hormones (usually progestational) early in pregnancy for obstetrical reasons—e.g., bleeding or repeated abortion. The pregnancy history and genetic background, therefore, are most important, the former in diagnosing abnormalities associated with the maternal use of hormones in early pregnancy and the latter in establishing the presence of congenital adrenocortical hyperplasia, which is inherited as an autosomal recessive characteristic. Since patients in Group II are masculinized females, they have chromatin positive buccal smears and normal female karyotypes. Elevated serum 17-hydroxyprogesterone and testosterone levels or urinary 17-ketosteroids (or pregnanetriol), or clinical evidence of salt-losing (most often not evident until the second week of life) establishes a diagnosis of congenital adrenocortical hyperplasia, and appropriate hormonal and fluid therapy is required. A history of the ingestion during early pregnancy of one of the hormones previously associated with virilization of female infants* is sufficient cause for development of abnormal external genitalia in a genetic female who has normal urinary 17-ketosteroid levels, although, in markedly virilized infants, demonstration of normal internal sex organs by x-ray or surgical exploration may be desirable to exclude a possible associated gonadal defect.

SURGICAL THERAPY

In patients with gonadal defects (Group I), surgical therapy consists either in correction of hypospadias and undescended testes with removal of inappropriate female organs or in removal of the phallus (and of the testes in male pseudohermaphrodites) and reconstruction of a satisfactory vagina, if one is not already present. The vaginal reconstruction is usually deferred until young adult life. If excessive breast development occurs at adolescence in male pseudohermaphrodites reared as males, the breast should be surgically removed, since testosterone therapy will not cause regression of the breast enlargement.

Female infants with congenital adrenocortical hyperplasia require surgical correction of the external genitals. Clitoral extirpation and a preliminary vaginoplasty are usually done between 6 and 12 months of age, if the infants have responded well to hormonal replacement therapy. Surgery is done at this age to remove the psychological distress of abnormal genitalia for the parents, and subsequently for the child, at the earliest time consistent with good surgical results and minimal risks. Further vaginal surgery is done, usually between 16 and 20 years of age. Female infants virilized by maternal ingestion of hormones undergo surgical correction of the external genitals only if the defect is sufficient to interfere with subsequent function.

HORMONAL THERAPY

Patients with *gonadal defects* do not require therapy until adolescence, although we have occasionally used human chorionic gonadotropin (500 I.U. 3 times a week intramuscularly for 1 to 3 months) or testosterone in infants to determine the ability of the testes and male external genitals to respond appropriately. At adolescence, those individuals reared as males who do not produce sufficient testosterone will require either gonadotropin (for patients with responsive testes) or testosterone therapy. Testosterone can be administered either orally (methyltestosterone or testosterone propionate buccal tablets, 5 to 30 mg. per day) or intramuscularly (testosterone cyclopentylpropionate, 25 to 100 mg. weekly; testosterone enanthate 50 to 200 mg. every 2 to 4 weeks). Testosterone is the hormone most often used for long-term treatment. Dosages of testosterone are increased over the adolescent period. In hypogonadal patients reared as females, estrogen therapy is begun usually at about 13 years of age using conjugated estrogens (0.3 to 0.625 mg./day). The dose may be increased to 1.25 to 2.5 mg./day and is used continually when female genital ducts are absent. If a uterus is pres-

---

* The following compounds have been reported to be associated with masculinization of otherwise normal female infants: testosterone, 17α-methyltestosterone, 17α-methylandrostenediol, 17α-ethynyltestosterone (Ethisterone, Pranone), 17α-ethynyl-19-nortestosterone (Norlutin), norethynodrel (Enovid), and diethylstilbestrol.

ent, cyclic therapy using the latter dosages (1.25 to 2.5 mg./day) for the first 21 days of each month, with medroxyprogesterone (10 mg./day) for the last 5 days of each estrogen cycle is begun. More recently, Enovid-E (norethynodrel, 2.5 mg.; mestranol, 0.1 mg.) daily for the first 20 days of each month has been used successfully by others for replacement therapy and may be preferable to the combination of estrogen and progesterone mentioned above.

Patients with congenital adrenocortical hyperplasia require replacement glucocorticoid and mineralocorticoid therapy. No gonadal hormonal therapy is necessary for female pseudohermaphrodites.

PSYCHOLOGIC FACTORS IN MANAGEMENT

Many unnecessary psychological problems can be avoided by appropriate management of patients with ambiguous genitalia in the neonatal period. The parents (and the patients when they are older) should be made tactfully and objectively aware of structural and functional limits of the abnormality in an understandable way, and they should be consulted and informed before all therapeutic procedures are undertaken. If all the facts concerning the cause of the abnormal genitalia are discussed and the origin of the abnormality is explained on the basis of a structural or functional developmental defect, the parents, and subsequently the patient, can obtain an appropriate and accurate understanding of the abnormality and of the necessary surgical and medical therapy for it. With such understanding, most patients are able to adjust satisfactorily to the significant defect in sexual function that sometimes is present. Occasionally, however, the patients become so disturbed in adolescence and young adult life that more intensive and formal psychiatric therapy is advisable.

Diagnosis and Management
of Ambiguous Sexual Development

JOHN W. HUFFMAN

Northwestern University Medical School,
Passavant Memorial Hospital, and Cook County
Graduate School of Medicine

> There once was a lady from Skye
> Who saw a young man passing by.
> With an envious eye,
> She said with a sigh:
> "There, but for a Y, go I."

The diagnosis of ambiguous genitalia in infants differs somewhat from the diagnosis in older girls and adults.

In infancy it is necessary to differentiate between the following conditions:

1. Ambiguous genitalia owing to androgenic substances received during early prenatal life.

2. Ambiguous genitalia owing to exposure to androgenic substances throughout antenatal life.

    a. Androgen-producing maternal tumors.

    b. Congenital adrenal cortical hyperplasia.

    c. Excessive maternal secretion of endogenous androgen (from ovary? from adrenal?).

3. Ambiguous genitalia owing to failure of normal development of the urogenital sinus and cloaca.

4. Ambiguous genitalia associated with gonadal dysgenesis in which the patient suffers from chromosomal mosaicism, with one cell line containing a Y chromosome.

5. Hermaphroditism.

6. The androgen intensitivity (testicular feminizing) syndrome.

7. Male pseudohermaphroditism.

The diagnosis begins in the delivery room or the nursery where the obstetrician or the pediatrician has a mandate to examine the genitalia of the newborn infant. At that time, the examiner notes the size of the clitoris, the location of the urethral meatus, the patency of the hymenal orifice, the appearance of the labia majora and minora and the presence or absence of masses suggestive of gonads in the inguinal canals or the labia majora.

This examination will differentiate between babies with morphologically normal genitalia, those with ambiguous genitalia, and those with gonads in the abdominal wall or vulva. It will not identify males with the androgen insensitivity syndrome who have intraabdominal testes. It may also fail to detect the individual who has essentially normal female external genitalia but who has anomalies of the internal genitalia and a Y chromosome in the karyotype; such individuals may not reveal their intersexual problem until puberty and some not even then.

The female child whose mother received a progestational or androgenic hormone during early pregnancy may be born with anomalous development of the external genitalia. The degree of deformity varies tremendously. Most infants have a large clitoris but one which *does not* reveal androgenic stimulation at birth (Figure 21–9). The phallus is long, lean, and flaccid, not plump and turgid. The vulva may be otherwise essentially normal, or a persistent urogenital sinus may have a minute, urethral-like opening at the base of the clitoris. Rarely, a urethral orifice may open on the shaft or at the tip of the glans of the phallus. The vagina, uterus, uterine tubes, and ovaries of these children are normal.

The child who received androgenic hormonal stimulation early in its antenatal life and developed ambiguous genitalia is a normal female with a normal percentage of Barr bodies in her buccal or vaginal smears, a 46,XX chromosomal constitution, and normal findings on endocrinological and biochemical assays.

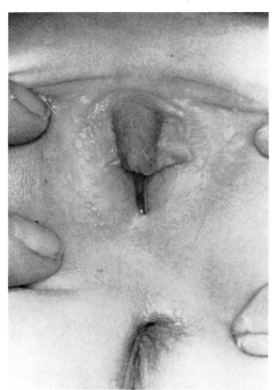

Figure 21-9. Iatrogenic pseudohermaphroditism. The mother of this infant received a progestin containing nortestosterone for threatened abortion during the early part of her pregnancy. The child's vagina and internal genitalia are normal. (From Huffman, J. W.: The Gynecology of Childhood and Adolescence. Philadelphia, W. B. Saunders Co., 1968).

The mother's history of receiving hormonal therapy, most often for threatened abortion, is very significant in making the diagnosis. Differentiation from gonadal dysgenesis, hermaphroditism, the androgen insensitivity syndrome, and male pseudohermaphroditism is established by examination of buccal or vaginal smears for chromatin bodies and chromosomal analysis.

There may be some difficulty in differentiating between the infant with ambiguous genitalia resulting from androgenic substances received in early antenatal life and one with ambiguous genitalia resulting from failure of normal development of the urogenital sinus and cloaca. However, the latter almost invariably has anomalies of the urinary and gastrointestinal tracts associated with a persistent urogenital sinus.

I have seen (and others have reported) girls with considerable clitoral enlargement strongly suggestive of antenatal androgenic stimulation (Figure 21–10). However, these patients' mothers did not receive any hormonal preparation during their pregnancies. The patients' histories were not notable, and endocrinologic assays were not enlightening. In several such cases, however, the patients' mothers stated that they had developed rather marked virilization during their pregnancies. It may be assumed that endogenous androgen produced by the mothers caused hypertrophy of the embryonic clitoris.

The external genitalia of the newborn female who has been subjected to androgenic stimulation through her antenatal life are entirely different in appearance from those described above.

A maternal ovarian androgen-producing tumor developing during pregnancy may produce a high titer of androgens. Not only does the mother develop

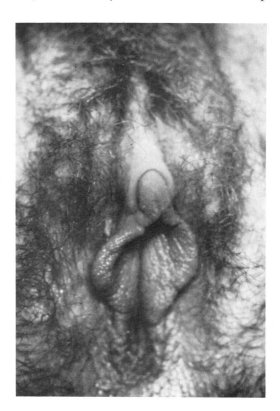

Figure 21-10. Idiopathic clitoral hypertrophy. Patient, 18 years of age, whose mother received no hormones during pregnancy but who did develop well-defined virilization during gestation, which disappeared after delivery.

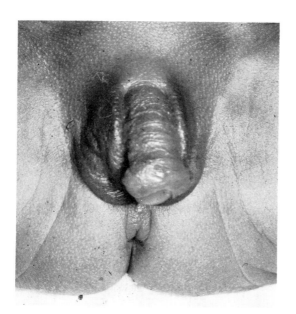

Figure 21-11. Virilization of a newborn female by a maternal masculinizing tumor. In this case the tumor was diagnosed as a luteoma. (Courtesy of Dr. Melvin E. Jenkins, Washington, D.C. From Huffman, J. W.: The Gynecology of Childhood and Adolescence. Philadelphia, W. B. Saunders Co., 1968.)

marked virilization but also the external genitalia of the embryo develop in a masculine direction. If the tumor is not removed before delivery, the infant is born with a large, plump phallus, which may be considerably larger than the penis of a normal newborn male (Figure 21–11). The urogenital sinus will have persisted, and the vagina and urethra open into it. Like the newborn who received androgen early in embryonic life, the baby is a chromosomal female with normal chromatin bodies in the buccal smear. Her endocrinologic and biochemical assay findings will be normal for her age.

The diagnostically significant factors in such cases are the mother's condition; the identification of increased androgenic hormone elaboration by the mother; and, in contradistinction to the child who has not been exposed to androgen for some time, the marked androgenic response in the clitoral tissues.

Ambiguity of the female external genitalia as a result of congenital adrenal cortical hyperplasia is the most frequently encountered problem of this type. There are several types of prenatal adrenal cortical dysfunction characterized by defective synthesis of cortisol. The type caused by failure to elaborate 21-hydroxylase, which converts 17-hydroxyprogesterone to cortisol, is the most common.

The babies are physically normal except for the condition of their genitalia. The labia minora are fused and the perineal body is thickened. The phallus is large and turgid. The fused labia, which resemble a wrinkled scrotum with a median raphe but without contained gonads, are often deeply pigmented. In addition, there may be some generalized skin pigmentation. An opening at the base of the phallus represents the orifice of the urogenital sinus (Figure 21–12). In most cases, the urethra and vagina open into the vestibule above the fused labia. Less commonly, the opening of the urogenital sinus may form a true penile urethra. In the latter instance, the vaginal orifice may be a minute aperture some distance above the perineal skin.

The turgid condition of the phallus, the skin pigmentation, the absence of gonads in the pseudoscrotum, and a mucoid (sometimes blood-stained) "urethral" discharge are significant findings. A mucoid discharge, especially if it is blood-

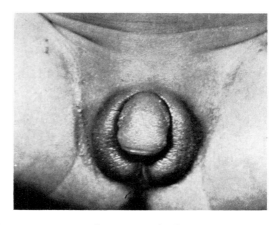

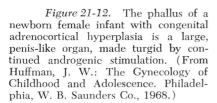
Figure 21-12. The phallus of a newborn female infant with congenital adrenocortical hyperplasia is a large, penis-like organ, made turgid by continued androgenic stimulation. (From Huffman, J. W.: The Gynecology of Childhood and Adolescence. Philadelphia, W. B. Saunders Co., 1968.)

tinged, is evidence that the child has a vagina and uterus which communicate with the urogenital sinus.

A buccal smear is, after the physical examination, the first diagnostic step. It is well to remember, however, that the percentage of cells containing chromatin bodies in the normal female may be relatively low during the first few postnatal days.

Endocrinologic tests determine the output of 17-ketosteroids in the urine and pregnanetriol in the urine or plasma. In a normal infant, the tests may be deceiving during the first few days after birth, when the levels of both 17-ketosteroids and pregnanetriol may be elevated. After the first week, however, the normal 24-hour excretion of 17-ketosteroids should not exceed 1 mg., and the urinary pregnanetriol excretion rate should not be more than 0.5 mg. per 24 hours. Plasma pregnanetriol levels are normally between 5 and 35 μg./100 ml. (the diagnostic levels of plasma pregnanetriol are from 80 to 550 μg./100 ml.). In an untreated infant with congenital adrenal cortical hyperplasia and excessive androgen output, two or more of these tests will reveal elevated titers.

Defective production of aldosterone in some cases of adrenogenital syndrome associated with congenital adrenal cortical hyperplasia may cause a marked increase in the urinary excretion of salt. This usually occurs during the latter part of the first week of life, but may develop precipitously at any time after birth. The child becomes listless and hypotonic, and develops vomiting, dehydration (Figure 21–13), and weight loss, and quickly succumbs unless actively treated. In the early stages of the salt-losing syndrome, the serum potassium level is elevated,

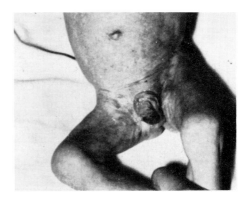

Figure 21-13. Salt-losing form of the congenital adrenogenital syndrome. Salt and fluid loss has caused obvious weight loss and necessitated intravenous fluid therapy. (From Dewhurst, C. J., and Gordon, R. R.: The Intersexual Disorders. Baltimore, Williams and Wilkins Co., 1969.)

the amount of blood urea nitrogen increases, and a sharp decrease in serum sodium level occurs. The presence of the salt-losing syndrome in a child with ambiguous androgen-stimulated genitalia is sufficient to make the diagnosis, without recourse to endocrinologic investigation.

Children with an 11-hydroxylase deficiency, which is uncommon, present with ambiguous genitalia, signs of androgenic stimulation, and elevated 17-ketosteroid and pregnanetriol titers. They have hypertension rather than a salt-losing syndrome.

Some cases of infants with ambiguous genitalia are grouped under the general heading of *gonadal dysgenesis*. The children are born with a moderately large phallus, which does not show prenatal androgenic stimulation, and a persistent urogenital sinus. The phallus is usually larger than a clitoris. The urogenital sinus is frequently an outlet for the urethra and a more or less well-formed vagina. There may or may not be a gonad in one of the labioscrotal folds. The internal genitalia consist of poorly formed female and male structures. Such infants are usually really pseudohermaphroditic males with an XO/XY karyotype. They may have a unicornuate uterus and a rudimentary uterine tube on one side, or paramesonephric structures may be absent. One or both gonads will be rudimentary testes or gonadal ridges with medullary elements in them. Most of these patients, but not all, will be chromatin negative. In infancy and childhood they are likely to be diagnosed as having the androgen insensitivity syndrome. As they grow older, they tend to be eunuchoid in habitus, of average or taller-than-average height, and, beyond the usual time for puberty, to show signs of virilization (Figure 21–14). They develop a large phallus, hirsutism, and virilism. After puberty they have a 17-ketosteroid titer lower than that for a normal male but higher than that for a normal female. Their pituitary gonadotropin titer may or may not be elevated.

The diagnosis of *hermaphroditism* cannot be made without histologic proof that the patient has both ovarian and testicular tissue. A child who has ambiguous genitalia which are not androgen-stimulated at birth, a chromatin positive smear, and XX karyotype and a normal 17-ketosteroid titer will be suspect. The external genitalia in true hermaphroditism, however, are not always anomalous; occasionally they are morphologically male or female, and heterosexual gonadal tissues are not found until an operation for some sexually unrelated cause exposes the patient's internal genitalia. In such cases a phenotypical female may have a normal ovary on one side and a fragment of testicular tissue with a portion of the

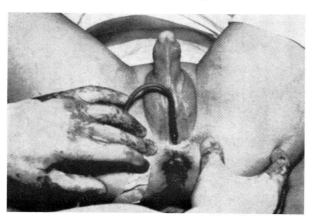

Figure 21-14. Androgenic type of gonadal dysgenesis. Phallus-like organ and vaginal orifice, below catheter inserted in urethra, of 14 year old patient. Laparotomy revealed a dysgenetic rudimentary streak of gonadal tissue on the left, a uterus, uterine tubes and a testicle on the right. Buccal smears were chromatin negative, and the karyotype was XO/XY. (From Greenblatt, R., *et al.*: Gonadal dysgenesis intersex with XO/XY mosaicism. JAMA *188:* 221, 1964.)

vas deferens persisting on the opposite side. A bisexed male may have an intra-scrotal testis on one side and, internally, a contralateral ovotestis and small uterine tube.

Nuclear chromatin tests are of relatively limited use in the diagnosis of hermaphroditism. Most of the patients are chromatin positive, with an XX chromosomal constitution when only one tissue is studied. If multiple tissues are examined, most of these individuals will be XX/XY. The chromatin negative patients are usually XO/XY.

During adolescence, deviation in the development of the secondary sexual characteristics may occur in either direction. Physical development deviates most often toward femaleness. As a result, a child who has been reared as a male may menstruate and develop breasts and at the same time acquire a beard and a low-ered vocal timbre. Since both gonadal tissues may have some hormonal function, the outcome in a specific case is unpredictable.

The *testicular feminizing* (or more correctly, the *total androgen insensi-tivity) syndrome*, a type of male pseudohermaphroditism, will usually not be discovered in childhood. The child has feminine external genitalia and intra-abdominal or inguinal testes. It may be suspected in the prepuberal patient if a buccal smear is negative for chromatin bodies and a vaginal blind pouch is dis-covered on vaginoscopy. In approximately 2 per cent of the cases of infants with apparently normal external female genitalia and a gonad in one or both inguinal canals, the gonads have been found to be testes. Biopsy of the gonad establishes the definitive diagnosis.

The familial character of the syndrome is well established. In an affected family, the females are normal but 50 per cent of the males, although they have XY chromosomal constitutions, are phenotypically female. There is usually a his-tory of sisters or aunts of the patient who suffered from primary amenorrhea.

The androgen insensitivity syndrome is most apt to be diagnosed when a patient comes because of primary amenorrhea. Typically, she has well-developed breasts, a feminine habitus (Figure 21–15), sparse pubic and axillary hair, infan-tile genitalia, and a short, narrow vagina without a cervix. The uterus cannot be palpated. The buccal smear is negative, and the karyotype is found to be 46,XY. Abdominal exploration by laparotomy or laparoscopy reveals a poorly developed minute uterus and intra-abdominal or inguinal testes. Hormonal assays indicate that the biosynthesis of testosterone by these individuals is normal. Dewhurst and his coworkers have unequivocally demonstrated (as has been suspected) that the syndrome results from a failure of end-organ response to androgen.

Male pseudohermaphroditism from other causes than the total androgen insensitivity syndrome manifests itself in a variety of ways. As a rule, these indi-viduals are born with ambiguous genitalia. In most cases, the patient has an enlarged phallus without evidence of androgen stimulation, and a urogenital sinus with an opening at the base of the phallus; testes are either in the abdomen, in the inguinal canals, or in the labioscrotal folds. A few have well-developed internal paramesonephric duct derivatives (Figure 21–16). At adolescence these persons may become virilized or feminized, or remain intersexed. Some inter-sexed males have normal masculine external genitalia, become virilized at puberty, and yet have well-developed uteri and uterine tubes.

The diagnosis of pseudohermaphroditism will be made when the infant with ambiguous genitalia is found to have a buccal smear which is negative for chroma-

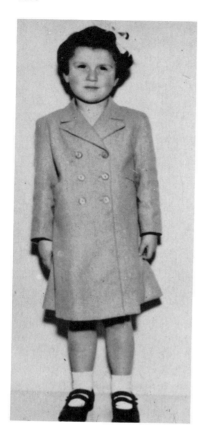

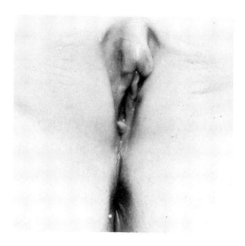

Figure 21-15. A case of the androgen insensitivity syndrome diagnosed during childhood. This patient has normal female external genitalia but had a testis in each groin. Her aunt and great-aunt have a similar abnormality. She is now 19 years of age and secondary feminization has occurred. (From Dewhurst, C. J., and Gordon, R. R.: The Intersexual Disorders. Baltimore, Williams and Wilkins Co., 1969.)

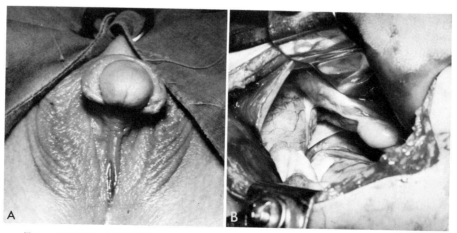

Figure 21–16. *A,* Ambiguous external genital in a male pseudohermaphroditic child. *B,* View of right side of the pelvis, showing a single abdominal testis with a uterine tube above it. (From Dewhurst, C. J., and Gordon, R. R.: The Intersexual Disorders. Baltimore, Williams and Wilkins Co., 1969.)

tin bodies and an XY chromosomal constitution. The virilized male pseudo-hermaphrodite with normal male external genitalia and rudimentary internal organs will not be diagnosed until an operation for some unrelated cause exposes their presence.

Summary

With few exceptions, intersex problems ought to be diagnosed in infancy. The exceptions are the patient with the total androgen insensitivity syndrome, the male pseudohermaphrodite with normal male external genitalia, and the hermaphrodite with normal female external genitalia. Infants with ambiguous genitalia who show signs of androgen stimulation at birth are almost certainly suffering either from congenital adrenal cortical hyperplasia or from the effects of a maternal masculinizing tumor.

Buccal smears are a primary step in the examination of individuals with ambiguous genitalia. A positive buccal smear with a normal complement of normal-sized chromatin bodies will exclude the total androgen insensitivity syndrome and male pseudohermaphroditism. A certain number of patients with ambiguous genitalia and gonadal dysgenesis will be mosaics, with chromatin positive buccal smears and an XX/XO karyotype; most such patients, however, are chromatin negative and have a Y chromosome in one of their genetic lines. In all of these individuals and in any other patient with ambiguous genitalia or who is of doubtful sex—other than those having congenital adrenal cortical hyperplasia—chromosomal analysis of one or more tissues is mandatory.

Hormone assays are of value in the diagnosis of congenital adrenal cortical hyperplasia but are otherwise not diagnostically helpful.

Laparoscopy is a useful diagnostic tool when the state of the internal genitalia is uncertain. Exploratory laparotomy with gonadal biopsy ought to be limited to those infrequent situations in which hermaphroditism is suspected. Inguinal or labial gonads in an infant with female genitalia should be biopsied.

For the most part, a careful history, the physical examination, chromatin-body determinations and chromosomal analysis will give the information which is needed to make a diagnosis when a patient presents with ambiguous genitalia.

Treatment

It is obvious that a plan for the treatment of a person with ambiguous genitalia should be made in infancy. Genetic females will be raised as females. If those suffering from congenital adrenal cortical hyperplasia are treated with cortisol from infancy, they will not be virilized; most of them will menstruate at puberty and a few will be able to conceive. Babies with the salt-losing syndrome are given desoxycorticosterone, cortisone, salt, and fluids. The infant with hyperplasia will respond to cortisone.

Females whose ambiguous genitalia are the result of fetal virilism caused by medication the mother received or by maternal endogenous androgen need no medical treatment other than, in some cases, excision of the large phallus, and division of the high perineal body.

It is most important that the parents of a female infant with ambiguous genitalia be impressed with the fact that their baby is truly female with normal female internal genitalia, that she will grow into a female adolescent and that relatively minor surgical procedures will correct her distorted external genitalia.

The clitoris should be excised in infancy, but I question the wisdom of performing a perineotomy in childhood because I have seen several patients who had been so treated who required additional plastic procedures for enlargement of the introitus before they could have coitus. I suggest that the same rule ought to hold for these patients as for those with vaginal agenesis: vaginoplasty should be delayed until they are nubile. The exception would be the girl with a very narrow urogenital sinus who might develop a mucocolpos after menarche. The technique of clitoral excision and perineotomy which is commonly used for the correction of the ambiguous genitalia of an intersexed female is shown in Figure 21–17.

Only broad generalizations can be advanced regarding the treatment of the infant with anomalous genitalia associated with other major urogenital anomalies because few cases are alike. Actually, correction of the genital abnormalities takes second place to that of the sometimes life-endangering deformities affecting the bowel or bladder. If there is fecal contamination of the urinary tract it is essential that this be eliminated as quickly as possible. Usually this can be done best by performing a colostomy. Obstruction of the urinary tract must be relieved; this may require cystostomy or ureterostomy. If the urogenital sinus cannot be used later for a urethra, a substitute will have to be created. If there is agenesis of the rectum, as there may be, an anus will have to be constructed.

The genetic male with the androgen insensitivity syndrome usually has

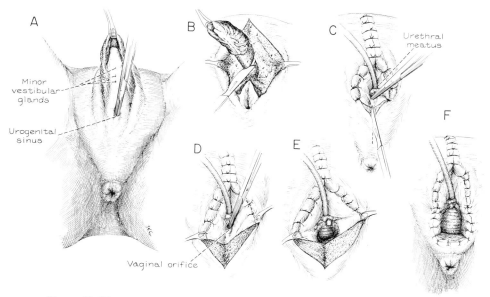

Figure 21-17. Surgical correction of the ambiguous genitalia of a pseudohermaphroditic patient consists essentially of excising the large phallus and opening the orifice of the urogenital sinus to expose the urethral and vaginal orifices. (From Huffman, J. W.: The Gynecology of Childhood and Adolescence. Philadelphia, W. B. Saunders Co., 1968.)

normal female external genitalia and is not likely to be seen until he comes as a female, complaining of primary amenorrhea or dyspareunia. Such an individual is anatomically adapted to the female role. It is much better if the patient is left in it. The possibility that the testes may undergo malignant change has been given as a reason for orchidectomy in such cases. There are varying opinions as to the likelihood of such a change occurring. Jones and Scott (1958) state that it occurs in less than 5 per cent of cases. Dewhurst and Gordon (1969) quote Polani's opinion that an ectopic testis carries a serious risk of malignancy even in the very young. Although the matter is debatable, it would seem better to convert the individual to an intersex state by orchidectomy and subsequently administer exogenous estrogens.

The sex which is assigned to an intersexed male with ambiguous genitalia depends on the size of the phallus and whether a functional penis can be created from it. Penis-consciousness is a factor in the male's sexual development, and unless he can identify with his peers, he will have major psychologic problems. The size of the penis, a penile urinary stream, and the ability to have erections are factors in gaining a masculine identity.

If it appears that a satisfactory penis cannot be constructed, the male pseudohermaphroditic child is preferably treated by orchidectomy and excision of the phallus, and then reared as a female. Estrogen administration is begun at the time of puberty.

The sex assigned to an hermaphrodite also depends on the structure of the external genitalia. The major consideration, as Dewhurst and Gordon note, is how well the genitalia can be made to conform to the sex in which the child is to be reared (or is living, if sex has already been assigned). Necessary surgical plastic procedures to alter the genitalia and reassignment of sex are justifiable in those intersexed persons who, upon becoming adolescents, find themselves uncomfortable in their assigned sex and discover sexual urges incompatible with it.

REFERENCES

Bishop, P.: Intersexual states and allied conditions. Brit. Med. J. 1:1255, 1966.

Boczkowski, K., and Teter, J.: Clinical, histological and cytogenetic observations on intersexuality. Obstet. Gynec. 27:7, 1966.

Clayton, G., et al.: Familial true hermaphroditism in pre- and postpuberal genetic females. Hormonal and morphologic studies. J. Clin. Endocr. 18:1349, 1958.

Dewhurst, C. J.: Sex chromosome abnormaliites and the gynaecologist. J. Obstet. Gynec. Brit. Comm. 78:1058, 1971.

Dewhurst, C. J., and Gordon, R. R.: The Intersexual Disorders. Baltimore, Williams and Wilkins, 1969.

Ferguson-Smith, M.: Karyotype-phenotype correlations in gonadal dysgenesis and their bearing on the pathogenesis of malformations. J. Med. Genet. 2:142, 1965.

Huffman, J. W.: Functional anomalies of the female genitalia. Pacific Med. Surg. 73:161, 1965.

Huffman, J. W.: The Gynecology of Childhood and Adolescence. Philadelphia, W. B. Saunders Company, 1968.

Jones, H., et al.: Pathological and cystogenetic findings in true hermaphroditism: A report of 6 cases and a review of 23 cases from the literature. Obstet. Gynec. 25:435, 1965.

Moore, K. (Ed.): The Sex Chromatin. Philadelphia, W. B. Saunders Company, 1966.

Morris, J.: Syndrome of testicular feminization in male pseudohermaphroditism. Amer. J. Obstet. Gynec. 65:1192, 1953. (Describes 80 cases; major contribution on subject.)

Slotnick, E. A., and Goldfarb, A. F.: Unilateral streaked ovary syndrome. Obstet. Gynec. 39:269, 1972.

Wilkins, L.: Masculinization of female fetus due to rise of orally given progestins. J.A.M.A. 172:1028, 1960.

Diagnosis and Management
of Ambiguous Sexual Development

Editorial Comment

When a patient is noted to have genital ambiguity it is understood that great care and compassion must be used in diagnosing and counseling the child and/or its parents. The authors noted the need to be alert for the possibility of salt-losing adrenogenital syndrome in the newborn period. Dr. Capraro noted the need for a team approach to the care of these individuals, with one physician acting as a spokesman. This physician is cautioned that he must use great care in choosing the words used in explaining sexual development or underdevelopment to the parents. The authors all agree that it is difficult to construct functioning male external genitalia, and the majority of these patients should be assigned the female sex. They stress the need for removal of an enlarged phallus during the first few months of life. In the past, it had been recommended that the vaginal reconstructive surgery be done just prior to the patient's marriage; the contributors, however, agree that this may now be done when the patient reaches early adulthood. Opinions have been expressed elsewhere that this might or even should be done earlier to maintain emotional equilibrium.

The authors agree that there is probable malignant potential in patients who have dysgenetic testes or intra-abdominal testes with the complete form of testicular feminization. They feel that when the diagnosis is made, these testes should be removed. However, there is some debate on this point—some authors believe that in the complete form of testicular feminization, the patient should be allowed to develop female secondary sexual characteristics and then have the intra-abdominal testes removed.

It is evident from these papers that with corrective surgical techniques, hormonal replacement, and careful and effective counseling, the individual with sexual ambiguity will reach adulthood with relatively normal appearing genitalia and with normal sexual function.

724

22

The Value and Limitations of Endocrine Assays Specifically for Obstetrical and Gynecological Conditions

Alternative Points of View:

By Dwain D. Hagerman and E. Stewart Taylor

By M. Wayne Heine

Editorial Comment

The Value and Limitations
of Endocrine Assays Specifically
for Obstetrical and Gynecological Conditions

DWAIN D. HAGERMAN AND E. STEWART TAYLOR

When we speak of "assays specifically for obstetrical and gynecological conditions" we generally mean special laboratory analyses which the clinician wishes to obtain on samples from his patients which the central hospital laboratory does not perform. Usually the tests involved are either too rarely requested or too complicated for the automatic analyzers now regularly used in such centralized laboratories to perform. It is inevitable that the cost per analysis of these special tests, which require the attention of highly skilled technicians and specialized equipment, will be very much greater than the cost for automated routine analyses, and the thoughtful clinician will not wish to request such expensive tests unless he is certain that they will be both of diagnostic value to his patients and reliably performed and reported by the laboratory. The reliability of the laboratory is particularly important in the case of endocrine analyses, for despite much technological progress in recent years, hormone analysis of biological samples remains an area filled with pitfalls for the inexperienced and often overconfident clinical pathologist or chemist, no matter how competent he may be in other areas. It may be that these complexities of a purely technical nature have unduly delayed application of endocrinologic analysis in obstetrics and gynecology, and that the most important point which can be learned by reading this chapter is to "beware of your analyst." At the same time, the recent rapid development of radioimmunoassay techniques for the determination of both small molecules such as steroids and larger species such as polypeptide and protein hormones may render this branch of clinical pathology as simple technically as much of the rest of the specialty has already become.[1,2] In either instance, providing some fairly detailed knowledge of the clinical status of the patient from whom the sample is

* Our laboratory work has been supported in part by Grant No. HD-05085, National Institute of Child Health and Human Development. We wish to thank K. L. Williams, P. A. Grey, and K. A. Isaacson for technical assistance. Dr. S. Vorawan, Population Council Postdoctoral Fellow (1970–1972) kindly permitted us to use some of his test results. Drs. George Betz and Sander Shapiro critically read our manuscript, but they cannot be held responsible for any errors of fact or opinion that remain in it.

727

derived, and giving the investigator some idea of the information desired from the analysis, very often greatly simplifies the task for the analyst, both in performing the test and in evaluating the validity of the results. Of course, it is the ultimate responsibility of the patient's physician to interpret the results of any procedure in the light of his full knowledge of his patient's condition.

Which Method to Use?

It is easy to set out a list of criteria for an ideal clinical laboratory method. The procedure should be chemically specific, accurate and precise to within a few per cent, and sensitive to within perhaps one tenth of the lowest value ever expected to be encountered in samples submitted to the laboratory. The method should also be theoretically sound from the physicochemical viewpoint: simple, convenient, and rapid in performance; inexpensive; and able to give results with clear-cut, critically diagnostic value to the clinician. In actual fact, the methods used rarely meet all of these criteria, and reasonable satisfaction can be afforded to all concerned if the method is rapid, possesses a generally clear empirical correlation between laboratory result obtained and the clinical condition of the patient, and is not so expensive or complicated that it cannot be employed by a majority of physicians who might find its results informative. This last specification may be quite variable, depending upon whether the practitioners involved spend their time doing full-time work in a university related hospital, contribute their services on a part-time basis to a large municipal hospital or similar institution, or operate a private practice with a small community hospital as their major health care facility.

As an example to illustrate these points, consider the determination of blood sugar. The original Folin-Wu method required a comparatively large blood sample, was technically and chemically unsatisfactory in a number of respects, and consistently overestimated the true value by about 20 mg. per 100 ml. Luckily, this inaccuracy (caused by inclusion of some nonglucose reducing substances) did not interfere with the interpretation of the results by physicians who had long since forgotten the existence of, much less the reason for, the excess, and only occasionally did it lead to minor confusion in discussions of unconsciousness related to hypoglycemia. That method was sufficiently good that it became a routine part of the initial workup of almost every hospitalized patient (as a screening test for diabetes mellitus), and it virtually replaced the earlier urinalysis for sugar content, in spite of the theoretical and practical deficiencies in the blood analysis. Only when chemists discovered methods which measured blood glucose itself, accurately and at no greater costs in time, effort, and money than the older method, was the blood sugar test replaced by the scientifically "better" method (with some initial confusion occurring in the minds of some clinicians when one of the "normal" values they expected suddenly decreased by about 20 mg. per 100 ml.

Just as the obstetrician or gynecologist will sometimes require consultation about his patients from other speciality areas, he will occasionally require endocrinologic analyses reflecting the function of glands not directly related to the reproductive system. Hopefully, his associates in general endocrinology will be able to provide these services, just as he may be able to assist them with the special analyses particularly related to obstetrics and gynecology. This chapter is organized from the viewpoint of the analyst, in terms of the chemistry of the molecules involved, rather than from the viewpoint of the careful clinician who considers the tests in terms of the organization of the organ systems involved (pituitary and hypothalamus, thyroid, adrenal cortex, ovary, placenta and fetus).

Hypothalamic Releasing and Inhibiting Factors

Perhaps the most exciting area of research in reproductive biology at the present time is that of the hypothalamic releasing or inhibiting hormones which apparently play the predominant role in the regulation of all of the secretions of the adenohypophysis.[3]* At least in the established cases, these compounds have all been found to be small polypeptides. They are released from as yet incompletely defined areas in the brain. These areas may be the conventional gross anatomical brain nuclei, but it is likely they are much more specifically delineated sites in the hypothalamus, which are under the control of (1) feedback information in the blood concentrations of the secretory products of ultimate target organs (i.e., the long feedback loop from the gonads), (2) perhaps the concentrations of the pituitary hormones which serve as intermediates in the signal transmission process (short feedback loop), and (3) the general or specific directions of higher centers in the central nervous system. Present in extremely minute quantities, these hormones have been measured by bioassay, and it is not yet clear whether or not there are separate LH and FSH releasing hormones, although currently it appears that a single releasing hormone regulates secretion of both FSH and LH by some kind of mechanism in which differential secretion is achieved by variations in sensitivity in the pituitary, depending on the overall hormonal status of the animal at the time. Additionally, both positive and negative feedback of the steroids on the pituitary may play a role in regulation. Likewise, it is not yet known whether prolactin is controlled by means of one inhibitory hormone or two hormones, one inhibitory and the other stimulatory. The hypothalamic hormones travel directly to the pituitary via the hypophyseal portal blood system, and radioimmunoassay methods for their determination are being developed. It is not yet known whether it will be possible to make meaningful measurements of their concentration in the peripheral bloodstream. Clearly, further experimental work is required in this area, particularly in relation to the role of dopamine and other neurotransmitters in the control of the releasing factors themselves, but the results of such experimentation will undoubtedly clarify some of the still mysterious interactions between the reproductive tract and the central nervous system, and might possibly point the way toward the development of improved methods of fertility control, both supportive and preventive.

Other Polypeptide Hormones

Another relatively small polypeptide hormone, oxytocin, and the chemically closely related compound vasopressin, have been known for some time to be

---

* As in many rapidly advancing fields, the nomenclature here is somewhat confusing because of repeated changes. The hypothalamic substance which causes release of luteinizing hormone from the pituitary has been successively referred to as LH releasing factor (LHRF), LH releasing hormone (LHRH), and LH regulating hormone (LHRH). The names of the other factors have evolved similarly.

synthesized in specific cells of the hypothalamus and to travel thence via axonal paths to the neurohypophysis (posterior pituitary). These hormones and a series of naturally occurring analogues found in various species of the Chordates probably arose during evolution from a common precursor, but in man they clearly serve separate functions and are independently released as required from the posterior pituitary. Despite our apparent ability now to measure blood oxytocin concentrations by radioimmunoassay,[4] no clinical trial of this measurement seems to have been validated. A variety of procedures for evaluation of "oxytocinase" activity in blood (which would remove the hormone and thus lower its concentration) have also been evaluated. Of these, measurement of cystine aminopeptidase activity in serum is probably the most specific in a group of rather nonspecific analyses. However, the clinical value of the procedure has never been clearly established.

Radioimmunoassay methods for measuring blood concentrations of the glycoprotein gonadotropins (luteinizing hormone, follicle stimulating hormone, and chorionic gonadotropin) have generally confirmed the deductions based on bioassays. The subunit structure of these hormones, with one common unit of constant composition and one variable composition fraction, complicated the preparation of specific antibodies, but these difficulties have been solved. Two interesting facts have been demonstrated by the new data: first, there is a large but brief (12 to 24 hour) increase in serum LH concentration just prior to ovulation, and second, the serum FSH concentration is closely synchronized with the corresponding LH concentration throughout the cycle. The LH/FSH ratio is not exactly constant, which accords with the idea that the functions of these hormones are separate and distinct, but the data require that their action be more closely coordinated and dependent on target organ sensitivity than heretofore believed. It would at present appear that a signal to the hypothalamus, consisting of a transitory rise in estrogen concentration, indicates to the hypothalamus that a follicle is in the last stages of preparation for ovulation and sensitizes the pituitary to hypothalamic LH releasing hormone (LHRH), that the LHRH relays this information to the anterior pituitary, that the latter in turn responds with the LH surge (which is accompanied by a similarly brief increase in serum FSH concentration), and that this sudden increase in gonadotropin concentration is the proximate cause of ovulation.[1] The concentrations of these hormones have been serially determined in many subjects and cycles, with highly consistent results, but nevertheless such measurements are probably not useful in determining the time of ovulation precisely in the ordinary clinical situation. The rise and fall in concentration of both LH and FSH is so brief that blood sampling—even when performed as frequently as daily—might easily miss the top of the ovulatory peak, giving an ambiguous result. Only further trial will settle this point. Other clinical situations in which LH determinations might be useful may appear as the test becomes more commonly available. Precise determination of FSH concentrations in blood do not seem to have any clinical usefulness at all as yet.[5] In principle, one should be able to distinguish among hypothalamic, pituitary, or ovarian dysfunction as the primary factor in failure to ovulate by determining concentrations of releasing hormone and gonadotropin in blood, but this possibility remains to be demonstrated as clinically feasible. The blood determinations certainly should replace the common total urine gonadotropin bioassay in the diagnostic routine for hirsute or mildly virilized women, or in the investigation of precocious puberty, and in the selection of patients for attempts at artificial stimulation of ovulation.

At least three and perhaps more protein hormones from the placenta, chorionic gonadotropin, chorionic somatomammotropin, and placental thyrotropin, make their appearance during pregnancy, and specific radioimmunoassay methods for the first two of these are now available. The bioassays for chorionic gonadotropin in urine, which have long been used as a basis for pregnancy testing, can now be abandoned, much to the relief of those who have in the past been responsible for their results.

The immunoassay for chorionic gonadotropin with a hemagglutination inhibition end point can be applied to urine for pregnancy testing and is far more reliable, quicker, and less expensive than any of the bioassays. It is available commercially in kit form to any practitioner who wishes to retain some laboratory work in his own establishment. The test is also sufficiently simple to be attractive, from the economic standpoint, to directors of central hospital laboratories and commercial clinical laboratories. It might be noted that not all the available radioimmunoassay antibodies distinguish clearly between pituitary LH and placental luteinizing hormone activity, but a discrete analysis of these hormones is readily possible.

The hemagglutination analysis for chorionic gonadotropin also can be carried out in a form which gives quite reasonable quantitative (as opposed to positive/negative, pregnant/nonpregnant) results and can thus be used to monitor the progress of patients under treatment for hydatidiform mole or choriocarcinoma. Unfortunately, the commercial kits presently available are relatively insensitive at the lower end of the scale, and values in this region should be verified by radioimmunoassay, since active disease may still be present. The management of such patients probably should be left to those specialists with considerable experience in the subject because of the relative rarity and possibly very serious outcome of a curable disease, but the laboratory analysis is essential in any event, and several centers have been established to provide consultation or full care, as the individual practitioner may wish.

Measurements of chorionic somatomammotropin (human placental lactogen) in maternal blood by radioimmunoassay at first seemed promising for the characterization of placental function or size, in the diagnosis of placental insufficiency, and so forth, but as more data are collected this possibility recedes.[6] The weight—and under ordinary circumstances presumably the function—of the placenta is rather highly correlated with the weight and (presumably again) the well-being of the developing fetus, but the blood concentration of the placental product, chorionic somatomammotropin, is not so highly correlated with the size of the placenta and seems to be even less closely related to the well-being of the fetus. Not all authors would agree with this conclusion and certainly if the analytical value is indeed very low, the fetus is in great danger, but the chances are that the physician would already be aware of such a serious situation from simple clinical observation. Interpretation of the results of this analysis and of several others would be simplified if one could decide whether the fetus regulates the growth of the placenta or the placenta regulates the growth of the fetus, but in fact there appear to be relatively few circumstances in which placental size or function is rate-limiting with respect to fetal development. Exceptions to this generalization would include rare cases of placental sulfatase deficiency,[7] the theoretically possible but as yet undescribed (presumably being lethal early) placental steroid aromatase deficiency, gross placental infarction, and partial separation of the placenta. Further clinical trial in the last two conditions might be warranted.

Accurate determinations of blood prolactin in the human have only recently become available. In fact, it is only the immunologic properties of the compounds that now finally permit one to conclude that prolactin is in fact a distinct secretory product of the human pituitary, unrelated to somatotropin, even though the hormones were directly separated from animal sources some time ago.[8] During pregnancy the prolactin concentration gradually increases from almost undetectable amounts at the time of conception to a maximum at term, and then gradually declines after delivery. Prolactin at least partially inhibits development of follicles and ovulation, presumably as the result of an interplay with the other hypothalamic/gonadotropin regulating hormones. Interruption of the pituitary portal circulation or central nervous system lesions which destroy or temporarily reduce function in the hypothalamic center responsible for the production of prolactin inhibiting hormone causes persistent lactation and anovulation. It soon should be possible to synthesize this small polypeptide hormone for use in treatment of the galactorrhea.

The recent demonstration that the human placenta does in fact secrete an active thyrotropin (a possibility which has been argued for many years) does not yet seem to have been tested for any possible relation to generalized placental function or fetal well-being, but undoubtedly such studies will appear.

Other Protein Tests

Although they are not endocrine assays, determinations of serum heat-labile alkaline phosphatase, an isoenzyme derived solely from trophoblast (when the assay is correctly performed), might be discussed in connection with the protein hormones. The serum concentration of the enzyme is weakly correlated with placental weight and with estrogen excretion in the urine of pregnant women. A sudden and dramatic increase in enzyme concentration during the last four weeks of pregnancy is sometimes suggestive of pending increase in the severity of preeclampsia or of the destruction of large amounts of placental tissue as by infarction, but the general impression seems to be that little useful information is to be gained by performing the test.[9] Likewise, evaluations of maternal serum α_1-fetoglobulin concentration has not yet been shown to be of any diagnostic value, although the amount of substance in the blood is correlated in a general way with gestational age and placental and fetal weight.[10]

With the exception of chorionic gonadotropin analysis, we therefore see that analysis of maternal urine or blood for polypeptides and proteins of specific maternal, placental, or fetal origin has not provided the clinician much in the way of useful information in the specific diagnosis of gynecologic disease nor in the evaluation of the status of the fetoplacental unit. This is probably not surprising when one considers the primitive nature of the analytical methods available prior to the quite recent development of the radioimmunoassay procedures. These latter methods were not possible until a large amount of "undirected" basic research on protein hormones had been completed by investigators without specific clinical interest. More rapid progress may be expected now that the foundations have been laid.

Steroid Hormones

With the steroid hormones, for which the beginnings of the transition from bioassay to chemical analysis took place rather earlier than for the polypeptide and protein hormones, one might expect to find the indications for the various analyses and the criteria for evaluation of the results to be more clear-cut, and such is in fact true.

Two classes of steroids must be considered as primary candidates for special analyses in obstetrics and gynecology—the progestins and the estrogens. In addition, androgens, including androstenedione, testosterone, and dehydroepiandrosterone, are also present in female blood, arising from both the ovary and the adrenal. In the ovary, they are intermediates in estrogen biosynthesis and in the adrenal they are by-products. Probably the adrenal predominates quantitatively in the secretion of androgens in the normal female, with androstenedione and dehydroepiandrosterone as the principal products. Androstenedione serves as a testosterone precursor in the periphery, but only small amounts of testosterone are secreted as such by either gland. In the normal female, pregnant or not, these hormones should probably be considered as incidental products escaping, as it were, from the physiologically important biochemical pathways of biosynthesis and degradation.

Some authors have regularly found increases in blood androgen concentration in association with polycystic ovary disease, but other investigators have found the association to be inconstant. The same may be said in general for female hirsutism. Distinct increases in blood androgen concentration, therefore, are strongly indicative either of a functioning gonadal tumor or adrenal hyperfunction from whatever cause. Measurement of production rates of these compounds might simplify the diagnoses, although they would not take into consideration end-organ sensitivity, but since the compounds do not have any predominant tissue of origin in the female (in contrast to the situation in the male) this suggestion probably is only wishful thinking.[11]

The major naturally occurring progestin is progesterone, synthesized in substantial amounts by the placenta as gestation proceeds. Progesterone is extensively metabolized into a large number of different compounds in both pregnant and nonpregnant women, about 30 to 40 per cent of the total secreted being converted to pregnanediol, which is excreted in the urine as the diglucosiduronate. Many different procedures have been described for the determination of the metabolite in the urine and more recently for the hormone itself in blood.[12,13]

In the nonpregnant woman, an increase in pregnanediol excretion in the urine or an increase in progesterone concentration in the blood during the second half of the menstrual cycle implies that ovulation has taken place or at least that a follicle has been stimulated to form a corpus luteum. Unfortunately, the increase does not occur immediately or dramatically following release of the oocyte but gradually, as the lutein cells increase in number, size, and function so that measurement in neither blood nor urine can specify precisely when ovulation took place—it can only show that it probably did some time ago. Measurement of blood progesterone concentration at intervals during the secretory phase of the cycle also should in theory establish or preclude the diagnosis of "inadequate luteal phase," which is sometimes used in describing patients with infertility. In practice, little use of the method has been made, perhaps because of difficulty in breaking habit patterns on the part of clinicians. A careful trial comparison of blood progesterone determination versus endometrial biopsy should be made.

If fertilization and implantation occur, the trophoblast cells of the developing embryo immediately begin the synthesis and secretion of progesterone in ever-increasing amounts, but at first the major fraction of the hormone is made by the corpus luteum of pregnancy, under the stimulating influence of chorionic gonadotropin and other factors. As the corpus luteum disappears, the placenta becomes quantitatively most important in progesterone production. Although the cells of the trophoblast, like most other animal cells, possess all the enzyme systems necessary for the complete biosynthesis of progesterone from acetate, quantitatively the most important precursor for progesterone biosynthesis by the placenta is cholesterol from the maternal circulation. Moreover, the human placenta is an incomplete endocrine gland (in addition to its other functions) and does not contain substantial amounts of any of the enzymes required for the further metabolism of progesterone except for reversibly reducing progesterone at the carbon 20 position to form 20α-dihydroprogesterone (pregn-4-ene-20α-ol-3-one). One might anticipate therefore that measurement of blood progesterone (or its urinary metabolite, pregnanediol) in the pregnant woman should give an excellent measure of the size and functional capabilities of the placenta when compared to appropriate normal values for the length of gestation involved. Or, alternatively, and assuming normal progress of the pregnancy, such data should give a useful assessment of the length of gestation already accomplished. Alas, such is not the case.

Regulation of biological function in the autonomous fetoplacental unit is apparently not so finely tuned as it is for many of the biochemical parameters of the adult, and the range of variation within and among normal individuals is so broad as to make deviations from normal undetectable by progestin analysis until the pregnancy is quite obviously in danger, as manifested by other, simpler signs and symptoms. In Figure 22–1 this point is illustrated by some of our own unpublished data on serum progesterone concentrations during pregnancy, in which the values from normally pregnant women show an extremely wide variability. The older urinary pregnanediol excretion data showed essentially the same thing. Obviously, all that can be concluded from these measurements is that the human placenta has a tremendous capacity for manufacturing progesterone and that rarely, if ever, is the pregnancy endangered by a deficiency in this capacity. This is *not* to say that in a large group of subjects with a specific condition there may not be differences in the average value found. In severe toxemia, there is some reduction in the average pregnanediol excretion rate from the expected value. However, the normal variability is so great that in a single subject the decrease caused by the disease is not sufficient to be diagnostic, even if serial determinations are done; the same is apparently true for other conditions which have been reported to alter the production and excretion of the progestins.

Estrogen determinations have been found to be somewhat more useful. The earlier determinations of urinary estrogen excretion in the nonpregnant

Figure 22-1. Representative serum progesterone concentrations in pregnancy. The data include serial analyses in a group of 16 women studied during the second half of pregnancy, using a protein binding method very similar to that of Neill and associates,[28] and individual analyses of samples from women earlier in pregnancy done by a specific radioimmunoassay procedure.[29] All the subjects produced an apparently healthy infant at term. Since no clear-cut trends in the patients studied serially were seen, and since the results given by the two methods were statistically indistinguishable, the data were pooled for presentation. The shaded area represents an approximation of the normal range.

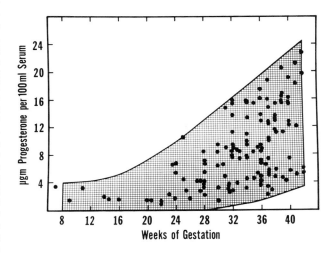

woman showed two peaks in most cycles, suggesting synthesis by some component of both the preovulatory follicle and the corpus luteum (perhaps mainly the theca interna and the theca lutein cells), but these measurements were not of great value unless very low and constant values were obtained, which suggested a quiescent ovary. When it became possible to measure estrogen concentrations in the blood accurately, the question immediately arose as to which one of the several present should be determined to obtain useful information. Of the 20 or more estrogens and estrogen metabolites that can be isolated from sources such as urine, estradiol-17β is biologically the most active in most assay systems. It is present in blood primarily in the free (i.e., not in a covalently conjugated) form but is largely bound nonspecifically to the serum proteins, especially albumin. Estrone, the second most active naturally occurring estrogen, circulates in the blood almost entirely in the form of its sulfuric acid conjugate, and only very small amounts of the other estrogens are present in the nonpregnant state. Both estradiol and estrone are secreted by the ovary and undergo interconversion in the somatic tissues; in addition, the adrenal secretes small amounts of both compounds, and to complicate matters still further, a small amount of the circulating androgen can also undergo aromatization in nonendocrine tissues. However, since estradiol-17β is by far the most potent biologically, most investigators have concentrated on its measurement in nonpregnant women.[14]

The small and transitory rise in estradiol-17β concentration that occurs a few days before ovulation and which is presumably the trigger for the ovulatory surge of LH is probably of greater scientific than clinical value, as is the larger postovulatory increase. But since the presence of circulating estrogen above a certain concentration in the blood reflects the action of FSH in stimulating the follicular apparatus to mature (and may indeed be involved itself in that maturation), measurements to make certain that the minimum is exceeded (and hence that follicles are ripening) are essential if attempts to induce ovulation artificially are to be successful in the treatment of infertility. Otherwise, prior treatment with preparations having follicle stimulating activity will be essential before ovulation can be induced. Estrogen measurements are useful in determining the dose of gonadotropin to be employed.

After fertilization and implantation, first the corpus luteum of pregnancy and later the fetoplacental unit synthesizes estradiol, and the concentration in the blood increases, as illustrated in Figure 22–2. Increases in concentrations of estrone and other steroids in the blood also accompany pregnancy (Figure 22–3). Other authors have described similar results for these and for other hormones, and, as has already been discussed for progesterone, the consensus seems to be that these measurements do not have any special diagnostic value. At least, we do not presently believe that any of them provide any clinically useful information during pregnancy that cannot be obtained more readily by measurement of total blood estriol concentration.[15-20]

In human pregnancy, the quantitatively predominant estrogen is estriol, which circulates in the blood almost entirely in conjugated forms, such as the 3-sulfate, the 16α-glucosiduronate, and the diconjugates. The kidney excretes almost exclusively the monoglucosiduronates, which arise by a complex pathway involving both the fetus and the placenta. Progesterone from the placenta is converted by the fetal adrenal into either dehydroepiandrosterone or its sulfate by removal of the two-carbon side-chain that is characteristic of the progestins. Some of this 19-carbon steroid is returned to the placenta, where it is reduced and aromatized to give estradiol-17β and estrone, which return to the maternal circulation, but a large fraction of the dehydroepiandrosterone is further hydroxylated at the 16α-position, probably in the fetal liver, before being returned to the placenta for aromatization, yielding estriol. A portion of the estriol (along with many other steroids) returns to the fetus to be excreted into the amniotic fluid, but the major portion of the estriol is captured by the maternal organs, where it is conjugated with glucuronic acid and then ultimately excreted. Some of the estriol in the maternal circulation is secreted via the bile into the gut in one or another form, where it may be further metabolized, but eventually most of this estriol is reabsorbed into the maternal circulation after its enterohepatic side trip.[21]

None of this complex metabolism would be of any clinical interest were it not for the fact that the rate-limiting enzymic step under most circumstances is

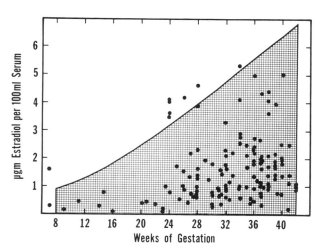

Figure 22-2. Representative serum estradiol-17β concentrations in pregnancy. The subjects are the same as those in Figure 22-1, and the same comments apply. Analyses for samples late in pregnancy were done by a protein binding method;[30] for samples earlier in pregnancy, a radioimmunoassay similar to that of Mikhail and co-workers[31] was used.

Figure 22-3. Representative serum concentrations of some other steroid hormones during pregnancy. The chart shows results of serial analyses for free (unconjugated) estrone (upper panel), 20α-dihydroprogesterone (middle panel), and 17α-hydroxyprogesterone (bottom panel) in a group of 16 women studied during the second half of gestation, all of whom gave birth to apparently normal infants. No definite trends with time were seen in the results from the individual subjects, so the data were pooled as representing a random sample for each hormone. The shaded areas represent approximate normal values for the data and show that as pregnancy advances there is a tendency for the concentrations of these steroids to increase in the blood. Analyses were done on a total extract of steroids from serum which was separated into phenolic and neutral fractions by base partition. These fractions were purified by paper chromatography, and the estrone was reduced chemically, repurified by thin layer chromatography, and assayed by protein binding displacement by a procedure very similar to that reported by Sybulski.[30] The dihydroprogesterone was oxidized chemically, repurified by thin layer chromatography, and assayed by protein binding displacement by a procedure similar to that of Neill and colleagues.[28] The latter protein binding displacement procedure was also used for assay of the 17α-hydroxyprogesterone fraction. Recoveries were monitored with radioactive standards added originally to the blood. These methods have been outmoded by the simpler radioimmunoassay procedures, but the results are recorded here to add to the rather small sample of normal values so far available.

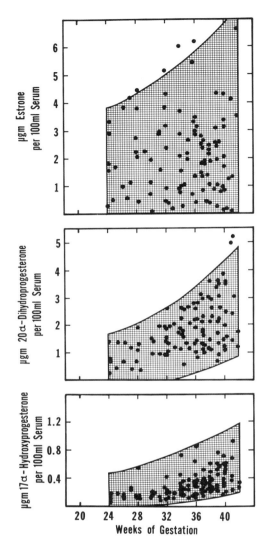

the final hydroxylation in the fetal liver. As long as this reaction remains the slowest step in the whole process, then the amount of estriol excreted into the urine or the total concentration of estriol in the maternal blood reflects the status of the fetus. Again, the wide range of normal values, encountered as the total amount excreted gradually increases in step with the advancing pregnancy, made interpretation of the analyses in urine difficult. At first, it was suspected that the methodology might be contributing to apparent variability, but eventually it became clear that in most cases it was indeed a biologic variation that was being observed. Early investigators attempted to set lower limits below which the fetus was at great risk of impending death but these limits varied both according to the details of the method being used for urinalysis and with the gestational age, and therefore they had to be set so low as to be almost useless to avoid unwarranted interference with a normal pregnancy in which the urinary estriol values were near the lower limits of normality.

Eventually, the utility of using the patient as her own control and observing the trend rather than the absolute magnitude of the urinary estriol excretion was recognized, and it is now generally accepted that serial values which do not rise at the rate expected for the particular method in use at the supposed gestational age should alert the obstetrician to possible fetal danger. Furthermore, steadily decreasing values suggest severe and imminent fetal hazard. If urinary estriol excretion is the measurement, questions then arise regarding how often samples should be analyzed and how specific a method the clinician should demand. There seems to be little or no diurnal variation in maternal blood total estriol concentration, but there is some diurnal variation in excretion, in addition to the already mentioned wide day-to-day variation in a single patient and the even wider patient-to-patient variation. Since the urinary estriol does *not* precisely parallel the urinary creatinine excretion, it would seem unwise to add yet another variable to this already complex situation and compromise for anything less than an accurately timed, careful, and complete 24-hour collection of urine for analysis. The only way in which such collections can be consistently obtained is for the physician himself or a highly motivated nurse or assistant to explain in detail to the patient what is required; no bottle label giving general instructions or directive in the nurses' order book can be expected to give consistently good collections. A satisfactory evaluation of the adequacy of the collections can be obtained from the total creatinine determinations, which should be routinely done for that purpose. Daily analyses are a luxury most patients in public hospitals cannot afford; thrice weekly determinations have been satisfactory in our experience in the management of most patients, even those who are critically ill, since the estriol determination is only a single piece of evidence in the total clinical picture to be evaluated in order to determine a course of action or inaction on the part of the physician.[22]

We shall not consider here details of the methodology except to emphasize that the determination is not as simple as some of the many recent publications in the clinical chemistry literature might lead one to believe. The issue as to whether a truly more specific (and therefore more expensive and more time consuming) method provides more information than a simpler approximation of "total" urinary estrogens is not resolved; some preliminary data would suggest that in certain complications of pregnancy, especially diabetes, the customary predominance of estriol-glucosiduronates (90 per cent or more of the total urinary estrogens) may not actually hold true. If this is indeed the case, then the more specific methods might give clearer clinical information, and identification and quantitation of the other abnormal metabolites might provide additional useful data.[23]

We have sidestepped this issue, as well as the problems involved in obtaining an adequate 24-hour collection of urine from the pregnant woman, by determining serum total estriol concentration by a complicated and difficult but entirely feasible published method which has been validated for specificity, accuracy, precision, and sensitivity.[24] Although this method has not been widely used because of its apparent complexity, it is in fact completely practical in any laboratory which is qualified to be doing any kind of steroid analysis. Figure 22–4 shows that the blood and urine results are reasonably well correlated in individual patients on a given day.

We have presented elsewhere some of our earlier experiences with this method, and other investigators have published similar data. It would appear that

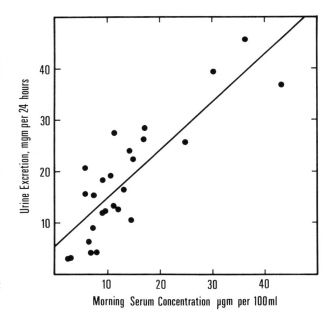

Figure 22-4. Correlation between serum and urine estriol. Morning serum samples and 24-hour urine collections from the same women were analyzed.[24, 32] The results show clearly the general agreement between the two methods and at the same time the random discrepancies that result from the wide biologic variation present in each of the procedures. Statistical analysis of these data shows that no better relationship between the results can be obtained by curvilinear regression; the regression equation for the line shown is:

Urine Estriol =
0.94 × Serum Estriol + 5.9 with a correlation coefficient of 0.83.

evaluation of serum estriol according to the principles already described for urinalysis provides as good or better clinical results as measurement of urinary excretion (failure to increase with time is a warning; consistently declining values indicate that a serious hazard exists for the fetus). Figure 22–5 shows some results of blood analysis obtained in a population of women suspected on other clinical grounds of carrying small for their gestational age fetuses. The data clearly show that many of these infants did in fact have lower than average capacity to maintain maternal serum estriol concentrations, and the majority of them were found to be small at birth. This is merely another way of saying that the capacity of the fetal liver to perform the rate-limiting step in the overall synthesis varies with the size and health of the liver, which in turn varies with the gestational age, size, and health of the whole infant.

In some circumstances—e.g., anencephaly below the level of the anterior pituitary, or corticoid therapy of the mother—other steps in the path may become rate-limiting; in these instances, slower side-chain cleavage by the fetal adrenal takes place. Only very rarely, as in the case of placental sulfatase deficiency already alluded to, does the placenta rather than the fetus become the controlling factor. Nor is renal disease (except of the most serious kind) any bar to the use of serum estriol concentration measurements in evaluating the status of the fetus.

When To Perform Tests

From the practical viewpoint, it is not ordinarily feasible to perform the present blood estriol measurement more than thrice weekly; the clinical situation appears usually not to vary so rapidly that more frequent determinations are necessary. In the general surveillance of patients with possible future complica-

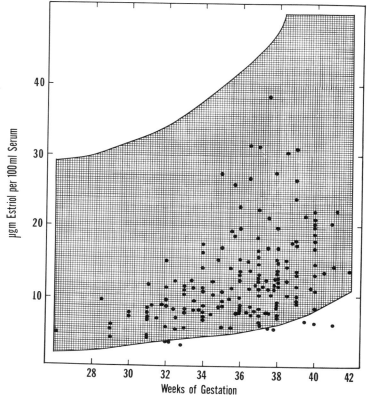

Figure 22-5. Random sample of serum estriol concentrations in samples submitted to the laboratory for "question of small for gestational age." See text.

tions, one determination per week has seemingly been useful to some of our colleagues.

A number of alternate procedures have been offered for evaluation. For example, a radioimmunoassay utilizing a nonspecific antibody might be used to measure total blood estrogen concentration.[25]

A small fraction of the estriol made during pregnancy is synthesized solely in the maternal compartment and might theoretically confuse interpretation of its measurement; a closely related steroid, estetrol (15α-hydroxyestriol) is apparently made *only* in the fetal liver. Its rate of synthesis and concentration is only about one-tenth that of estriol and its analysis is therefore more difficult. The clinical usefulness of determining its level remains to be evaluated.[26]

Application of the apparently more attractive radioimmunoassay methods to these problems likewise remains to be proved. Antibodies with sufficient specificity to distinguish the several estriol conjugates without prior chemical separation unfortunately are not available as yet. Nor does there seem to be any *a priori* reason to favor the determination of any one of the conjugates over the others, so that further empirical testing will be essential. Radioimmunoassay of other estrogens in the maternal blood seems even less rational because a smaller proportion of these are made in the fetoplacental compartment, compared to estriol, and because of their extensive interconversion; however, since such a method is available for measuring blood estradiol-17β, some values have been enthusiastically reported; should the observed clinical correlations withstand further testing, this procedure might become one of choice because of its simplicity.[18]

Analyses of amniotic fluid estrogen content have been tried because they might be more closely related to the status of the fetus; the synthetic and physiologic pathways already described make this seem unlikely and the clinical usefulness of such analyses remains to be demonstrated.[27] Functional tests such as the infusion of estriol precursors or other specific compounds to be metabolized by the fetus remain experimental but promising.

In discussing the tests available and giving our opinion of their possible worth, we have avoided as far as possible describing the laboratory technicalities involved because of their lack of immediate importance to the physician; we would emphasize again here that no endocrine assay is of any value whatsoever unless the limitations of the methodology used are clearly understood and appreciated by the analyst, and appropriately transmitted by him to the clinician. Unfortunately the clinician has often been conditioned either to accept without further thought any test result from the laboratory, or to completely disregard any value which does not fit precisely into his preconceived notion of the status of the patient. In either of these unfortunate but all too common occurrences, nobody benefits from the laboratory work except possibly the sponsoring institution's finances.

REFERENCES

1. Diczfalusy, E.: Immunoassay of Gonadotrophins. Stockholm, Karolinska Sjukhuset, 1969.
2. Diczfalusy, E.: Steroid Assay in Protein Binding. Stockholm, Karolinska Sjukhuset, 1970.
3. Schally, A. V., Arimura, and Kastin, A. J.: Hypothalamic Regulatory Hormones. Science 179:341, 1973.
4. Chard, T., Boyd, N. R. H., Forsling, M. L., McNeilly, A. S., and Landon, J.: The development of a radioimmunoassay for oxytocin: the extraction of oxytocin from plasma, and its measurement during parturition in human and goat blood. J. Endocr. 48:233, 1970.
5. Friedman, S.: Clinical uses of serum FSH and LH measurements. Obstet. Gynec. 39:811, 1972.
6. Letchworth, A. T., and Chard, T.: Human placental lactogen levels in pre-eclampsia. J. Obstet. Gynaec. Brit. Comm. 79:680, 1972.
7. Fliegner, J. R. H., Schindler, I., and Brown, J. B.: Low urinary oestriol excretion during pregnancy associated with placental sulphatase deficiency or congenital adrenal hypoplasia. J. Obstet. Gynaec. Brit. Comm. 79:810, 1972.
8. Arai, Y., and Lee, V. H.: A double-antibody radioimmunoassay procedure for ovine pituitary prolactin. Endocrinology 81:1041, 1967.
9. Aleem, F. A.: Total and heat-stable serum alkaline phosphatase in normal and abnormal pregnancies. Obstet. Gynec. 40:163, 1972.
10. Seppala, M., and Ruoslahti, E.: Radioimmunoassay of maternal serum alpha fetoprotein during pregnancy and delivery. Amer. J. Obstet. Gynec. 112:208, 1972.
11. Osburn, R. H., and Yannone, M. E.: Plasma androgens in the normal and androgenic female: a review. Obstet. Gynec. Surv. 26:195, 1971.
12. Klopper, A. I.: An evaluation of the contribution of GLC techniques for the estimation of progesterone and pregnanesteroids. Clin. Chim. Acta 34:215, 1971.
13. Neill, J. D., Johansson, E. D. B., and Knobil, E.: Patterns of circulating progesterone concentrations during the fertile menstrual cycle and the remainder of gestation in the Rhesus monkey. Endocrinology 84:45, 1969.
14. Lloyd, C. W., Lobotsky, J., Baird, D. T., McCracken, J. A., and Weisz, J.: Concentration of unconjugated estrogens, androgens and gestagens in ovarian and peripheral venous plasma of women: the normal menstrual cycle. J. Clin. Endocr. Metab. 32:155, 1971.

15. Fisher-Rasmussen, W.: Plasma oestrogens and the fetal outcome. Acta Obstet. Gynec. Scand. 50:301, 1971.
16. Jorgensen, P. I., and Frandsen, V. A.: The clinical value of oestrone-oestradiol estimation compared with that of oestriol estimation in pathological pregnancies. J. Steroid Biochem. 2:355, 1971.
17. Tulchinsky, D., and Korenman, S. G.: The plasma estradiol as an index of fetoplacental function. J. Clin. Invest. 50:1490, 1971.
18. Sybulski, S., and Maughan, G. B.: Maternal plasma estradiol levels in normal and complicated pregnancies. Amer. J. Obstet. Gynec. 113:310, 1972.
19. Tulchinsky, D., Hobel, C. J., Yeager, E., and Marshall, J. R.: Plasma estrone, estradiol, estriol, progesterone and 17-hydroxyprogesterone in human prgenancy. I. Normal pregnancy. Amer. J. Obstet. Gynec. 112:1095, 1972.
20. Tulchinsky, D., Hobel, C. J., Yeager, E., and Marshall, J. R.: Plasma estradiol, estriol, and progesterone in human pregnancy. II. Clinical applications in Rh-isoimmunization disease. Amer. J. Obstet. Gynec. 113:766, 1972.
21. Diczfalusy, E., and Mancuso, S.: Oestrogen metabolism in pregnancy. In Klopper, A., and Diczfalusy, E., eds.: Foetus and Placenta. Oxford, Blackwell, 1969.
22. Klopper, A.: The assessment of placental function in clinical practice. In Klopper, A., and Diczfalusy, E. (eds.): Foetus and Placenta. Oxford, Blackwell, 1969.
23. Cohen, S. L.: The excretion of labile oestrogens during human pregnancy. II. Diabetic pregnancy. Acta Endocrinol. 67:687, 1971.
24. Nachtigall, L., Bassett, M., Hogsander, U., Slagle, S., and Levitz, M.: A rapid method for the assay of plasma estriol in pregnancy. J. Clin. Endocr. Metab. 26:941, 1966.
25. Gurpide, E., Giebenhain, M. E., Tseng, L., and Kelly, W. G.: Radioimmunoassay for estrogens in human pregnancy urine, plasma, and amniotic fluid. Amer. J. Obstet. Gynec. 109:897, 1971.
26. Fishman, J., and Guzik, H.: Radioimmunoassay of 15α-hydroxyestriol in pregnancy plasma. J. Clin. Endocr. Metab. 35:892, 1972.
27. Klopper, A.: Estriol in liquor amnii. Amer. J. Obstet. Gynec. 112:459, 1972.
28. Neill, J. D., Johansson, E. D. B., Datta, J. K., and Knobil, E.: Relationship between the plasma levels of luteinizing hormone and progesterone during the normal menstrual cycle. J. Clin. Endocr. Metab. 27:1167, 1967.
29. Thorneycroft, I. H., and Stone, S. C.: Radioimmunoassay of serum progesterone in women receiving oral contraceptive steroids. Contraception 5:129, 1972.
30. Sybulski, S.: Determination of free estradiol-17β levels in pregnancy plasma by competitive protein-binding method. Amer. J. Obstet. Gynec. 110:304, 1971.
31. Mikhail, G., Wu, C. H., Ferin, M., and VandeWiele, R. L.: Radioimmunoassay of plasma estrone and estradiol. Steroids 15:333, 1970.
32. Hagerman, D. D., and Isaacson, K. A.: Comparison of ammonium sulfate precipitation and resin adsorption methods for routine measurements of total urinary estrogens in pregnancy. Gynecol. Invest. 3:195, 1972.

The Value and Limitations
of Endocrine Assays Specifically
for Obstetrical and Gynecological Conditions

M. Wayne Heine

University of Arizona College of Medicine

Introduction

The advances in laboratory endocrine analysis that have been made in the past two decades have been phenomenal. Initially, only bioassay methods were available, but these were laborious and of limited sensitivity. These bioassay methods were followed by colorimetric, fluorimetric, and gas liquid chromatographic methods. Immunoassay procedures have now been added. Each of these techniques was of improved sensitivity and sometimes specificity. They can measure hormones in extremely small quantities of body fluids, and this has allowed a delineation of the interplay of hypothalamic-pituitary, gonodal, placental, and the other endocrine gland factors. A greater understanding of the reproductive cycle and of the endocrinology of pregnancy has allowed development of various methods of contraception and improved fetal salvage. Regardless of the several endocrine assays now available, many endocrine problems have yet to be elucidated. We shall discuss the major endocrine assays that the obstetrician-gynecologist may utilize in the daily care of patients.

Gonadotropins

The development of radioimmunoassay techniques has permitted determinations of the pituitary gonadotropins luteinizing hormone (LH) and follicular stimulating hormone (FSH) from small amounts of serum with reasonable rapidity and ease, and this has led to a more complete understanding of the physiology and control of the human menstrual cycle. Previous techniques, including bioassay, were not able to separate FSH and LH completely.

The majority of the patients in whom serum pituitary gonadotropin levels will be useful (and therefore tested) are those with primary and secondary

743

amenorrhea. In evaluating a patient with primary amenorrhea, elevated FSH levels may suggest ovarian failure, while low levels (below 3 milliunits) would indicate hypogonadotropic hypogonadism. In patients with secondary amenorrhea repeated elevated FSH serum (above 60 milliunits) may mean premature ovarian failure. If, however, the serum levels are low, hypothalamic or pituitary disease must be given strong consideration. In the majority of cases, however, one or more determinations of serum pituitary gonadotropins may fall with the normal range and be of little aid in determining the cause of the amenorrhea. The FSH and LH serum determinations are most useful, however, in the evaluation of patients with precocious sexual development. Should the levels of these pituitary gonadotropic hormones be within the adult range (3 to 30 milliunits), it would certainly suggest that the origin of precocious puberty can be traced to the central nervous system. If the serum FSH and LH levels are low or nearly absent, one should consider the possibility of a functioning ovarian tumor.

It has been over 40 years since Aschheim and Zondek[1] described the reaction of ovaries of immature mice to a substance now known as chorionic gonadotropin (HCG), which is present in the urine of pregnant women. Numerous bioassays utilizing rabbits, mice, rats, frogs, and toads have subsequently been described. It was not until the mid-1940's that human chorionic gonadotropin was noted to be antigenic. In the 1960's, it was found that an antibody to HCG could be produced in rabbits, and this material could be used for a complement fixation test in determining the presence or absence of pregnancy.

Innumerable commercial pregnancy test kits are now available and are being utilized in both commercial laboratories and physicians' offices. Although these tests are extremely useful in diagnosing early pregnancy, the physician should know that there may be interfering factors that limit the sensitivity and reliability of the test. Kerber and associates[2] recently compared the various immunologic tests for pregnancy and noted that the range of sensitivity varied from 7000 international units (I.U.) to 3500 I.U. per liter of urine. Of two of the more commonly used tests, the Dap test is sensitive to 2000 I.U. and the pregnosticon slide test is sensitive to 1000 I.U. per liter of urine, respectively.

It should be kept in mind that the human chorionic gonadotropin cross-reacts with luteinizing hormone. During the LH surge of ovulation, up to 400 I.U. of this hormone can be found in a 24 hour urine specimen. The amount of luteinizing hormone is also elevated in the amenorrhea of menopause, with values as high as 800 units per liter of urine being reported. However, as already stated, the commercial tests are sensitive to 1000 I.U. or greater, and at this level cross-reaction with LH that might otherwise give a false positive test at the peak rise in ovulation or in menopausal women will not be likely to occur. Proteinuria on occasion may give a false positive reaction. Psychotropic drugs, such as phenothiazine, antidepressants, and anticonvulsant agents, may also interfere and produce false negative results. It is therefore important that a drug history be obtained or included with a urine sample submitted for a pregnancy test. It has been our experience that women with ectopic gestations may give a false negative reaction in approximately 40 to 50 per cent of the cases; therefore, it is important not to exclude the diagnosis of ectopic pregnancy on the basis of a negative immunologic pregnancy test alone.

The immunologic pregnancy test kits may be useful in identifying trophoblastic disease, but owing to limitations of sensitivity to HCG, its value is restricted to a screening procedure. Approximately 25 per cent of patients with persistent trophoblastic disease will have a negative immunologic pregnancy test. In order to obtain an accurate assessment of the status of trophoblastic disease, it is necessary to use the more sensitive bioassay or immunoassay methods for human chorionic gonadotropin. It is now accepted that by either of these methods the effectiveness of chemotherapy can be followed by the disappearance of chorionic gonadotropin titer. As elsewhere in medicine (and most other areas), there is an exception. We recently encountered a patient in whom chemotherapy appeared to be effective in reducing the HCG titer, but vaginal examination revealed irregularity and enlargement of the uterus. Subsequent surgery showed chorionadenoma destruens, which had penetrated the myometrium to the serosal surface of the uterus. Despite improvement in levels of chorionic gonadotropin titers, the clinical evaluation revealed progression of the disease.

While the newer immunologic methods of measuring chorionic gonadotropins are extremely useful in making the diagnosis of early pregnancy, it would be well to recall the different sensitivities and the factors that may interfere with the various tests. Hence, the physician must be familiar with the accuracy and type of test being used either in his office or consulting laboratory and interpret these tests in conjunction with the clinical data.

ESTROGENS

It has been almost two decades since Brown[3] described his modifications of a colorimetric method for measuring urinary estrogens. Subsequent methods have become more refined and sensitive, utilizing such techniques as fluorescence, gas chromatography, and radioimmunoassay. Techniques have become so sensitive that picograms of hormones may now be measured in serum. Most of the present knowledge has been obtained, however, from measuring the three major estrogens—estrone, estradiol, and estriol—in urine. With the more recent techniques it now is possible, within limits, to relate estrogen values to a disturbance in the menstrual cycle. However, the values found in ovulating women and women with anovulatory cycles are not too different, so a single or even two urine or serum values have limited usefulness. By utilizing the progesterone provocation test one can determine whether there are physiologic amounts of estrogens present or not.

In the evaluation of the estrogen status of patients with precocious puberty we have found it simpler, less expensive, and just as informative to determine the vaginal pH and the appearance of the vaginal cytology. It is more important to assess the presence or absence of FSH and LH and thus determine whether the source of the estrogens is hypothalamic-pituitary ovarian stimulation or a functioning ovarian neoplasm.

Serum or urinary estrogen assays probably have their greatest value in monitoring exogenous gonadotropin therapy. The sequence used by Brown and Beisher[4] showed that by starting with a low dose of FSH and gradually increasing the dose in 30 per cent increments until a rise in urinary estrogen is obtained, then utilizing the chorionic gonadotropin, the incidence of ovarian hyperstimulation can be reduced. This regimen does not, however, reduce the incidence of multiple ovulations, but it is possible, by using more sensitive serum methods to adjust the dose level, that this can be done. Unless the laboratory has the ability

to perform daily urinary or serum estrogen determinations, exogenous gonadotropin therapy probably should not be attempted.

The estrogen assay which has probably received the greatest assessment is
that of estriol in pregnancy. Estrogen secretion in early pregnancy doubles
approximately every 2½ weeks until the eighteenth week. A drop in levels of
either estrogens or pregnanediol or both may precede an abortion by a few days
or even a few weeks in cases of missed abortion. The use of cytologic methods is
often misleading. Also, estriol determinations are not helpful in following patients
thought to have trophoblastic disease. Although the chorionic gonadotropin levels
may be very high, the serum or urinary estrogen levels will not be elevated.

It does appear that repeated estriol assays, with determinations of lecithin/
sphingomyelin ratio of the amniotic fluid, contribute to reducing the perinatal
mortality rate. Certainly estriol determinations in late pregnancy are helpful in
deciding on the appropriate time for delivery. Some of the complications of late
pregnancy in which estriol determinations may be used are toxemia, essential
hypertension, chronic renal disease, prolonged pregnancy, or history of prior stillborn delivery. The assessment of estriol levels in diabetic pregnancy is less clear.

In the evaluation of the patient with preeclampsia, one is often tempted
to procrastinate, especially if the pregnancy is of less than 36 weeks' duration. If
the serum estriol values stay within normal range it may be safe to wait. However, if there is a fall in estriol values, the fetus will probably fare better with
immediate delivery by the most expeditious means. In following patients with
third trimester complications, it is important that estriol levels be determined two
to three times per week or even daily, since we have observed fetal death within
72 hours after the first fall in estriol levels. Estriol determinations have not proved
to be of value in patients who are carrying fetuses with erythroblastosis fetalis.
The evaluation of the amniotic fluid for bilirubin pigments has been found to be
more accurate in evaluating the fetal status. Amniotic fluid estriols have been
measured, but there is a large overlap in results between those afflicted fetuses
who have minimal problems and those who succumb to erythroblastosis in utero.

The usefulness of estriol determinations is now limited mainly to certain
complications of the third trimester pregnancy. The availability of rapid, low-cost
urinary or serum estriol determinations may allow all patients to have this procedure done sometime early in the third trimester of pregnancy. At present there is
some debate as to what a low estriol level means in many patients. Wallace and
Michie[5] state that there is a 35 per cent incidence of mental retardation in infants
of 14 patients who were found to have low estriol values. Greene and co-workers,[6]
however, have not been able to substantiate this finding. As with any laboratory
value one should keep in mind that certain medications do interfere with determinations. Mandelamine lowers urinary estriol values without actually affecting
the pregnancy. Corticoids and ampicillin have been found to lower both serum
and urinary estriol values without interfering with pregnancy.

ANDROGENS

Much information has accumulated about androgen production in both
the adrenal gland and the ovary since Zimmermann[7] first described his colorimetric reaction between meta-dinitrobenzene and C-19 steroids. However, despite
the more refined colorimetric techniques of measuring either C-19 steroids or the

separation and measurement of various androgens by gas chromatography, and despite even the various sensitive immunoassay measurements of serum androgens, many of the questions of diagnosis and treatment of the hirsute or virilized women are yet to be clarified. Many of these procedures are laborious, time-consuming, and still relatively expensive. Even when all of these various androgens are measured in either urine or serum, their origin in many cases cannot be precisely stated. However, measurement of serum or urinary androgens is diagnostically important in the virilized woman. In the majority of anovulatory women who are not hirsute, serum or urine androgen measurements are of limited value. As will be seen, a differentiation is possible between a functioning ovarian neoplasm and adrenal hyperplasia or neoplasia.

The colorimetric Zimmermann reaction and its refinements measure androgens such as androsterone, etiocholanolone and dehydroioosoandrosterone. The normal female excretes approximately 5 to 15 milligrams of 17-ketosteroids per 24 hours, of which approximately 75 per cent is secreted by the adrenal. Many drugs interfere with the laboratory values, and the medications which may result in an increase in urinary 17-ketosteroids are meprobamate, triacetyloleandomycin, spironolactone, penicillin, phenaglycodol, phenothiazines, ethinamate, and nalidixic acid. Other medications which may result in a decrease of urinary 17-ketosteroids determinations are chlordiazepoxide, etryptamine acetate, and reserpine. In evaluating a patient with evidence of virilization, if the baseline values of ketosteroids are elevated to 13 milligrams or above, a diagnostic dexamethasone suppression test is next in order. Dexamethasone (1.25 mg. per 45 kilograms of body weight) is given daily for a period of five to seven days. If one is concerned about the possibility of Cushing's syndrome, a graded dose suppression test of 2 mg. for two days and 8 mg. for two days, with the 24 hour urine being collected on the second day of each dose, is performed for ketosteroid and hydroxysteroid determinations. Depending on the degree of refinement of the Zimmermann technique used, the ketosteroids will decrease to between 2 and 4 mg. per 24 hour urine collection. This indicates that the excess ketosteroids are adrenal in origin. Failure to respond completely suggests that the excess androgen is ovarian in origin.

For years, many practitioners felt that when a sensitive, relatively simple method for measuring urinary or plasma testosterone became available, many of the diagnostic and therapeutic questions concerning the virilized female and hirsutism would be answered. Now these tests are available, but the problem of the source of excesses of this androgen hormone still exists. This is a result of the large overlap between baseline testosterone values in the normal female and in those with polycystic ovaries or idiopathic hirsutism. In our laboratory, normal serum testosterone values range between 20 and 40 nanograms per 100 ml. Patients with idiopathic hirsutism show values that range between 30 and 50 nanograms per 100 ml., with those thought to have polycystic ovaries exhibiting values in the 30 to 80 nanograms per 100 ml. range. In order to get a true picture of the actual amount of testosterone present, it is necessary to obtain production rates and metabolic clearance rates, as well as serum concentrations. Even then the exact site of excess androgen production or stimulation may not be elucidated. With a large overlap in testosterone values, it is hardly practical to perform these tests.

However, by utilizing the 17-ketosteroid values together with those of serum testosterone, further information may be obtained. Patients with polycystic ovaries often have high normal, or only slightly elevated 24 hour urinary ketosteroid levels, and the serum testosterone values are usually slightly above normal. The patient with adrenal virilization will often have higher levels of urinary 17-ketosteroids. This is a generalization that may give the gynecologist some idea of whether to start his treatment with suppression of the adrenal gland or suppression of the ovary.

In the child with virilization or the adult female whose 24 hour urinary ketosteroid levels are markedly elevated, the possibility of adrenogenital syndrome should be kept in mind. This syndrome is usually associated with elevation of pregnanetriol, which may be measured either directly or by measuring ketogenic steroids. This value is obtained by oxidizing a portion of the urine, causing the C-21 steroids to lose their C-20,21 side chain and become C-19 ketosteroids. The Zimmermann reaction is then tested for. This procedure can measure cortisol, cortisone, and their tetrahydro derivatives, as well as pregnanetriol. If the patient has signs and symptoms suggestive of Cushing's syndrome, 17-hydroxysteroid values should be obtained from the same urine collection from which 17-ketosteroid values were determined. The physician should take care to bear in mind that, as already mentioned, numerous medications do interfere with the colorimetric procedure of measuring urinary 17-hydroxysteroids. Such drugs include chloral hydrate, meprobamate, triacetyloleandomycin, spironolactone, chlordiazepoxide and hydroxyzine. Drugs which may cause a decrease in the uterine values of 17-hydroxysteroids are phenathiazines and reserpine. The obese patient may have a slightly elevated 24 hour urinary 17-hydroxysteroid value. It is sometimes difficult to differentiate marked obesity from Cushing's syndrome by this test alone. Sensitive serum methods of measuring cortisols, such as immunoassay methods, will allow for a more accurate diagnosis by measuring the A.M. and P.M. cortisol values and looking for the diurnal variation which will be present in the obese patient but absent in the patient with Cushing's syndrome.

If the patient is thought to have decreased adrenal function, it may be necessary to obtain both a 24 hour urine sample for 17-hydroxysteroid determination, as well as A.M. and P.M. plasma specimens for serum cortisol determinations.

Summary

The newer techniques of hormonal evaluation are certainly an important addition to the armamentarium of the gynecologist. Their limitations, however, must be constantly kept in mind. In this day of automated laboratory analysis and mass screening, it must be remembered that laboratory data are meant to aid clinical judgment, not replace it.

One of the areas in which the new techniques are particularly useful is in the diagnosis of early pregnancy. With the change in abortion laws and the importance of counseling and doing surgery during the first 10 to 12 weeks of pregnancy, the new pregnancy test kits have been extremely helpful. It should be remembered that the sensitivity of these kits is limited and that it is important to use the more sensitive immunoassay or bioassay methods in following patients with trophoblastic disease. Sensitive pituitary gonadotropin assays will reinforce the diagnosis of idiopathic precocious puberty over that of a possible functioning ovarian tumor. They also aid in the diagnosis of ovarian or hypothalamic-pituitary failure in patients with amenorrhea, but they have not been found to be too practical in the evaluation of patients with anovulatory cycles. The various estrogen assays have not proved to be particularly useful in the day-to-day care of most endocrine problems. They are valuable tools, however, in determining the dose of exogenous gonadotropins to be used in patients with low or absent gonadotropins who desire pregnancy. Estriol, however, has been found to be valuable in determining the best time for delivery in many high-risk patients. As less expensive and faster serum methods become available, it may be possible to do routine serum estriol determinations on all patients early in the third trimester of pregnancy.

Although refined laboratory techniques certainly improve our diagnostic accuracy, it is well to keep in mind the various limitations and factors which may interfere with the results, and make sure the tests aid, not replace, good clinical evaluation.

REFERENCES

1. Aschheim, S., and Zondek, B.: Die Schwangerschafts diagnose aus dem Harn durch Nachweis des Hypophysenvorderlappenhormones. Klin. Wchschr. 7:1404, 1928.
2. Kerber, I. J., Inclan, A. P., Fowler, E. A., Davis, K., and Fish, S. A.: Immunologic tests for pregnancy. Obstet. Gynec. 36:37, 1970.
3. Brown, J. B.: A chemical method for the determination of oestriol, oestrone, and oestradiol in human urine. Biochem. J. 60:185, 1955.
4. Brown, J. B., and Beischer, N. A.: Review: current status of estrogen assay in gynecology and obstetrics. Part I. Estrogen assays in gynecology and early pregnancy. Obstet. Gynec. Surv. 27:205, 1972.
5. Wallace, S. J., and Michie, E. A.: A follow-up study of infants born to mothers with low oestriol excretion during pregnancy. Lancet 2:560, 1966.
6. Greene, J. W., Beargie, R. A., Clark, B. K., and Smith, K.: Correlation of estriol excretion patterns of pregnant women with subsequent development of their children. Amer. J. Obstet. Gynec. 105:730, 1969.
7. Zimmermann, W.: Eine Farbreaktion der Sexualhormone und ihre Anwendung zur Quantitativen Colorimetrischen Bestimmung. Ztschr. Physiol. Chem. 233:257, 1935.

The Value and Limitations of Endocrine Assays Specifically for Obstetrical and Gynecological Conditions

Editorial Comment

Many of the laboratory procedures considered in this chapter relate to entities discussed in other chapters in this book, particularly Chapters 20 and 21. Unless the clinician is directly and deeply involved in the management of large numbers of patients with deviations in embryonal development and disturbed endocrine function of the female reproductive tract system, he must rely in large measure on those who are. The plurality and relative newness of many laboratory procedures reflect the vigorous research activity in this area of human biology. These tests and procedures demand periodic and authoritative scrutiny of their validity and limitations. From this background, the clinician must select those with clinical relevance and those which might be regarded as relating primarily to research.

Not only are these determinations useful to the clinician in arriving at the correct diagnosis, but they may dictate the correct therapy as well. As suggested by one of the contributors, the assay may furnish strong evidence for or against certain modalities or methods of therapy. The prime example cited is the case in which progesterone values in normal pregnancy vary over a wide range. Advocacy of progesterone replacement therapy in treating certain pregnancy complications therefore appears to be based on rather tenuous grounds and strongly challenges the view that this medication is ever indicated during gestation.

The sophisticated nature of many of the procedures and the demand for accuracy raises doubts whether only speciality laboratories should be involved in performing these determinations. Unquestionably, not having any information at all is to be preferred to inaccurate or false information. Certainly the clinician and laboratory investigator should both desire that the tests be specific and the results fall within a reasonable range of accuracy.

23

Evaluation and Preferred Management of Premenstrual Tension–Pelvic Congestive Syndrome and Allied States

Alternative Points of View:

    By Michael J. Daly

    By Mary Anna Friederich and Anthony Labrum

    By John B. Josimovich

Editorial Comment

Evaluation and Preferred Management of Premenstrual Tension—Pelvic Congestive Syndrome and Allied States

MICHAEL J. DALY

Temple University

The present-day controversy over woman's role in society has not only intrigued both men and women, young and old, but has also attracted the attention of serious investigators from such varied disciplines as economics, anthropology, psychology, medicine, and political science. The reevaluation of feminine roles, expectations, potentials, and needs has been vigorously undertaken by many. Some of these investigators have been men, but the majority have been women. They have offered a variety of views, one extreme suggesting that the human female differs from the male only in her anatomical structure. In the active feminist movement, as in all political and social movements, the strongest voices are those of the more extreme or radical elements. One of the areas that has received considerable attention is the effect of the menstrual cycle on woman's behavior and her ability to perform effectively at all phases of the menstrual cycle.

A review of medical history reveals that this concern is not new. Many myths, superstitions, and fears have their basis in the menstrual cycle. Some of these fantasies were incorporated into religion as in Jewish law, under which women were isolated and considered "unclean" at the time of the menstrual flow. We can identify in various cultures through the centuries mass awareness of the behavior disturbance associated with the menstrual cycle. The Greeks, for instance, associated menstrual distress with a "wandering uterus." The developing European cultures suggested a link between the psychological disturbances of the menstruating female and supernatural causes. Careful scrutiny of the symptoms recorded in the past shows the similarity to the modern woman's complaints of premenstrual tension. This term was coined for a syndrome first described by Frank[1] during this century and characterized by irritability, anxiety, depression, and edema. Twenty-five per cent of women will admit to having such symptoms during four days prior to menstruation or during the first four days of their menstrual period. An evaluation of these symptoms is appropriate here.

SYMPTOMS

IRRITABILITY.   The most common complaint is irritability, which usually begins about four days prior to the onset of menstruation. Most women will have a degree of this restlessness or hyperactivity feeling; some will not. To those patients who seek medical help, this feeling may bring about behavior in which they "hate themselves." The basis of this irritability may be either biochemical, psychological, or, more commonly, a combination of both. The outlet for the feeling may be by excessive work, increase in sexual activity, or anger.

ANXIETY.   Anxiety is less frequently recognized as such by women but may be observed by an astute physician. It is a symptom of the ego conflict or the conflict of basic drives wrought by one's image of one's self. Because of this, it is much more apt to be psychologically stimulated. Anxiety can often be recognized in the dream content of these patients, which is usually related to fears of death, mutilation, and separation. It has been reported that significant dreams at this time can reduce the degree of anxiety present.

DEPRESSION.   Depression is not always present in this syndrome, and usually occurs later, in the mood swings that occur from time to time. The mood of the patient is frequently separated from her behavior pattern. Mood can be felt but may not be manifested through behavior. Depression results from a feeling of anger coupled with guilt, which may or may not be associated with reality behavior. Depression is most likely to be seen in those women who find it most difficult to express anger or who allow themselves to become constantly frustrated.

EDEMA.   Edema has been classically described as a premenstrual symptom, and it is an interesting phenomenon both from an investigative standpoint as well as from a therapeutic approach. It is the most readily measurable of the premenstrual symptoms. Many women may complain of the other symptoms described in premenstrual tension without discernible edema or any great change in body weight.

ETIOLOGY

At present there is no definite answer to the etiology of the premenstrual syndrome. Southam and Gonzaga,[2] in an extensive review of literature, stress the physiological alterations such as hypoglycemia, sodium and water retention, and excessive amounts of antidiuretic hormones, all of which have been considered causative mechanisms, but none of which are consistently manifested. Psychogenic factors have also been hypothesized as being etiologic, partly because of a lack of consistent organic findings and partly because there is a high incidence of psychologic disturbance and neurosis in women who suffer from premenstrual syndrome. It seems likely that the etiology is a combination of physiological and psychological factors.

In a "basic" personality, these symptoms are triggered by a biochemical process which is related to the pituitary-ovarian-hypothalamic axis, with the suggestive possibility of adrenal involvement. Melody[3] has reported, as have others, that premenstrual syndrome does not occur in anovulatory cycles. Janowsky and associates,[4] in studying the biochemical changes in women complaining of premenstrual tension, hypothesized that cyclic behavior changes may be induced by some substance that varies in parallel with aldosterone. This, they suggest, may be angiotensin, which like aldosterone is activated during the luteal phase of the cycle, or after progesterone administration, and during pregnancy. Angiotensin is also known to influence animal behavior through the central neurotransmitters and the action of the autonomic system. Central cholinergic activity, initiated by angiotensin, may account for emotional changes during the premenstrual period. Although Janowsky and his co-workers were not able to collect any direct evidence, their studies on the renin-angiotensin-aldosterone system and the ovarian hormones suggest a new perspective in the total picture of the premenstrual tension syndrome.

PSYCHOLOGICAL IMPLICATIONS.   The premenstrual syndrome is of considerable psychological significance, since the mood variations can be demonstrated to affect the degree of psychologic disturbance occurring throughout the menstrual cycle. Deutsch[5] many years ago suggested that the menstrual flow intensified a female's preexisting unconscious and conscious conflicts about pregnancy, sexuality, childbearing, fears of mutilation and death, uncleanliness, competitiveness, aggression, and masturbation. It was Deutsch's belief that in the presence of a weak ego structure, neurotic and psychotic reactions can be related to the menstrual cycle. Benedek and Rubenstein[6] demonstrated that the relationship of moods and behavior patterns were predictable based on the phases of the menstrual cycle. There are many reports in the literature to indicate that the more unstable woman—that is, the woman who feels insecure, who has little ability to make decisions, and who also has difficulty in achieving her needs—is more apt to develop the symptoms of this syndrome than a more stable woman. This suggests that progesterone or its releasing factors may act like a tranquilizer on the hypothalamus.

ATTITUDES AND BEHAVIOR.   Human behavior depends on biochemical programming. This is the result of genetic influences, early experiences, social and cultural training, and disease states, among other factors. The premenstrual state most often affects only behavior, but in a few women it may produce psychotic behavior. Hormonal-biochemical factors may contribute to psychological distress in women. Jeniger (see Luce[7]), in studying different ethnic and social groups, found that the hormone fluctuation was more important in the onset of premenstrual symptoms than familial taboos, although some of the words chosen by these groups would imply a negative attitude toward menstruation. Such common expressions as "getting hit," "unwell," "falling off the roof," convey a dread of the menstrual flow, whereas, "my friend" would suggest a more welcome attitude relative to menstruation—more precisely, that pregnancy had not occurred.

These extreme attitudes toward menstruation may add to premenstrual stress, and to marital and family maladjustments, so that tensions may be less well tolerated at this time of the cycle. It seems reasonable to suppose that the psychosexually less mature woman will be more prone to premenstrual tension.

PSYCHOPHYSIOLOGY

Premenstrual tension may be considered to depend on three major elements which contribute to the observed pathology. They are personality, environmental stress, and cyclic hormonal balance.

1. *Personality.*   The neurotic or psychotic woman who functions on a thin edge will not be able to cope with even minimal distress.

2. *Environmental Stress.*   Obviously this will vary, but it takes its toll over a period of years.

3. *Cyclic Hormonal Balance.*   Anovulatory women do not develop premenstrual tension. Progesterone may secondarily bring about fluid retention by initially decreasing the extracellular fluid volume, followed by a renin-angiotensin-aldosterone activation. This may produce vascular involvement and account for many of the symptoms of this syndrome, such as a feeling of tension and often headache.

DIAGNOSIS

The diagnosis of premenstrual syndrome should be made on the basis of positive findings. They are:

1. The presence of irritability, anxiety, or depression occurring with or without edema, within four days prior to or during the menstrual cycle, or four days midcycle.

2. The existence of these symptoms for four consecutive menstrual cycles.

3. The fact that the patient is incapacitated enough to warrant medication or the services of a physician.

These criteria are usually found in women between the ages of 30 and 40 years. The premenstrual syndrome should be differentiated from "spasmodic dysmenorrhea" with its accompanying menstrual pain. In this case, progesterone levels are usually high, whereas in premenstrual tension there is usually an abrupt fall in progesterone levels premenstrually.

MANAGEMENT

The management of premenstrual tension often taxes the acumen of the clinician. The physician may need to employ psychotherapy, drugs, dietary restrictions, or a combination of these.

PHARMACOLOGIC

1. *Edema.*   When the symptoms are primarily related to edema, chlorothiazides should be given in dosages of 250 mg. to 500 mg. in the morning for two weeks prior to menstruation, at the same time instituting a low sodium diet with adequate potassium intake.

2. *Anxiety.*   Anxiety may be controlled until better adjustments can be made by the use of diazepam (Valium) in doses of 10 mg. three to four times per day.

3. *Depression.*   Many of the more potent antidepressant drugs may produce severe side-effects and must be used with caution. Meprobamate and benactyzine hydrochloride (Deprol) may be used with relative safety and will usually be effective.

When depression is associated with manic behavior, lithium carbonate (300 mgm., t.i.d.) is of value. This drug should not be used in women with renal or hepatic disease, and care should be taken to avoid causing lithium toxicity.

4. *Progesterone-Estrogen Ratio.*   Anovulatory women do not develop premenstrual tension but women who ovulate and suffer an acute drop in proges-

terone levels do. In these women, administration of progesterone in the second half of their cycle may prove helpful in relieving all their symptoms except edema.

5. *Castration.* I do not feel that surgical or irradiation castration has a place in the management of premenstrual tension.

PSYCHOTHERAPY

Even though many of the symptoms of premenstrual tension can be controlled by diuretics, improved dietary intake, and inducing anovulatory cycles, very little success will be reached without treating all the patient's problems. Psychotherapy begins with the patient discussing her frustrations, possible pent-up anger, and any guilt feelings, and this will help her find better outlets for her emotions. Whenever possible, negative environmental influences should be eliminated.

The opportunity to express her feelings may be therapeutic and helpful in allowing the patient to see the amount of unexpressed anger she may have. Usually this has built up over many years, in many cases resulting in a lack of emotional growth by the patient.

Certainly the patient's early memories and attitudes concerning menstruation, sexuality, and pregnancy should be explored. Most women who have premenstrual tension will usually have a concomitant sexual problem. Frequently these women are not able to respond sexually through orgasm. Misconceptions should be corrected and, when appropriate, sexual counseling should be given.

For those women who are married, involving the husband in therapy sessions may be helpful. Frequently he has no concept of the problems or of his wife's feelings. If the spouse allows his wife to learn to express anger, but at the same time control it, both will come closer and their marriage will be given more meaning. In this way anger may be released and guilt prevented.

When possible, the physician should explore dreams with his patient and allow her to give her interpretation. The dream patterns may be most therapeutic in the release of pent-up emotions. The physician will be genuinely rewarded by having provided true comprehensive care.

Vascular Congestion and Hyperemia

In 1949, Taylor[9,10,11] brought to the attention of the gynecologists of this country a syndrome which he felt was due to chronic pelvic vascular congestion and hyperemia. Prior to this publication, European physicians had referred to such conditions as "pelvic congestion," "chronic parametritis," or "broad ligament neuritis." According to Taylor, these patients complain of tension, fatigue, headaches, insomnia, dyspareunia, and frigidity. He further states that they have disturbances in moods and attitudes, and have related psychosomatic symptoms of the gastrointestinal tract as well as of other body systems. It was his opinion that these symptoms were brought about by fibrosis of the pelvic organs, which resulted from changes secondary to chronic vascular congestion. Equally important was his concept that the pelvic changes produced discomfort and increased the psychological problems that seemed to be a common denominator in his patients.

ETIOLOGY

The work of Masters and Johnson[12] has shown that there are two principal physiologic responses to sexual stimulation. The first is vasocongestion and the second is increase in myotonia. Any male who has had sexual stimulation without ejaculation, such as from petting, usually will feel pain in the testicles from vasocongestion. A similar occurrence may be produced in the female when she is stimulated to some degree, such as to the plateau phase, but does not achieve orgasm. Whether this can produce permanent pathological changes in the pelvic organs is open to debate, but that such episodes can produce pelvic discomfort, and that this pain may further irritate the psyche of these women, is quite obvious.

MANAGEMENT

The management of pelvic congestion should be directed at eliminating the cause, which may be both emotional and physical. These include:

1. Increasing psychosocial growth.
2. Relieving the impediments to full sexual response, such as fear, guilt, or disgust.
3. Manipulation of the environment when appropriate.
4. Desensitization when indicated.
5. Correction of pelvic relaxation.
6. Appropriate treatment of chronic pelvic infection.

Summary

The varied syndromes that are ascribed to chronic tension in women are the result of multiple factors—psychological, environmental, biochemical, and anatomical changes owing to disease states. These factors may become a vicious circle thereby decreasing the woman's functional capacity. The proper management requires the identification of the problem and correcting as many of the components of the complex as possible. This requires the appropriate pharmacological regimen, psychotherapy, behavior therapy, and, rarely, surgical intervention. The physician should primarily direct his efforts to relieving the tension state that exists with the patient, whether this can be traced to her personality or environment or, more commonly, both. Negative or unfounded statements such as "It is your nerves or imagination" should be avoided. In this way many women who might have become "pelvic cripples" will not be subjected to needless drugs or surgery.

REFERENCES

1. Frank, R. T.: Arch. Neurol. Psychiatry 26:1053, 1931.
2. Southam, A. L., and Gonzaga, F. P.: Systemic changes during the menstrual cycle. Amer. J. Obstet. Gynec. 91:142, 1965.
3. Melody, G. F.: Behavioral implications of premenstrual tension. Obstet. Gynec. 17:439, 1961.
4. Janowsky, D. S., Gorney, R., Castelnuovo-Tedesco, P., et al.: Premenstrual-menstrual increases in psychiatric hospital admission rates. Amer. J. Obstet. Gynec. 103:189, 1969.

5. Deutsch, H.: The Psychology of Women. New York, Grune & Stratton, 1944.
6. Benedek, T., and Rubenstein, B. B.: Correlations between ovarian activity and psychodynamic processes; ovulative phase. Psychosom. Med. 1:245, 401, 1939.
7. Luce, G.: Body time: Physiological Rhythms and Social Stress. New York, Pantheon Press, 1971.
8. Lauritzen, C.: Bull. Schweiz. Akod., Med. Wisc. 25:463, 1970.
9. Taylor, H. C., Jr.: Vascular congestion and hyperemia; their effect on structure and function in female reproductive system; physiologic basis and history of concept. Amer. J. Obstet. Gynec. 57:211, 1949.
10. Taylor, H. C., Jr.: Vascular congestion and hyperemia; their effect on function and structure in female reproductive organs; clinical aspects of congestion-fibrosis syndrome. Amer. J. Obstet. Gynec. 57:637, 1949.
11. Taylor, H. C., Jr.: Vascular congestion and hyperemia; their effect on function and structure in female reproductive organs; etiology and therapy. Amer. J. Obstet. Gynec. 57:654, 1949.
12. Masters, W. H., and Johnson, V. E.: Human Sexual Response. Boston, Little, Brown & Co., 1966.

Evaluation and Preferred Management of Premenstrual Tension—Pelvic Congestive Syndrome and Allied States

Mary Anna Friederich and Anthony Labrum

University of Rochester School of Medicine and Dentistry

Introduction

After a long review of the literature on premenstrual tension, the authors have come away with feelings of confusion and exhaustion. The first time the term "premenstrual tension" was used in the United States literature was in 1931, when Frank reported on 15 patients he had seen with this "syndrome."[23] Long before this, however, there were references in the French and English literature to the "menstrual wave" theory, as it was called by Jacobi in 1877, for example.[34] Culturally speaking, we know that various societies, both primitive and not so primitive, have had feelings of awe about the menstruating woman and have built up a large variety of cultural rites to neutralize their fears and concerns. The menstruating woman has been so powerful and frightening a figure that certain cultures have banished her and her family from group activities at the menstrual time. Jewish customs of purificatory baths are just one example of this. We wonder if these cultural rites are not a reflection of a universal unconscious knowledge that powerful psychic and physiologic forces are at work in women around and during the menstrual period. We still have much to learn about these forces. We must admit that much of what we will present here may be incorrect, owing to the fragmentary knowledge that now exists.

Culturally speaking, men and women are conditioned from early childhood to accept physical and psychological changes around the menstrual period. The terms "sick" and "unwell" for menstruation common in everyday language are such examples. This makes it very difficult to weed out cultural factors from psychosomatic ones in a given patient. It is equally difficult to interpret the body of English literature. Very few authors have reviewed any of the cultural rites in this area. Women may discern certain secondary gains to be had from cultural traditions which tell them that they are supposed to have premenstrual symptoms, thus excusing them from their usual duties. They also may feel freer to let under-lying feelings come to the fore premenstrually—i.e., depression, anger, sexual libido, and so forth—because society is more permissive of this in the premen-strual period. This is a complicated cultural, psychologic, and physiologic prob-lem, with each factor playing an important role in so-called premenstrual tension.

DEFINITION OF PREMENSTRUAL TENSION

What about the term "premenstrual tension"? There is much debate in the literature as to whether the condition should be called "premenstrual tension," "premenstrual syndrome," "toxemia of menstruation," or none of these. This com-plex does occur in women who are not menstruating and has been described in pubertal and premenarchal years, immediate postmenopausal years, amenorrheic women on human gonadotropic hormone therapy, and women after hysterectomy and oophorectomy. The only common denominator is that symptoms occur regu-larly and cyclically. We will use the term "premenstrual tension."

What are the symptoms of premenstrual tension and what percentage of women suffer them? This all depends on whose report one reads. The incidence has been reported to be between 5 and 95 per cent of all women! The age distri-bution is 10 to 60 years. In the early literature, the percentage was small and only patients who had come for help were reported. More recently, as larger groups of women are surveyed who do not come to physician attention, the per-centage has been expanded to 95 per cent. This, of course, depends on the spe-cific symptoms one includes as comprising premenstrual tension—obviously, the more symptoms one lists the greater will be the percentage of women who have them. Here is a partial list of symptoms: irritability, nervousness, fatigue and exhaustion (or its counterpart, increased physical and mental activity), crying spells, depression, inability to concentrate, craving for sweets, increased appetite, weakness or fainting, trembling of the fingers, low abdominal pain or bloating, headache, generalized aches and pains, gain in weight, edema, painful swelling of the breasts, nausea, vomiting, diarrhea, and constipation. Questionnaire studies of women in non-Western cultures also indicate a comparable prevalence of these premenstrual symptoms. One way out of the confusion is to determine with each given patient which symptoms are painful and troublesome. Many women may be aware of some breast or abdominal swelling, but don't look upon this as a bother. Others may be aware of some vague nervous tension premenstrually but are capable of performing quite as usual. These are physiologic changes, not symptoms. Why are these considered normal cyclic changes by some women and painful symptoms by others? Certainly the psychologic growth and development of the individual, her current environmental stresses, and possible physiologic aberrations may all make a difference. We wonder if the many questionnaire surveys of populations of women have accomplished anything more than collect-ing a long list of changes which occur cyclically.

EPIDEMIOLOGY OF PREMENSTRUAL TENSION

There is some evidence, however, that women may be more vulnerable to a variety of problems in the premenstrual period. Dalton has made several obser-vations on this in the British literature. In 1960, she reported on 124 women involved in accidents and seen in four London general hospital accident wards.[16] She interviewed women between the ages of 15 and 55 years admitted as a result of an accident. She divided the 28-day menstrual cycle into seven four-day periods, three of which turned out to be significant: days 1–4 (menstruation), 13–16 (ovulation), and 25–28 (premenstruum). Of the 84 regularly menstruating women, 52 per cent were involved in accidents during menstruation or the four days preceding it. With purely random distribution, 28.5 per cent of the accidents would have been expected to fall within these days.

Also in 1960, Dalton reported on the weekly scholastic marks of 217 menstruating schoolgirls, ages 11 to 17, and found that for one of every four girls there was a drop in the weekly school mark during the premenstruum, followed by a rise after menstruation.[15] She concluded from this that "on occasions of important examination, the handicap imposed by menstruation will be proportionately increased." This was contradicted by Wickham in 1958,[69] who surveyed aptitude test performances in 1525 young women and found no significant differences in any of the tests on the basis of phase of the menstrual cycle. Sommer did a similar study in 1972 and found no differences in scores on the Watson-Glaser Critical Thinking Appraisal Test in college women or in their actual examination scores in their course in psychology.[58] Since no statistical tests were made on Dalton's data, but were on the other studies, it seems unlikely that intellectual functioning is affected to a significant degree by the phase of the menstrual cycle in schoolgirls or young college women.

Later in 1960, Dalton reported an increase in misbehavior during menstruation in a group of schoolgirls, as reported by their teachers.[19] This included "unpunctuality," "forgetfulness," and "avoiding games." Unfortunately, the teachers' own menstrual cycles were not recorded. A more serious aspect is her report in 1961 of an increased incidence of crimes committed during the premenstrual and menstrual days.[18] Over a six month period, she interviewed 386 newly convicted prisoners. Of these, 284 were menstruating regularly. Forty-nine per cent of the crimes were committed during days 25–28 or 1–4. Fifty-six per cent of the crimes of theft were committed at this time, and 54 per cent of the alcoholics and 44 per cent of the prostitutes were sentenced in these phases. In 1945, Cooke indicated that 84 per cent of all crimes of violence committed by women in Paris were perpetrated during the premenstrual and early menstrual phases.[12] Morton and associates[48] in 1953 found that 62 per cent of violent crimes were committed in the premenstrual week and 17 per cent during menstruation by the inmates of the Westfield State Farm. All of this probably indicates that certain women who have tenuous control over hostile impulses may lose this control premenstrually.

In 1970, Dalton reported that 54 per cent of all children attending a clinic for minor upper respiratory infections did so during their mothers' four premenstrual and four menstrual days. This shows that the mother's menstrual cycle may have an effect on her family as well.[13]

Belfer and associates reported in 1971 that a significant percentage of 34 acknowledged alcoholic women they worked with related their drinking to the menstrual cycle and indicated that drinking usually began or increased in the premenstruum.[6]

Wetzel and colleagues, in a review of the literature on suicide in the menstrual cycle, showed a probable increased incidence of attempted and completed suicide during the luteal and menstrual phases.[67] Two studies of women calling a suicide prevention center found that increased numbers of calls occurred in the menstrual and luteal phases. Another report, by Wetzel and McClure, on Hindu women who committed suicide by immolation, stated that 19 of 22 were menstruating at the time.[68]

In investigating the time of admission of 276 patients for acute psychiatric episodes, Dalton found that 46 per cent of all admissions occurred during days 25–28 or 1–4 of the cycle.[17] Fifty-three per cent of attempted suicides, 47 per cent of patients with depression, and 47 per cent of schizophrenic patients were admitted during this time. These figures have been confirmed by Janowsky and co-workers in 1969 in a study of consecutive female admissions to the psychiatric in-patient service of the Harbor General Hospital.[36] Also, Kramp has confirmed this for the mental hospital in Viborg, Denmark.[73] Essentially the same statistics were obtained by Jacobs and Charles in 1970 in a study of 200 outpatients who presented themselves for psychiatric help.[35] They concluded that physicians should be aware that menstruation serves as a monthly stress and is a time of increased vulnerability, which may precipitate or augment underlying psychiatric symptoms, particularly anxiety. Unfortunately we could not find any report on a longitudinal study of psychotic or neurotic patients that records at what times of the menstrual cycles they became ill during a given period of time. One questionnaire study indicated that about 45 per cent of neurotic and psychotic women report no change in symptoms with the menses. In summary, this seems to indicate that some women do have increased psychiatric symptoms with menses, but others do not. Prevention of premenstrual and menstrual exacerbation of symptoms requires that the physician know his patients well and understand how they respond to premenstrual and menstrual changes.

One last example, again an epidemiologic study from England,[44] reports on 131 consecutive necropsies performed on women aged 18 to 46 at a London mortuary. Of 102 cases that could be evaluated (not menopausal or diseased), 89 deaths occurred during the luteal phase and 13 during the menstrual and follicular phases. Death was significantly more frequent in the mid-luteum. Suicides and accidents accounted for more than 50 per cent of the deaths in this series.

CLINICAL STUDIES OF PREMENSTRUAL TENSION

From our review of the literature, it is apparent that some women are more vulnerable to serious problems in the premenstrual and menstrual periods. What do we know about psychologic changes in a given group of women during the menstrual cycle? Benedek and Rubenstein did the pioneer work in this field in the 1930's. Benedek, a psychoanalyst, analyzed a group of women with psychiatric problems and had them take daily vaginal smears. Rubenstein, working in another city, dated the menstrual cycle from the smears. Benedek tried to predict the phase of the cycle from the content of the therapy discussions and later correlated them with Rubenstein's findings. Since an entire book was written on this,[7] we are oversimplifying the results in saying that they found that passive receptive tendencies correlated with progesterone production and active heterosexual strivings correlated with estrogen production. Benedek characterized the premenstruum (when both estrogen and progesterone levels are low) as being high in feelings of fear about mutilation and death, in anxiety and depression, and in sexual fantasies and drives. Since then, several investigators, using different modalities of study, have confirmed much of this. For instance, Shader and his associates (1968) administered various psychological tests to a group of 76 female graduate students and found that marked changes in libido occurred with the menstrual cycle.[56] The more highly anxious women had the most marked changes.

There are many studies in which a group of women, usually nurses or students, have been asked to check off psychologic symptoms such as irritability, depression, anxiety, tension, nervousness, and fatigue, and to rate the seriousness of these symptoms. Moos Menstrual Distress Questionnaire is one of the better studies.[46] This was performed at one arbitrary point in time. The investigators felt, however, that the test results would not have been different if the women filled out the questionnaire during a menstrual period or other times in the cycle. Despite commonly held ideas, young women as well as women in their 30's and 40's have symptoms around the time of their menstrual periods. Moos and associates found that women in their teens and 20's complained more of dysmenorrhea, autonomic reactions, water retention, and negative affect during their menses, with fewer complaints being made premenstrually.[46] In contrast, women in the later 20's and over had more symptoms premenstrually than menstrually. This shift in emphasis and phase was related to age, and Moos could not separate parity from age and degree of symptoms. Others would agree. Several studies equate degrees of irregularity of menses with degrees of menstrual and premenstrual symptoms. Likewise, several studies show that there is a correlation of menstrual traits between girls and their mothers—if the mother has premenstrual tension or dysmenorrhea, the daughter is very likely to have it also. This is not a hard and fast rule, however. Some girls may be free of symptoms and yet have mothers with symptoms, and conversely. Though this characteristic may be passed from mother to daughter psychologically, it may also indicate an inherited organic foundation.

Other investigators have attempted to follow women both with and without symptoms of premenstrual tension over a period of time. The purpose is to determine if there are mood changes throughout the cycle. Some have had women check off a daily list of symptoms for several menstrual cycles. Others have done repeated interviews at various points in a cycle, and still others have analyzed five minute segments of free-associated speech at different points in the cycle. All agree that there are mood fluctuations. Hostility, directed both inward and outward, anxiety, and depression are at peaks premenstrually and then ebb, usually at the time of ovulation, A given person seems to show consistent changes from cycle to cycle, but there is individual variation—some women have less anxiety premenstrually, for example. Level of anxiety tends to correlate with psychologic development. There have been relatively few symptomatic women followed by these methods over a period of time and then compared to an asymptomatic control group. The numbers are so small that the results are probably not valid. Results imply that symptomatic women have a more negative affect—i.e. depression, anxiety, and hostility—at all times in the cycle than asymptomatic women. There is no agreement as to the psychosexual background of these two groups, but, as noted, the group is much too small to be representative.

There are studies in the literature comparing groups of normal, neurotic, and psychotic women with respect to incidence of premenstrual tension. The earliest one was by Rees in 1953.[53] In these studies, often the investigator gives some sort of personality inventory test to a group of women to determine how so-called "neuroticism scores" compare to the severity of premenstrual symptoms. As you might expect, women with high "neuroticism scores" are more likely to have symptoms of premenstrual tension. One study found neurotics to have more menstrual pain than controls, patients with affective disorders to be the same as controls, and schizophrenic patients to have less pain than controls. Symptoms of premenstrual depression, anxiety, and so forth, likewise were increased in neurosis, normal in affective disorders, and decreased in schizophrenia. All point out that normal controls may have severe symptoms and severely ill neurotics and psychotics may have no symptoms. All these facts serve to emphasize that physical factors may be involved and that one cannot generalize about any given patient.

Pathophysiology

The occurrence of premenstrual changes in women of different cultures, at different ages, and indeed even in other primates suggests some basic biological mechanisms for the changes, with perhaps some additional factor related to stress that can precipitate or exacerbate the symptoms.

Frank suggested that premenstrual symptoms were related to cyclic variations in "sex hormone" and assumed that excess secretion of estrogen affecting "the sympathetic and cardiovascular systems" caused the premenstrual symptoms.[23] Although pregnanediol was first isolated from pregnancy urine in 1929, its relation to progesterone was not clear for some years. At the time Frank wrote his paper, estrogen was the only measurable ovarian hormone; progesterone had not yet been isolated from the ovary. In 1938, Israel, on the basis of endometrial curettings from women with premenstrual tension, argued that this syndrome was due to defective luteinization which in turn produced relative hyperestrinism.[33]

Quite early in the history of premenstrual tension, it was thought to be associated with excessive salt and water retention, which led to edema, edema of gut wall (bowel distention), edema of breasts (breast tenderness), and cerebral edema (premenstrual headache, mood changes, and epilepsy). It was assumed that estrogen and progesterone caused salt retention, except for those who incriminated estrogen alone and assumed there was a deficit in progesterone production to account for the relative hyperestrinism. For the last 40 years, salt and water retention, with their associated edema and premenstrual weight gain, has been widely accepted as the basis for premenstrual tension and has led to "rational therapy" of salt restriction and diuretic medication. Generalized edema associated with menstruation was reported by Thomas in 1933.[63] A study of body weight variation during the menstrual cycle by Thorn and associates in 1938 indicated an average weight gain of 1 kg. or more during the premenstrual phase of the cycle, but also showed that 76 per cent of the 50 subjects gained up to 1 kg. at the time of ovulation.[65] This was confirmed by Chesley and Hellman in 1957.[11] Thorn and colleagues made the important observation that although abnormal swelling, increased appetite, and thirst occurred in two-thirds of the subjects who gained weight, these symptoms were also experienced by one-third of women with no significant premenstrual weight gain. Clearly, premenstrual fluid retention seemed to be an independent variable in relation to other premenstrual changes. Many studies of weight gain and of salt and water balance have been published, but we feel that only studies of patients on a metabolic ward setting with fixed sodium intake are helpful in clarifying the relation of fluid retention to premenstrual symptoms. Bruce and Russell in 1962 studied 10 women complaining of premenstrual tension on a metabolic ward.[9] Five gained some weight premenstrually, but similar changes occurred at the midcycle. Three patients developed premenstrual tension, but their weight gains were no different from those of women who remained symptom-free. Klein and Carey in 1961 found no significant difference between total exchangeable sodium (Na_e) in the various phases of the menstrual cycle.[38] This was confirmed by Gray and colleagues in 1968 and by Michelakis and associates in 1971.[28,45] The original belief that excess estrogen production might be a factor in premenstrual tension was studied by Prill and Kruger in 1963.[52] They measured estrogen excretion (Ittrich method) in nine women with premenstrual tension and 10 matched controls. No difference in total estrogen or estriol, estrone, or estradiol excretion was found.

Thorn and colleagues in 1937 studied the effects of progesterone on dogs and concluded that a sodium retaining effect had been demonstrated.[64] Landau and associates showed that progesterone had salt excreting properties,[41] and in 1961 Landau and Lugibihl demonstrated that progesterone has an anti-aldosterone effect at the level of renal tubules.[40] The natriuretic action of progesterone has been demonstrated in men and in postmenopausal women. Various models have been used to demonstrate this salt excreting effect, including measurements of the sodium content of sweat and saliva. The body responds to this natriuretic action of progesterone in a complex way. Sodium loss leads to a decrease in exchangeable body sodium and a fall in total body water. Shrinkage of extracellular fluid leads to activation of the juxtamedullary mechanism in the kidneys, with release of renin, which initiates the conversion of renin substance to angiotensin II, which in turn evokes secretion of aldosterone. This, acting on the renal tubules, prevents sodium excretion, and a new sodium balance is established and maintained by increased levels of aldosterone. All these changes are thus secondary to the sodium excreting effects of progesterone, and after a brief disequilibrium, a new sodium balance is established by means of increased aldosterone production.

To summarize, we can say that some women do manifest edema during the menstrual cycle, but that there is no evidence that fluid retention is related to premenstrual affect changes. Variations of body sodium are brief and quickly restored to normal by the renin-angiotension mechanism. Furthermore, in conditions in which excess salt and fluid retention do occur, such as primary hyperaldosteronism, there are no changes in affect comparable to those found premenstrually, nor do such changes occur in association with the edema of nephrosis, cardiac failure, or hepatic disease.

The failure of diuretics when tested in double-blind trials to reduce premenstrual symptoms (to be discussed later), is further evidence that sodium and water retention are not related in a cause-and-effect way to the emotional changes and some other symptoms occurring in the premenstrual phase.

Symptoms compatible with hypoglycemia are experienced by some women during the premenstrual phase, including fatigue, faintness, or shaking attacks, which are relieved by eating sweets. In 1950, Morton showed that some women with premenstrual tension have a flat glucose tolerance curve in the premenstruum.[49] Progesterone itself does not affect the glucose tolerance test, but the possibility that changes in other hormones (growth hormone, glucocorticoids) might affect the test has not yet been clearly determined. Yalow and Berson in 1965 described functional hypoglycemia, occurring 24 hours after a meal, in essentially unstable, tense, anxious women with gastric hypermobility and increased gastric acidity.[71]

NEUROPHARMACOLOGICAL EFFECTS OF PROGESTERONE

Gillman in 1942 administered progesterone intramuscularly to women in the follicular phase of the cycle.[25] Two of 16 subjects complained of one or more of the symptoms of lassitude, depression, or irritability. Hirst and Hamblen (1942), during a study of the excretion products of injected progesterone in humans, record "a sudden onset of acute depression, with psychomotor retardation and associated feelings of impending calamity" in one subject.[32]

One possible mechanism of the manner in which this progesterone effect is produced is via action on the brain. Also in 1942, Selye recorded frank hypnotic effects after administration of progesterone in partially hepatectomized animals.[55] Intravenous progesterone inhibits neurons related to the general arousal system (reticular activating system, reticulo-neocortical pathways, and hypothalamic-limbic pathways), depresses single-unit firing, decreases response to all forms of stimuation, and blocks propagated action potentials. Electroencephalograms show sleep changes. Whereas estrogen lowers the arousal threshold to environmental stimuli, progesterone appears to block or reverse these effects.

Neurochemical studies indicate that progesterone decreases levels of brain norepinephrine in rats, particularly in the midbrain. Progesterone increases 5-hydroxytryptamine levels of the midbrain and hindbrain of rats. At a biochemical level, progesterone accelerates the rate of hydrolysis of ATP, uncouples oxidative phosphorylation, and, by direct action on the electron transport chain, inhibits mitochondrial respiration. It also affects membrane permeability, preventing influx of sodium ions across the membrane. Progesterone, in connection with estrogen, produced marked deterioration of a prelearned, conditioned avoidance response in cats. Progesterone causes decreased activity, increased food intake, increased body weight in intact female rats, and decreased wheel running activity. Locomotor activity is a powerful factor in energy balance, and a reduction in level of activity could easily lead to increase in weight.

The neurochemical hypothesis of affective disorders holds that increased levels of norepinephrine (NE) in the brain (or certain areas of the brain) lead to tension, agitation, or mania, and decreased activity is associated with depression. Serotonin (5-hydroxytryptamine, or 5-HT) seems to deviate from a mean level, in depression and mania, without an obvious correlation. Carlsson (1969) believed that NE increase is related to excitation and changes in 5-HT were more important in depression.[10] Ladisich and Bauman in 1971 discussed the relationships of progesterone to premenstrual tension and puerperal psychoses and suggested that both conditions are associated with falling levels of progesterone.[39] Tange and Greengrass (1971) also studied the role of neuroendocrine changes in the brain in relation to depression in the premenstrual phase, postpartum, and the climacterium.[61] They showed that a significant increase of NE occurs in the cortex in female rats given estrogen or progesterone, whereas a significant decrease of NE occurs in the hindbrain. Only progesterone produces any significant increase in brain 5-HT content, in both the midbrain and the hindbrain.

The problem with animal studies of this kind concerns interpretation of gross tissue levels of neuroendocrine transmitters. The evidence from several recent studies suggests that very complex interactions occur within the nerve ending and in the interneuronal space, which cannot be evaluated by measurement of total tissue levels of neurotransmitters.

Recently, Maas and associates suggested that understanding of changes in affect may only come through the study of interactions between steroid hormones, electrolytes, and catecholamines.[42] Studies on disposition of catecholamines have shown that if sodium or potassium is omitted from the incubation or perfusion media, there is a marked decline in uptake and an increased efflux of NE from neural tissue. Adrenal cortical steroids control ATPase activity either directly or via Na^+ and K^+ levels. Increased adrenocortical secretion ("stress") would be expected to be associated with an increase in ATPase activity, an accelerated uptake of NE, and a decreased rate of synthesis of catecholamines. This would lead to depression. The fact that progesterone will support life in an adrenalectomized dog seems to have been forgotten. It seems that progesterone can act as a corticosteroid and may have the same effect on NE uptake, leading to depression. It is interesting to note that depression is the one side-effect of oral contraceptives which has consistently shown up in double-blind trials, and the bloating, breast changes, and weight gain associated with use of oral progestins in some women are comparable to the premenstrual syndrome. It seems that only some women respond this way to oral progestins and perhaps, as in those women who exhibit severe premenstrual changes, we have to look for some metabolic—perhaps neuroendocrine—anomaly, which results in this possibly excessive response to progesterone.

There has been much interest recently in the "switch" phenomenon, in which manic-depressive patients swing from one affect to the other. It is possible that a woman may "switch" from a normal or a depressed phase to a tense, anxious (hypomanic) phase as progesterone levels fall. We have seen other patterns. Explanation of these must await a clearer understanding of neurochemistry and particularly of the interaction between basic neurochemical states and an individual affect or behavior pattern.

The possibility that progesterone may *cause* some forms of premenstrual distress, particularly depression, is advanced as a basis of some of the problems in some women. The recent demonstration by Adamopoulos and associates, that more than half of a small group of patients were anovulatory during the "switch" period and had premenstrual tension during this time implies, as we have suggested elsewhere in this chapter, that "premenstrual tension" may be a group of disorders with different etiologies.[1] Oral contraception seems to help some women. The medication might work by raising the level of progestin, by preventing the production of natural progesterone, or by changing the level of anxiety or depression in patients related to fear of pregnancy.

TREATMENT

We are impressed with the lack of accurate or consistent descriptions of premenstrual tension in the literature. Some women seem to be depressed through the luteal phase, and then swing into a very tense, agitated phase during the last few days of the cycle or the early days of the menstrual flow. Others have different sequences of change in affect. Before we can seriously discuss treatment, we need to describe this disorder in detail as it occurs in many patients. Are we dealing with variants of one disorder, or are there different kinds of premenstrual disorders? Only after we have obtained data to answer these questions may rational therapeutic intervention be possible.

HISTORY OF THERAPY

The belief that excessive estrogen production was the cause of premenstrual tension led Frank to suggest irradiation of the ovaries. This was performed on many women "with improvement for two or more years." Israel utilized irradiation of the pituitary in his regimen of treatment. He also employed progestins to oppose the presumed hyperestrinism, still working on the assumption that excess estrogens were responsible for premenstrual distress. Freed (1945) used androgens in doses which would lead one to expect that hirsutism and voice changes would be produced in at least some patients.[24]

In 1953, Greene and Dalton achieved impressive success with monthly injections of progesterone.[30] Although some women responded well to the oral progestins, Dalton believed that only "natural" progestins would be maximally effective.[14]

Frank suggested the use of diuretics as well, and these have been employed in various forms for 40 years. Greenhill and Freed, in 1940, used ammonium chloride and low sodium intake.[31] Winshel used chlorothiazide.[70] A summary of the results of various treatments is shown in Table 23–1. None of these were double-blind studies.

How is it that so many different medications have been so "effective" in treating this disorder? In the first place, all patients will respond to some degree if you show interest in them as individuals. The more dynamic the personality of the investigator is, the greater this psychological effect is likely to be. If medication is also given, a significant number will respond on the basis of the placebo effect. The incidence of premenstrual symptoms according to various studies ranges from 5 to 95 per cent, so clearly there may be significant differences in the population of patients selected for study in different series. The criteria for whether or not therapy was successful are always based on the patient's self-evaluation. The duration of follow-up is important, partly because premenstrual symptoms may vary from cycle to cycle, and partly because, as Goldzieher and colleagues have shown in 1971, placebo effects can continue at a diminishing rate of effectiveness for several months.[27] Evaluation of therapy requires the following:

1. All studies must be of a double-blind nature.

2. Selection of subjects must be based on clearly defined objective criteria, such as time away from work, visits to a physician, days in bed, or performance in various psychological tests or psychoendocrine studies.

3. The duration of the study must allow for variations from cycle to cycle, and for the possible prolonged duration of a placebo effect.

4. Criteria for cure must also be objective (see No. 2).

5. Only one treatment should be given. In contrast to this, several of the studies have combined progestins, diuretics, salt restriction, vitamins, and tranquilizers.

No study has achieved all these criteria, but some double-blind studies are avail-

TABLE 23–1. *Results of Types of Therapy Suggested For Premenstrual Tension*

AUTHOR	TREATMENT	GOOD OR VERY GOOD RESULTS (PER CENT OF TOTAL CYCLES OF TREATMENT)
Appleby[4]	Meprobamate	53%
	Chlorothiazide	33%
	Dimethisterone	10%
	Lactose (placebo)	7%
	Ethisterone	10%
Barfield and associates[5]	Cytran (progestin-diuretic-tranquilizer)	87.4%
Block[8]	Vitamin A	60%
Fortin and associates[22]	Psychotherapy	56%
Greenblatt[29]	Reserpine	72%
Greene and Dalton[30]	Progesterone	90.1%
	Ethisterone	65.3%
Greenhill and Freed[31]	Ammonium chloride and low sodium intake	85%
Jordheim[37]	Medroxyprogesterone acetate	17.1%
	(Series A) Medroxyprogesterone acetate and hydroflumethiazide	25.5%
	(Series B) Medroxyprogesterone acetate and hydroflumethiazide	24.31%
	Placebo	22.21%
Pennington[51]	Meprobamate	78%
	Placebo	3%
Reeves and associates[54]	Control patients	12.3*
	Placebo	9.5*
	Potassium chloride	12.6*
Stokes and Mendels[59]	Pyridoxine	30.7%
	Placebo	38%
Swyer[60]	Mephenesin	60.8%
	Mephenesin and ethisterone	61.9%
	Ethisterone	56.5%
	Placebo	40%
Warfield[66]	Cytran (progestin-diuretic-tranquilizer)	96.3%

* Average number of symptoms, last five days of cycle.

able. Morton, in his prison study, obtained improvements on placebo therapy of 15 per cent and 39 per cent, the higher figure being obtained in women on a high protein diet.[48] The corresponding figures for ammonium chloride therapy were 61 per cent and 79 per cent, respectively. In a study by Swyer, good or very good results were obtained in 60 per cent of women treated with mephenesin, 56 per cent of women in ethisterone, and in 40 per cent of patients on the placebo.[60] Stokes and Mendels obtained an improvement in 11 per cent of patients on pyridoxine, whereas 55 per cent of patients improved on the placebo.[59] Jordheim found no difference between progestins plus diuretic and progestins alone in an uncontrolled comparison.[37] When he compared the progestin-diuretic combination with a placebo, he again found no difference, obtaining a good or very good response in 21.4 per cent of study patients, and in 19 per cent of patients on the placebo. Good or very good response to the placebo was noted in 15, 19, 39, 40, and 55 per cent of patients in the various studies quoted above. Pennington's study, using meprobamate and a placebo, showed only a 3 per cent improvement on placebo compared with 78 per cent improvement for meprobamate, results which are difficult to interpret.[51]

The use of lithium carbonate in the treatment of severe premenstrual tension was advocated by Sletten and Gershon in 1966[67] and by Taylor in 1970. Lithium was originally believed to act as a competitive inhibitor of sodium. The mode of action is probably more complex, including increased deamination of norepinephrine and inhibition of tyrosine hydroxylase, thereby decreasing the amount of norepinephrine available to receptor sites. It may also affect membrane permeability in the neurons.

Frank was perhaps farsighted when in discussing treatment of patients with premenstrual tension he suggested "patients can be helped psychologically to utilize their increased sexuality through gaining a better understanding of themselves."

OUR RECOMMENDATIONS FOR THERAPY

At this stage we still do not know the cause of premenstrual changes, hence we cannot suggest specific therapy. Understanding of this condition lies in part in the area of psychopharmacology. We are impressed with the frequency with which stressful life events precipitate the onset of severe premenstrual symptoms among our own patients. Salt restriction and diuretics have been used for many years without obvious success.

The guidelines for treatment we feel we can recommend are:

1. Discussion of the setting in which the premenstrual distress started or became worse. Can this be related, as Donovan[20] suggested, to a life-long pattern of response to difficulties?

2. Evaluation of sources of tension present from month to month. If appropriate, advise reduction of tension, particularly during the premenstrual week.

3. Discussion of the marital-sexual problems. Does sexual intercourse during the premenstruum help relieve tension, or does anger with the husband at this time inhibit sexual response? Is this a time of the month when multiple orgasms might fully reduce tension?

4. Elimination of a high carbohydrate diet. Ultimately a high-protein, high-fat intake will prevent the premenstrual hypoglycemic attacks which are a problem for some women.

5. A trial of oral contraceptives may be justified in order to depress endogenous progesterone. Some women will improve, some will remain unchanged, some will become worse. A rebound effect after the active oral progestin is finished may occur, and a few women get very much worse at this time.

6. Meprobamate is effective for some women, but it should only be considered as a temporary expedient. If the possibility of many more years of treatment for symptoms exists, some non-drug therapy should be the goal.

7. Lithium carbonate may be considered in women who do not respond to any of the above approaches and are severely incapacitated by the premenstrual changes. This is applicable only to a very small group of patients.

8. We must critically evaluate the effect of salt restriction and use of diuretics. The evidence accumulating suggests that we may be harming rather than helping our patients with premenstrual tension as well as missing the point

that this condition may be associated with an abnormally *low* rather than raised body or tissue sodium level.

We feel that rather than playing pharmacopoeial roulette, we should take the harder approach of accumulating data about the condition by listening to our patients—what are the circumstances of their lives, what was the setting for the onset of the premenstrual distress, and what is bringing this patient to her doctor at this time? Often a supportive relationship allows the patient to talk about her feelings and is the only therapy needed.

ASSOCIATED CONDITIONS

PELVIC CONGESTIVE SYNDROME.   This condition is accepted as an entity by some gynecologists and not by others. Taylor in 1949 described the history and his views of the physiological basis of this disorder.[62] He considered arterial dilatation, venous engorgement, and local increase in extravascular tissue fluid as being important findings in this disorder. He also considered the natural history of the disorder, which progresses from predominantly vascular congestion to pelvic fibrosis. In an impressive, and we think neglected paper, Duncan and Taylor in 1952 presented an intensive study of 36 patients with the pelvic congestive syndrome.[21] The symptoms and physical findings are clearly described. Duncan and Taylor also studied children, parent-child relationships, sexual behavior and attitudes, and life setting at the time of onset. The authors found that their patients had had no secure family life experience in childhood, and particularly that they lacked a satisfactory relationship with their mothers or a mother substitute. Inability to function adequately as a woman either sexually or maternally was displayed by most. In 34 of the 36 patients, the onset of the pelvic symptoms was related to stressful life situations. Some preliminary evidence of changes in pelvic blood flow with affect states was also demonstrated. Most of the women in this study were found to have significant emotional disorders, an association which has also been found by others. These women are psychologically ill and difficult to help. Frequently they have no insight or interest in psychotherapy and resist referral to a psychiatrist. Their pattern of life for many years has involved physical suffering as a means of dealing with psychologic and social conflicts. To take away the physical pain may leave them with such intense psychic pain that acute psychosis or even suicide may result. Ordinarily, physicians see themselves as persons who relieve pain. However, with insight into the character structures of these women, physicians should try and sustain them as much as possible, perhaps attempting to modify their social situation. In this instance, pain relief should not be the major goal of therapy.

As we learn more about visceral conditioning using bio-feedback, it may be possible to teach these patients how to vary their pelvic blood flow by conditioning techniques. Perhaps the psychobiologic connection is that psychic stress somehow activates increased pelvic blood flow, which these patients interpret as pain.

UNIVERSAL JOINT SYNDROME. Allen (1955) and Allen and Masters (1971) have described the bilateral broad ligament tear as the "universal joint syndrome" and recommended surgical intervention to correct this.[2,3] There have been no long-term follows-ups of their patients to learn how they function generally. Surgery should be considered very carefully and utilized infrequently. We have all seen women subjected to multiple surgical interventions who are still complaining of pain, dyspareunia, or premenstrual congestive feelings.

IDIOPATHIC CYCLIC EDEMA.   We mention this for completeness' sake. The prime manifestation is periodic brawny, nonpitting edema of the face, hands, abdomen, and feet. The patients are usually middle-aged, obese, menstruating women. The edema is unrelated to the menstrual cycles. Women may gain 12 lb. in weight in a few days' time. Often edema is accompanied by anxiety and depression. Patients are aware of increased oral fluid intake with small urinary output during bouts of edema. The disease seems to be self-limited, but may recur periodically over a period of several years. There are no known serious sequelae.

The etiology of this condition is obscure. Excessive aldosterone secretion, difficulty in adjusting to rapid change in salt intake, exaggerated orthostatic effect, and increased capillary permeability have all been suggested.

REFERENCES

1. Adamopoulos, D. A., Loraine, J. A., Lunn, S. F., Coppen, A. J., and Daly, R. J.: Endocrine profiles in premenstrual tension. Clin. Endocr. *1*:283, 1972.
2. Allen, W. M.: Chronic pelvic congestion and pelvic pain. Amer. J. Obstet. Gynec. *109*:198, 1971.
3. Allen, W. M., and Masters, W. H.: Traumatic laceration of uterine support. Amer. J. Obstet. Gynec. *70*:500, 1955.
4. Appleby, B. P.: A study of premenstrual tension in general practice. Brit. Med. J. *1*:391, 1960.
5. Barfield, W. E., Jungck, E. D., and Greenblatt, R. B.: The premenstrual tension syndrome: A comprehensive approach to treatment with a progestin-diuretic-tranquilizer combination. South. Med. J. *55*:1139, 1962.
6. Belfer, M. L., Shader, R. I., Carroll, M., and Harmatz, J. S.: Alcoholism in women. Arch. Gen. Psych. *25*:540, 1971.
7. Benedek, T., and Rubenstein, B. B.: Studies in Psychosomatic Medicine: Psychosexual Functions in Women. New York, Ronald Press Company, 1952.
8. Block, E.: The use of vitamin A in premenstrual tension. Acta Obstet. Gynec. Scand. *39*:586, 1960.
9. Bruce, J., and Russell, G. F. M.: Premenstrual tension. A study of weight changes and balances of water, sodium, and potassium. Lancet *2*:267, 1962.
10. Carlsson, A.: Pharmacology of synaptic monoamine transmission. Progr. Brain Res. *31*:53-59, 1969.
11. Chesley, L. C., and Hellman, L. M.: Variations in body weight and salivary sodium in the menstrual cycle. Amer. J. Obstet. Gynec. *74*:582, 1957.
12. Cooke, W. R.: The differential psychology of the American woman. Amer. J. Obstet. Gynec. *49*:457, 1945.
13. Dalton, K.: Children's hospital admissions and mothers' menstruation. Brit. Med. J. *2*:27, 1970.
14. Dalton, K.: Comparative trials of new oral progestogenic compounds in treatment of premenstrual syndrome. Brit. Med. J. *2*:1307, 1959.
15. Dalton, K.: Effect of menstruation on schoolgirls' weekly work. Brit. Med. J. *1*:326, 1960.
16. Dalton, K.: Menstruation and accidents. Brit. Med. J. *2*:1425, 1960.
17. Dalton, K.: Menstruation and acute psychiatric illnesses. Brit. Med. J. *1*:148, 1959.
18. Dalton, K.: Menstruation and crime. Brit. Med. J. *2*:1752, 1961.
19. Dalton, K.: Schoolgirls' behavior and menstruation. Brit. Med. J. *2*:1647, 1960.
20. Donovan, J. C.: Psychologic aspects of the menopause. Obstet. Gynec. *6*:379, 1955.
21. Duncan, C. H., and Taylor, H. C.: A psychosomatic study of pelvic pain. Amer. J. Obstet. Gynec. *64*:1, 1952.
22. Fortin, J. N., Wittkower, E. D., and Kalz, F.: A psychosomatic approach to the premenstrual tension syndrome: a preliminary report. Canad. Med. Ass. J. *79*:978, 1958.
23. Frank, R. T.: The hormonal causes of premenstrual tension. Arch. Neur. Psych. *26*:1053, 1931.
24. Freed, S. C.: The treatment of premenstrual distress with special consideration of the androgens. J.A.M.A. *127*:377, 1945.

25. Gillman, J.: The nature of the subjective reactions evoked in women by progesterone with special reference to the problem of premenstrual tension. J. Clin. Endocr. 2:157, 1942.

26. Goldzieher, J., et al.: Nervousness and depression attributed to oral contraceptives: a double-blind placebo controlled study. Amer. J. Obstet. Gynec. 111:1013, 1971.

27. Goldzieher, J., et al.: A placebo controlled double-blind cross-over investigation of the side-effects attributed to oral contraceptives. Fertil. Steril. 22:609, 1971.

28. Gray, M. J., Strausefeld, K. S., Watanabe, M., Sims, E. A., and Solomon, S.: Aldosterone secretory rates in the normal menstrual cycle. J. Clin. Endocr. 28:1269, 1968.

29. Greenblatt, R. B.: Use of reserpine (serpasil) in certain gynecologic disorders. Ann. N.Y. Acad. Sci. 59:133, 1954.

30. Greene, R., and Dalton, K.: The premenstrual syndrome. Brit. Med. J. 1:1007, 1953.

31. Greenhill, J. P., and Freed, S. C.: The mechanism and treatment of premenstrual distress with ammonium chloride. Endocrinology 26:529, 1940.

32. Hirst, D. V., and Hamblen, E. C.: Vasomotor effects of progesterone. J. Clin. Endocr. 2:664, 1942.

33. Israel, S. L.: Premenstrual tension. J.A.M.A. 110:1721, 1938.

34. Jacobi, M. P.: The Question of Rest for Women During Menstruation. New York, G. P. Putnam's Sons, 1877.

35. Jacobs, T. J., and Charles, E.: Correlation of psychiatric symptomatology and the menstrual cycle in an outpatient population. Amer. J. Psych. 126:1504, 1970.

36. Janowsky, D. S., Gorney, R., Castelnuovo-Tedesco, P., and Stone, C. B. L.: Premenstrual-menstrual increases in psychiatric hospital admission rates. Amer. J. Obstet. Gynec. 103:189, 1969.

37. Jordheim, O.: The premenstrual syndrome. Acta Obstet. Gynec. Scand. 51:77, 1972.

38. Klein, L., and Carey, J.: Total exchangeable sodium in the menstrual cycle. Amer. J. Obstet. Gynec. 81:223, 1961.

39. Ladisich, W., and Bauman, P.: Influence of progesterone on norepinephrine metabolism in connection with amphetamine and stress. Neuroendocrinology 7:16, 1971.

40. Landau, R. L., and Lugibihl, K.: The catabolic and natriuretic effects of progesterone in man. Rec. Progr. Hormone Res. 17:249, 1961.

41. Landau, R. L., Berganstahl, D. M., Lugibihl, K., and Kascht, M. E.: Metabolic effects of progesterone in man. J. Clin. Endocr. 15:1194, 1955.

42. Maas, J. W., Fawcett, J. A., and Dekirmenjian, H.: Catecholamine metabolism, depressive illness and drug response. Arch. Gen. Psych. 26:252, 1972.

43. MacKinnon, P. C. B., and MacKinnon, I. L.: Hazards of the menstrual cycle. Brit. Med. J. 1:555, 1956.

44. MacKinnon, I. L., MacKinnon, P. C. B., and Thomson, A. D.: Lethal hazards of the luteal phase of the menstrual cycle. Brit. Med. J. 1:1015, 1959.

45. Michelakis, A. M., Stant, E. G., and Brill, A. B.: Sodium space and electrolyte excretion during the menstrual cycle. Amer. J. Obstet. Gynec. 109:150, 1971.

46. Moos, R. H.: The development of a menstrual distress questionnaire. Psychosom. Med. 30:853, 1968.

47. Moos, R. H., Kopell, B. S., Melges, F. T., Yalom, E. D., Lunde, D. T., Clayton, R. B., and Hamburg, D. A.: Fluctuations in symptoms and moods during the menstrual cycle. J. Psychosom. Res. 13:37, 1969.

48. Morton, J. H., Addison, H., Addison, R. G., Hunt, L., and Sullivan, J. J.: A clinical study of premenstrual tension. Amer. J. Obstet. Gynec. 65:1182, 1953.

49. Morton, J. H.: Premenstrual tension. Amer. J. Obstet. Gynec. 60:343, 1950.

50. Morton, J. H.: Premenstrual tension. Clin. Obstet. Gynec. 2:136, 1959.

51. Pennington, V. M.: Meprobamate in premenstrual tension. J.A.M.A. 164:638, 1957.

52. Prill, H. J., and Kruger, E.: Estrogen excretion in women with premenstrual tension. Endokrinologie 44:34, 1963.

53. Rees, L.: Psychosomatic aspects of the premenstrual tension syndrome. J. Mental Science 99:62, 1953.

54. Reeves, B., Garvin, J., and McElin, T.: Premenstrual tension: symptoms and weight changes related to potassium therapy. Amer. J. Obstet. Gynec. 109:1036, 1971.

55. Selye, H.: Correlation between the chemical structure and pharmacological actions of the steroids. Endocrinology 30:437, 1942.

56. Shader, R. I., DiMascio, A., and Harmatz, J.: Characterological anxiety levels and premenstrual libido changes. Psychopharmacology Research Laboratory of the Harvard Medical School and the Massachusetts Mental Health Center, Boston, Massachusetts. July–August, 1968.

57. Sletten, I. W., and Gershon, S.: The premenstrual syndrome: a discussion of its pathophysiology and treatment with lithium ion. Comp. Psych. 7:197, 1966.

58. Sommer, B.: Menstrual cycle changes and intellectual performance. Psychosom. Med. *34*:263, 1972.
59. Stokes, J., and Mendels, J.: Pyridoxine and premenstrual tension. Lancet *1*:1177, 1972.
60. Swyer, G. I. M.: Treatment of premenstrual tension. Brit. Med. J. *1*:1410, 1955.
61. Tange, S. R., and Greengrass, P. M.: The acute effects of estrogen and progesterone on the monoamine levels of the brain of rats. Psychopharmacology *21*:374, 1971.
62. Taylor, H. C.: Vascular congestion and hyperemia. Their effect on the structure and function in the female reproductive system. Amer. J. Obstet. Gynec. 57:211, 1949.
63. Thomas, W. A.: Generalized edema occurring only at the menstrual period. J.A.M.A. *101*:1126, 1933.
64. Thorn, G. W., Garbutt, H. R., Hitchcock, F. A., and Hartman, F. A.: The effect of cortin on the sodium, potassium, chloride, inorganic phosphorus and total nitrogen balance in normal subjects and in patients with Addison's disease. Endocrinology *21*:202, 1937.
65. Thorn, G. W., Nelson, K. R., and Thorn, D. W.: A study of the mechanism of edema associated with menstruation. Endocrinology *22*:155, 1938.
66. Warfield, C. I.: Cytran therapy in premenstrual tension. Obstet. Gynec. *17*:49, 1961.
67. Wetzel, R. D., Reich, T., and McClure, J. N., Jr.: Phase of the menstrual cycle and self-referrals to a suicide prevention service. Brit. J. Psych. *119*:523, 1971.
68. Wetzel, R. D., and McClure, J. N., Jr.: Suicide and the menstrual cycle: a review. Comprehensive Psych. *13*:369, 1972.
69. Wickham, M.: The effects of the menstrual cycle in test performance. Brit. J. Psych. *49*:34, 1958.
70. Winshel, A. W.: Chlorothiazide in premenstrual tension. Int. Rec. Med. *172*:539, 1959.
71. Yalow, R. S., and Berson, S. A.: Dynamics of insulin secretion in hypoglycemia. Diabetes *14*:341, 1965.
72. Taylor, W. J.: Current trends in clinical pharmacology in the USA. Int. Z. Klin. Pharmakol. Ther. Toxikol. *4*:21, 1970.
73. Kramp, T. L.: Studies on the premenstrual syndrome in relation to psychiatry. Acta Psychiat. Scand. Suppl. *203*:261, 1968.

Evaluation and Preferred Management of Premenstrual Tension—Pelvic Congestive Syndrome and Allied States

JOHN B. JOSIMOVICH

University of Pittsburgh School of Medicine and Magee-Women's Hospital

Two decades have passed since the description of the pelvic congestive syndrome (PCS) by Taylor.[1] Earlier studies suggesting the distinctiveness of this syndrome were well described by Gauss,[2] who retained the original diagnostic term, *pelipathia vegetativa*, denoting the overwhelming impression of psychomotor-autonomic dysfunction. The progressive yearly decrease in bibliography items on the subject of PCS would apparently testify to increasing disenchantment with this diagnosis. In fact, this syndrome is not mentioned as a cause for surgical intervention in two recent textbooks of obstetrics and gynecology,[3,4] while a third doubts its existence.[5] It would seem that surgeons, too, often fully expecting to catch a glimpse of the characteristic flushed, blood-engorged organ lying in a pool of amber fluid in the cul-de-sac, in patients who suffered agony on cervical manipulation in the surgeon's office, were frustrated by normal-appearing pelvic viscera at operation. On occasion, a variant of the clinical syndrome, in which adnexal areas were felt to be soft to touch preoperatively, except for pulsating blood vessels, would reward the surgeon at operation by revealing unilateral or bilateral defects in the broad ligament, as first reported by Allen.[6] Other cases of chronic pelvic pain, often accompanied by marked dyspareunia, have proved to be attributable to venous varicosities demonstrated by radiography, presumably owing to incompetence of the left ovarian vein valve at the entrance into the left renal vein.[7] The impression that there is no residual category of PCS may be deceptive, however. In most cases of PCS, when pelvic visualization or pathologic examination of pelvic viscera, or both, have permitted study, varicosities, endopelvic fascial laxity, or ligamentous defects have not been found. What, then, are the components of this syndrome, which are found repeatedly enough to suggest that it truly represents a distinct entity?

1. A feeling of pressure, "heaviness," and steady discomfort, usually of

bilateral nature, is noted by almost all patients. Such discomfort often radiates to the sacral area posteriorly and to one or both inner thighs.

2. Aggravation occurs premenstrually, with emotional tension and physical fatigue. Relief occurs with menses, or by spending time in the recumbent position.

There may be accompanying vulvar or perianal pruritus, other psychosomatic colonic distresses, unusual premenstrual breast tenderness, headaches (migraine or "tension"), and often a poor psychological image of self or spouse.

Possible Pathophysiology

ORGANIC DYSFUNCTION. The careful description of vascular superficial flush, cul-de-sac transudate, and visceral vascular congestion described so carefully by Masters and Johnson,[8] conjuring up the remembrance of adolescent reproductive tract agony in the male gynecologist, taken in conjunction with the frustrated sexual drives of many of the patients with PCS,[1,9,10] has led to expectations that orgasmic dysfunction is the basis of the disorder. This has not been found in many cases of the disorder, including the Columbia University series.[1] Inability to always find orgasmic dysfunction is not surprising, since the Masters and Johnson series shows that there is a gradual stepwise reduction in vascular and extravascular fluid shifts following coitus that is not terminated by orgasm. However, whether the occurrence of orgasms with sufficient frequency, resulting in more rapid decreased engorgement, might alleviate the uterine symptoms of this syndrome, is still to be determined.

HORMONAL CHANGES INDUCED BY PREGNANCY OR BY ORAL CONTRACEPTIVE STEROIDS. Stearns and Sneeden[11] reviewed their findings of subserosal myometrial and subepithelial edema, telangiectasia, and lymphangiectasia, allegedly supported by camera lucida drawings by Benson of specimens derived from such patients. They concluded that these pathologic changes induced by pregnancy were a cause of a chronic pelvic pain syndrome that had many symptoms in common with the PCS. Permanent distortion of pelvic arteries or veins from pregnancy is suggested in only two-thirds of cases in the PCS group.[1] More recent clinical evaluations suggest that this syndrome worsens in the fourth and fifth decades (rather than the second and third decades, as originally described by Taylor and colleagues), but is not, however, closely related (i.e., within one year) to the last pregnancy. The progestational steroids used for oral contraception have not been found, to date, to cause vascular congestion of the pelvis.[12]

AUTOIMMUNE DISEASE. Lazlo and Gyorgy[13] have presented compelling evidence that there is a reproducible pathology associated with PCS: in 82 per cent of 80 patients with chronic pelvic pain, relatively marked blood vessel and parametrial connective tissue pathology was found, as opposed to a lesser degree of such changes noted in only 17 per cent of 30 control patients. The authors found a characteristic fragmentation of the collagen fibers and reaggregation of the elastic fibers with both light and electron microscopy. Histochemical studies also revealed increased neutral polysaccharides in the parametrial connective tissues, as well as significant augmentation of both acid and neutral polysaccharides in the subendothelial tissue of the blood vessels. These microscopic pathologic features were noted to be the same as those seen in certain collagen diseases, suggesting an autoimmune process to the authors.

PROSTAGLANDINS.   A more recently proposed theory for the etiology of the condition postulates a role for the prostaglandins. Prostaglandins have already been implicated as the cause of dysmenorrhea,[14] since arterial and venous tone are altered by these tissue products,[15,16] but it remains to be seen whether these compounds mediate the vascular changes in the pelvic viscera noted in certain cases of PCS.

Future Study Aims

The singular lack of consistent abnormal pathologic findings in PCS have, it must be admitted, prevented it from consideration as a legitimate clinical entity. It must be remembered, however, that the varying procedures of vessel ligation and the length of the procedure would make the pathologist's assessment of the blood volume of the uterus impossible. It is not clear whether or not the syndrome is characterized by edema without alteration in blood volume, resulting at times in transudation into the peritoneal cavity, or, on the other hand, whether there is merely an increase in vascular volume. Increased fluid loss outside the vascular space would presuppose a defect in fluid return at the level of the venous capillary veins or lymphatics. Analyses for edema *could* be carried out by measuring the wet weight of the uterine specimen relative to protein or collagen hydroxyproline, whereas vascular engorgement would have to be estimated with radioactive scanning after systemic injection of radio-labeled material retained by the vessels (e.g., ^{131}I-labeled albumin). Thermography of the vaginal vault has been used previously in a small series of evaluations of the syndrome, and the results suggest excessive pelvic visceral blood flow in patients, particularly during periods of induced nervous tension.[9] Further histochemical studies similar to those reported by Lazlo and Gyorgy[13] on the tissue removed from PCS patients and those with other indications for surgery must be carried out, recognizing that a real need for publication of the findings exists.

It is clear from an epidemiological viewpoint, however, that different groups of pathologists must confirm a reproducible pathologic description of the syndrome, *including* demonstration of a correlation with pelvic distress and incidental operative findings of "congestion" in patients operated on for *other* reasons.

Clearly the confusion over psychiatric diagnoses of maladjustment noted in such a high percentage of PCS patients and in primigravid controls[10] has perhaps obscured the syndrome and its accompanying signs. Thus, a prospective study based on the preoperative scanning and postoperative determination of relative water content from a large number of abdominal or vaginal hysterectomy specimens obtained after surgical sterilization or endopelvic fascial repair procedures must be carried out. In the past, only patients seriously disturbed physically and psychiatrically by pelvic pain have been considered in this series of PCS.

In summary, rightful doubt exists as to the reality of the syndrome as a distinct clinical entity. Because most gynecologists occasionally see patients having the symptoms and signs already described, without good correlation with psychological or sexual pathology, it is fitting for us to retain the idea of its existence and develop the necessary diagnostic tests to permit confirmation, so therapy can be planned. I shall believe PCS exists unless or until such studies make it no longer a tenable diagnosis. Until such time, I do not choose to believe that an engorged, cyanotic uterus, with surrounding fluid transudate, can be any more asymptomatic than would be a congested gallbladder, appendix, lung, bursa, or other body organ.

The treatment of PCS, once the diagnosis is entertained, still consists first of all of reassurance that psychosexual aberrations or other organic pathology need not necessarily be feared. If the symptom persists, and other pathologic conditions are excluded by pelvic examination, anesthesia examination, or laparoscopy, a trial regimen of contraceptive steroids may be started to alleviate the premenstrual aggravation so often seen in this syndrome. In very rare cases, surgical ablation of the uterus, particularly when other indications exist, may still be carried out, provided that the procedure is deemed unlikely to worsen the self-image of the patient as determined by the surgeon, often with the help of a psychiatric consultation.

REFERENCES

1. Taylor, H. C., Jr.: Pelvic pain based on vascular and autonomic nervous system disorders. Amer. J. Obstet. Gynec. 67:1177, 1954.
2. Gauss, C. J.: Eine häufig vorkommende, mehrfach beschriebene, meist verkannte und oft operativ umsonst angegangene Erkrankung: die Pelipathia vegetativa. Deutsch. Med. Wchnschr. 74:1288, 1949.
3. Willson, J. R., Beecham, C. T., and Carrington, E. R.: Obstetrics and Gynecology. 4th Ed. St. Louis, C. V. Mosby, 1971.
4. Kistner, R. W.: Gynecology: Principles and Practice. Chicago, Year Book Medical Publishers, 1971.
5. Novak, E. R., Jones, G. S., and Jones, H. W., Jr.: Novak's Textbook of Gynecology. 8th Ed. Baltimore, Williams & Wilkins, 1970.
6. Allen, W. M.: Chronic pelvic congestion and pelvic pain. Amer. J. Obstet. Gynec. 109:198, 1970.
7. Edlundh, K. O.: Pelvic varicosities in women: a preliminary report. Acta Obstet. Gynec. Scandinav. 43 (Suppl 7):118, 1965.
8. Masters, W. H., and Johnson, V. E.: Human Sexual Response. Boston, Little, Brown & Co., 1966.
9. Duncan, C. H., and Taylor, H. C., Jr.: Psychosomatic study of pelvic congestion. Amer. J. Obstet. Gynec. 64:1, 1952.
10. Gidro-Frank, L., Gordon, T., and Taylor, H. C., Jr.: Pelvic pain and female identity: a survey of emotional factors in 40 patients. Amer. J. Obstet. Gynec. 79:1184, 1960.
11. Stearns, H. C., and Sneeden, V. D.: Observations on the clinical and pathologic aspects of the pelvic congestion syndrome. Amer. J. Obstet. Gynec. 94:718, 1966.
12. Feste, J. R., and Kaufman, R. H.: Pelvic congestion resulting from 19-nortestosterone with ethinyl estradiol. South. Med. J. 58:945, 1965.
13. Lazlo, J., and Gyorgy, G.: Pathogenesis of pelvic pain. Amer. J. Obstet. Gynec. 85:141, 1963.
14. Pickles, V. R., Hall, W. J., Best, F. A., and Smith, G. N.: Prostaglandins in endometrium and menstrual fluid from normal and dysmenorrhoeic subjects. J. Obstet. Gynaec. Brit. Comm. 72:185, 1965.
15. Anggard, E., and Bergström, S.: Biological effects of an unsaturated trihydroxy acid (PGF2α) from normal swine lung. Acta Physiol. Scand. 58:1, 1963.
16. DuCharme, D. W., Weeks, J. R., and Montgomery, R. G.: Studies on the mechanism of the hypertensive effect of prostaglandin F2-alpha. J. Pharmacol. Exp. Ther. 160:1, 1968.

Evaluation and Preferred Management of Premenstrual Tension–Pelvic Congestive Syndrome and Allied States

Editorial Comment

Few subjects are more controversial than premenstrual tension, the pelvic congestion syndrome, and the assessment of pelvic discomfort in the absence of demonstrable pathology. In their careful review, Drs. Friederich and Labrum suggest that these somewhat nebulous clinical states, although difficult to define, are frequently encountered in the overall clinical care of the female.

Patient complaints have been subject to various interpretation. Emotional patterns have been described that occur at different times in the menstrual cycle. There has been much speculation as to the possible cause-and-effect relationship of the endocrine and metabolic changes in the course of the menstrual cycle and the emotional response of the patient. The introduction of the laparoscope has provided a means of assessing the patient's symptoms; that is, it is now possible to visualize the internal organs directly to see whether or not there is any pelvic pathology. Also, as one contributor remarks, in seeking to determine the etiology of these controversial syndromes, laparoscopic examination will provide information on the appearance of the reproductive organs at various periods in the menstrual cycle, which possibly may be correlated with the patient's complaints and physical findings—i.e., edema.

The neuroendocrine system is now being investigated fruitfully, and we are beginning to recognize that the neurochemical effects are subject to emotional influences. There is the hope that this research approach will clarify the etiology(ies) and will lead ultimately to rational patient management. For the present, however, there should be agreement that treatment is purely empirical, to say the least, and is all too often based only on clinical impressions. Often the diagnosis is stated with a certainty that suggests an unawareness on the part of the physician of some degree of bias in how his decision is arrived at. We must admit that we are hardly free of this defect ourselves.

A word of caution might be appropriate: whereas there may be much speculation as to the role of the emotions in these clinical states, the physician must be aware that mental illness may be lurking in the background in the diagnosis of premenstrual tension or its related states. Certainly, he must have some concept of what is meant by anxiety neurosis, neurocirculatory asthenia, nervous exhaustion, hysteria, a conversion reaction, and manic-depressive disease. Admit-

Pros and Cons of Estrogen Therapy for Gynecologic Conditions

WILLARD M. ALLEN

University of Maryland School of Medicine

When estrogens first became generally available (about 1932), physicians had already become accustomed to the dramatic effects of desiccated thyroid and insulin in the treatment of hypothyroidism and diabetes. It was natural for them to look upon the new female sex hormone as treatment for the most widespread deficiency disease of all, the menopause. Estrone (Theelin) was introduced first. Later, estradiol was prepared from estrone and marketed as estradiol benzoate and estradiol dipropionate. Extensive clinical investigation quickly established the effectiveness of these natural estrogens.

Orally effective estrogens soon became available. Ethinylestradiol (Ethinyl) was used extensively by 1940. This extraordinary compound was found to be more potent (i.e., in activity per milligram) orally than any of the natural estrogens were when administered intramuscularly. This compound is used very little today except in combination with progestogens in oral contraceptives. Diethylstilbestrol (DES) has been around a long time too. These two orally active estrogens were found to have one unpleasant side-effect: they produced nausea in some patients. Oldtimers were not mystified by the nausea produced by oral contraceptives; they had encountered the same nausea in their patients treated with ethynylestradiol or stilbestrol. It is quite probable that the success of Premarin, which was introduced in 1942, was in large measure a result of its lack of side-effects. These three orally effective estrogens—ethynylestradiol, diethylstilbestrol, and Premarin—are the ones used today, the same as 30 years ago.

During the 1930's and 1940's clinical investigators were so busy studying the general effects of estrogen that they gave little thought to the possible hazards connected with this glorious new phase of medical practice. This oversight is easily understood. The compounds which they used initially were true hormones in every sense, and estrone, estradiol, progesterone, and testosterone occur naturally. The advent of such synthetic estrogens as ethynylestradiol and diethylstilbestrol caused no ripple of apprehension, for, after all, these were compounds which seemed to have all the biological properties of the natural estrogens and, since they were effective orally, they were more convenient to use.

It is difficult and perhaps impossible for the present generation to appreciate the long history behind the ban of DES in cattle feed—if they know anything about it at all! Years ago, stilbestrol pellets were placed in the necks of small chicks to caponize the males, and they proved very effective, too. However, when the heads and necks of these birds were fed to minks, the fur business suffered a temporary decline; there was enough residual stilbestrol in the necks of these birds to serve as an oral contraceptive. Stilbestrol subsequently was deliberately added to cattle feed for purposes of breeding control. We now know, however, that DES accumulates in the liver and kidneys of these animals, and it surely would be a hazard for those rare individuals who look upon liver and kidney as delicacies to be enjoyed day after day. Even so, it is unlikely that stilbestrol in the necks of chickens or in the liver and kidneys of cattle would be enough of a hazard to deny the pleasure of eating the good meat of DES-treated cattle, which is more tender. The hard truth is that stilbestrol, and natural estrogens too, causes cancer in susceptible animals.

The "pros" for estrogen were well established 30 years ago. The "cons" for estrogen usage, on the other hand, are not so clear. I will attempt to clarify some of the indications and contraindications for the use of estrogen in clinical medicine.

One of the very first uses of estrogen was in the treatment of gonococcal vaginitis in children, which may seem nonsensical. However, it was well known at the time that gonococcal vaginitis did not occur in sexually mature women and the question was: why was the vagina of the child susceptible? Why not mature the vagina of the child with estrogen and see what happens? The result was eminently satisfactory—the atrophic, infected vaginal epithelium of the child matured, the gonococcus disappeared from the smears, and the vaginitis was cured. An unexpected byproduct of the oral treatment with estrogens, development of the breasts and growth of pubic hair, was observed. Because of this undesirable side-effect, vaginal suppositories containing estrogen were produced and found to be effective. The use of estrogen-containing suppositories, jellies, and creams is seldom considered today for the treatment of vaginitis in children. Actually there is no better or safer method for the treatment of annoying vaginitis in children, whether the cause be poor toilet habits, residual infection from foreign bodies (which should first be removed), or possibly even gonorrheal vaginitis (in which case the drug should be combined with oral antibodies). A dose of about one-tenth to one-fifth of the adult dose is sufficient.

The use of estrogen for postmenopausal vaginitis is too well known to warrant more than casual comment. Some patients prefer oral medication, whereas others prefer local treatment. Either method is satisfactory, but rejuvenation of the vaginal mucosa is more rapid when the estrogen is applied locally. Also, local treatment seldom stimulates the breasts and nipples, whereas oral treatment usually does. During the years of good ovarian activity, the use of estrogen, either orally or locally, is probably never indicated for the treatment of vaginitis.

The postmenopausal woman frequently has symptoms involving the urinary tract. Urethral and meatal epithelia suffer from estrogen deficiency just as does the vaginal epithelium. Symptoms of burning and frequency, especially if there is a urethral caruncle, are usually relieved by estrogen. In fact, in elderly patients who have frequent attacks of cystitis there may be marked improvement from administration of oral or vaginal estrogen.

A much more difficult problem arises in older women with dyspareunia.

The vagina may appear to be adequate when, in fact, there is so little elasticity at the introitus that intercourse is painful. A good rule to follow is that the older woman with dyspareunia should be treated with both oral and vaginal estrogen before corrective vaginal operations are seriously considered. In fact, estrogen should be given to virtually all postmenopausal patients for two or three weeks prior to and following most vaginal operations.

The classic indication for the use of estrogen is the "menopausal syndrome," and therein lies a tale of success, frustration, and uncertainty. Certainly many, if not most, of the symptoms which occur during the menopausal period result from sex hormone deficiency. One might suppose that estrogens would specifically relieve the symptoms, but any experienced clinician knows all too well that estrogen does not always achieve a dramatic change in all patients. This should not be surprising, since waning ovarian activity is accompanied by the loss of other sex hormones besides estrogens, yet usually only estrogen is given as replacement therapy. The advent of new methods for studying levels of FSH and LH, as well as estradiol, estrone, progesterone, and testosterone (plus others), makes it possible to investigate once again and in more depth the many vagaries of the menopausal syndrome with the hope that more rational methods of therapy can be instituted now than in the past.

The lush advertisements for estrogens convey the message that estrogens are a cure-all for the anxious, wrinkled, sexually frustrated older woman who has to compete in this era of cocktail parties, sexual freedom, and errant husbands. How nice it would be if this were true. However, the ads do serve a useful purpose no matter how exaggerated the subtle implications may be. They emphasize one truth: menopausal women do have a multitude of problems, some of which are remarkably improved by estrogen.

Several facts regarding the menopausal syndrome have emerged. Vasomotor symptoms such as hot flushes and excessive sweating are relieved dramatically by estrogens. Depression is usually improved but not abolished. Involutional melancholia is present in many women and sometimes to such a degree that "something has to be done." If estrogen really did eliminate all the unpleasantries of the climacterium in all women, there would be no need for the various psychotropic drugs which are so extensively used. As a matter of fact, combinations of estrogen and a tranquilizer have been available and in use for many years. Failure to achieve success with estrogen is likely to be the result of inadequate dosage. Young surgically castrated women require much more estrogen than older women during the natural menopause. The young woman may need 2.5 mg. or more of Premarin daily, whereas the older woman seldom needs more than 1.25 mg. daily and frequently will feel quite well on 0.625 mg. Only when adequate dosage seems to have failed should psychotropic drugs be used.

When the symptomatic patient has achieved good relief from estrogen therapy an important question arises. How long should therapy be continued? In general, estrogen therapy should be continued so long as symptoms remain. Actually, many women are able to "diagnose" their own needs and administer their own medication quite effectively; when symptoms return, estrogens are resumed. No one can predict how long symptoms will persist. Some women need estrogen for only a year or two, whereas others may need estrogen for several years. Estrogen should be used for the symptomatic patient in the fifth as well as the sixth decade of life.

Laboratory tests have little practical significance in establishing the need for estrogen therapy during the climacterium. This may seem heretical when it is so well known that estrogen deficiency raises the level of FSH and produces regressive changes in the vaginal smear. However, the postmenopausal patient without symptoms also has an elevated FSH level and an atrophic vaginal smear. These laboratory tests establish a state of estrogen deficiency, but they do not establish the need for therapy. Nevertheless, the vaginal smear does help in assuring that an adequate dosage of estrogen has been achieved.

There seems little doubt that estrogens will continue to be used as the primary treatment for the menopausal syndrome. Clinicians have already had a good deal of experience with other steroids. Testosterone and methyltestosterone have been used as adjuncts to estrogen therapy for many years, but there is little evidence that these combinations are of much value except in the occasional patient. They may improve a patient's vigor, or stimulate her sexually, but it is important to realize that the androgen contained in the combinations is virilizing. Most women don't like to have hair on the face or a deep or hoarse voice.

During the past 10 years, a somewhat different approach to the menopausal syndrome has been possible as a result of the advent of the oral contraceptives. We might suppose that these tablets would prove to be the answer to the problems of the menopause. Indeed, they have provided a remarkable boon to menopausal patients. Most of the dysfunctional bleeding which occurs so frequently as ovarian activity begins to wane is controlled by one or two cycles of oral contraceptive therapy. They provide a regular source of estrogen when ovarian estrogen is produced irregularly and they induce regular, albeit artificial, menstrual cycles, which give some women a feeling of youth. However, the same hazards from the pill exist for the menopausal woman as for younger women. Although the dangers are slight, most menopausal and postmenopausal women can be treated with other estrogens when the danger of pregnancy is over.

The menopausal syndrome is not limited, of course, to women going through the natural processes of aging. The surgical menopause is returning once more to plague countless numbers of young women. World-wide epidemics of gonorrhea cause tragedies that become personal disasters to women who develop tubo-ovarian abscesses, many of whom are scarcely out of childhood. The "pelvic sweep" has returned again to challenge the judgment and test the surgical skills of the gynecologist. The perennial use of estrogens is a tremendous blessing for these unfortunates.

The long-term use of estrogens in young women deprived of ovarian function for any reason is generally accepted. However, long-term use for the prevention of aging in the postmenopausal woman is a much more controversial topic. "Estrogens forever" enjoys the status of a cult. Popular and successful books extol the advantages of long-continued use of estrogens after the menopause. There is much to be said in favor of this cult. There is no doubt that the pelvic organs (excluding the ovaries) are rejuvenated by estrogen. Administration of estrogen to elderly women restores the vagina and uterus to the status of the young adult and when progesterone is added intermittently the endometrium is indistinguishable from that of the young uterus. It is relatively easy to reestablish a "normal" menstrual cycle in older women with estrogen and progesterone. Opponents of "estrogens forever" base their objections on the possibility that cancer of the uterus or breast may be induced.

Most of the uncertainty regarding estrogens grows out of experience with and publicity about the oral contraceptives. Before the pill, there were few worries about the hazards of estrogens. Gynecologists knew, of course, that estrogens produced withdrawal and breakthrough bleeding, and that overdosage suppressed ovulation, and most physicians also knew that estrogens produced cancer in certain experimental animals. These facts regarding estrogens have been known for over 30 years. During all these years, clinicians did not become aware of any increase in cancer of the breast or uterus or of phlebitis in women receiving estrogens. Then, in 1962, a few deaths from thromboembolism occurred in young women taking the pill. These tragedies, whether due to the pill or not, alerted the populace to the possible dangers of estrogens in general and oral contraceptives in particular.

Numerous clinical studies in the past 10 years seem to indicate that taking of oral contraceptives does increase the likelihood of phlebitis and thromboembolic disease. However, the risk is so slight that millions of women continue to use oral contraceptives. The prevailing view is that the vascular problems arising from the pill are traceable to the estrogen rather than the progestogen contained in them. However, there are some objections to this view. Large doses of stilbestrol have been used over the years in the treatment of endometriosis and in certain types of advanced breast cancer without any reports of phlebitis or thromboembolism coming to light. Massive doses were used during pregnancy without anyone becoming aware of any hazards. Likewise, in more recent years, large doses of the progestogens (principally Delalutin, Provera, and Norlutate) have been used in the treatment of both endometriosis and endometrial cancer without any cases of phlebitis or thromboembolic disease being reported. It might be more logical to suppose that the vascular effects of the pill are due to the combination of hormones rather than to either the estrogen or the progestogen alone.

Apprehension over the hazards of oral contraceptives has only minor bearing on the validity of "estrogens forever." The real question is whether or not long-continued use of estrogens benefits the patient or causes harm. Certain benefits are obvious. The vagina stays young, healthy, and more supple. The skin is probably kept in a more youthful state. Some experienced investigators have demonstrated that the appearance of both osteoporosis and vascular disease is delayed. Surely, these are desirable facets of the aging process. Best of all, the evidence seems to indicate that no harm is done. Several of the advocates of "estrogens forever" have amassed data from patients treated for many years which indicate that long use of estrogens (chiefly Premarin and stilbestrol) has not been accompanied by any increase in the incidence of cancer of the breast or endometrium or any other form of cancer. No one knows, of course, whether better rejuvenation would be accomplished by using estrogen combined with progestogen (for example, sequential oral contraceptives), since no long-term studies in postmenopausal patients have been reported.

One can find little fault with the widespread use of physiologic doses of estrogen in the treatment of the menopausal syndrome, prepubertal and postmenopausal vaginitis, and in women with nonfunctioning ovaries. On the other hand, occasionally a patient is deliberately treated with overdosage with estrogen. Is this effective and safe?

The medical treatment of endometriosis with large doses of stilbestrol was introduced about 30 years ago. The general principles of therapy were simple:

stilbestrol was given orally in gradually increasing dosage until 50 to 100 mg. was taken daily. Ovarian activity was suppressed. Menstrual periods ceased and most patients were relieved of pain. After several months, treatment was discontinued. Spontaneous cycles resumed in four to six weeks and occasionally previously infertile patients became pregnant. Surprisingly, these larger doses of stilbestrol produced few side-effects other than nausea, occasional breakthrough bleeding, and some cystic hyperplasia of the endometrium. Certainly few, if any, patients demonstrated hypertension or phlebitis. The treatment was seldom curative. Most patients had a recurrence of symptoms after the menstrual cycle was reestablished.

Today most patients with endometriosis are treated medically either with progestational agents (Provera, Norlutate, and so forth) or combination type oral contraceptives. All of these agents suppress ovulation and perhaps assist in "burning out" the misplaced endometrium. As a matter of fact, oral contraceptives are usually beneficial even when given cyclically. It would not be accurate to say, however, that stilbestrol no longer has a place in the treatment of endometriosis. The chronicity of this disease is such that all available methods of ovarian suppression should be considered.

The prevalent use of overdosage of estrogens in treating dysfunctional uterine bleeding is much less easily evaluated. Cystic hyperplasia occurs for the most part during adolescence and during the premenopausal years. It has been known for more than 50 years that the ovaries of young women with cystic hyperplasia and bleeding contain many medium-sized follicles and no corpora lutea. Even though there is continuous bleeding, sometimes severe, the endometrium is remarkably healthy in appearance. There are small areas of necrosis which presumably are the source of the bleeding. Since a similar type of cystic endometrium is produced when large doses of either stilbestrol or natural estrogen are given, it is commonly supposed that cystic hyperplasia results from "too much estrogen for too long a period of time." This supposition provides the rationale for the use of progesterone or the progestational agents. The results are predictable. A single injection of Delalutin (125 to 250 mg.) or injections of progesterone (50 mg. for three consecutive days) or the use of oral progestogens such as Norlutate or Provera (10 to 15 mg. for five days) produces "chemical curettage." There is only one disadvantage to this treatment: withdrawal bleeding may be excessive when the hyperplasia is marked. It seems absolutely irrational to give estrogen for this condition but in actual practice immediate overdosage with estrogen (5 mg. of stilbestrol orally every hour for several hours or Premarin intravenously) will frequently stop excessive bleeding. Today many patients, both the young and those nearing menopause, are treated successfully with a single course of oral contraceptives.

Adenomatous hyperplasia is somewhat different. It is not clear what hormonal factors are responsible for this lesion. It would seem that some steroid in addition to estrogen is probably required. Many pathologists believe that this is a precancerous lesion. Since the lesion is seldom found in women who desire more children, hysterectomy is logical, satisfactory, and curative. However, experimentally oriented gynecologists have successfully treated adenomatous hyperplasia with progestational agents. In any case, there seems little reason to use estrogen for the treatment of this lesion.

The multitude of women who have occasional episodes of abnormal bleeding fall into a different category. They usually do not have hyperplasia or endometrial cancer. When abnormal bleeding occurs in younger women who have been having normal cycles, one should suspect pregnancy rather than dysfunctional bleeding. Many women do have occasional anovulatory cycles, with a menstrual period appearing at the wrong time in the cycle. It is seldom necessary to treat such patients as nature usually corrects the problem.

A special problem arises in patients with a cystic ovary, either with or without abnormal bleeding. It is common practice to give such patients a trial with either stilbestrol or oral contraceptives to see what will happen. There is no harm in this providing a careful evaluation of the findings is made in a month or two. As a matter of fact, abnormal bleeding associated with a cystic ovary increases the suspicion that the cyst is a functional cyst rather than a true tumor. Ovarian tumors, both benign and malignant, do not usually disrupt the menstrual cycle unless they are hormone-secreting. It is helpful to recall that all 15 cm. ovarian tumors were small initially. A simple rule to follow is that the 5 cm. ovary which has not disturbed the cycle should not be treated with estrogen or other sex steroids unless there is a strong suspicion of endometriosis. If the cyst is accompanied by abnormal bleeding, ovarian suppression with stilbestrol or oral contraceptives is fully justified.

The turmoil which exists now over the carcinogenic potential of stilbestrol is a result of the surprising finding that some female offspring of women treated with stilbestrol during pregnancy have developed a rare type of cancer of the vagina. Studies now in progress indicate that some of the female children whose mothers received stilbestrol during early pregnancy have dysplasia of the vaginal covering of the cervix which looks grossly like congenital erosion. In many cases, the dysplasia extends to the upper vagina. The seriousness of these findings is obvious.

The mechanism behind this effect of stilbestrol on the embryo and growing fetus is obscure. However, a few aspects of the problem seem to be clear. First, stilbestrol, or a metabolic product of stilbestrol, must have reached the fetus and by some means have altered the development of a very small segment (the cervicovaginal junction) of the reproductive tract. Second, the remainder of the reproductive tract appears to be normal. Third, no adverse effect on the hypothalamus or pituitary seems to have occurred, since the young women appear to have normal, cyclic ovarian function. It is tempting, of course, to assume that a similar carcinogenic effect would not have occurred had natural estrogens rather than stilbestrol been used during pregnancy. However, it is well known that both natural estrogens and synthetic nonsteroidal estrogens produce cancer of the breast in susceptible animals.

No one really knows how many women have received stilbestrol during pregnancy. The idea that larger doses of stilbestrol (up to 200 mg. daily) were beneficial in threatened abortion, habitual abortion, and pregnancy complicated by diabetes was so thoroughly ingrained in the minds of obstetricians that many of them used the drug almost prophylactically. Even though controlled studies using placebo failed to demonstrate the benefits of stilbestrol, its use was continued because it was inexpensive, presumed to be safe, and "it might help." Fortunately, very few pregnant women have received stilbestrol in recent years. However, the epidemic of vaginal adenosis and vaginal cancer may continue for several years since stilbestrol was used extensively for at least 15 years.

These extraordinary findings will without doubt be used to strengthen the conjecture that estrogens may be responsible for both endometrial and breast cancer in women. As a matter of fact, a few cases of endometrial cancer have been reported in women with ovarian agenesis who have been treated with stilbestrol for many years. If numerous additional cases of endometrial cancer are discovered in patients with stilbestrol-treated ovarian agenesis the supposition would be fairly strong that stilbestrol, at least, is carcinogenic in women under special circumstances. However, several investigators have observed no increase in the incidence of either breast cancer or endometrial cancer in women treated for many years with physiologic doses of either stilbestrol or Premarin.

The concept that endometrial cancer may be caused by unremitting stimulation of the endometrium by estrogen is certainly not new. At one time, this supposition was so strong that some gynecologists advised women who were continuing to menstruate after age 50 to either undergo a hysterectomy or permit induction of menopause by use of radium. Today, women over 50 who are menstruating are congratulated for being still young. When we consider that most women are under the influence of their own estrogens for about 40 years, it seems illogical to suppose that a few more years of ovarian function would be harmful or, for that matter, that a few years of estrogen therapy could be harmful.

The belief that estrogen may cause breast cancer has been expressed so many times by physicians, surgeons, and the news media that many doctors, and their patients too, honestly believe that estrogens do cause cancer. The idea came into being over 30 years ago, when it was found that estrogens in high dosage did induce cancer in susceptible animals. The vital statistics of breast cancer indicate that the incidence, curability, and death rate have remained unchanged throughout the whole era of estrogen therapy. If estrogen therapy really did induce cancer of the breast in women, a dramatic increase in the incidence should have become apparent by now.

Some breast cancers seem to be estrogen-dependent, which is why ovariectomy is performed for recurrent disease. This does not mean, of course, that estrogens caused the cancer. On the other hand, soft-tissue metastases in postmenopausal women temporarily regress when large doses of estrogen are given. The dose used is usually 15 mg. of stilbestrol daily, but why this dose? This dose was recommended by a committee because stilbestrol was available in 5 mg. tablets and because 15 mg. daily was obviously enough to suppress the gonadotropic output of the pituitary gland. When this recommendation was made, there was evidence that stilbestrol was helpful but there was none that this dose was ideal.

It is obvious that the "pros" of estrogen therapy remain about the same as they were when estrogens were introduced. Estrogen continues to be the primary agent for treatment of the menopausal syndrome. It is indicated in virtually all young women deprived of ovarian function (except those castrated because of breast cancer). Estrogen is helpful too in the prevention of osteoporosis and arteriosclerosis in aging women, and it is useful in the suppression of ovulation. In the treatment of dysfunctional bleeding, estrogen has largely been replaced by oral contraceptives. Likewise, progestational agents are probably more effective than estrogen in the medical treatment of endometriosis. In general, estrogens are useful in those conditions in which there is estrogen deficiency, and oral contraceptives rather than estrogen are used when suppression of ovulation is indicated.

The "cons" of estrogen usage are quite different now from what they were

in the early years of estrogen therapy. Certainly estrogens, in the form of stilbestrol at least, should not be used during pregnancy. When estrogens were first
introduced, there was a legitimate fear that they might induce breast cancer in
women. Up to this time, however, no sound evidence has appeared to support this
fear.

Pros and Cons of Estrogen Therapy for Gynecologic Conditions

The Climacterium (The Menopause and the Postmenopause): Clinical Implications and a Rationale for Estrogen Replacement Therapy

Nathan Kase

Yale University School of Medicine

In women, after three decades of ovulatory menstrual function accompanied by full biologic estrogen maintenance of dependent tissues, at approximately 40 years of age the frequency of ovulation decreases. This event initiates a period of waning ovarian function called the climacterium, which may last as long as 20 years, and will carry the woman through decreased fertility, menopause, and manifestations of progressive tissue atrophy and aging. It is likely that the major factor in this picture of multisystem involvement is the diminution of estrogen production associated with this period of life.

Clinical symptoms may be associated with this estrogen withdrawal. A policy supporting replacement therapy, consistent with cautious medical practice, is offered to compensate for this hormonal loss.

THE CLINICAL IMPLICATIONS OF PROGRESSIVE ESTROGEN WITHDRAWAL

Although waning of estrogen secretion is not plotted as a straight line, its progressive diminution over time leads to a sequential loss of estrogen-dependent functions (ovulation, menstruation, vaginal and vulvar tissue strength), and also causes generalized atrophy of all estrogen dependent tissues.

This estrogen loss results from the continued attrition in the numbers of residual ovarian follicle units in the fifth decade of life. Since fewer follicles are available, progressively less estrogen production is possible. These oldest follicle units have remained in the ovary unstimulated by gonadotropin, perhaps not entirely by chance, but possibly owing to their inherent refractoriness to otherwise appropriate gonadotropin stimulation. When these are finally activated, the degree of differentiation each is likely to experience is limited. Thus, each follicular growth period will be increasingly shortened and blunted, and less estrogen is produced. Eventually, even these older and more sluggish follicles are exhausted. Estrogen production will then be at a lower level of efficiency, resulting almost entirely from indirect resources, such as the peripheral conversion of ovarian stromal and adrenal precursors to active estrogen in nonendocrine tissue sites.

Finally, the gonadal resource becomes defunct, and the ovary shrivels to an atrophic mass of fibrous tissue. Estrogenicity, now at marginally sustaining levels, is the sum of inadvertent dietary intake and adrenal activity. As peripheral tissues age (in the seventh, eighth, and ninth decades), even these low levels decrease still further.

The symptoms frequently seen and related to estrogen loss in this protracted climacterium include:

1. Disturbances in menstrual pattern, including anovulation and reduced fertility, hypo- or hypermenorrhea, and irregular menses.

2. Vasomotor instability (hot flushes and sweats). Hot flushes (or hot flashes) are not well understood but are claimed to be the result of instability in the hypothalamus and the autonomic nervous system, brought about by a decline in estrogen. Hot flushes are wave-like sensations of heat that involve the upper chest, neck, and face, which are frequently followed by profuse perspiration. The flushes may last a few seconds or as long as 30 minutes or an hour. They are especially disturbing at night.

3. Psychological symptoms, including anxiety, increased tension, mood depression, and irritability.

4. Atrophic conditions: atrophy of vaginal epithelium, urethral caruncles, dyspareunia, pruritus owing to vulvar, introital, and vaginal atrophy, general skin atrophy, and urinary difficulties, such as urgency and cystitis.

5. A variety of other complaints, such as headaches, insomnia, myalgia, changes in libido, and palpitations. Lower back pain may be a nonspecific effect of osteoporosis, a condition which occurs in about 25 per cent of postmenopausal women.

A precise understanding of the symptom complex which any individual patient may display is often difficult to achieve. Some patients will show severe multiple reactions that may be disabling, whereas others will show either no reactions or minimal reactions which go unnoticed until careful medical evaluation. The majority of patients (50 to 60 per cent) require medical assistance and support for intermittent difficulties of moderate severity.

It appears that three factors are at work in all climacteric women. The symptomatic reaction is the sum of impact of these three components:

1. The amount of estrogen depletion and the rate at which estrogen is withdrawn.

2. The collective inherited and acquired propensities to succumb to or withstand the impositions of the overall aging process.

3. The psychologic impact of aging and the individual's reaction to the emotional implications of "a change of life."

Although menopause—i.e., the last menstrual period—is only a single point in the protracted unfolding of the climacterium, only the most stoical, objective, and rationally composed women dismiss it as a minor physiologic event. For most women, it signals an end to the known, the accustomed and expected, and the beginning of an era of insidiously diminishing competence, leading irretrievably to aging and death. Add to this gloomy prospect the almost obsessive cultish pursuit of youthful sexual femininity that our society espouses, and one can only wonder why more postmenopausal women have not complicated their physiologic deficits with great emotional burdens.

Clearly, good medical practice obligates the concerned physician to support patients in all aspects of the prolonged and possibly difficult climacteric period. I have found it helpful to classify these needs according to events of the "early" and "late" climacterium.

THE SYMPTOMS OF THE EARLY CLIMACTERIUM (PERIMENOPAUSE)

The degree of symptoms experienced by women and the resulting non-physiologic reactions as they proceed through early estrogen withdrawal appear to depend on the speed of that withdrawal. If it is occasioned by surgical or radiation castration, the resulting abrupt estrogen loss is often very symptomatic. The worst expressions of vasomotor flushes and sweats, globus hystericus, formication, palpitations, and so forth, may be displayed in these circumstances. The accompanying emotional reactions, depressions, anxiety, and irritability also appear to be the most virulent under these conditions.

If estrogen loss is very slow, vasomotor reactions are minimal, but abnormal and often prolonged uterine bleeding becomes the worrisome factor. Appropriately, both the patient and her physician will be concerned about an underlying malignant process resulting in this abnormal expression. Reassurance on this score may require operative investigation.

A large group of women who do not belong in either extreme undergo depletion of estrogen at an intermediate rate, so that menopause is accompanied only by mild periodic flushes.

Obviously, the factors which influence the slope of estrogen withdrawal are unknown. Gonadotropin sensitivity, number of follicles, the degree of peripheral estrogen production, the amount of retained ovarian stromal activity, and the physical and emotional health of the patient are certainly all involved.

THE SYMPTOMATOLOGY OF LATE CLIMACTERIUM

The clinical effects of the late climacterium (extremely low estrogen production) depend on many factors, including the general resistance to aging of the target tissues, the patient's overall health, quality of diet, level of physical activity, and so forth. Also important is the amount of estrogen produced by the peripheral nonendocrine routes.

With extremely low estrogen production, not enough estrogen is available to sustain even marginally any estrogen-dependent tissue. Pruritus, vaginitis, dyspareunia, urinary difficulties (dysuria, urge incontinence, urethritis), and osteoporosis are the likely results of this situation. Somewhat greater degrees of function may sustain tissues marginally. It is not infrequent to find estrogenized cervical mucus and vaginal epithelium in a woman 10 to 15 years post menopause. Finally, periodic stress may yield spikes of estrogen production that may produce sufficient endometrial activity to cause breakthrough bleeding. It is a clinically accepted experience that late menopause bleeding may arise following stresses, such as death of loved ones, anniversaries, or emotional upheavals.

In view of these considerations, it is my practice to advise almost all post-

menopausal women to begin hormonal replacement therapy for symptoms of the early climacterium and for prophylaxis against development of the problems of late climacterium. In practice, I exclude from therapy: (1) those patients in whom low doses of estrogen are specifically contraindicated, such as estrogen-dependent tumors, impaired liver metabolism, and, as a matter of clinical judgment, patients with thromboembolic problems or conditions predisposing to thromboembolism, and (2) women who exhibit bleeding as a reflection of early or late climacteric dysfunction. After appropriate investigation, however, patients with bleeding may also be candidates for therapy with estrogen.

Postmenopausal Estrogen Replacement Therapy

ADVANTAGES OF ESTROGEN THERAPY

1. CONTROL OF VASOMOTOR REACTIONS.   Although there is some evidence to implicate autonomic nervous system dysfunction in the production of the vasomotor reactions, the immediate and sustained response of these symptoms to estrogen replacement is clinically very impressive and persuasive.

2. REDUCTION OF EMOTIONAL REACTIONS TO THE CLIMACTERIUM.   Whether directly related to estrogen withdrawal or indirectly stemming from the implications of the menopause, estrogen replacement has reduced anxiety, depression, and mood swings in my patients. Therapy has not eliminated these issues, and additional sedation or psychotropic drugs may be required, although infrequently.[1]

3. PREVENTIVE MEDICINE.   As a result of these immediate responses in early climacteric symptoms, the patient enters the climacterium more confident of herself emotionally, sexually, and physically. In my view, this establishes good patient–physician interchange. The follow-up of the patient on effective estrogen replacement therapy is more secure and certain. The practitioner offering estrogen replacement has a better, more reliable opportunity to act as the primary physician for these aging women. Monitoring of all health systems will be improved as a result of this single-system involvement. Intestinal, mammary, cardiac, and various metabolic functions are scrutinized periodically, consistent with good medical practice.

4. OSTEOPOROSIS.   An example of the specific prophylaxis accomplished by estrogen replacement is its beneficial preventative effect on the development of osteoporosis. Undoubtedly, this process, which occurs in both males and females, begins before the climacterium. Furthermore, the rate at which osteoporosis develops is based on a variety of metabolic conditions, exercise, diet, inherited constitution, etc. All of these may be more important to the overall process affecting bone density than estrogen replacement. Nevertheless, the observations on castrated and gonadal dysgenesis patients, as well as postmenopausal women with prolonged unreplaced estrogen deficit, lead to the conclusion that the presence of estrogen does retard the rate of demineralization typical of this process. Estrogen cannot reverse osteoporosis (i.e., replace lost bone), but it does have prophylactic values and acts as a defense against the worsening of an established, inevitable process. Estrogen does not displace diet, exercise, calcium, vitamin D, or fluorides in the specific treatment of this disorder, but it adds to the long-term quality of the response to whatever combination of therapy is used.

5. ATHEROSCLEROSIS.   Although the question of estrogen effect on athero-sclerosis is not resolved, atherosclerosis is reported to be more common and more severe in women who undergo premature menopause.[2,3] On the other hand, the use of estrogen in the prevention of recurrent myocardial infarction has been disappointing. Indeed, with higher doses of estrogen, there has been an increased incidence of arterial occlusion and thromboembolism. Furthermore, administration of estrogen does not revert the serum lipid pattern of a postmenopausal woman to that of a premenopausal woman.[4] At this time, therefore, it cannot be said that prevention of atherosclerosis is a clear-cut advantage of estrogen therapy. Indeed, at higher doses, there may even be a deleterious effect.

THE DISADVANTAGES OF ESTROGEN REPLACEMENT THERAPY

1. FEAR OF CANCER.   Probably the greatest disadvantage of estrogen therapy is the irrational but significant fear on the part of the patient (and sometimes enhanced by the physician's own nagging doubts in this matter) that by using estrogen therapy she is tampering with nature's plan. Often the patient will believe she will pay a penalty for this self-determination through some dreadful punishment—mainly the development of cancer. There are no data of which I am aware that implicate estrogen replacement therapy, in the method of administration which I recommend, in the development of breast,[5] reproductive tract, or any other malignancy in the human patient.

2. SIDE EFFECTS OF ESTROGEN.   Despite careful support of the patient, often the appearance of side-effects (usually owing to injudicious dosage) restimulates the fears and concerns of the patient. These side-effects include breast tenderness, intermittent uterine breakthrough bleeding, an increase in vaginal discharge, edema, and weight gain. Each requires careful responses in terms of concern, investigation, revision of dosage and, where necessary, specific ancillary therapy.

3. METABOLIC EFFECTS.   Estrogens, again particularly when used in injudicious dosages, may have serious impact on total health. Major concerns include diabetes, hypertension, and atherosclerosis. The details of the manner by which high doses of synthetic estrogens affect the metabolic process involved are of major concern, as estrogen is an important component of the steroidal contraceptives. Furthermore, the ratios of potency between equine urinary estrogen conjugates when compared on a weight basis to synthetic estrogens are: *50 μg. ethynyl-estradiol = 80 μg. mestranol = 1 mg. diethylstilbestrol = 5 mg. conjugated estrogens.* It is my opinion that the usual dose formulations (0.625 mg. or 1.25 mg. daily) used in the climacterium are probably below provocative synthetic estrogen contraceptive concentrations. Nevertheless, careful medical history, family history, and follow-up surveillance are necessary for all patients on estrogen replacement. My practice involves an annual visit, including: general history, physical examination, and PAP smear, with emphasis on breast, pelvic, and rectal examinations, blood pressure, urinalysis, and complete blood count.

METHOD OF ESTROGEN REPLACEMENT THERAPY

WHAT DRUG SHOULD BE USED?   I favor the use of conjugated estrogens, a mixture of the sodium salts of the sulfate esters of estrogens, principally estrone and equilin, excreted in the urine of pregnant mares. Not less than 50 per cent is sodium estrone sulfate, and not less than 20 per cent is sodium equilin sulfate. In my experience, I have encountered far fewer problems with these conjugated estrogens.

WHEN SHOULD TREATMENT BEGIN?   My policy, which advocates initiation of therapy in the early climacterium, is to begin estrogen treatment in any woman who is one year postmenopausal and who does not show withdrawal bleeding when challenged with progestin administration.

HOW TO TREAT?   Estrogens are administered on a cyclic basis, either three weeks on, one week off, or as a convenient method to remember, from the first through the twenty-fourth days of each month. If the uterus is present, continuous estrogen therapy may induce tissue proliferation and uterine bleeding, even atypical endometrial changes, owing to constant stimulation. Many practitioners do not see the need to use cyclic administration in the absence of a uterus, and therefore advise daily estrogen therapy in the patient who has had a hysterectomy. Owing to the lack of data, a definitive statement cannot be made on this issue. However, in my practice I use cyclic treatment for all patients.

The dose of estrogen utilized is that which will provide sufficient estrogen to sustain physiologic functions, yet will stop short of provoking a return of menstrual flow. An important principle of treatment is that relief of symptoms can almost always be achieved by submenstrual doses of estrogen. For the *early climacterium*, when there is still considerable endogenous estrogen present, the usual effective dose is 0.625 mg. of conjugated estrogens per day. In *late climacterium*, when endogenous estrogen may be very low, at best, higher doses (1.25 mg. or, at most, 2.5 mg. daily), may be necessary, depending on symptoms. The addition of progestin medication should be unnecessary since the dose of estrogen should be deliberately chosen to avoid endometrial stimulation.

Spotting and bleeding require evaluation to rule out uterine malignancy. This entails discontinuation of estrogenic medication, appropriate examination, and office biopsies (endometrial and endocervical), and, if bleeding continues, diagnostic dilatation and uterine curettage.

I find no need to monitor dosage by any means other than by symptoms; assessments of vaginal cytology are not useful.

Occasionally a patient will continue to have symptoms, particularly involving decreased libido. I have found that the addition of androgen (methyltestosterone, 5 mg. daily) may provide an increased sense of well-being, along with an increase in libido. The patient should be cautioned that hirsutism may develop on this dosage after prolonged (three to six months') administration.

In summary, no one can hope to stay young forever, and hormones certainly won't prevent aging. There should be no misconceptions here. Some of the difficulties of aging, however, can be softened with estrogen therapy, and several potentially disabling problems can be avoided. In my view, the benefits of carefully monitored estrogen replacement therapy far outweigh the risks.

REFERENCES

1. Tramont, C. B.: Cyclic hormone therapy: a report of 305 cases. Geriatrics *21*:212, 1966.
2. Parrish, H. M., Carr, C. A., Hall, D. G., and King, T. M.: Time interval from castration in

premenopausal women to development of excessive coronary atherosclerosis. Amer. J. Obstet. Gynec. 99:155, 1967.

3. Higano, H., Robinson, R. W., and Cohen, W. D.: Increased incidence of cardiovascular disease in castrated women. New Eng. J. Med. 268:1123, 1963.
4. Furman, R. H.: Gonadal steroid effects on serum lipids. In Salhanick, H. A., Kipnis, D. M., and Vande Wiele, R. L. (eds.): Metabolic Effects of Gonadal Hormones and Contraceptive Steroids. New York, Plenum Press, 1969.
5. Burch, J. C., and Byrd, B. F., Jr.: Effects on long-term administration of estrogen on the occurrence of mammary cancer in women. Ann. Surg. 174:414, 1971.

Pros and Cons of Estrogen Therapy for Gynecologic Conditions

HILTON A. SALHANICK

Harvard School of Public Health and Harvard Medical School

Estrogenic drugs are among the most potent drugs in the pharmacopeia. Effective in microgram dosages, they are available for oral, intramuscular, and intravenous administration as well as in long-acting and short-acting preparations. With the advent of estrogen-containing contraceptive medications, estrogens, in one form or another, have become one of the most common drugs in current use.

Our ignorance often matches our knowledge of potential usefulness. We do not have simple methods of evaluating proper dosages, of separating the various effects, or even of assessing toxicity. Consequently, because our knowledge is imprecise, there is considerable controversy and often opposing sides hold strong views. In the past such controversies have been settled by gains in new knowledge. One purpose of this article is to point out the need for such new information in certain areas.

Since almost all effective drugs have the potential to do some sort of harm, drug therapy is based upon the concept of benefit-risk ratio. Thus, while it may be appropriate to use exceedingly toxic drugs for the treatment of very serious illness, it may not be appropriate to use drugs of minimal toxicity for casual purposes. Estrogens fortunately have a wide range of safety—for example, as much as 100 times a therapeutic dose is associated with a low incidence of serious consequences. On the other hand, some of the morbid effects such as thromboembolism which are not obviously associated with "predisposing conditions" can be demonstrated only by sophisticated epidemiologic techniques and consequently are often impossible to predict. Nevertheless, these effects are real and deserve careful and continuous consideration. An estimate of the risk-benefit ratio by the physician is of critical importance.

In therapy it is difficult to conceive of biological effects which are not dose-related. Undoubtedly there are apparent threshold dosages, but this is, at least in part, related to our inability to measure certain kinds of minimal or graded responses. (The very concepts of illness, health, and morbidity are difficult to define and probably vary with individuals. Recently, even the definition of death has required refinement.) The significance of this concept of graded responses in establishing principles of therapy is obvious. For example, in the case of estrogens, I believe that one should use the lowest dose which achieves the desired response. A "standard" dose applied to all patients must certainly be an excessive dose for some patients. Furthermore, the concept of the dose-response curve also implies that there is a certain time beyond which the duration of therapy should not be prolonged needlessly. Whether time has a cumulative effect on subthreshold responses or whether it increases the statistical probability for a catastrophic effect, there is reason to expect that long-term therapy is beset with more complications than short-term therapy. Unfortunately, in this area, also, our knowledge is not secure.

I believe, therefore, that the following principles should govern therapy with estrogens as well as with many other drugs:

1. Estrogens should be used in minimal effective dosage.
2. They should be used for specifically defined indications.
3. The benefits and risks should be weighed carefully by the physician.
4. Therapy should not be prolonged beyond the period required to achieve the therapeutic goals.

UNDESIRABLE EFFECTS OF ESTROGENS

As experience with estrogens administered in large amounts to large numbers of women for contraceptive purposes has accumulated, a myriad of biological effects have been noted. These effects have been serious (e.g., thromboembolism), bothersome (e.g., nausea), and often of unknown potential (e.g., hyperlipidemia). A number of very serious associations have been suggested but without adequate substantiation. In this last group are breast and cervical malignancy. Recent data would indicate that, if anything, the estrogens may diminish the incidence of breast carcinoma. The implications that cervical malignancy may be related to estrogen therapy are highly controversial, and it might be fairly stated that we simply do not have adequate information at this time.

There has been considerable clinical experience with, and a great deal of experimental data has been compiled on, the effects of estrogens on the endometrium. Estrogens cause uterine growth and modify or cause uterine bleeding, depending on the state of the endometrium. There have been claims that estrogens can effect premalignant change in the endometrium, but to my knowledge no one has conclusively demonstrated a causal relationship with metastatic carcinoma of the endometrium. A number of cases of endometrial carcinoma in women treated with estrogens have been reported, but no properly controlled study has been conducted.

Estrogens effect a number of metabolic changes. These include decreased glucose tolerance, elevated lipids, especially triglycerides, and increased synthesis of certain proteins, such as thyroid binding globulin and corticosteroid binding globulin. The interpretation of these data are extremely complex.

In the case of the decrease in glucose tolerance, there have been diverse reports, including the suggestion that some of the estrogens modify the tolerance "beneficially" and that the effect is not permanent. (There are also reports that the effect is continued after estrogenic treatment is discontinued.) The basic problem, however, is the interpretation of the modestly changed tolerance. Since there are no demonstrable symptoms or immediate consequences of the altered curves, the important question to be resolved deals with the long-term consequences. In analysis of insurance data, it is not possible to demonstrate that there is greater mortality risk over a 10-year period for persons who do not require insulin and have no associated symptoms.

The abnormal lipid changes are often equally subtle, but in my opinion have more serious implications. To best demonstrate the effects of the estrogens one should perform "before and after" determinations rather than relying upon a single determination while the patient is still on therapy. The reason for this is the wide range for "normal" levels. Thus, a young healthy girl may have as much as a doubling of triglyceride levels and still have plasma levels in the "normal" range. Since few symptoms are immediately attributable to the lipid changes, the real concern is the long-range effect of the lipid alterations on a person's cardiovascular system.

Such long-range consequences are very difficult to demonstrate without an extraordinarily complicated epidemiologic study of such scale that it probably would be impossible to carry out. Thus, the implications of the alterations in lipid metabolism also remain inferential at this time.

In the case of the protein changes, interpretation is even more complicated. Although elevated binding proteins may increase the blood levels of adrenal steroids or thyroid hormone, there is little if any actual increase in free hormone. Evidence of increased hormonal effects is not detectable by current technology.

Other changes are more familiar to clinicians. Hepatic changes include decreased biliary excretion, altered metabolic patterns, and the induction of enzymes of the endoplasmic reticulum. The altered metabolic patterns relate to the changes in carbohydrate, amino acid, protein, and lipid metabolism, which have already been commented upon. The decreased biliary excretion is of small magnitude unless there has been evidence of previous impairment of the excretory system (e.g., jaundice of pregnancy). It is well known that alkylated steroids may impair excretion of bile, and thus estrogens like ethynylestradiol may exert their effects in two ways: by virtue of the estrogenicity of the steroid or through action of the ethynyl side-chain. The enzymes of the endoplasmic reticulum are noted for their roles in detoxification. Thus, the accumulation of these enzymes increases the rate of inactivation of both natural and exogenous substances, including drugs such as barbiturates, narcotics, and even DDT. The significance is difficult to interpret—one might even postulate a beneficial effect.

Of more serious nature, in my opinion, are the changes in blood pressure. If distribution curves of blood pressures are compared for a group of women before and after the administration of contraceptive dosages of estrogens, there is a shift of about 15 mm. Hg for the systolic pressure and a corresponding but smaller shift for the diastolic pressure. This implies that most women undergo some small increase in blood pressure when estrogenic steroids are administered. Since it is usually young, healthy women who take contraceptive pills, almost all of these pressures remain within what are usually considered to be normal limits. Nevertheless, a small percentage of women have alarming elevations—often to systolic levels as high as 170 mm. Hg—and these findings have now been replicated in many clinics. The reason for this response to estrogens is not clear, but it is known that there is increased retention of both sodium and fluids, increased renin substrate activity, and increased aldosterone levels in patients treated with contraceptive steroids. Hypertension of this sort is usually symptomless; if not sought out, it will not likely be discovered. Again, data that might show that the modest increases in blood pressure have serious impact are not available; intuitively, however, most clinicians would be concerned with the small group of patients with elevations outside the "normal" limits.

Finally, there are many other systems which respond in unusual ways to estrogenic substances. Included in the list of undesirable effects are increased severity of headaches, certain dermatologic changes, possible changes in porphyric patients, and so forth. Considering the millions of women being treated with more than physiologic dosages of estrogen, what is surprising is not the complication rate but the infrequency of more dramatic complications. One might even suspect that a hidden selection process is occurring whereby those women who respond more sensitively with untoward effects withdraw more or less unnoticed from therapy because of minor or unreported symptoms, such as nausea, general malaise, or changes in mood and libido.

USES OF ESTROGEN

The potential risks from estrogen therapy should be balanced against the benefits. Estrogen therapy is specific for a number of conditions or situations and in some of these is clearly the drug of choice, if not the only drug.

Contraception

Undoubtedly, the most common use for the estrogenic steroids is as a component of contraceptive medication. Two estrogens are used almost interchangeably: mestranol and ethynylestradiol. There have been long discussions about their relative potencies, but the problem is probably not resolvable, for they do not behave in precisely the same way in many assay systems. In more technical terms, the dose-response relationships are not parallel, so that it is difficult to assign relative potencies to the substances. Furthermore, the detection of estrogenic activity in the human is a crude measurement at best.

Mestranol and ethynylestradiol provide very effective contraception. They provide better control than the totally synthetic steroids, such as diethylstilbestrol. In fact, unless a separation between effectiveness and side-effects is clearly demonstrated in the future, the introduction of new estrogens into our therapeutic regimens is difficult to support. The differences among the various contraceptive agents are limited, therefore, to dosage and progestational agents involved. These last have very diverse activities and are offered in a wide range of biological doses.

So far we do not know how to individualize contraceptive therapy. Estrogen dosages have declined considerably in the past decade and probably will continue to do so. Recent data from Australia[1] indicate that for women under 25 years of age, 30 μg. of ethynylestradiol would suppress ovulation just as well as the 50 μg. currently present in the lowest dosage pill combination therapy. This is not the case for older women, however, who required larger amounts to suppress ovulation.

Irregular Bleeding and Amenorrhea

Estrogens are often used either to control menorrhagia or to institute rhythmic episodes of bleeding in women with amenorrhea. Most commonly, they are used in the forms available for contraception. It should be recognized that there are few diseases whose etiologies are changed by this form of therapy. While the characteristics of a bleeding period may be modified beneficially by the administration of the estrogenic hormones, the basic pathology, with the possible exception of a few endometrial lesions, is not altered by such therapy. Furthermore, abnormal uterine bleeding of endocrine etiology is almost always associated with adequate estrogen secretion, so that simple monthly therapy with progesterone would suffice. In cases of amenorrhea, both primary and secondary, the use of estrogen modifies only the manifestations of the problem, and does not affect the etiology.

Nevertheless, there is a place for the judicious and occasional use of controlled cycles. For example, in a young girl with irregular bleeding at the time of menarche, most often the problem will solve itself. Cyclic therapy with estrogen or progesterone or both permits the patient, her family, and her physician to procrastinate for several months until further maturation of the endocrine system occurs.

On the other hand, abnormal bleeding in premenopausal and menopausal women should not be treated with estrogens until the possibility of malignancy has been ruled out.

Cosmetic Effects of Estrogens

Estrogens obviously have important effects on secondary sex characteristics and can be useful therapeutic agents for problems of acne, hirsutism, excessive stature, and breast development. Acne responds quite promptly to artificial cycles and estrogen is therapeutically useful in conjunction with other local and systemic therapy. Moderate dosages are reasonably successful.

The treatment of hirsutism is more complex because it requires higher dosages and longer treatments and is not always successful. The mechanism of action is probably twofold: estrogens inhibit gonadotropins and thus may decrease androgenic secretion from the ovary, and estrogen has a target effect on the skin and its accessories. Dosage levels as high as 5 mg. of stilbestrol per day may be necessary, and side-effects are common. Improvement is slow—often being most evident on the back and arms rather than on the face—and, as a consequence, hirsute patients become easily discouraged. In my experience, some patients do not seem to respond at all. Needless to add, such therapy is not a substitute for proper diagnosis and therapy of the basic lesion.

For the excessively tall girl with eunuchoid appearance, estrogens may be helpful in stopping skeletal growth. These patients usually have amenorrhea, are in their middle teens, and show little secondary sex development. After proper study to eliminate the various pathologic etiologies of primary amenorrhea, growth curves should be reconstructed, and x-rays of wrists and knees for bone age and epiphyseal closure should be obtained. Moderate doses of estrogen over a period of about a year will result in increased closure of the epiphyses and also some increase in breast development. It should be recognized that therapy of this sort over a prolonged period of time is a source of controversy, especially since normal processes of puberty may be occurring simultaneously.

Finally, the use of estrogens for stimulating breast development has been disappointing. One frequently reported effect of oral contraceptives has been a general increase in breast size for women on the medication. My experience has been that continued therapy over a prolonged period of time is moderately successful. Effects are disappointing in various genetic syndromes, and when artificial estrogens (e.g., stilbestrol) are used, they tend to darken the nipples more than the steroid estrogens do. Patients with greater needs or expectations should probably consider mammoplasty.

Dysmenorrhea

The literature of the 1940's contains a wealth of information on the use of estrogen, its biological effects, and dosages to be given as an effective therapy for dysmenorrhea. It is of interest that the recommended dosages of these clinical trials were in the range of 40 μg. of ethynylestradiol—a dose also found to be suppressive of ovulation when oral contraceptives were developed several decades later. There is no doubt that the treatment is effective, but it is temporary, and cessation of therapy results in return of symptoms when ovulatory cycles resume.

Endometriosis

The treatment of endometriosis (and often its diagnosis as well) is the subject of intense polemics. On one side, the claim is made that estrogens taken in high doses for long periods of time are curative. On the other side, some believe that estrogens have only limited effect, and that the effect which does occur is only symptomatic. The data available cannot resolve this difference, because, among other reasons, the diagnosis is inferential, even when based upon biopsy. The presence of small foci of endometriotic tissue is not so rare that it is sufficient for accurate prognosis. "Spontaneous" cures occur in many cases. On the other hand, some clinically diagnosed cases of severe endometriosis may appear to be associated with minimal pathologic findings upon laparotomy.

Without doubt, estrogen therapy is effective in the treatment of the discomfort associated with endometriosis. Were it not for the fact that infertility is the other common complaint in endometriosis there would be no question about the utility of estrogen therapy. Because treatment with estrogens guarantees infertility, the therapeutic benefit for infertile women desiring children requires intermittent therapy. Therein lies the paradox. Given a patient with demonstrable endometriosis and infertility, should she be treated with (1) additional periods of infertility caused by moderate doses of estrogen, or (2) large doses of estrogen in an attempt to decrease the extrauterine endometrial growth, (3) surgery, or (4) optimistic therapeutic inactivity until the patient chances to become pregnant or decides against it? It is clear that if an unquestionably effective therapy were available for endometriosis, this dilemma would not exist. My own point of view is that estrogen therapy in moderate doses is indicated to alleviate symptoms, but that it should not be used repeatedly or for *prolonged* periods of time with the hope that the patient will become pregnant when it is discontinued. When dealing with the infertility aspects of endometriosis one such trial should be sufficient. Even so, therapy with progestational agents may offer many advantages.

Menopause

No discussion of estrogen therapy would be complete without discussion of the use of estrogens for menopausal symptoms. Though this topic is one of considerable controversy, I find less reason to be perplexed with the use of estrogens in menopause than with almost any other condition. Most menopausal patients are not difficult to diagnose. Estrogen levels are low, menses are decreased or absent, vasomotor symptoms may be present, and the vagina and other target tissues confirm the lack of estrogenic stimulation. Alterations in emotional stability may occur for many reasons, and one should not be surprised that, in some cases, estrogens, psychotropic drugs, psychotherapy, and even placebos are equally effective (or ineffective). The important point is that when the symptoms result from a lack of estrogen, they respond to small amounts of estrogen in a manner dissimilar to any other treatment. The treatment is sensitive and specific.

The use of estrogens for menopause necessitates several important cautions. First, the therapist should be certain that there is no evidence of malignancy, since the use of estrogens may obscure the diagnosis and quite possibly complicate the treatment. Second, the physician should have "ongoing" control of the patient with this as with any other medication given over a prolonged period of time. A physician seeing for the first time a postmenopausal patient treated with estrogens and complaining of bleeding has the obligation to rule out malignancy. It is important that the patient and physician agree to regular follow-up examinations during this course of therapy. Third, if prolonged treatment is contemplated, the patient should be treated with low dosages. The problem of assessing dosages for individual patients is difficult in theory but simple in practice. The indices for estimating the sensitivity of the end-organs are not good and therefore one must rely upon such methods as vaginal cytology. The vaginal epithelium can be used to titrate dosages to an adequate level. Therapy is often given for three weeks and withdrawn for one week, but this procedure is more a matter of custom designed to avoid unscheduled bleeding than a demonstrably preferred method.

The most controversial question relates to the "routine use after menopause." Given the conditions already mentioned, it is clear that not all women should be treated continuously with estrogens, because some are not in frequent contact with their physicians, and because some have histories which contraindicate such treatment. In my opinion, however, most women do find small doses of estrogens beneficial, and in the absence of contraindications, I recommend this treatment to my patients. I have measured the height of my patients over a period of many years and found no significant changes in height in either treated or untreated patients, and in several cases no changes in height in the presence of increasing osteoporosis. With the recent rebuttal of the benefit of estrogens in preventing osteoporosis, one of the last bulwarks of the proponents of estrogenic treatment was lost. I do, however, retain the impression (or maybe the prejudice) that estrogens in menopause are beneficial to the general well-being of the patient.

Other Conditions

Estrogens have been used for many conditions for which I am unaware of either good data or rationale. Included in this group are the maintenance of pregnancy, various skin lesions, and metabolic conditions, among others. They have been used for prostatism, arteriosclerosis, and various types of malignancy, including breast cancer. I shall not attempt to evaluate such therapy; it is outside my current experience. In the case of pregnancy, however, it should be emphasized that diethylstilbestrol has been demonstrated to be a transplacental carcinogen and should not be used. There is evidence that large doses of stilbestrol might be useful as an implantation inhibitor, but these data are derived from limited trials.

Choice and Doses

The choice of estrogens formerly was more difficult than it now is. The evidence that stilbestrol has undesirable actions on the fetus (and perhaps the adult) greatly reduced the usefulness of the drug. One expects that similar reservations should hold for the other estrogens, at least for the artificial ones. Contraceptive agents are packaged conveniently, but in these formulations estrogens are usually accompanied by an androgenic or progestational agent or are provided in excessive dosages. Consequently, the conjugated estrogens or the ethynyl-estrogens remain available, and the relative disadvantages and advantages of these preparations probably balance each other.

Summary

Estrogens are potent, effective drugs with considerable usefulness and potential for harm. Patients should be carefully selected for treatment, treated with minimally effective doses, and followed carefully. It may well be that there is more controversy surrounding the diagnosis of the conditions to be treated than the merits of the treatment itself. As the former problems are resolved, one can predict that estrogen treatment will become less controversial.

REFERENCES

1. Carey, H. M., and Pinkerton, G. D.: The antifertility effectiveness of low doses of ethinyl-oestradiol. Med. J. Aust. 1:512, 1972.

Pros and Cons of Estrogen
Therapy for Gynecologic Conditions

Editorial Comment

The late Professor Frederick Hisaw, in a conversation concerning his experimental studies on the effect of the various hormones on the uterus,[1] admonished the researcher and clinician that "the trouble is that both appear to hold the view that any old estrogen will do." He would be pleased to know that this undiscriminating attitude no longer prevails. Certainly the contributors have indicated that despite the efficaciousness and clinical use of estrogen therapy there are distinct indications and contraindications to its application.

There seems little question that the natural estrogens are preferable to synthetic forms—more precisely, to diethylstilbestrol. Additional evidence is accumulating of the adverse effect of diethylstilbestrol on the fetus when the mother has received this agent during pregnancy. That adenosis and clear cell carcinoma of the vagina are produced in the female offspring of mothers receiving diethylstilbestrol during pregnancy is now more than a possibility, but this finding will be a source of controversy and speculation for years to come.[2] Such findings may reveal relationships that are basic to the etiology of cancer or at least some cancers. Apparently there is no adverse effect on the male offspring and the fact that males escape or reveal no evidence of malignancy supports the suggestion that gonadal secretion participates in sex differentiation, a theory that was introduced in the classical studies of Lillie (circa 1917). In short, the endocrine activity of the fetal testes may negate any stilbestrol effect.

Whether excessive estrogen therapy (namely, large doses of Premarin) contribute to adenomatous hyperplasia of the endometrium is also subject to controversy. Nevertheless, unopposed estrogen administration in the postmenopausal female (i.e., Premarin, 1.25 mg. daily) often results in uterine bleeding, which is disconcerting to both the patient and her physician. Many such patients are elderly, and both operative manipulation, however minor, and the risks entailed in the administration of anesthesia in such patients are undesirable and to be avoided. The policy of watchful expectancy, hoping that the bleeding will cease following withdrawal of estrogen therapy, is the usual procedure to be followed. However, the length of time one should wait for the bleeding to cease is not well established. Presumably one should not procrastinate beyond a few weeks after the medication has been withdrawn, after which further investigation is indicated.

Contraindications to the use of estrogen therapy are increasing as data accumulate on the adverse cardiovascular effects in patients on contraceptive medication. Besides deep vein thrombosis and pulmonary embolism, increased risks has been found for thrombotic stroke as well.[3,4] Hyperlipidemia is a well-known metabolic alteration and may be related to myocardial infarction, which has also been implicated in estrogen therapy. When these data are extrapolated to older women well beyond the menopause, whose cardiovascular system is perhaps already compromised, the risk of long-term estrogen therapy cannot be minimized. Certainly dosages should be minimal and the patient carefully monitored regarding blood pressure and other parameters. The agent used must be carefully selected and in the proper dosage, keeping in mind that no longer will any one estrogen suffice to meet all clinical needs.

REFERENCES

1. Hisaw, F. L., Velardo, J. T., and Goolsby, C. M.: Interaction of estrogen on uterine growth. J. Clin. Endocr. *14*:1134, 1954.
2. Reid, D. E.: A controversy in fetal ecology. Amer. J. Obstet. Gynec. *114*:419, 1972.
3. Collaborative Group for the Study of Stroke in Young Women: Oral contraception and increased risk of cerebral ischemia or thrombosis. New Eng. J. Med. 288:871, 1973.
4. Oral contraceptives and stroke (editorial). New Eng. J. Med. 288:906, 1973.

25

Vaginal Versus Abdominal Hysterectomy

Alternative Points of View:

By Robert H. Barter

By Milagros A. Macasaet and James H. Nelson, Jr.

Editorial Comment

Vaginal Versus Abdominal Hysterectomy

ROBERT H. BARTER

The George Washington University School of Medicine

> Hysterectomy is a relatively easy operation to perform and is often easiest when least necessary.—T. N. A. Jeffcoate.[1]

Historically, vaginal hysterectomy was performed more than 250 years prior to the first abdominal hysterectomy. According to one source, vaginal removal of the uterus was done first by Berengarius of Bologna in 1507.[2] This first operation was on a patient who had fungating carcinoma of the cervix, and like most other vaginal hysterectomies for the next two centuries, was performed primarily for this reason or for complete prolapse of the uterus. An abdominal hysterectomy (perhaps the first) was performed by Langenbeck in 1825, but his patient did not survive.[3] Apparently subtotal cesarean hysterectomy, which was first performed successfully by Porro in 1876,[4] opened the way for the abdominal approach. Wertheim performed his first abdominal hysterectomy in 1898.[5] From that time on, unfortunately, abdominal hysterectomy has been done more frequently than the vaginal, except for a few dedicated vaginal hysterectomists, who through the years have continued to use the vaginal approach whenever possible.

In 1971, hysterectomy was second only to appendectomy in the number of operations performed. Last year it was estimated that there were 678,999 hysterectomies performed in the United States. A recent statistical survey of some 12,000 hysterectomies has provided some statistics which have to be accepted as being of significance.[6] According to these data: (1) The mortality rate for patients undergoing hysterectomy was less than half that for patients having an appendectomy and less than one-eighth the rate for patients undergoing cholecystectomy. (2) Abdominal hysterectomies were performed in 70 per cent of all patients, whereas only 30 per cent were vaginal operations. (3) Antibiotics were given to 48 per cent of all hysterectomy patients. (4) There was a greater risk of postoperative infections in women undergoing vaginal hysterectomy, and significantly more of those patients had fevers and received antibiotics. (5) There has been a steady downward trend in the use of transfusions, from 80 per cent in the late

1950's to a figure of 3.9 per cent in the mid-1960's. (6) The longer any patient had been in the hospital prior to her surgery, the greater was her morbidity following elective hysterectomy. (7) When patients were cared for by residents, there was a higher incidence of serious postoperative infections.

Abdominal Hysterectomy

There are instances in which the abdominal approach is preferable to the vaginal operation. These are: (1) Patients who have uterine or pelvic tumors too large to be removed vaginally; (2) most patients with carcinoma of the endometrium in whom removal of the ovaries at the time of the hysterectomy is mandatory; (3) patients who have had multiple pelvic operations previously and in whom it might be expected that there would be pelvic adhesions; (4) patients in whom there is absolutely no descensus of the uterus under anesthesia (as in some nulliparous patients and even in some multiparas); (5) occlusion of the cul-de-sac by endometriosis or by some other intra-abdominal condition; (6) radical surgery for carcinoma of the cervix or endometrium; (7) the inability of the operating surgeon to perform the vaginal operation expeditiously.

Vaginal Hysterectomy

Conversely, the vaginal procedure is certainly to be preferred under the following circumstances: (1) in any patient who has a significant degree of uterine prolapse when symptoms are such that removal of the uterus is desirable; (2) when there is significant pelvic relaxation so that a repair of a cystocele or rectocele is necessary in conjunction with the hysterectomy; (3) when the operation is for sterilization purposes;[7,8,9] (4) in markedly obese patients in whom the removal of the uterus, if technically possible, can be done much more easily than by means of the abdominal approach; (5) in most patients who have carcinoma in situ of the cervix; (6) for abnormal uterine bleeding, premenstrual tension, and symptomatic fibroids up to the size of a 14 week pregnancy;[7] (7) generally, in any patient when hysterectomy is indicated if the vaginal operation is technically possible.

Comparison of Abdominal and Vaginal Hysterectomies

The reason that 70 per cent of the hysterectomies in the United States are being done abdominally is the result of several factors. They are: (1) the fact that general surgeons and gynecologists untrained in vaginal surgery still do a significant number of the hysterectomies performed in the United States; (2) the fact that some of the residency programs in obstetrics and gynecology are, or have been, directed by those who are not "vaginally oriented" as pertains to gynecological surgery; (3) in many hospitals, lack of surgical assistants makes it preferable or necessary to perform the abdominal operation.

In recent years, two very significant advances have made the vaginal type of hysterectomy even more acceptable. The first of these is the introduction of a synthetic absorbable suture material, polyglycolic acid. With the elimination of catgut, there is much less postoperative edema, and with less tissue edema, there is less morbidity and less postoperative pain. The second factor has been the use of intra-operative and postoperative antibiotic therapy.[10,11] If there is no history of drug sensitivity, the patient is given intravenous ampicillin during and immediately after the surgery. The antibiotic is continued intravenously for the first 24 hours, after which the patient is given ampicillin by mouth for several days. If the patient is sensitive to penicillin or its derivatives, she is given intravenous, and later oral, tetracycline.

Advantages for the vaginal operation are that it can be done more quickly, thus requiring less anesthesia, and the blood loss and postoperative discomfort should be minimal. Early ambulation is the rule following vaginal hysterectomy. With the combined usage of prophylactic antibiotics and the synthetic absorbable suture material, patients may be discharged from the hospital as early as the second or third day following vaginal hysterectomy. Obviously, this gives the vaginal operation some superiority, for few patients following abdominal hysterectomies are discharged in less than a week postoperatively. All of the above implies that the operator has been well trained in vaginal surgery.

Without question, at least 50 per cent of the hysterectomies now being done abdominally could be done more safely, more easily, and with less blood loss and with less morbidity if the surgery were being performed by capable vaginal hysterectomists. If the reported, but regrettable, ratio of 70 per cent abdominal to 30 per cent vaginal hysterectomies is to be altered, more emphasis must be placed on training of residents in the proper use of vaginal surgery, and particularly vaginal hysterectomy. Unless such is done, the majority of hysterectomies in this country will continue to be done abdominally.

REFERENCES

1. Jeffcoate, T. A.: Principles of Gynaecology. 3rd Ed. New York, Appleton-Century-Crofts, 1967.
2. Kennedy, J. W., and Campbell, A. D.: Vaginal Hysterectomy. New York, F. A. Davis, 1944.
3. Langenbeck, C. J. M. (ed.): Beschreibung zweier, vom Herausgerber verrichteten, Exstirpation krebshafter, nicht forgefallener Gebarmutter. Neue Bibliothek fur die Chirurgie und Ophthalmologie. Hanover, Hahn, 1828, Vol. 4, p. 698–728.
4. Speert, H.: Obstetrics and Gynecologic Milestones. New York, Macmillan Co., 1958, p. 587.
5. Speert, H.: Obstetrics and Gynecologic Milestones. New York, Macmillan Co., 1958, p. 673.
6. Child, M. A., and Ledger, W. J.: Personal communication.
7. Nichols, D. H.: Vaginal hysterectomy versus tubal ligation. Obst. Gynec. 34:881, 1969.
8. Van Nagell, J. R., Jr., and Roddick, J. W., Jr.: Vaginal hysterectomy as a sterilization procedure. Am. J. Obstet. Gynec. 111:703, 1971.
9. Laufe, L. E. and Kreutner, A. K.: Vaginal hysterectomy: a modality for therapeutic abortion and sterilization. Am. J. Obstet. Gynec. 110:1096, 1971.
10. Goosenberg, J., Emich, J. P., Jr., and Schwarz, R. H.: Prophylactic antibiotics in vaginal hysterectomy. Am. J. Obstet. Gynec. 105:503, 1969.
11. Allen, J. L., Rampone, J. F., and Wheeless, C. R.: Use of prophylactive antibiotic in elective major gynecologic operations. Obstet. Gynec. 39:218, 1972.

Vaginal Versus Abdominal Hysterectomy

Milagros A. Macasaet and James H. Nelson, Jr.

State University of New York Downstate Medical Center

The title of "Vaginal Versus Abdominal Hysterectomy," unqualified as it
is, strongly implies that both procedures are electively and simultaneously available to a gynecologist regardless of the indication for surgery. This has no doubt
led Hawksworth, an ardent advocate of vaginal hysterectomy, to have said in
1965, "There is no place for gymnastic exercise, nor expertise just to show that a
uterus can be got out from below," and yet, since the first successful vaginal hysterectomy by Langebeck in 1813, there is this uncertainty about vaginal versus
abdominal hysterectomy.

Strangely enough, this seemingly continuing question is not only the surgeon's concern, but the patient's as well. Gray had noted that often, on the basis
of hearsay, patients fear the vaginal approach. In our experience at Kings County
Hospital, the majority of patients proposed for vaginal hysterectomy welcome the
approach, although it is not infrequent to encounter one or two a year who are
reluctant, if not outrightly opposed, to vaginal hysterectomy.

What follows is essentially a comparison of the two methods of hysterectomy in all its facets, including indications and contraindications, advantages and
disadvantages, and morbidity and mortality. If all these aspects are considered in
depth, perhaps there is no controversy at all. Instead, an intelligent and knowledgeable selection of approach may be made by the surgeon.

Indications

Vaginal hysterectomy is performed frequently today, and is a safe gynecological procedure. The primary indication is uterine prolapse. This covers a
wide spectrum of different degrees of descensus and pelvic relaxation. Different
clinics and various authors have different criteria for these, and only if the uterus
prolapses completely out of the vagina is there universal agreement. In our own
clinic a classification system of four degrees is used. Hawksworth has cautioned
that if there is no descent of the uterus when traction is applied to the cervix

higher incidence of febrile morbidity after vaginal hysterectomy is no doubt related to hematoma formation.

There is a much higher incidence of the use of antibiotics and longer postoperative fever (100.4° F. on three consecutive postoperative days), following vaginal hysterectomy. Pelvic abscess is also more frequent.

Abdominal wound infection occurs with varying frequency after abdominal hysterectomy. Even if meticulous hemostasis is effected, the occurrence of abdominal wound infection is proportional to the thickness of the abdominal wall —that is, the thicker the panniculus adiposus, the more likely are wound infection and breakdown to occur postoperatively. Although evisceration is rare after uncomplicated abdominal hysterectomy, it is a potentially grave complication.

5. DISTURBANCE OF BOWEL FUNCTION. This may vary from adynamic ileus to mechanical intestinal obstruction. This occurs after abdominal hysterectomy, in which there is more manipulation of the intestine. Intestinal obstruction of the mechanical type is a serious complication of abdominal hysterectomy, sometimes requiring a second laparotomy.

On the other hand, paralytic ileus not responding to conservative management, or mechanical obstruction, if it occurs following vaginal surgery, is a very serious complication, and definitely needs abdominal exploration to effect treatment.

Another intestinal complication possible during the performance of hysterectomy is rectal injury. There is more likelihood of injuring the rectum via the vagina than via the abdominal route.

6. PULMONARY AND VASCULAR COMPLICATIONS. These occur more often after abdominal than after vaginal hysterectomy. There is a higher incidence of atelectasis, pneumonitis and pulmonary embolism following abdominal hysterectomy. Because of the abdominal discomfort postoperatively, patients tend to have shallow respiratory excursions, and Sjostedt demonstrated a decrease in tidal volume after abdominal hysterectomy. Phlebitis is also less common after vaginal hysterectomy.

Pulmonary embolism occurs less commonly following vaginal hysterectomy, although it must not be discounted. This is one of the definite advantages of vaginal hysterectomy. The incidence of pulmonary embolism after abdominal hysterectomy is estimated to be about 1 per cent (that is, anywhere from 1 to 1.4 per cent), and after vaginal surgery about 0.3 to 0.4 per cent.

LATE POSTOPERATIVE COMPLICATIONS

This topic is more pertinent to vaginal hysterectomy patients.

1. Prolapse of vaginal vault, although not normally encountered, often does occur in patients following vaginal hysterectomy and usually in the elderly patient. The more severe the degree of prolapse and inversion of the vagina at the time of the original surgery, the more likely it is to occur.

2. Recurrent cystocele and rectocele. Although these are not always symptomatic, recurrent cystocele or rectocele is a real problem to the patient and a source of some embarrassment for the surgeon.

3. Enterocele. Either recurrent or primary enterocele may occur after vaginal hysterectomy. Enterocele is a fairly common occurrence and numerous

papers have been written on how to prevent or repair it. It is most important that enterocele be diagnosed, for failure to recognize it dooms the patient to recurrence of the pelvic relaxation. It is more apt to be missed during vaginal hysterectomy than during hysterectomy via the abdomen, but it may be corrected quite easily by either route.

4. Vaginal evisceration. Rupture of the vaginal vault followed by evisceration of bowel through the vagina had been reported 16 times in the world literature, and recently another seven cases have been reported. One such case was seen by one of us (Dr. Macasaet) in a 54 year old obese black female four months after vaginal hysterectomy. The common denominator in this complication is the atrophic tissues of postmenopausal women. Most of these patients have had several operative procedures for uterine prolapse, and enterocele was present in the majority.

5. Prolapse of the fimbrial end of the fallopian tube through the apex of the vaginal vault. This may happen after either type of hysterectomy and may be a source of bleeding. The omentum has also been found at the apex of the vaginal vault.

FAILURES

These are more pertinent after vaginal hysterectomy.

1. Shortening of the vagina. This is especially annoying to sexually active women. To a greater extent, this is influenced by repair of cystocele.

2. Stenosis of vagina. This is rare, except when vaginectomy has been done.

3. Fallopio-vaginal fistula. This is also a very rare situation.

CONCLUSION

The mortality rate after hysterectomy remains low, comparatively lower than after cholecystectomy or appendectomy. Complications still occur, however, with disturbing frequency.

More hysterectomies are done today, for the indications have increased. An example is the performance of vaginal hysterectomy for purposes of sterilization. Greenhill has said that it is heartening to see the increased use of vaginal hysterectomy, for there is a definite place for this operation. Hence, every gynecologist should be able to perform a vaginal hysterectomy with as much ease as an abdominal hysterectomy. It should be added, however, that the vaginal route should be used only when clearly indicated and when it can be accomplished with safety.

REFERENCES

1. White, S. C., Wartel, L. J., and Wade, M. G.: Comparison of abdominal and vaginal hysterectomies. Obstet. Gynec. 37:530, 1971.
2. Toit, P. F. N.: The prevention of complications in vaginal hysterectomy. South African Med. J. 45:99, 1971.
3. Hochuli, E., Fankauser, B., and Bollinger, J.: Die stellung der vaginalen hysterektomie. Schweiz. Med. Wschr. 100:1071, 1970.
4. Gray, L. A.: Vaginal Hysterectomy. Springfield, Ill., Charles C Thomas, 1961.

5. Lash, A. F.: Vaginal surgery for non malignant gynecological conditions. Illinois Med. J. *137*:499, 1970.
6. Copenhaver, E. H.: Vaginal hysterectomy. Amer. J. Obstet. Gynec. *84*:123, 1962.
7. Hawksworth, W.: Indications for vaginal hysterectomy. J. Obstet. Gynaec. Brit. Comm. *72*:847, 1965.
8. Lewis, T. L. T.: The William Hawksworth Memorial Lecture 1970. Aust. N.Z. J. Obstet. Gynaec. *11*:1, 1971.
9. Howkins, J.: Total abdominal hysterectomy. J. Obstet. Gynaec. Brit. Comm. *70*:20, 1963.
10. Smith, R. D., and Pratt, J. H.: Serious bleeding following vaginal or abdominal hysterectomy. Obstet. Gynec. *26*:592, 1965.
11. Rolf, B. B.: Vaginal evisceration. Am. J. Obstet. Gynec. *107*:369, 1970.
12. Zacharin, R. F.: Stress Incontinence of Urine. New York, Harper & Row, Publishers, 1972.
13. Allen, E., and Peterson, L. F.: Versatility of vaginal hysterectomy technic. Obstet. Gynec. *3*:240, 1954.
14. Papaloucas, A., Mantis, C., and Zervos, S.: Management of the vaginal vault after vaginal hysterectomy. Int. Surg. *54*:458, 1970.
15. Mac Leod, D., and Howkins, J.: Bonney's Gynecological Surgery, 7th Ed. New York, Harper & Row, Publishers, 1964.
16. Gwillim, C. M.: Hysterectomy. Proc. Roy. Soc. Med. *43*:972, 1950.
17. Sjostedt, S.: Pulmonary ventilation after vaginal and abdominal hysterectomy. Acta Obstet. Gynec. Scand. *39*:39, 1960.
18. Greenhill, J. P., Ed.: The Year Book of Obstetrics and Gynecology. Chicago, Year Book Medical Publishers, 1971, p. 330.
19. Krige, C. F.: Vaginal Hysterectomy and Genital Prolapse Repair. Johannesburg, S. Africa, Witwatersrand University Press, 1965.
20. Campbell, A. D.: In Meigs, J. V., and Sturgis, S. H. (eds.): Progress in Gynecology, Vol. II. New York, Grune and Stratton, 1950.

Vaginal Versus Abdominal Hysterectomy

Editorial Comment

Although we cannot express excessive enthusiasm for the procedure, undoubtedly there are many patients whose pelvic symptoms can best be resolved by a vaginal rather than an abdominal hysterectomy. At the same time, vaginal hysterectomy, like any other surgical procedure, demands competent assistants and ample exposure of the operative field. The latter may not be possible if there is a narrow pubic arch. Hence, when a vaginal hysterectomy is contemplated and indeed initiated, on rare occasions it may have to be abandoned for the abdominal approach if pelvic exposure is inadequate or adnexal disease or uterine enlargement proves to be of greater magnitude than was initially appreciated.

The contributors have assessed the pros and cons of these procedures. One (Dr. Barter) has especially favored the vaginal approach, which is understandable, since he has contributed substantially to improving the technique of the operation. There seems little doubt, however, that the complications and morbidity rate are somewhat higher in vaginal hysterectomy, which relate mainly to the need to perform a colporrhaphy. Even so, the morbidity rate can be reduced by careful attention to preoperative preparation of the patient, the use of antibiotic therapy, careful hemostasis, and minimal blood loss in the course of the operation.

Certainly in those patients who require attention for the correction of urinary incontinence, the vaginal approach is preferable. This is not to say that occasionally there may not be a patient with incontinence to some degree who cannot be cured by abdominal hysterectomy followed by a Marshall-Marchetti-Krantz procedure. Assuming it is technically feasible, vaginal hysterectomy alone may be the procedure that will best serve the patient's immediate and more remote needs. In fact, in cases where sterilization is at issue, a vaginal hysterectomy must be weighed against vaginal tubal ligation. In fact, bringing the tubes into view often is a procedural matter not far removed from that required for a vaginal hysterectomy. In the event that the patient has an IUD in situ, it would be well to remove it and postpone the operation until two or more weeks after the subsequent menses (see Chapter 10).

Despite the fact that the vaginal operation, when hysterectomy is indicated, is regarded as safer than the abdominal approach in the elderly poor-risk patient, vaginal hysterectomy is frowned upon by some experienced gynecologists. Rather than expose the peritoneal cavity and upper vagina to possible infection, a La Forte or Manchester procedure must be considered.

824

Finally, it should be realized by those in training that when total prolapse is present, a vaginal hysterectomy may be more difficult or at least more lengthy than when lesser forms of prolapse occur. The bladder must be dealt with cautiously. Establishing the line of cleavage of the endopelvic fascia overlying the bladder and cervix is the key to success.

Index

Page numbers in *italics* refer to illustrations; (t) indicates tables.

827